The dentist and his assistant

The dentist and his assistant

Edited by

Shailer Peterson

B.A., M.A., Ph.D., F.A.C.D. (Hon.), F.I.C.D. (Hon.)

Associate Dean and Professor of Dental Education, The University of Texas Dental School at San Antonio, Texas; formerly Dean and Professor of General Dentistry, University of Tennessee College of Dentistry, Memphis, Tenn.; Assistant Secretary for Educational Affairs of the American Dental Association, Secretary of the Council on Dental Education and Council of the National Board of Dental Examiners of the American Dental Association; affiliated with the Chicago College of Dental Surgery, the University of Chicago, the South Dakota State College, the University of Minnesota, and the University of Oregon

Third edition

With 987 illustrations, in 302 figures

The C. V. Mosby Company

Saint Louis 1972

Third edition

Printed in the United States of America

International Standard Book Number 0-8016-3819-4

Library of Congress Catalog Card Number 72-176385

Distributed in Great Britain by Henry Kimpton, London

VH/VH/VH 9 8 7 6 5 4 3 2

Contributors

JAMES T. ANDREWS, B.A., D.D.S., F.A.C.D.

Chairman and Professor, Department of Operative Dentistry, and Director of Dental Auxiliary Utilization Program, University of Tennessee College of Dentistry, Memphis, Tennessee

ROGER E. BARTON, D.D.S.

Associate Dean for Administrative Affairs, formerly Director of Auxiliary Dental Education Programs, University of North Carolina School of Dentistry, Chapel Hill, North Carolina

MARILYN MOSS BECK, B.S., R.D.II.

Assistant Professor of Dental Hygiene, Marquette University School of Dentistry, Milwaukee, Wisconsin

CHARLES M. BELTING, B.A., M.S., D.D.S., F.A.C.D.

Chief, Dental Service, Veterans Administration Hospital, Sepulveda, California; Lecturer in Periodontics, University of California at Los Angeles School of Dentistry, Los Angeles, California

HARRISON M. BERRY, Jr., M.Sc., D.D.S., F.A.C.D.

Associate Dean and Professor of Radiology, formerly Director of Courses in Oral Hygiene, University of Pennsylvania School of Dental Medicine, Philadelphia, Pennsylvania

CHARLES O. CRANFORD, D.D.S.

Chief, Manpower Dental Branch, U. S. Public Health Service, Department of Health, Education, and Welfare (On leave for graduate study at the University of Texas at Austin–The Lyndon B. Johnson School of Public Affairs, Austin, Texas)

TILLIE D. GINSBURG, R.D.H., B.A., M.Ed.

Director and Associate Professor of Dental Hygiene, Marquette University School of Dentistry, Milwaukee, Wisconsin

KATHRYN S. GOLLER, R.D.H., C.D.A.

Clinical Associate, Department of Community Dentistry, and Co-Director, Dental Therapist Training Program, University of Alabama in Birmingham School of Dentistry, Birmingham, Alabama

ROSS C. HUNTLEY, D.D.S.

General Practitioner in Sherman Oaks, California; Lecturer, University of Southern California and University of California at Los Angeles, Los Angeles, California

RICHARD E. JENNINGS, D.D.S., M.S.D.

Chairman and Professor, Department of Preventive Dentistry (Pedodontics), The University of Texas Dental Branch at Houston, Houston, Texas

LOIS K. KRYGER, C.D.A.

Dental Assisting Consultant, Education Development Branch, Division of Dental Health, National Institutes of Health, Department of Health, Education, and Welfare, Bethesda, Maryland

JACK C. MILLER, B.A., M.S.W.

Professor, Practice Relations, The University of Texas Dental Branch at Houston, Houston, Texas

WALTER J. PELTON, B.S., D.D.S., M.S.P.H., F.A.C.D.

Assistant Dean and Chairman, Department of Community Dentistry, The University of Alabama in Birmingham School of Dentistry, Birmingham, Alabama; formerly Chief, Division of Dental Resources, United States Public Health Service, Health Education, and Welfare, Bethesda, Maryland

JAMES E. PHILLIPS, A.B., M.Sc., D.D.S.

Associate Professor of Radiology, University of Pennsylvania School of Dental Medicine, Philadelphia, Pennsylvania

RALPH W. PHILLIPS, M.S., D.Sc., F.A.C.D.

Assistant Dean for Research and Research Professor of Dental Materials, Indiana University–Purdue University at Indianapolis School of Dentistry, Indianapolis, Indiana

BILLY E. RIGSBY, D.D.S.

Chairman and Professor of General Practice, and Director, Dental Auxiliary Utilization Program, The University of Texas Dental School at San Antonio, San Antonio, Texas

GERTRUDE M. SINNETT, B.S., R.D.H.

Administrative Assistant to Dean, Associate Professor of Dentistry, and Director, Dental Auxiliary Utilization Program, The University of Alabama in Birmingham School of Dentistry, Birmingham, Alabama

MILTON SISKIN, B.A., D.D.S., F.A.C.D. F.I.C.D.

Chairman of Endodontics and Professor, Department of Operative Dentistry, University of Tennessee College of Dentistry, Memphis, Tennessee

WADE B. WINNETT, D.D.S., M.S.D.

Associate Professor of Operative Dentistry, Meharry Medical College School of Dentistry, Nashville, Tennessee; formerly Chairman, Department for Education of Auxiliary Dental Personnel, University of Tennessee College of Dentistry, Memphis, Tennessee

ARTHUR H. WUEHRMANN, A.B., D.M.D., F.A.C.D.

Professor of Dentistry and Director, N.I.D.R. Dental Radiology Research Training Grant, The University of Alabama in Birmingham School of Dentistry, Birmingham, Alabama

Preface

The first edition of *The Dentist and His Assistant* was published in 1961 and the second edition in 1967; therefore, work on the first edition began more than 10 years ago. It became one of the first textbooks designed for formal courses in dental assisting. A major revision took place in the second edition, and another major revision can be seen in this third edition.

Every instructor of dental assisting students should read the preface of each new book in the field in order to be able to judge whether it can be used effectively as the major textbook to be required of all students or whether it will be used as a reference along with other books and journal articles. Most students, whether they be in a classroom or be dental assistants in an office reading to keep up with the profession, should also carefully read the preface of new books written for dental assistants. Both instructors and students need to know the authors' philosophy so that they may determine how the book is intended to function. Also, they need to know what the book does not claim, so that neither the instructor nor the student will seek for something that is not there.

In the first edition, it was reported that there were 76,000 dental practitioners in 1955 employing 82,500 persons as auxiliary personnel, 62,000 of whom were dental assistants. Just a handful of schools offered formal programs at that time, so nearly every dental assistant had been educated by her own dentist-employer. Also at that time graduates of dental schools had not been given much, if any, training in how to make the best use of trained dental assistants or even what to expect of them. Now, approximately 15 years later, great changes have taken place. Nearly a third of all practicing dentists have received training in dental school on how to use a chairside assistant. Instead of a handful of schools, about 141 have now been accredited or provisionally approved and another 35 are making application.

In 1967 the total number of dentists and auxiliary workers rose to 235,700 and 92 percent of all dentists employed auxiliaries. In 1971 there were approximately 150,000 dental assistants, about 18,900 of whom were members of the American Dental Assistants Association—another statistic that will grow rapidly in the next few years.

The profession of dental assisting requires and demands excellent textbooks both for use in the schools and as reference books in the dental office. The dental assisting profession is on the threshold of a whole new era for expanding duties; completely new and different responsibilities are being added to the curriculum in each school. This means that the dental assistant of the future and the instructor who teaches her will need to have available the best books possible. One cannot teach for tomorrow's dental practice with yesterday's textbooks and references.

Every instructor and student should examine first of all a textbook's coverage; that is, whether it includes all courses or subjects found in the dental assisting curriculum and how completely. From the outset of planning for *The Dentist and His Assistant,* the philosophy of the editor and the many collaborators has been as follows:

1. A profession such as dental assisting could never use a *single* textbook that would attempt to include everything required in the dental assisting curriculum. If all of the dental assisting curriculum could be encompassed in a single book, then dental assisting would not hold the important place that it now occupies in the health professions.
2. Dental assistants and their educators need a basic textbook that covers the topics and subjects required in the curriculum but not provided by other single books written specifically for the future dental assistant.
3. The book should be written by persons who have the dental assistant's interest strongly in mind and who have taught them or worked with them in their association.
4. The book should not include a summary of course work in such areas as chemistry, English, speech, or typing, although these are customarily a part of the dental assisting curriculum. There are other excellent books devoted specifically to these subjects which the dental assisting instructor can assign as library references.
5. The book should emphasize that dental assisting is a profession and should direct the thinking and the attitude of prospective dental assistants so that they will be assets to their profession and to the dental office in which they are employed.
6. The book should include material on dental office practice whether it be in the reception room or the operatory.
7. The book should stimulate the student to be watchful and anticipate changes taking place in the whole dental profession as well as in the special field of dental assisting.
8. The book should prove useful to keep as a reference and to be placed in the dental assistant's office.
9. The book should provide the dentist-employer with information that will make him appreciate what dental assistants are being taught today and what they are competent to perform for him. It also should show the relationship and responsibilities between the dental assistant and the office.
10. The book should provide the dentist with a reference in which he can assign reading material for new employees so that they can be brought up to date on what is expected of dental assistants in an office today.
11. While not originally written for any purpose other than for teaching dental assistants about their duties and responsibilities, previous editions of *The Dentist and His Assistant* have proved to be excellent sources for explaining to someone such as a prospective dental student or a dental supply salesman what dentistry is all about.

Instructors who have used *The Dentist and His Assistant* previously will note that the organization and sequence of chapters have been completely revised. An instructor realizes that the assigned textbook in a curriculum for a "whole profession" must be used differently than a textbook in chemistry, algebra, English, or a foreign language. In these and other courses, the authors develop the chapters so that the student is expected to follow from the first through the sequence to the final chapter.

Any deviation from this assignment order is usually detrimental to the success of that course.

In *The Dentist and His Assistant,* the instructor and students must realize that they will be studying in all parts of the textbook at any one time. For them to pursue the book from Chapter 1 to the end would be a mistake. A student of dental assisting will need to be studying material in all *four* of the following parts of this textbook:

PART I **Professional background**
PART II **Office practice**
PART III **Scientific background**
PART IV **Supporting the office practice**

These are the four areas that make up the total education of a dental assistant. The chemistry assignments in other books and also the lectures will contribute to Part III, Scientific Background. The English and speech will reinforce Part IV, Supporting the Office Practice. These four areas are practical topics that the instructor can use throughout the entire length of the curriculum. This supports the topic teaching approach and integrative curriculum.

The editor and the contributors to the twenty chapters comprising these four parts hope that they have given every director of dental assisting and instructor in these schools a useful instrument to adopt as a basic textbook around which to plan their approach to the instruction of dental assistants.

The joking statement is often made that no one should ever publish his first edition but instead should start with his second or third. There is much truth in this statement. However, we are glad that more than 10 years ago we did focus attention on the need for a *new profession of dental assisting* and provide one of the first books that would help give status and importance to this new group. We have talked with instructors who have used previous editions as textbooks and as reference books. We have talked with those who have chosen to use the textbooks of other authors. We have listened to the philosophies of directors who claim that they will never use a single textbook. Through all of this, we have learned many lessons and we have tried our best to provide for the dental assistant and her instructors a book that will meet their needs and of which they can be as proud as we are.

Most of the twenty contributors to this textbook were my colleagues when I was asked by The C. V. Mosby Company to undertake the first edition of *The Dentist and His Assistant.* It would require space beyond that available here to detail the experience that each has had in teaching dental assistants, teaching dental students how to utilize dental assistants, working with expanded duty education, directing DAU programs, writing articles for dental assistants, working with the Education and Certification Committees of the ADAA, judging table clinics for dental assistants, and so on. All of these twenty contributors and myself are extremely proud of the role that each of us has played in the field of education and certification of the dental assistant.

The citation of academic positions does not communicate the past services rendered to dental assistant education. My position with the American Dental Association gave me the unusual opportunity to help create the first formal educational requirements for dental assistants and to work with the early ADAA Certification Board when it was first trying to develop examinations and create the first program for proving continuing competence. I worked with many of my contributors on the DAU Committee; every contributor has made successful efforts toward establishing and reinforcing the importance of the dental assistant in the dental health team of today and tomorrow.

The contributors to this textbook are responsible for many important developments in the history of dental assisting. They helped write the specifications for the requirements of school accreditation by the ADA's Council on Dental Education and helped write the first Certification Board Examinations. They were involved in the struggle that won full recognition from the ADA for the activities and aspirations of the American Dental Assistants Association. They constructed some of the first courses for dental assistants both in and outside of schools, developed the DAU programs that permitted all dental schools to receive funds in order to educate their dental students in the use of the chairside assistant, and have toured the country teaching four-handed dentistry to the faculties of these schools.

If there were a *Who's Who for Dental Assisting Education,* you would find all of these educators listed with their array of accomplishments. Dentistry owes them all a tremendous debt of gratitude for their help and their leadership in this important field.

Shailer Peterson
Editor

Contents

PART I PROFESSIONAL BACKGROUND

CHAPTER 1 HISTORY AND ORIENTATION

WALTER J. PELTON, B.S., D.D.S., M.S.P.H.

The woman who chooses dental assisting as a career becomes a part of one of the oldest, most honored, and at times most colorful of the world's great professions. Like other sciences, dentistry had its beginnings in the crude efforts of early man to find an immediate solution to an immediate problem of pain or disease. Like many others, dentistry advanced slowly, its history marked by the incantations of magicians and witches, by the amulets of the superstitious, by the chartings of planetary influences by medieval astrologers, and by the taboos and rituals of both pagan and modern religions. During the Middle Ages, the treatment of teeth, as well as the treatment of other human diseases, offered a profitable field to many an enterprising charlatan, and during the years of the Renaissance and Restoration, it proved a worthwhile sideline for blacksmiths, barbers, and wigmakers.

It was from this diversified background that modern dental science, with its widescale research and its advanced methodology and instrumentation, slowly emerged. No short account can adequately deal with so large a subject, but even a cursory review of some of the highlights of dentistry's history should provide the student dental assistant with a greater knowledge and understanding of the scope and direction of her new profession.

THE BEGINNING OF DENTISTRY

Man is generally believed to have inhabited the earth for at least 25,000 years, or more probably for 100,000 years. Earliest archaeologic findings suggest that perhaps from man's first appearance on earth he has been plagued by dental diseases, and that for a good part of his existence he has been trying to do something about them. Skulls dating back to the Neolithic, or New Stone Age, show that prehistoric man practiced the removal of teeth by knocking them out, and that by at least 5000 B.C., he was drilling holes (trepanation) in the facial bones to treat disease.

Attempts at diagnosis also appeared early. In several cultures, dental decay was ascribed to tooth worms. The Babylonian god Ea, the first diety known to be associated with the healing arts, was often invoked as the enemy of tooth worms, and the ancient Chinese sought to eradicate tooth worms by prescribing a pill that was 50 percent arsenic. (It is interesting that this use of arsenic in one of the earliest known attempts at preventive dentistry has a modern counterpart in the arsenic pastes that are still being used to devitalize teeth.)

According to both archaeologic findings and written records, advances in instrumentation and preventive dentistry slowly continued over the ages. By 3000 B.C., the toothpick had been developed, and the cruder tools of the New Stone Age had been replaced by instruments especially designed for the extraction of teeth. By 1000 B.C., the scientists had turned their attention to dental problems. Among the teachings that Cicero ascribed to Aesculapius, the mythical Greek god of medicine, are those recommending the extraction of teeth and the practice of oral hygiene. To the Greeks also goes the credit for an early mouthwash—a concoction consisting in part of the ashes of hares and mice, marble dust, and water.

Although most of the early speculations concerning the nature and treatment of dental diseases are amusing to us today, some ancient practitioners made blind guesses that came surprisingly close to scientific truths. For example, several centuries before the Christian era a court physician in Nineveh, the city to which the Biblical Jonah was sent, suggested that certain bodily ills of his sovereign might be cured by treatment of the teeth. Although his theory unfortunately failed in practice, it was at least a crude approximation of the modern concept of the systemic nature of certain diseases.

In combining the practice of dentistry with the practice of medicine, however, the physician from Nineveh was not unique, because the recognition of dentistry as a completely separate branch of the healing sciences and the growth of specialization within dentistry are relatively recent developments. Yet even in these respects, modern practice was to some extent foreshadowed by ancient peoples.

The first dentist of whom there is a record lived in Egypt, where the practice of medicine as a special art is believed to have developed in the centuries between 3000 and 500 B.C. His name was Hesi-Ré, which meant "Great One (Chief) of the Toothers and the Physicians"; he was evidently a dentist-physician. The second known dentist, also Egyptian, was named Neferiret-es, which meant "Treater or Maker of Teeth." This name at least suggests a dental specialty.

The fact that the Egyptians considered the extraction of a lawbreaker's front tooth an especially severe and degrading form of punishment is another indication of the emphasis they placed upon good teeth.

Although the Egyptians may have developed some prosthetic devices, the credit for making the first denture should probably be given to the Etruscans, a people who from about 800 to 500 B.C. inhabited a part of Italy roughly corresponding to modern Tuscany. Even now, comparatively little is known about the Etruscans or their civilization, but among the artifacts discovered by archaeologists are 12 examples of fixed or removable bridgework. These appliances, which are made of gold, can be seen today in Italian museums.

During the height of their empire, the Romans, borrowing heavily from the Etruscans and the Greeks, made marked progress in the field of dentistry. Their dead, also, yield evidence of gold bridgework. By the first centuries of the Christian era, some forms of dental treatment and the use of prosthetic devices had apparently become fairly common. Both the Babylonian and Palestinian Judaic *Talmuds* list rules regarding the wearing of artificial teeth, and the Moslem *Koran* gives instructions in the practice of oral hygiene.

It was also in the early Christian era that dentistry gained a patron saint. She was Apollonia, the Christian daughter of a heathen official of Alexandria, Egypt. During one of the periods of persecution of Christians, Apollonia's teeth were broken and torn out one by one in an effort to make her deny her new faith. Refusing to recant, she was burned at the stake, praying the while that those who invoked her name might be spared the pain of dental diseases, especially toothache. She was canonized in the third century as Saint Apollonia.

Perhaps the comfort that she offered kept sufferers in good stead, because in the years that followed, much of the skill that had been gained in dentistry was lost in the return to magic and superstition that marked the Middle Ages. It was from the witch's cauldron and the astrologer's chart that men of the Middle Ages received their "cures." In the years that followed, magicians were succeeded by the tradesmen—the blacksmith, the barber, the wigmaker—who pulled and "fixed" teeth with great profit but little knowledge.

THE BEGINNING OF MODERN DENTISTRY

Although a few forward steps continued to be made, especially in the sixteenth and seventeenth centuries, it was not until the eighteenth century that a French dentist laid the lasting foundation for what may with any accuracy be called the modern science of dentistry. The dentist was Pierre Fauchard (1678-1761), and his great contribution to the science was a 2-volume work entitled *Le Chirurgien-Dentiste (The Surgeon-Dentist)*. Published in Paris in 1728, this book was a well-organized and intelligent account of everything that Fauchard had learned about teeth, either from the teachings of others or through his own research. So thorough was Fauchard's work that it covered, to some degree, almost every phase of dentistry, even as it is known today. So advanced were Fauchard's facts and theories that his book continued to be used as an authorative guide for more than 100 years.

Fauchard was the originator of metallic bands and ligatures for moving teeth to correct irregularities in alignment. He developed a surgical treatment for pyorrhea that still serves as the basis for the more radical treatments of today. In the course of time, many of his theories and procedures have been improved upon or replaced, but the influence of his treatise was so great that Pierre Fauchard is universally known as the father of modern dentistry.

Modern dentistry began in Europe, but for more than a century it has had its center in the United States. For example, it was an American dentist, Horace Wells, of Hartford, Connecticut, who first used laughing gas (nitrous oxide) during a dental operation. Wells, who had witnessed an exhibition in which several young men were put under the influence of laughing gas, was convinced that the gas could be used to reduce the pain and shock of surgery. He therefore inhaled laughing gas himself, and while he was unconscious, an associate extracted one of his teeth. The date was December 11, 1844. After that operation came widescale use of general anesthesia, not only by dentists, but by members of the medical profession as well.

The introduction of general anesthesia was important, but it was not the only innovation of American dentistry in the 1840's. Four years before Wells experimented with laughing gas, another event occurred that was to change the whole direction of the dental profession in the United States—the founding of the world's first dental school.

Prior to 1840, dental practitioners had received all their training through apprenticeships. The first of these apprenticed dentists probably came from England to America in colonial times. Two of them, James Reading and James Mills, became the first "tooth drawers" to practice in New York, and perhaps the first to practice anywhere on the North American continent. Another apprenticed dentist, William Baker (1755), served as surgeon-dentist to George Washington. A third practitioner, John Baker, M.D., (1763) of Boston, is now recognized as the first man in this country to qualify for the title of *dentist.*

It was by the efforts of these men and those who followed them that the American dental profession expanded through the apprenticeship system. Under this system, a young man associated himself for a period of training with an established practitioner, who taught the apprentice all that he himself knew. Throughout the eighteenth and most of the nineteenth centuries, dentists continued to learn their skills from individual practitioners or small groups of surgeon-dentists who gave lectures, offered courses, and provided on-the-job training. Indeed, many dentists are still learning in this fashion. One form of apprenticeship that continues is that which qualifies a dentist for the practice of a specialty, such as orthodontics. The difference is that today the student aspiring to become a specialist must first obtain his basic dental degree from an accredited college before entering upon his apprenticeship. That difference was made possible by the establishment in 1840 of the Baltimore College of Dental Surgery, the world's first dental school.

The 4 teachers who made up the faculty of the Baltimore College during its first year provided instruction to a total of 5 students. It was a small beginning to a great movement. By 1969, 53 American schools, staffed by some 8,300 teachers, were providing professional educations for 16,008 undergraduate dental students. If graduate, postgraduate, and special dental students, and students enrolled in schools for dental assistants, dental hygienists, and laboratory technicians are added to that figure, there are about 26,000 students enrolled in full-time educational programs devoted to dentistry. In 1971, there were 52 dental schools in full or partial operation and accepting beginning freshman students; there were also an additional 5 dental schools that had been established and that plan to begin accepting students in the next few years.

MODERN DENTAL EDUCATION

The establishment of a dental school with its own curriculum and with a staff of teachers who were experts in dentistry had two immediate and lasting results. It irrevocably separated the science of dentistry from that of general medicine. In so doing, it also created in the United States two major healing professions, medicine and dentistry, which were to remain separate and distinct. This advance is yet to be reached in many countries.

The scientific growth and development made possible by this separation of functions were in time enhanced by the organization of dental associations (such as the American Dental Association in 1859), by the establishment of state dental practice acts and dental licensing boards, and by the publication of an increasing number of journals devoted exclusively to the profession and practice of dental science. Dentistry grew both in knowledge and in number of practitioners.

Success, however, brought its own problems. As the several states began to pass laws regulating the practice of dentistry, demands for a formal dental education grew, and as they grew, men with more business acumen than dental knowledge began to take an active interest in educational problems. The result of their interest was the institution known as the proprietary school.

Proprietary schools, as a rule, were organized and operated for the purpose of making money. Since the dental profession had not yet established accreditation requirements, schools set their own standards. Too many of the proprietary schools emphasized the quantity of tuition-paying students they trained, rather than the quality of training that they provided. Consequently, individual schools passed on and off the scene with amazing rapidity. For example, of the 29 dental schools founded between 1840 and 1884, only eight were in continuous operation throughout that period. Between 1883 and 1902, the state of Illinois alone chartered some 28 schools, but by the turn of the century, only 57 dental schools were operating throughout all the United States. Those fifty-seven represented the largest number to be open at any one time in the entire history of American dental education.

Despite the high death rate among individual institutions, the proprietary schools found a ready following, since they offered the degree that many states required before licensing a practitioner. As a group, they prospered for the better part of a century. That the substandard schools among them no longer exist to plague the profession is largely because of the efforts of William J. Gies, a scientist and educator.

In 1926, at the urging of professional leaders within dentistry, and under the auspices of the Carnegie Foundation, Gies published the result of a 5-year study entitled *Dental Education in the United States and Canada*. In his scholarly and objective analysis, Gies was highly critical of the proprietary schools as they then operated. He urged that dental education be made a function of the university. Although he emphasized the importance of close and continued cooperation between the dental and medical professions, he insisted upon the autonomy of dental teaching and practice. He underscored the value of integrating the clinical with the biologic sciences, and he pointed out the importance of research associated with teaching. He made a strong plea for more adequate public support of dental education.

The dental profession had fully cooperated with Gies in his study. Partially as a result of his recommendations, and partially as a result of its own analysis of the educational situation, the profession acted to correct the existing inadequacies. Licensing laws were strengthened, and accreditation standards for dental schools were made more stringent. The standards and educational requirements enforced by the Dental Education Council of America and its successor, the American Dental Association's Council on Dental Education, were largely responsible for the improvements in dental education and indirectly responsible for the subsequent improvements in dental service.

One by one, substandard schools were forced to close their doors. Schools with acceptable academic standards were put under public control. Finally, in 1929, the problem dissolved for good, when the last of the proprietary schools became a public institution. By 1930, there were 38 surviving dental schools, all of which met or surpassed the new and more exacting educational standards. Their degree requirements were far different from those of the Baltimore College of Dental Surgery, which in 1840 had asked its students to attend 2 full courses of lectures lasting from the first of November to the last of February, to write a thesis, and to take a practical examination. Even so, standards were to become more strict.

By 1916, rather narrow and rigid requirements for dental schools had been adopted, because in the 1917-1918 session, the dental curriculum had to be 5 years in length, each year consisting of 32 weeks, with 6 days each week. In 1934, it was recommended that every student have at least 2 years of predental education plus a full 4-year professional course in dental college before being granted his dental degree. Two years of predental education became a requirement in 1939 and remains the minimum requirement today. However, only 6 percent of the students are admitted to dental college with this minimum standard. Two-thirds have a bachelor's or other degree, and the remainder have 3 or 4 years of study without a degree before gaining admission to a dental college.

By 1970, however, the press for more dentists caused the accrediting agencies to relax the time requirement of 4 years for a dental degree, and a few leadership institutions began to implement experimental curriculums, which were 3 calendar years in length. Nonetheless, dental education in the United States today is truly a university discipline.

THE DENTAL HEALTH TEAM

In order for dentistry to attain its present preeminent position among the health sciences, the enforcement of higher educational requirements was not only desirable but also necessary. However, it also contributed to a problem that may have serious repercussions in the future, since nothing has yet fully compensated for the subsequent reduction in the number of dental schools. Our current total of 53 dental schools is still four below the number of those operating at the beginning of the century. Today we are barely able to train enough dentists to keep pace with the nation's steady growth in population.

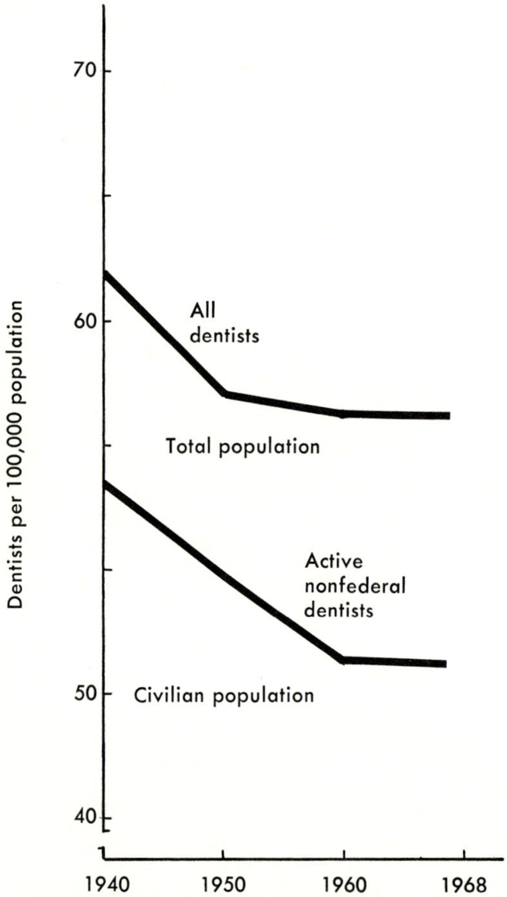

Fig. 1-1. Trend in supply of dentists, ratio of all dentists to total population, and ratio of active nonfederal dentists to civilian population, 1940 to 1968. (Compiled from data supplied by Division of Dental Health, United States Public Health Service, as reported in Dental Manpower Fact Sheet, 1965, and Health Resources Statistics 1969, Washington, D.C., 1970, Department of Health, Education, and Welfare.)

Fig. 1-1 indicates that the ratio of all dentists to the total population began to plateau in the 1950's, but the number of private practitioners available to the civilian population continued to proportionally decline until the 1960's. The marked decline in the proportionate number of dentists has apparently been halted by the impact of the Health Profession's Educational Assistance Act of 1963. New dental schools and the renovation and expansion of old ones began to increase the number of graduates by 1967. By March, 1971, the planned expansion of dental school enrollments was seriously threatened by the lack of federal funds to match those of institutions ready to build `or remodel.

In order to avoid a breakdown in the present system of delivering dental services, we must not only struggle to increase the number of dentists trained each year, but we must also begin to ultilize their professional skills more effectively. It is possible that disaster has been averted up to this point by the greater and greater dependence on laboratory assistance, especially that provided by the commercial laboratories. This practice has permitted the dentist to devote a large part of his workday to clinic activities. Even through improved materials and better equipment have been helpful, one of the most promising ways of making more effective use of professional skills is through the wide-scale adoption of a practice that is relatively new to dentistry —the dental health team.

The pivotal member of the dental health team is the dentist himself. Completing the team are a group of specially trained and highly skilled persons whom the dentist employs and supervises in the performance of certain clearly defined duties. As it is used in this chapter, the term *auxilliary personnel* refers neither to manufacturers and distributors of dental instruments and materials nor to the commercial dental laboratory technicians. Rather, it refers to the dentist's office staff. The term includes the secretary or receptionist, who keeps the appointment book and performs the clerical duties in the dentist's office, the dental hygienist, who performs prophylaxis and educates patients in oral health practices, and the dental laboratory technician, who fabricates appliances at the direction of the dentist and under his authorization and prescription. In this chapter, it refers most specifically to the dental assistant.

The concept of the dental health team may prove to be one of the most significant innovations in the history of modern dentistry. What it means to the present pattern of dental practice can be seen by comparing the dental manpower supply that existed in 1950 with that of 1967. The total number of dentists and auxiliary workers rose from 161,100 in 1950 to 235,700 in 1967, a relatively large increase. As Fig. 1-2 suggests, the number of active dentists increased by 27 percent in the same period, and the number of auxiliaries rose by 65 percent, accounting for 58 percent of the total dental work force. Although some dental assistants and laboratory technicians enter the labor force without formal training, there has been a phenomenal growth of educational programs between 1965 and 1969, resulting in about an 80 percent increase in the number of dental auxiliary graduates. An even more substantial increase is expected to occur in the next few years, when graduate totals reflect training programs that are continuing to be established, largely outside of dental school environments.

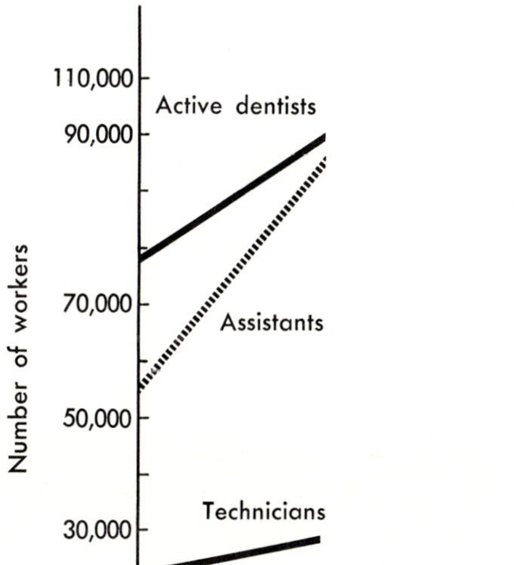

Fig. 1-2. Estimated number of active dentists (including 8000 in federal services), dental assistants, dental laboratory technicians, and dental hygienists in 1950 and 1967. (Division of Dental Health: Health Manpower Source Book, Section 21, Allied Health Manpower, 1950-80, Washington, D.C., 1970, Department of Health, Education, and Welfare.)

Fig. 1-2 also seems to substantiate the finding of the 1968 Survey of Dental Practice that 92.4 percent of the participating dentists employed auxiliaries in 1967; this figure is up 2.5 percent since the survey 3 years earlier.

Although the employment of every type of allied personnel is common throughout the United States, the regional patterns in the dental health team vary. Moreover, regional patterns have changed with time. For instance, in New England, where the first school for dental hygienists was founded, the employment of dental hygienists was the highest in the nation for many years. In the Survey of Dental Practice, full-time hygienists were found to be more frequently employed by dentists in the Southeast and Southwest. It is also interesting to note that full-time dental assistants were more frequently employed by dentists in the Far West, Southwest, and Southeast, in that order. Full-time dental laboratory technicians were more frequently employed by dentists in the Southwest and Far West.

FUTURE DEMANDS OF THE DENTAL HEALTH TEAM

Important as it has been in reducing the impact of the current downtrend in dental manpower supply, the development of the dental health team is neither a stopgap nor an emergency measure. The auxiliary aide cannot replace the dentist; the aide's skills augment his. The employment of auxiliary personnel, particularly the dental assistant, has proved to be highly efficient and economically desirable step. Undergraduate students in dental colleges today are being taught to work with assistants. These facts mean that the closer we come to meeting the future requirements for dentists, the greater will be the demand for auxiliary personnel.

The problems of supplying dental care to the greater numbers of people who will be living in the United States in the future is presented in Figs. 1-1 and 1-2. Fig. 1-2 indicates that the absolute number of dentists is greater than ever before, but, as Fig. 1-1 shows, even though the dentist-to-population ratio has remained constant during the 1960's, the ratio still remains considerably below the 1940 levels. In other words, even though more dentists are available than ever before, they are graduating from dental schools in sufficient numbers only to replace those who die or retire and to keep pace with the increasing population. The key issue is whether a static dentist-to-population ratio can satisfy the rising expectations and demands for dental care. The problem is further complicated by the changing character of the population.

Urban people get more dental care than rural people. In addition, educational attainment and income levels are directly associated with the receipt of dental care. A trend toward greater urbanization than ever before, enrollment in schools and programs of higher education breaking records each year, and unprecedented economic growth throughout all sections of the United States are major factors contributing to increase the demand for dental services.

Consider, for example, the dental care received by children under 14 years of age as related to the education of their fathers. If fathers (considering only those between 25 and 54 years of age) have had less than 5 years of formal schooling, 16 percent of their children receive dental care. Of those fathers who finished elementary school, 34 percent of their children receive dental care. Of the fathers with some high school training, 54 percent receive dental care, and of those that went beyond high school, 73 percent. Thus, under today's pattern of educational attainment of fathers, the overall average of children under 14 years of age who see a dentist is 48 percent.

However, more and more people are finishing elementary school and going on to high school and college. If the same percentages are applied to the children of the better educated fathers of 1980 (that is, the 1960 rates of 16, 34, 54, and 73 percent, as mentioned), the overall average becomes 56 percent. Hence, instead of 48 percent of 35 million youngsters as in 1960, the dentists of 1980 will see 56 percent of 57 million, even at today's rates of utilization.

This same kind of change in demand will affect parents and every other group in the population. Obviously, if the ratio of dentists to population continues along present trends, some vast changes will have to be made in the methods of supplying dental care in order to keep up with automatic increases in demand associated with better standards of living.

Another assessment of what the future may bring can be estimated from the amount of money private patients spend for dental care. Consumer expenditures for dentistry in 1950 were about $1 billion, and by 1967 they had risen to approximately $3.2 billion. During this period, dentists increased their fees somewhat, and, after adjusting for the increase, the conclusion is that private spending by a larger population was considerably more than the 1950 level. Conservative projections for private expenditures for dental care in 1980 exceed $5 billion.

If dental schools can graduate enough dentists to maintain the present dentist-population ratio, the average private practitioner in 1980 will have to be even more productive than today's 3 chair operator (who uses from 2 to 3 auxiliaries), in order to satisfy an expected $5 billion demand for private dental care.

The tremendous growth in health insurance plans indicates another changing characteristic of the population. Prepayment for hospital and physicians' services has become a way of life in the United States during the last 25 or 30 years. The trend toward the inclusion of dental services as a fringe benefit in labor-management negotiations, however, is just now being felt. Currently, about 3 in every 4 persons have some form of health insurance, while about 1 in 20 are enrolled in prepaid dental care plans.

Still another change, public attitudes toward dental care as a wanted service in public programs, is looming even larger with each passing day. A good example of changing attitudes is the emphasis placed on dental health needs in community action programs, which have emerged from the "war on poverty." Undoubtedly, as the dental profession understands more fully that it is concerned with a health service that must be made available to all, and as the public seeks to acquire such health services, there can be only one result—a still greater demand than ever before, mostly by the less privileged groups, who have received little dental care in the past.

Therefore, if we do more than keep pace with population growth, the nation will need 139,700 practicing dentists by 1980. These dentists, in turn, will need to employ far more auxiliary personnel than the numbers already given for the present time. In fact, they will need 168,000 assistants and 39,200 dental hygienists. They will also have jobs for nearly 50,000 secretaries and receptionists. At least 39,000 laboratory technicians will be needed, although the majority of these will continue to be employed in commercial laboratories rather than in private offices.

Only through a wide-scale expansion of training facilities, both for dentists and for all types of auxiliary personnel, and through continued improvement of our educational methods can dentistry meet the challenge before it. Tomorrow's dental health team must not only be larger, but it must be even more highly skilled than it is today. In the last half-century, advances in technology, research, and methodology have been so great that they are changing the whole approach to dental practice.

FUTURE TRENDS IN DENTAL PRACTICE

The full impact of the great technologic advances in dental science has not yet been felt in dental practice. Some new developments, such as ultrasonic cutting tools, have not been perfected for widespread clinical use, and lately attention has been diverted to the possible effects and ways of using laser beams on tissues and materials related to dentistry. Still others, such as the high-speed instruments and the diamond rotary cutting instruments that are made possible by the use of water as a coolant during grinding, are already widely employed. Improved cements and impression materials are already at hand, and some day, perhaps, adhesive plastic filling materials that are stronger, better, and more aesthetic will be available. All of these improvements will make it possible for the dentist and his staff to give better care with less discomfort to the patient.

Closely allied to improved instrumentation is an equally important, if less dramatic, change that is taking place in the physical environment of dental practice. Dental offices and dental equipment are being redesigned.

Careful study has led to the designing of offices in which efficiency is combined with comfort. Proper seating arrangements, correct lighting, and the convenient placement of hand-washing facilities, instrument cabinets, supply storage, and ancillary dental equipment are making it possible for the dental team to work better and faster, to see more patients, and to experience less fatigue in doing so. It is of special interest that the planning of the new dental office has been based on the realization that the dentist at the chair is working with an assistant rather than alone.

Perhaps the greatest technologic change in dental practice is yet to be felt. Research concerning the duties of auxilliaries began in the federal dental services and dental schools following an American Dental Association (ADA) resolution urging such projects. By 1970, it had been demonstrated that dental assistants could be successfully trained in 1 year to perform tasks in the mouth previously reserved for the dentist only. Also by 1970, many states had revised or were considering revising their respective dental practice acts to accommodate the expanded role of dental auxiliaries.

As helpful as this development may be, many questions will have to be answered before the idea is widely adopted. For instance, the cost-effectiveness of such auxiliaries has yet to be determined. Then, too, will the average dentist be willing to expand the number of operatories in his office; if an expanded-duty chairside assistant can be taught to perform well in 1 year, what is to become of the dental hygienists who are trained in 2 years to perform only limited functions; and will the public accept this new type of auxiliary?

In short, tomorrow's dental health team may not only be larger and more skilled, but the duties of each member of the future team may be different than they are today.

DENTAL SCIENCE IN MODERN HISTORY

Technologic advances and improved office environment are the facets of modern dental practice that possibly make the greatest impression upon the patient. Members of the dental health team, however, are perhaps more deeply aware of the even greater importance of increasing knowledge of the nature of dental diseases, a knowledge made possible by the greatly expanded research programs of this century.

Fluoride research is an excellent example. The discovery that the addition of fluorides to public water supplies reduces the incidence of dental caries has meant improved dental health for millions. As it gains universal acceptance, fluoridation may make great changes in the pattern of dental care. Yet it will not reduce the total demand for care. Fluoridation means that the dentist of the future will see more and more patients whose teeth have not been utterly destroyed by rampant caries. These will be persons whose teeth can be saved and whose mouths can be rehabilitated. There will perhaps be a greater need for bridges and partial dentures and a smaller need for full replacement. There will be greater stress on orthodontics and periodontics. There will also be a greater public awareness of the need for adequate care and a greater appreciation of it.

A more recent preventive practice available to the dental profession is the exfoliative cytologic examination for detecting oral cancer. Based on Papanicolaou's method of detecting uterine cancer by examining cells scraped from the vaginal tract, researchers have shown that the method is of value in diagnosing malignancies of the nasopharynx and the oral cavity.

Knowledge of new drugs, tranquilizers, and particularly antibiotics has given the dental profession more tools for greater usefulness than ever before possible. These advances in technology and research will bring other historic changes. Like medicine, dentistry will undoubtedly move toward the establishment of more group practices. Group practice will mean not only the economic advantages of shared facilities and multiple-chair offices, it will also mean greater economy in the use of skills—greater emphasis on specialization and more intelligent delegation of responsibilities to all members of the dental health team. Also like medicine, dentistry is moving toward organized methods of prepaying dental services. More and more states have seen fit to use their legal machinery to permit dental service corporations to function. A dental service corporation is the dental counterpart of Blue Cross or Blue Shield, which are nonprofit organizations through which one may purchase insurance for hospital or physicians' services. Although dental prepayment plans will go a long way toward removing the financial barrier for many, the dental profession will have to find other ways to finance all the dental care needed by those unable to pay their way.

Change brings challenge and opportunity. Dentists of tomorrow will possess even greater knowledge and even higher skills. So will the auxiliary personnel they employ to assist them. The young dentist in training now is being taught to work well and efficiently with a chairside assistant. Soon they will be taught how to use expanded-duty assistants. When he enters practice, the instruments that he uses and even the office that he works in will make the services of auxiliaries indispensable. The job opportunities for young women in dentistry will therefore multiply, especially for those who are highly trained. The assistant trained on the job by her employer will soon be augmented by a formally trained graduate of an accredited school of dental assisting, a skilled auxiliary aide capable of making a substantial contribution to the advancement of dental health.

Following is a list of some of the most interesting and important events that took place in the fields of dentistry and dental assisting between 1839 and 1971. A study of these milestones will give the dental assistant a number of clues as to what the future holds for her and for the dental health team.

1839: American Society of Dental Surgeons, first dental society, was founded.

1839: *American Journal of Dental Science,* first dental periodical was published.

1840: Baltimore College of Dental Surgery, first dental college, opened with 4 teachers and 5 students.

1841: First dental law was passed (Alabama).

1844: Prevention of diseases of teeth through good oral hygiene was advocated in editorial in *American Journal of Dental Science.*

1844: Horace Wells used nitrous oxide as anesthetic in dental operation.

1844: N. W. Kingsley advocated employment of women as dental assistants.

1859: American Dental Association was organized.

1865: Lucy Hobbs was admitted to Ohio Dental College; she was the first woman graduate of a dental school.

1866: James Truman advanced idea of admitting women into dentistry.

1889: First international congress was held in Paris.

1902: In January, C. M. Wright proposed a subspecialty in dentistry—polishing of teeth and care of the mouth—to be practiced by women. He made suggestions concerning length of training, subject matter, and when training should be given. He recommended that a certificate be presented at graduation and that the subspecialty be legally controlled.

1902: In August, F. W. Law advocated "a new profession—odontocure—a girl with an orangewood stick, some pumice, and possibly a flannel rag, who shall go from house to house."

1903: M. L. Rheim made recommendation to Stomatology Section of American Medical Association (AMA) concerning training and state board requirements of the "dental nurse" experienced in dental prophylaxis. The AMA commended it, and New York State Dental Society attempted to amend The Dental Practice Act. (Law was amended in 1916.)

1905: A. C. Fones trained office assistant in prophylactic procedures.

1913: A. C. Fones organized and sponsored 6-week training course for dental hygienists to staff preventive dental clinic in Bridgeport, Connecticut.

1916: First dental hygiene school was established at Hunter College, with prescribed requirements for admission. Formal courses also offered at Rochester Dental Dispensary in Rochester, New York, and at Forsyth Dental Infirmary for Children in Boston, Massachusetts.

1917: Dental hygienists were licensed in Connecticut for first time.

1918: First dentist was employed by North Carolina State Department of Health to head dental health activities.

1919: Dentists were employed in United States Marine Hospital to provide dental care for merchant seamen. Dental care authorized for World War I veterans.

1921: New Zealand established program to provide dental care for preschool and elementary school children by specially trained auxiliaries.

1922: California hygienists requested American Dental Association to promote organization of American Dental Hygienists' Association.

1923: American Dental Association fostered establishment of American Dental Hygienists' Association and American Dental Assistants Association.

1923: American Dental Hygienists' Association was organized by 46 dental hygienists representing 11 states.

1924: American Dental Assistants Association was organized under auspices of American Dental Association; it was composed of a number of previously established city and state organizations.

1927: Decision was made to establish *Journal of the American Dental Hygienists' Association.*

1928: National Board of Dental Examiners was created by American Dental Association.

1930: Stainless steel alloys were developed and chrome alloys were used as prosthetic materials.

1930: Regular Corps status was obtained for dentists in United States Public Health Service.

1931: North Carolina passed first law making a dentist a member of every board of health in the state.

1933: First issue of official publication of American Dental Assistants Association was published. It evolved from a publication started in 1931 by dental assistants of the First District, New York City.

1935: Social Security Act strengthened state and local health organizations and provided for better programs, including dentistry.

1939: American Association of Public Health Dentists was established.

1942: Diamond cutting instruments were fostered as substitute for steel burs, which became scarce during World War II.

1943: Dental Health Section was created in American Public Health Association.

1946: Council on Dental Education, American Dental Association, established 4 years of high school and 2 years of college training as minimum requirement for dental hygiene training.

1946: Aptitude tests for dental students were authorized by House of Delegates, American Dental Association.

1947: Accreditation requirements for schools of dental hygiene were adopted by House of Delegates, American Dental Association.

1947: American Dental Association authorized Examining Board for Dental Specialties.

1947: Certification Board was organized by American Dental Assistants Association, permitting members to pursue correspondence courses.

1948: Topical applications of sodium fluoride were demonstrated nationwide as a method of controlling dental caries in permanent teeth of children.

1948: Accreditation requirements for dental technicians' schools were adopted.

1948: First conference of state dental directors with United States Public Health Service and Children's Bureau was held. Association of State and Territorial Dental Directors was formed.

1948: National Institute of Dental Research was established as part of United States Public Health Service.

1949: Central office and an executive secretary were established by the American Dental Hygienists' Association in Washington, D. C.

1950: Dental hygienists attained legal status in all states and territories.

1950: Fluoridation of public water supplies to control dental caries was advocated by American Dental Association and United States Public Health Service.

1952: Formal accreditation program of hygiene schools was begun by American Dental Association's Council on Dental Education.

1954: First statewide dental service corporation was organized by State Dental Association in Washington.

1956: Six dental schools using federal funds started to experiment with methods of training dental students to use chairside assistants.

1958: Central office and executive secretary were established for American Association of Dental Schools.

1958: Congress included $3.7 million in United States Public Health Service appropriation for construction of building for dental research.

1960: American Dental Association approved educational standards for dental assisting.

1960: American Dental Association approved basic standards for conduct of certification program for dental assistants.

1960: American Dental Association House of Delegates passed resolution urging dental schools and federal dental services to undertake experimentation and research in the training of dental assistants and dental hygienists in order to expand their duties.

1960: Federal funds were made available to all dental schools for training dental students to use assistants.

1960: American Dental Assistants Association collaborated with American Dental Association to help United States Public Health Service produce first movie to be used for recruiting dental assistants for training in accepted schools.

1960: Dental caries was shown to be a transmissible disease in laboratory animals.

1960: General Dental Council in Britain inaugurated experimental 2-year training courses for auxiliaries who would perform certain dental operations under dentist's direction.

1960: The Social Security Act was amended to help aged persons who did not need public assistance to meet routine requirements, but who did not have resources available to cover their health needs. The program, Medical Assistance for the Aged (MAA), was popularly known as the Kerr-Mills Bill. Dental services were to be provided under the program in certain states.

1961: First official list of schools having accredited dental assistant education programs was published by American Dental Association.

1961: National Dental Health Center was established in San Francisco by Public Health Service to be concerned with applied research and for training dental public health workers.

1961: *Survey of Dentistry,* a 3-year study by American Council on Education, outlined ambitious program for future growth and development of the dental profession. The *Survey of Dentistry* is the most comprehensive evaluation of American dentistry since the William J. Gies study of 1926.

1961: Dentists in Saskatchewan, Canada, recommended a new type of dental auxiliary be trained to take over some of the technical operations performed by dentists. Alberta and Manitoba already were engaged in such pilot training programs.

1962: Joint Commission on Accreditation of Dental Laboratories received approval of the American Dental Association.

1962: Dental laboratory technicians, hygienists, and assistants were offered scholarships for the first time by the American Fund for Dental Education.

1962: Arrangements approved the previous year came to fruition when the National Board for Dental Hygienists held its first nationwide examination just 29 years after the establishment of the National Board of Dental Examiners.

1963: Health Professions Educational Assistance Act providing grants-in-aid for construction of dental teaching facilities and student loans was signed by President Kennedy.

1963: Fluoridation was finally approved by New York City officials.

1963: A 1960 law requiring mandatory fluoridation of all piped water systems in Ireland was upheld by Irish supreme court after long court battle (67 days of testimony) involving many witnesses for and against from the United States and other foreign countries.

1964: The American Dental Association took steps to create an independent agency, the National Association of Dental Service Plans, to coordinate contracts for group dental care plans in more than 1 state, to assist in developing dental service corporations, and to provide for an interchange of information.

1965: A combination correspondence and residence course for dental assistants equivalent to 1 academic year of college study was established at the University of North Carolina with financial assistance from the W. K. Kellogg Foundation.

1965: The Connecticut Public Health Council unanimously approved a statewide regulation requiring the addition of fluorides to public drinking waters.

1965: The Office of Economic Opportunity undertook Operation Head Start as part of the War on Poverty program to prepare 60,000 children from needy families to enter kindergarten or first grade by offering to finance up to 90 percent of total cost of the program, which included dental care. Approximately $100 million was allocated for the total program.

1965: Medicare, the first major change in the Social Security Act of 1935, became law. Among other things, it provided hospital and medical expenses for persons 65 years of age or older, optional voluntary hospital insurance plans, and dental care for certain children by financing the programs through increased Social Security payments rather than by direct appropriations as in the Kerr-Mills Bill (1963).

1965: The Health Professions Educational Assistance Act of 1965 extended for 3 years the grant-in-aid program for construction of dental teaching facilities. Also provided were scholarship grants to students and basic and special improvement grants to dental schools to relieve the financial stringencies of schools and to improve the quality of education.

1966: Congress provided grant funds for medical and dental library research, training programs, resources, special scientific programs, and biomedical publications that were authorized by the Medical Library Assistance Act of 1965.

1966: American Dental Association recommended that individual practitioners proceed with studies and legislative action concerning the identification of additional functions which can be delegated to auxiliary personnel working under the direct supervision of a dentist.

1967: American Dental Association

urged dental societies and dental examining boards to support revision of dental practice acts to obtain more effective use of dental assistants and dental hygienists.

1970: Division of Dental Health (PHS) announced that funding for Dental Auxiliary Utilization Program would be phased out and that interested dental schools could apply for funds to support programs for training in expanded auxiliary management (TEAM).

1970: The American Association of Dental Schools and American Dental Association initiated steps to relax accreditation standards to permit dental students to graduate after less than 4 years training.

Suggested readings

Bremmer, M. D. K.: The story of dentistry, from the dawn of civilization to the present, ed. 3, Brooklyn, 1954, Dental Items of Interest Publishing Company.

Fones, A. C.: The origin and history of the dental hygiene movement, J.A.D.A. **13**:1809, 1926.

Gies, W. J.: Dental education in the United States and Canada, New York, 1926, Carnegie Foundation for the Advancement of Teaching.

Gurley, J. E.: The evolution of dental education, St. Louis, 1960, American College of Dentists.

Hollinshead, B. S., and others: The survey of dentistry, Washington, D. C., 1961, American Council on Education.

Horner, H. H.: Dental education today, Chicago, 1947, University of Chicago Press.

McCluggage, R. W.: A history of the American Dental Association, Chicago, 1959, American Dental Association.

Peterson, S., editor: Clinical dental hygiene, ed. 4, St. Louis, 1972, The C. V. Mosby Co.

Prinz, H.: Dental chronology, Philadelphia, 1945, Lea & Febiger.

Weinberger, B. W.: An introduction to the history of dentistry, vol. II, St. Louis, 1948, The C. V. Mosby Co.

Young, W. O., and Striffler, D. F.: The dentist, his practice, and his community, Philadelphia, 1964, W. B. Saunders Co.

CHAPTER 2 THE DENTAL ASSISTANT AND HER ASSOCIATION

SHAILER PETERSON, B.A., M.A., Ph.D.

RECOGNITION

Everyone appreciates possessing a title or some special recognition of his position or accomplishments. The dentist has the title *doctor* that he has earned through his education and experience, and he is justifiably proud of this degree and title. More than 13,000 dental assistants have earned the right to be called Certified Dental Assistants, and they are privileged to wear a pin or insignia with the CDA emblem. Also, these girls can place the abbreviation CDA after their names when they appear on programs of the local and state meetings and when signing business letters.

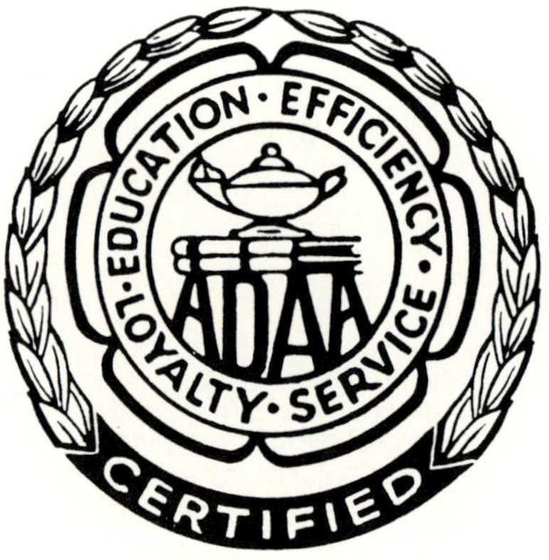

Fig. 2-1. Emblem worn by the certified dental assistant. (Courtesy University of Tennessee College of Dentistry.)

Both the dentists and the dental assistants have recognized the desirability of developing a program that would provide for this identification of CDA. It is significant that it was the dental assistants who actually developed the first certification program in the late 1920's. Although the program prospered, it was not until it became more formalized and became the joint project of both the American Dental Association and the American Dental Assistants Association that the program began to grow rapidly and attract a great amount of attention.

Titles and special recognition come in a variety of ways. In every dental office the personnel are given special titles that describe their activities or responsibilities. For example, there are the receptionists, the bookkeepers, the secretaries, the chairside assistants, the roving assistants, and persons with other such descriptive titles. These titles reflect the responsibility the dentist has assigned to the girl, and this responsibility represents the special qualifications she possesses to hold this position.

The dentists refer to one another by the type of practice each has. Some who treat a variety of different cases are called general practitioners, and those who tend to restrict their practices are the orthodontists, oral surgeons, prosthodontists, pedodontists, periodontists, oral pathologists, endodontists, and those in the dental public health service. These titles are descriptive of the type of work each dentist performs for the patient, but in recent years it has become increasingly important and essential that the dentist who limits his practice be specialized through certain formal courses. In other words, the title that had been descriptive now indicates special education and experience.

The dental assistant who has qualified as a Certified Dental Assistant has received the highest formal recognition that can be given to a dental assistant. As dentistry has grown and developed as a profession, the requirements for the dentist have become more complicated. Similarly, as dentistry has grown, it has become necessary for the well-qualified dental assistant to know more and more about the many additional facets of dentistry. Just as it is a longer and more strenuous program of education for the young man who wants to earn a dental degree today than it was 50 years ago, so is it now increasingly more difficult for a dental assistant to earn the title of CDA than it was 30 years ago.

The dental assistant who wants to possess and earn the CDA title is now required to take a formal program of education and to take a comprehensive examination to prove her competence. Of the approximately 120,500 dental assistants in practice today, only a small percentage of the girls will be able to take the time to return to school and take these formal programs. In the future, it is possible that the aggregate of short courses and the accumulation of credits through correspondence courses may become the method for obtaining the qualifications for taking the certification examinations. As of March 3, 1971, there were 13,330 dental assistants who have passed the certification examination and, hence, are eligible to be called Certified Dental Assistants. During 1970, 2,800 dental assistants took the examination; this shows the increasing number who are eligible with formal training to earn this title.

Dentists have a high regard for certification and what it means. On the other hand, the dentist-employer values more highly the ability, the competence, the skill, and the loyalty of a skillful dental assistant, since he would much rather employ a girl with these attributes and qualifications than employ a less capable girl, even though she may have acquired the CDA degree.

This is not to say that certification is not important. Certification is extremely important, and it will undoubtedly become more important in the years to come. Also, certification in itself provides evidence of a specific high level of proficiency. However, it is important to recognize that there will always be a great number of highly competent dental assistants who are not certified through formal education and examination.

Dentists have continued to educate and train their own dental assistants for many years, and a few will continue to prefer to do this than to hire girls who have received formal education. There will, of course, be many dentists who will find it impossible to hire fully trained girls who have been exposed to formal educational programs, and these dentists will need to train their own assistants or employ girls who have been trained by other dentists and by short courses.

All graduates of dental schools today are being educated and practiced in the use of chairside assistants. This phase of their education has resulted in a large proportion of graduates wanting to employ dental assistants immediately after graduation. Nearly all of these recent graduates are entering dental practice fully convinced that they need to employ a dental assistant.

They believe that the dental assistant is essential for the dental office. This means that these new dentists are seeking well-qualified dental assistants.

Dentists will always seek the best-qualified dental assistant, and he will make use of many criteria. Dentists seek those who are known to be qualified; this means that they prefer to seek those who have become Certified Dental Assistants, all other qualifications being equal.

A dental assistant can also earn special recognition through her attendance at workshops and seminars and continuing dental education programs. Some of these programs are designed for the dental assistant and the dentist to accompany one another and learn together about the new techniques in dentistry and about improving the efficiency in operating a dental office.

CERTIFICATION

Certificate

Certification is granted individually to persons who earn a passing grade in dental assisting on an examination conducted by the Certification Board. This certificate is evidence to its owner, to the dental profession, and to all members of the dental health team that a particular level of skill and knowledge of dental assisting has been successfully attained. Thus, certification is an emblem of personal accomplishment and attainment in a chosen field of work.

Board

The Certifying Board of the American Dental Assistants Association is responsible for conducting the Certification Program. The examination or tests that must be taken to become certified are prepared and conducted by a group of experienced and informed dental assistants who make up the agency (or board) that develops and administers the certification program. Certification is done by people, fellow dental assistants, who dedicate a great deal of time and effort to the establishment of proficiency standards by which Certified Dental Assistants are evaluated and judged.

Examination

Both written and practical examinations have been developed by the Certifying Board to measure achievement in knowledge and skill of those who desire to be recognized as Certified Dental Assistants.

The planning of formal training programs for dental assistants developed slowly. In the 1920's and 1930's, dental assistants, more quickly than a majority of dentists, readily accepted and responded to early organizing for the attainment of educational goals through the formulation of formal courses in the art of dental assisting. From the students who enrolled in the first available courses sponsored by the American Dental Assistants Association came the recommendation that training programs conducted at the national level produce standards of proficiency and competence in dental assisting that should be promulgated at the national level. The goals of certification on the basis of national standards of ability and achievement were, thus, logically evolved by a group of earnest and industrious extension-study students, who, of their own accord, dedicated themselves to an ideal of education. The certification examination subsequently developed was established as a guarantee that the body of knowledge, then identified as dental assisting, and the skills needed by trained dental assistants would be uniform from state to state and region to region. The first American Dental Assistants Certification Board accordingly was established in 1948. This board operated continuously from that date until the fall of 1960, when it was replaced by the Certifying Board of the American Dental Assistants Association, operating under the purview of both the American Dental Assistants Association and the American Dental Association.

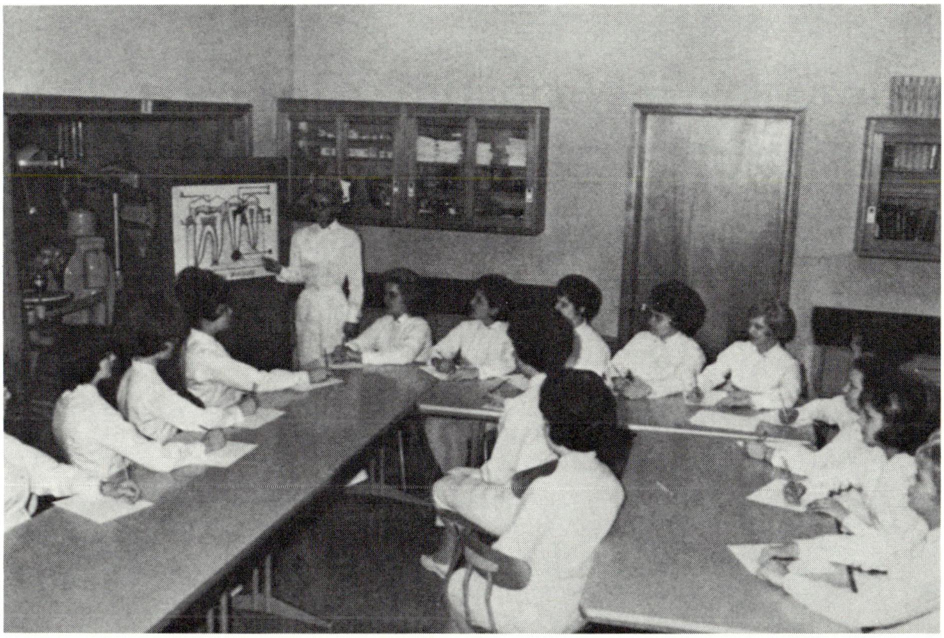

Fig. 2-2. Future dental assistants attending class. (Courtesy Chattanooga Technical Institute.)

The first certifying board was a national agency sponsored by the American Dental Assistants Association. It conducted operations from 1948 to 1960 under policies of this association and, with its examination program, played a prominent role in creating standards of dental assisting practices, which are now quite universally accepted. During the period of time that the American Dental Assistants Certification Board was operative, the full cooperation of the Council on Dental Education of the American Dental Association was extended to its members to the degree that in the latter part of the 1950's the dental profession began to give serious attention to the adoption of education and certification standards for dental assistants. In other words, the dental profession—although somewhat slowly at first—became impressed enough with the efforts to educate and certify dental assistants to want to give recognition and status to this essential auxiliary service of dentistry. Thus, the certification program has earned the respected and official endorsement of the dental profession in the 2 decades during which it evolved from no more than an idea into a full-scale national program of major significance. Certification is a serious program, conceived by dental assistants and dentists to raise the standards of dental assisting to the status of an important auxiliary dental service.

Everyone has some worries and concern over the prospects of taking an examination. Information about the test will always allay one's apprehension. About 3,000 candidates each year qualify and take the certification test prepared by the Certification Board of the American Dental Assistants Association, in consultation with The Psychological Corporation of New York. Ordinarily, about 88 to 90 percent of the candidates earn passing grades on both the written and practical examinations. Since the Certification Board conducts its program nationally, it seems evident that the 2-part testing program has been carefully constructed to reflect the type and amount of formal training in dental assisting that candidates must have experienced before they are eligible to take the board examinations.

If a candidate has had formal training or, better still, formal training and dental assisting experience, she should not be worried that she might fail the certification examination.

PROFESSIONALISM

Nearly 90 percent of all dentists are members of the American Dental Association. This is the highest percentage of persons from any group to belong to its own society or association. At the present time, only about 15 percent of the 120,500 dental assistants in practice today hold membership in the American Dental Assistants Association. However, this percentage is growing every year, because the practicing dental assistant who fully recognizes the importance of her profession wants to be a member of her professional organization.

The dentist and his assistant are both members of important health professions. When they chose this career, they selected it from many other kinds of jobs or business. Dentists have the American Dental Association to represent them, just as physicians have the American Medical Association. Similarly, the dental assistant has her national association, the American Dental Assistants Association, along with state and local associations and societies to help her.

Because professional health associations are very exclusive organizations, and because their membership is open only to those who practice the profession, dentists, dental assistants, and dental hygienists should take advantage of their opportunity to hold membership in their own organizations.

Professional organizations help to maintain high standards in many ways. They help to establish educational requirements for the preparation of the professional person and to arrange for continuing education programs. These programs help its members to keep up to date and to be worthy of advancements and promotions. They help to promote sound programs of dental health care for the public, and in so doing, they represent both the public's welfare and the welfare of their members.

Professional organizations such as the American Dental Assistants Association can accomplish many things for its members, and it looks for guidance and suggestions from the practicing dental assistants. The association can do many things for each of its members; however, what all of these members can do to make the organization strong and effective is also important.

All candidates for certification are required to take 2 separate examinations: one is called the practical and the other the written examination. The structure of the complete examination, then, is similar to examinations dentists must take before they receive a license to practice dentistry. The practical examination is given at testing centers established by the Certification Board, and the examiner is a local dentist, appointed by a state representative of the American Dental Assistants Association.

Although part of the practical examination includes "paper and pencil" test questions, it also requires that each candidate demonstrate abilities dental assistants must have to satisfactorily perform duties in a dental office. The practical examination, therefore, includes exercises similar to those that must be performed for a practicing dentist; for example, candidates are expected to demonstrate the preparation of an instrument tray setup before a root canal operation. Or the candidate may be required to assist the dentist at the chairside and to pass instruments as the dentist treats or simulates treatment of the patient.

The written part of the certification examination is intended to sample the candidate's understanding and competence in applying the skills and abilities considered essential for dental assistants to know before they will be able to function effectively in a dental office. The areas of knowledge covered by the written examination, a multiple choice type test, include all kinds of information that the dental profession has determined to be minimum and essential.

The test is not constructed so that it will be difficult to pass. Rather, it is designed to test a candidate's knowledge of the names of dental instruments, how to use dental materials, the classification and proper names of the teeth, the anatomy of the head and neck regions of the body, the basic techniques of mixing amalgam and other filling material, and the role of the dental assistant on the dental health team. The assistant who is not familiar with these and similar fundamentals of dental assisting is probably not a very successful or efficient dental assistant—and effective and efficient service is the basic reason for having the certification program.

Certified dental assistants are expected to annually attest to having made certain contributions and undertaken specific activities that indicate a personal and constructive involvement in dental and dental assistance organizations. In a broad sense, claims of participation in the affairs of local, state, and national organizations are indicative of an active interest in dental assisting and dentistry. Reading the *Dental Assistant,* the official journal of the American Dental Assistants Association, indicates interest to be informed and involved actively in the affairs of dental assisting and dentistry. Presentation of clinics before dental assistant groups, or in connection with dental society meetings, also suggests that abilities and skills in dental assisting of the participants are of a higher order than the average nonparticipant in this auxiliary service of dentistry.

These activities and involvements are the essence of what the Certification Board has called its renewal "point system." It is this same kind of a point system that is now being considered by the medical and dental professions as a means of checking to see if their members are keeping up-to-date. Several state dental licensing boards are working on suggestions that will provide a mechanism so that the public will be assured that the dentist it chooses is going back to school periodically.

Making rules that require dentists and dental assistants go back to school periodically or to attend continuing education courses may seem unnecessary. Most persons feel that a truly professional person will take it upon himself or herself to read the literature and to take refresher courses and so on. As a matter of fact, the percentage of persons who take such courses voluntarily now is very high. But, in spite of this, licensing boards and certifying boards feel that those who already want to keep up-to-date will not object to such rules and regulations; those who fail to keep updated need to be encouraged or even forced to do so.

The dental assistants can be proud of the fact that it was their own organization that took the first official steps toward making rules and regulations that require its members to take continuing educational work if they are going to remain eligible to be certified.

CHAPTER 3 THE DENTAL ASSISTANT AND HER EMPLOYER

SHAILER PETERSON, B.A., M.A., Ph.D.
WADE B. WINNETT, D.D.S., M.S.D.

The purpose of this chapter is to demonstrate that the dentist needs the dental assistant in his office, and the dental assistant needs her supervising dentist-employer. Throughout this textbook, emphasis is on the utilization of the dental health team. The dentist depends upon his dental assistant, his dental hygienist, his dental laboratory technician, and all of the other persons who keep his office operating with top efficiency.

It is, of course, true that every employer and employee should have a mutual respect for one another and be able to work together in a cooperative fashion, regardless of the kind of business that they are in. However, when the life and the safety of a patient is at stake, the team that is responsible for this very special health service must have a much closer relationship than mere cooperation and mutual respect. The same kind of teamwork and allegiance is needed when a special combat troop goes out on a mission. While each has his or her job to perform, there must be 1 person who is responsible for directing and supervising the total activity, or, in this case, the service to the patient.

One must not forget that the employer who directs and supervises the work that is done by the team is also the one who elects to take all of the responsibility for the work of the entire team. If the patient dies, or if the tooth cannot be saved, it is the dentist-employer who takes this responsibility. If one of the team members does anything that in itself makes the operation fail, even though it is that team member who is really at fault, the dentist-employer must still assume the blame and the responsibility.

Therefore, the dentist-employer does his best to hire for his team only those persons who are dependable and who will be a credit to his office and his practice. The dentist knows that the success of his practice depends not just on his own judgment and skill, but also upon the supporting activities that his team members will provide as each does his or her work at the proper time.

There are many patients who have had the experience of being in a dental office where the members of the dental team performed as if they were well-trained members of an acrobatic team, aware of the importance of each motion to success or failure. There is today no position of any importance that is not supported by a team of workers. Whether it be the motor car racer who depends upon his pit crew, the Air Force pilot who depends upon his ground crew to keep his plane in top condition, or the orchestra conductor whose music depends completely upon the coordinated efforts of each member, the "name of the game" is *teamwork.*

The fact that the dental assistant is a member of a team does not detract from her importance or from her indispensability. Furthermore, being a team member does not detract from the dental assistant's individuality or from her responsibility to make professional decisions. However, the team approach does mean that while the dentist-supervisor plans and directs the overall treatment plan and is responsible for the rules of the office, he must have the assurance from his staff that they will function as a unit at all times. In other words, no individual member can be permitted to go off on a tangent and decide to execute her job at a different pace than everyone else or to disregard the rules of the office.

A professional person is one who has the wisdom and judgment to be able to take the responsibility for making decisions. Every dental assistant has been given knowledge that makes it possible for her to make judgments, just as the dentist must make judgments about patients and treatment. The dentist and the physician who see any of their patients in the hospital must also work as a team, for they must render their professional judgments within the framework of the rules and regulations of the hospital; they cannot work at cross purposes to the hospital administration and the team of hospital personnel.

The dentist and the dental assistant will have certain sets of rules and customs that are used in their private dental office; they work with another set of rules when they are working on patients in a hospital; and they may work with still another set of rules when they are demonstrating in a dental school. In a similar way, a dentist and his team members may perform certain operations in 1 state, but they would have to abide by new rules if the dentist were to practice in another state. It is the responsibility of the dentist and his dental assistant to learn the rules and regulations wherever they are working.

In other chapters in this book, attention is given to the dentist and his dental assistant studying the patient in order to know as much as possible about him. The better they know the patient, the better the dentist and his dental assistant can cope with any of his or her fears. Just as it is vitally important to know if the patient is allergic to certain medications, it is essential that one knows whether the patient has been unduly frightened in a dental office or hospital situation previously.

Just as it is important for the dental assistant to study and understand her patients, and just as every dental student tries his best to understand his instructors, the dental assistant must also study her dentist-employer and the other members of the dental health team. It is easy to misunderstand a person if one does nothing to understand him. It is easy to misinterpret the behavior of a person when one does not fully understand him.

It is perfectly normal and desirable for a person to want to be liked by her employer and by her associates. Therefore, it is also natural for her to want to understand what it is that her employer expects of her and how he expects her to work with the other employees. This point is being emphasized, because all too often, the employer is either too busy to explain all of the things that he expects to be done, or he may think that his employees can figure these things out for themselves.

If one were to try to list the things that a member of the dental team should do, it might at first seem like a very peculiar list. Many of the items and the precautions would seem so natural and commonplace that most persons would think it completely unnecessary to even mention them. For example, the most important rules of behavior for the members of a team are as follows:

1. Be considerate of others.
2. Think before acting.
3. Try to use best judgment at all times.
4. Do not jump to conclusions.

No book can teach an employee to get along with her employer or with all of the people who work in her office. There are some employees who seem to get along well in any office situation, and there are others who have one problem after another. There is probably no position that does not have some problems; in general, the best advice is that the employee should keep in good communication with her employer, so that when she senses that there is a problem, she will find it easy to discuss it with him. It does no good to discuss one's personal problems with the other employees, for it will ultimately be an understanding between the dental assistant and her employer that will correct the misunderstanding or problem that she has in the office.

Every dental assistant, in choosing her career, has realized that there is prestige in being a part of a health team, and that the environment of a dental office is much more pleasant than that most of other kinds of positions. Everyone in a prestigious position wants to work hard to hold that position and to grow in value to the entire team. Perhaps there are some positions that are "just jobs," and if one loses his position, there may be many others equally as good readily available. This is not true in the case of a dentist, a dental assistant, or any other member of the dental health team. These positions are valuable, and they are sought after. Those who are fortunate to obtain them, work hard to make themselves an indispensable part of that dental office team. Furthermore, they find that they must continue to work hard to maintain their position of importance. A worthwhile, prestigious position is worth working to obtain, and it is worth working to retain. A dental assistant has reason to be proud of her position.

CHAPTER 4 THE PROFESSION AND EXPANDING DUTIES

SHAILER PETERSON, B.A., M.A., Ph.D.
WADE B. WINNETT, D.D.S., M.S.D.

DIFFERENCES OF OPINION

On any subject there can undoubtedly be two or even more different opinions, or points of view. Some dental assistants say that they have enough to do now, and they don't want any more responsibilities. Others say they want to be permitted to perform more duties and to have greater responsibilities. Some dentists also want to have the duties and responsibilities of their dental assistants to be expanded or enlarged, and still others think that they now have all of the responsibilities that they should be given.

A similar statement could be made about the dental hygienists. Some dental hygienists want to have their duties enlarged, and still others feel that they have enough things to keep them busy, and they do not wish to have any more expected of them. Some dental hygienists want the dental assistant to be given more responsibilites, but they wish their own duties to remain unchanged. There are all combinations of opinions on this problem of duties that should be delegated to the dentist and to the different members of his office team.

In dental school, a dentist is educated and given experience so that he will be equipped to treat all of the usual kinds of problems that he will encounter in his patients. In other words, a dentist could perform all of the functions in an office. For example, he could make the appointments, receive the patient, and perform the office and secretarial work that is usually done by the dental assistant. The dentist could perform the oral prophylaxis and talk to the patient about oral hygiene, which is usually done by the dental hygienist. The dentist could also do all of the laboratory work that is done either by the dental laboratory technician in his office or by a commercial dental laboratory. The dentist could also repair his dental equipment, which is normally done by the serviceman from the dental dealer. The dentist could sterilize his own instruments, sharpen them, and keep his office spotless.

It would be wasteful of the dentist's time and education if he were to perform all of these duties, for these can be done by dental assistants, dental hygienists, and dental laboratory technicians. The dentist should be left with plenty of time to devote to diagnosing the patients problems, planning the total treatment of the patient, performing the surgery, restoring the teeth, treating the patient, designing the dental appliances, and doing all of the other highly technical duties that only the dentist is qualified to perform.

DUTIES OF DENTAL HYGIENIST

When one lists all of the different activities that take place in the dental office, the reception room, the operatory, the business office, and the laboratory, there is a comprehensive list of all of the duties that someone on the dental health team must perform and for which someone must take the prime responsibility. Over the years, there has been some general agreement upon what things it seemed practical to assign to the dental hygienist, for example. She has been given the responsibility of scaling and polishing the teeth (dental, or oral, prophylaxis). She has also been given an educational background so that she understands what needs to be taught to patients about a sound dental health education program. The dental hygienist is also trained to give topical applications of fluoride. Normally, it has not been expected that the dental hygienist work as a receptionist, a chairside assistant, a bookkeeper, or a laboratory assistant.

DUTIES OF DENTAL ASSISTANT

On the other hand, the dental assistant has been expected by most dentists to act as a chairside assistant, secretary, and receptionist. Some have also been trained to work as bookkeepers, to pour study models, and to take and process dental x-rays. As a dental practice becomes busier, and more patients are being served, additional dental assistants are then employed. When that happens, the dentist-employer begins to assign special responsibilities to each of the added dental assistants and to the dental hygienists. Sometimes a dental assistant will be given special education and training, so that she will become very adept at duties that were not always assigned to a dental assistant.

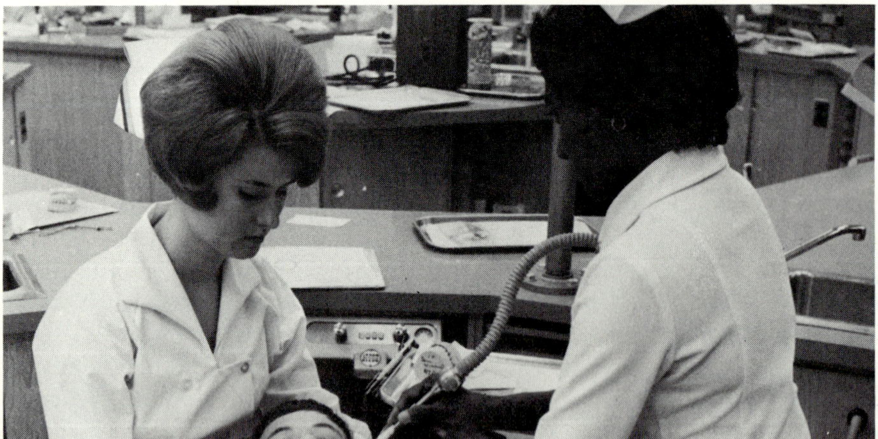

Fig. 4-1. An expanded-duty dental assistant utilizing the services of a chairside assistant in a patient care situation. (Courtesy Dental Manpower Development Center, Louisville, Kentucky.)

NEW EVALUATION

To prepare for the increasing demand for dental services, several methods are being used. New dental schools are being constructed, and present dental schools are being expanded to enroll larger classes. Also, studies are being conducted to decrease the length of the dental school program, in order to produce practicing dentists in a shorter length of time. Increasing the number of dentists, however, is not enough. Therefore, the dental profession is advocating that the dentist reevaluate his own function and his own duties in his office, so that he will make the very best use of his talents and delegate to other persons the responsibilities that he can let them perform under his supervision. The dentist needs to delegate to his helpers those duties that they are either equipped to perform or that they can be trained to do. With a team approach, his office team can provide an optimum of dental service to his patients.

It has been suggested that as long as the dentist is responsible for the safety of the patients in his office, he should be encouraged to authorize his auxiliary personnel to perform any and all operations in that office that he feels they are qualified to perform and for which he is willing to be responsible. This is basically the way that professional men view the operations in their offices, for they surely will not permit any of their personnel to perform duties that they are not qualified to perform. This would endanger the patient, and the dentist would be responsible.

However, it is really not enough that every dentist and every office have its own set of rules and regulations. Lists of responsibilities need to be agreed upon so that the schools that educate the dental assistant and dental hygienist can properly provide the education and the experience for those responsibilities that the dentist expects personnel to accept. Dentists do not have time to educate their own personnel, although all of them give freely of their time to add to the education of each person on their staffs. The state boards of dental examiners needs to recognize that there are certain groups of responsibilities that the practicing dentists and the schools agree are appropriate

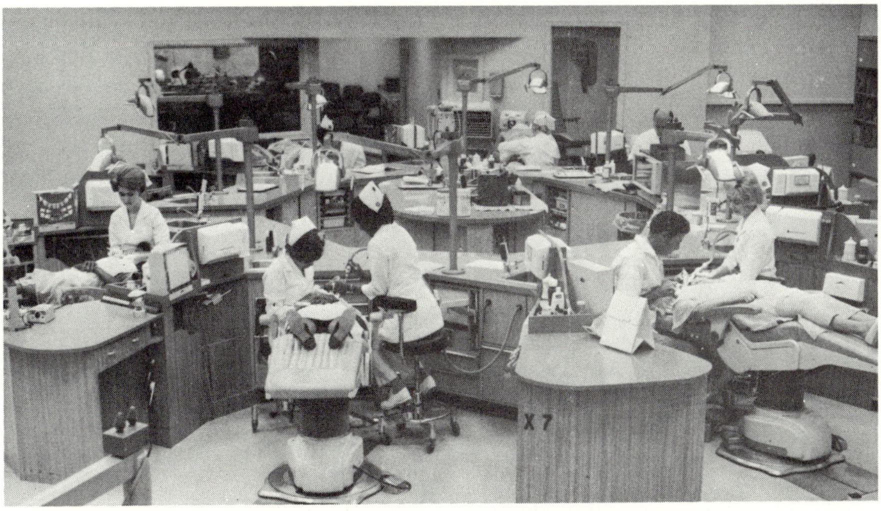

Fig. 4-2. Dentist at the Dental Manpower Development Center working at the "wheel" of operatories, assisted by 3 expanded-duty dental assistants and 1 roving assistant. (Courtesy Dental Manpower Development Center, Louisville, Kentucky.)

for the curriculum of these trained personnel.

The task of listing responsibilities is very complicated, because a dental assistant who was educated in a formal program 5 or 10 years ago was not given formal education in the responsibilities that are included in the curriculum today. The same is true for the dental hygienist. However, many dental assistants and dental hygienists who were educated years ago, and even dental assistants who did not take a formal program years ago, have enrolled in short, refresher courses, and others have had expert training from their own dentists and by constructive study. Therefore, some may know as much or more than a student who completes a program in a modern school today.

LEVELS OF PREPARATION

Not everyone who calls herself a "dental assistant" is qualified or competent to perform all of the items in any comprehensive list of responsibilities. There are great variations in the duties of different dental assistants. This is not a criticism, for a woman working in a dental office in which her total responsibility is in the reception room does not need to be expert in chairside assisting and in taking radiographs. On the other hand, there are some offices in which only 1 assistant is employed, and, therefore, the responsibilities she is given will undoubtedly encompass quite an array of duties. It is, therefore, the responsibility of the dentist-employer to determine what he can permit her to do, for he realizes that he is ultimately responsible for any mistakes that she may make and for the welfare of the patients who come in contact with that assistant.

Not all dental assistants have come out of the same mold; not all of them are alike. Not all of them possess the same talents, abilities, and judgments. Not all schools have had the same curricula, and those that have had similar programs have given different emphasis upon its various parts. In other words, the graduates of one school are not identical, and sometimes not even similar, to those of another. Similarly, the needs of one dental office as established by one set of dental partners is different from that of another office.

At one time, many studies were conducted to determine what things a dental assistant could be trained or educated to do. This was a rather foolish exercise, for it could have been anticipated that a dental assistant can be trained and educated to perform nearly any kind of a duty, providing she possesses the innate ability and is allowed enough time to receive this training and education. All that these studies pointed out was the fact that if one wanted to educate the woman to perform all of the duties that could be outlined for her, it might be such a lengthy program that end results would not justify spending either the time or the effort. These studies did make one realize that there is not enough time in any dental office for a dental assistant to perform all of the various jobs that she has been trained to do. Even the dentist does not make use of all of his talents and expertise in his practice. He may be a general practitioner, but even then he will specialize to a degree and devote most of his time to those services and operations that he finds satisfaction in doing. Therefore, the dental assistant really needs a basic education and acquaintance with the dental office as a general background for her services. In addition to this, she requires specialized instruction in those areas of responsibility that she will be given. Instead of expecting to take every dental assistant out of a common mold, one should instead tailor-make the dental assistant for the job that her dentist or her group of employers want her to assume in their office.

The next few years will witness the establishment of many generalized dental assisting programs, but the big change will be that an increasing number of schools will also offer short courses or special programs through which the dental assistant can become an expert in those skills that will be required by her future boss. It is likely that the new curricula will make it possible for students to acquire special certificates or diplomas to attest to the fact that they have been enrolled in a specific course for a period of time and have achieved a certain level of competence. Such a method would provide the employing dentist with a type of certificate from an institution attesting to the training of the dental assistant, and he would not always be required to judge competency himself.

Many studies have been conducted to demonstrate to the dentist and his auxiliary personnel the various responsibilities that can be delegated to the dental assistant and the amount of time that this will save the dentist. Studies have also been conducted to demonstrate the length of education that is required to provide the level of competence that is judged essential, or minimal.

LOUISVILLE PROJECT

One of the most extensive research and teaching programs of this type that has been conducted was the so-called Louisville Program, conducted by the staff of the Division of Dental Health of the United States Public Health Service. Officially, the program was called the "Dental Manpower Development Center in Louisville." It was conducted for 5½ years under the direction of Dr. William J. Simon, formerly Dean of the University of Iowa College of Dentistry; the research was conducted under the direction of Dr. Harry Bruce, who was at that time Associate Director of the Division of Dental Health. The reports* by Dr. Stanley Lotzkar provide important information about the concept of so-called expanded duties. Every dental assistant and every dentist who employs auxiliary personnel should study these reports and those listed as suggested reading at the end of this chapter.

The first report of Dr. Lotzkar discusses the skills and responsibilities that are normally or traditionally performed by only the dentists and that were taught to a group of dental assistants during a 1-year educational program. These included such tasks as: (1) alginate impression, (2) matrix placement, (3) amalgam and synthetic placement, (4) carving and polishing of amalgam restorations, and (5) finishing of synthetic restorations. It is reported that while the auxiliaries took more time to perform the same operation as the dentist, the quality of each procedure was very acceptable.

There have been other studies in which the auxiliary has taken on more difficult tasks and tasks that are not reversible. For example, some auxiliaries have been taught to cut hard tissue, such as in the preparation of cavities. However, most members of the profession are of the opinion that the auxiliary should only be given responsibilities that can be reversed, or that can be brought back to normal and redone if first done incorrectly. Obviously, if tissue is cut and damaged, or if a nerve is exposed during the preparation of a cavity, there is no way that the actual damaged tissue or part can be returned to its original state and the cavity prepared without the nerve exposed.

NEW ZEALAND PROGRAM

The dental nurse in New Zealand does prepare cavities in childrens' teeth and, hence, is permitted to perform operations that are irreversible. When the discussions were first begun concerning the expanding functions of a dental assistant and a dental hygienist, there were some who were very fearful that any change in duties

---

*Lotzkar, S., Johnson, D. W., and Thompson, M. B.: Experimental program in expanded functions for dental assistants: phase 1 base line and phase 2 training, J. Amer. Dent. Ass. 82(1):101, Jan. 1971.

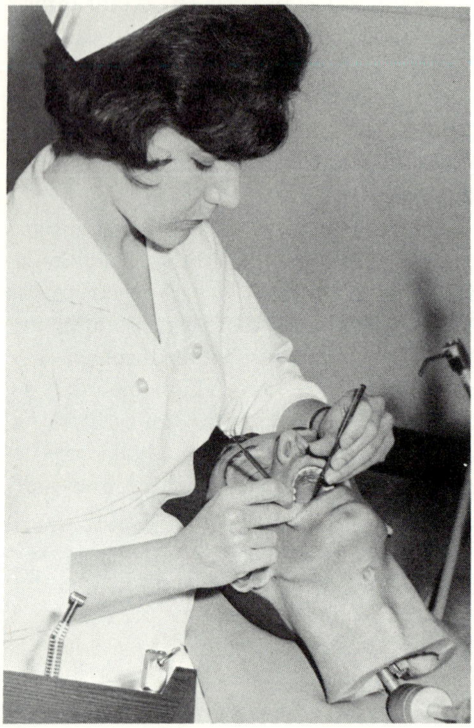

Fig. 4-3. An expanded-duty dental assistant practicing placement and carving of an alloy in a simulated head. (Courtesy Dental Manpower Development Center, Louisville, Kentucky.)

would create serious problems. People sometimes forget that everyone makes changes and adjustments in the way that they do things all of the time. The dentist adjusted from his old conventional handpiece to the air turbine and high-speed handpiece, and by now he has probably forgotten that this change ever took place. Every dental assistant learned to adapt to the new dental equipment when her dentist discarded the old "gasoline pump" type dental unit and replaced it with a modern mobile unit with all of its new gadgetry. It is really just another transitional step for the dental assistant who has never taken an x-ray to acquire this skill. Also, the dental assistant who assists at the chair and passes instruments to her doctor has taken her first step when she passes the amalgam to the dentist. The next step is for her to place the amalgam itself, and the next step is to carve and polish the restoration. These new additions become rather natural steps that really should not frighten anyone quite as badly as they have frightened some persons.

INEVITABILITY OF CHANGE

Some persons will say that it is still a matter of choice as to whether the dental assistants and dental hygienists will decide to take on the new and added responsibilities that update their usefulness. Perhaps this is true, but as long as the dental profession has made the decision that the dentists must be relieved of some of these duties that can be performed efficiently by auxiliary personnel, it is only a question of who will perform them. If the dental assistant and dental hygienist should resist or turn down this opportunity to become more adaptable, then the profession will immediately begin to educate and train a new auxiliary, called the "dental nurse," or a "dental therapist," or any other new name to distinguish him or her from the present members of the team.

The nurse in the medical profession has gone through and is going through a history of learning new skills, adapting herself, and expanding her functions; in addition, new kinds of auxiliary personnel have been created. New kinds of nurses have been created to divide the numerous tasks that the physicians and the public require, and this is exactly the same procedure that is now becoming a new milestone in the progress of dentistry. Therefore, it is really not a question of whether the dental assistant should learn new skills so that she can in effect expand her functions and responsibilities. Instead, it is a question of how fast we can decide what new tasks should be assigned to the dental assistants and how fast educational programs can be set up to provide these skills for practicing dental assistants and students.

There are some dental assistants who have resisted any expansion of duties, due to the fact that they probably misunderstand the urgency of this problem and the effect that it will have upon them. Expanding duties and responsibilities means permitting the dental assistants to be eligible to perform a greater variety of tasks than they are now trained and now permitted by law to do. Expansion of duties does not mean that every dental assistant is going to work hours that are twice as long and have twice as many different kinds of things to do during the day. For example, the fact that a prespective employee has the skill to use the typewriter does not mean that she will spend any significant amount of time typing or being a secretary. This skill is useful for even the chairside assistant to possess in emergencies, just as it is useful for the dentist himself when he is working on a paper to deliver to his local dental society.

Added skills provide the dental assistant with more attributes that will make her useful and valuable in a dental office, particularly in a dental office that already has a staff that has become accustomed to do all of the ordinary and usual things that dental assistants have been doing for years. Also, just as dentists now tend to specialize, the dental assistant will also find that she will be able to specialize. The dentist will now employ her because she possesses a special combination of talents, in which she has become very expert. She will not be hired just because she has learned to do a hundred things in a mediocre manner.

DENTAL ASSISTING SPECIALISTS

The young women who are learning to become dental assistants today are being educated at a very exciting period of time. They will have the unusual opportunity of being among the first dental assistants to have the unusual opportunity to take on new and real responsibilities, responsibilities that have never been done before by anyone other than the dentist himself. They will be among the first to become dental assisting specialists and to work as essential members of the dental office team.

DAU PROGRAMS

Every dental assistant who completes her education wonders what kind of an employer she will have and what kind of an office she will be working in. If she works for a dentist who has graduated within the last 10 years, she will be working for one who has had a special Dental Auxiliary Utilization (DAU) Program included in his curriculum. He has learned to work on patients while being assisted at the chair by a well-trained and experienced dental assistant. About one third of all practicing dentists have had this formal kind of training in their dental schools.

However, the wise use of dental assistants is certainly not restricted to recent dental graduates, for it is a well-known fact that practically all dentists use one or more dental assistants. Some of these dentists have gone back to take refresher courses on how to use auxiliary personnel efficiently; others have read articles on the subject, and many have taught courses for dental assistants as part of their own local dental society program. Every dentist today is well aware of the importance of using dental assistants in his office as chairside assistants, receptionists, secretaries, and so on. At all of the meetings that dentists attend, they are being told how they can make even better use of auxiliary personnel and how they can improve their practice by the use of new and modern dental equipment. The dental assistant needs to assist her dentist in selecting the new equipment and in helping to place it in the office (see Chapter 8).

Dental societies and state boards of dental examiners are all becoming very concerned about the duties that need to be given to all of the auxiliary dental personnel. More than half of the states have already liberalized their state dental practice acts, and the rest are all working on it.

The dental assistants need to be alert to the changes that are coming about in the new duties and responsibilities that will be assigned to them. They need to see that it is important for them to be able to take on these new tasks, and they should be glad that these opportunities for advancement do exist. It is in this way that dental assisting will become even more important, and it is in this way, too, that the dental assistant can show to her employer that she is increasingly valuable to the delivery of the dental health services of that office.

Suggested readings

Abramowitz, J.: Expanded functions for dental assistants: a preliminary study, J. Amer. Dent. Ass. **72**:386, Feb. 1966.

Baird, K. M., Covey, G. R., and Protheroe, D. H.: Employment of auxiliary clinical personnel in the Royal Canadian Dental Corps, J. Canad. Dent. Ass. **33**:183, April 1967.

Baird, K. M., Shillington, G. B., and Protheroe, D. H.: Pilot study on the advanved training and employment of auxiliary dental personnel in the Royal Canadian Dental Corps: preliminary report; J. Canad. Dent. Ass. **28**:627, Oct. 1962.

Baird, K. M., Purdy, E. C., and Protheroe, D. H.: Pilot study on advanced training and employment of auxiliary dental personnel in the Royal Canadian Dental Corps: final report, J. Canad. Dent. Ass. **29**:778, Dec. 1963.

Fulton, J. T.: Experiment in dental care; results of New Zealand's use of school dental nurses; Geneva, 1951, World Health Organization.

Hammons, P. E., and Jamison, H. D.: Expanded functions for dental auxiliaries, J. Amer. Dent. Ass. **75**:658, Sept. 1967.

Law, F. E., Johnson, C. E., and Knutson, J. W.: Studies on dental care services for school children; first and second treatment series, Woonsocket, Rhode Island, Public Health Rep. **68**: 1192, Dec. 1953.

Law, F. E., Johnson, C. E., and Knutson, J. W.: Studies on dental care services for school children; third and fourth treatment series, Woonsocket, Rhode Island, Public Health Rep. **70**: 402, April 1955.

Lefcowitz, M. J., and Signorile, V.: Chairside task inventory: self-measuring checklist of assistant utilization, J. Amer. Dent. Ass. **70**:94, Jan. 1965.

Rosenzweig, S., Egelhoff, C., and Webb, N.: An evaluation of the dental auxiliary utilization program, J. Dent. Educ. **35**:169, March, 1971.

Waterman, G. E., and Knutson, J. W.: Studies on dental care services for school children; first and second treatment series, Richmond, Indiana, Public Health Rep. **68**:583, June 1953.

Waterman, G. E., and Knutson, J. W.: Studies on dental care services for school children; third and fourth treatment series, Richmond, Indiana, Public Health Rep. **69**:247, March 1954.

Waterman, G. E.: Effective use of dental assistants, Public Health Rep. **67**:390, April 1952.

PART II OFFICE PRACTICE

CHAPTER 5 A TOUR THROUGH A MODERN DENTAL OFFICE

CHARLES M. BELTING, B.A., M.S., D.D.S.
ROSS C. HUNTLEY, D.D.S.

EDITOR'S INTRODUCTION

There is no better way for a future dental assistant to be oriented to the work ahead of her than to be given a tour through a modern dental office and see the layout of the office, the basic parts of thc total office, the different members of the dental health team and what they do, the equipment and supplies that are required in dentistry, what the patient sees in a modern office, and how the business affairs are handled. In this orientation, the dental assistant will be looking for all of the places where a dental assistant functions. She will see herself as a part of this dental team and as a part of the complex office structure. She will begin thinking about the role that she will play and how she will fit into the team.

This chapter does not elaborate upon any single part of the tour. It is only an introduction to these factors, so that as one reads other chapters in this book that do explain them in more detail, these chapters will have more meaning than if they were read without an overview. Together they will provide a description of how a modern dental office functions with a modern dental assistant to make this possible.

• • •

OVERVIEW OF OFFICE

Office design

Traffic flow

The flow of traffic through the dental office should be arranged so that the patients do not have to enter and exit through the same door. Patients should be welcomed at a window in the waiting room, ushered through an inner door to the appropriate operating room as soon as possible, and dismissed through a separate door to the business office. If possible, a service exit also should be provided, preferably in the laboratory, for delivery of supplies and as an auxiliary exit for personnel.

Note: We would like to acknowledge the skillful assistance of A. A. Caputo, Ph.D., in the taking of the photographs used in this chapter, and the secretarial assistance of Helen G. Gallagher in preparing the manuscript. Dr. Caputo and Miss Gallagher are on the staff of the Veterans Administration Hospital at Sepulveda, California. The contributors also want to thank the staff members of Dr. Huntley's office for their many helpful suggestions. The staff includes Jarilee Jones, Mildred Houston, C.D.A., Nancy Huntley, C.D.A., Jeanne Ward, C.D.A., Tina Fisher, C.D.A., Inace Bounty, C.D.A., Kay Lupo, R.D.H., and Karl Clajus, C.D.T.

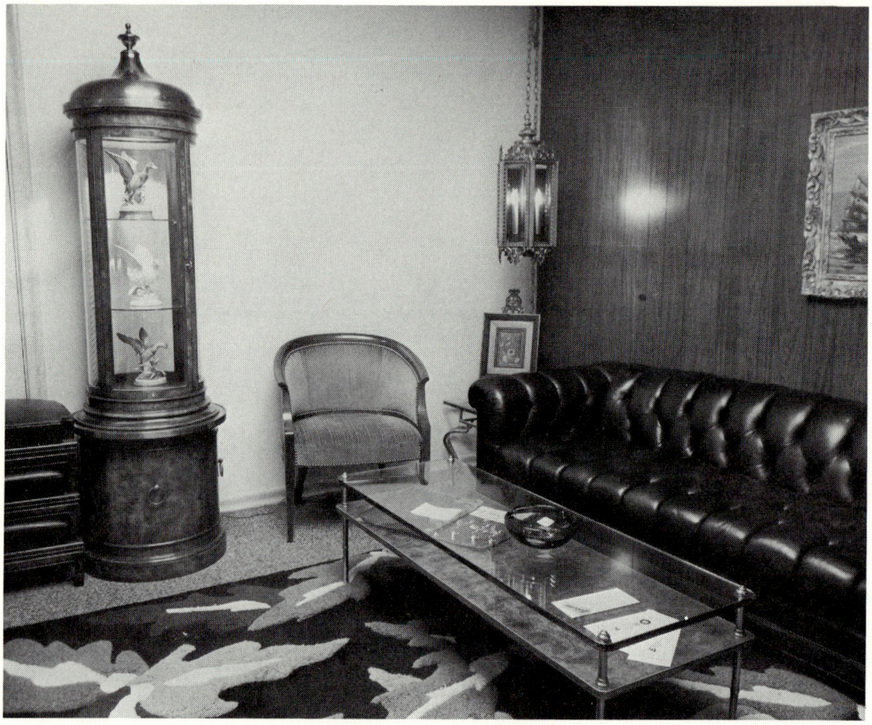

Fig. 5-1. Waiting room.

Waiting room (see Fig. 5-1)

The decor of the waiting room should reflect the high quality of the service rendered in the office and be furnished with the same meticulous care with which one furnishes his home. Careful selection should be made of wall treatments, book shelves, works of art, lamps, sofas, tables, and reading material. Use of mirrored walls should also be considered. The waiting room should be large enough to accommodate seating capacity for at least 2-hours of patients. Lighting should be sufficient to permit reading anywhere in the room. A speaker with controlled music and air conditioning should be connected to the waiting room, just as it is to each other room in the office. A large, ceiling-to-waist-high clear glass with a sliding partition should separate the waiting room from the business office. Too often, such glass partitions are too low for a tall person, who has to stoop to talk to the receptionist. Skimpy openings also create a shut-out feeling.

Business office (Fig. 5-2)

The area behind the desk in the business office should be large enough to accommodate 3 people—2 persons working at the desk and 1 person at the reception window. In front of the desk, the area through which the patient leaves the office should be raised, with a counter top at waist-high level. This provides a convenient surface on which the patient may write and make appointments with the receptionist. Ample lighting over the desk area should be provided to reduce eye fatigue during prolonged periods of desk work.

Doctor's private office

A private office where the doctor can review radiographs, make case presentations, discuss financial arrangements, and

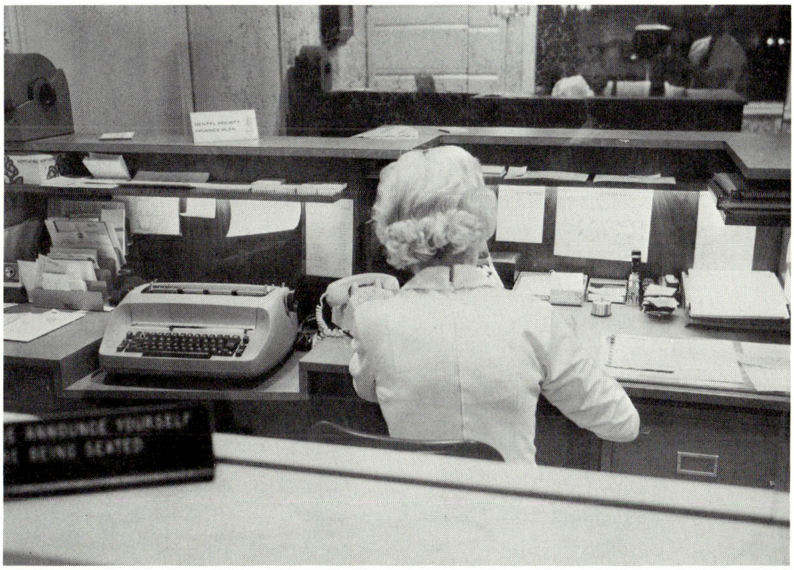

Fig. 5-2. Business office, as seen through window in waiting room. Patients are dismissed to the business office through a door on the right and exit from the door on the left, by-passing the waiting room.

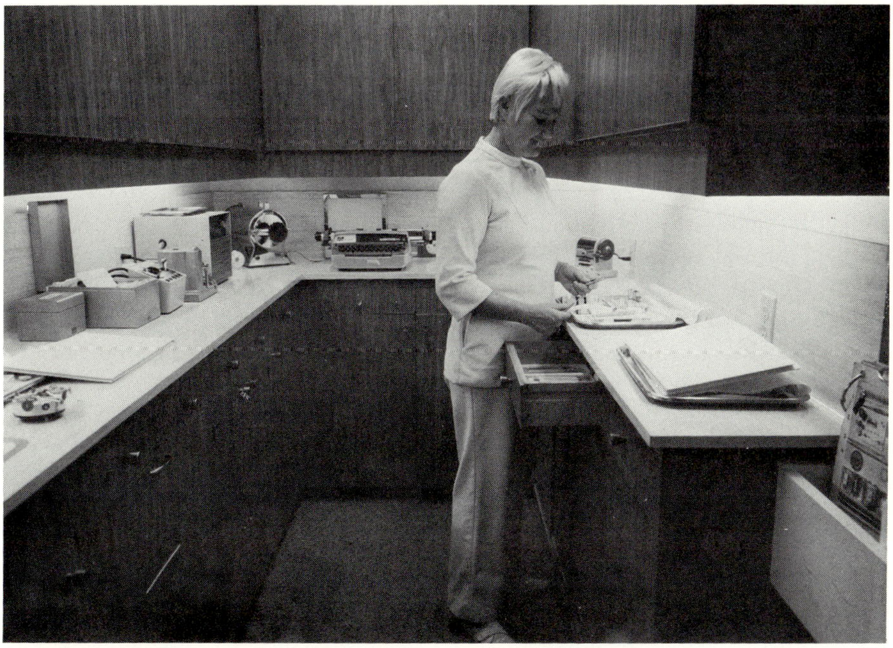

Fig. 5-3. Central dispensary. Note dental assistant assembling tray preparation. To the right is a patient's folder on top of a prepared tray.

hold private conversations is essential. The office may be small, but it should be large enough to have seating capacity for at least 2 people in addition to the dentist's own chair and desk.

X-ray section

Panoramic x-ray equipment can be located in a small auxiliary area, such as in the dressing room. Conventional x-ray machines should be located in each operatory to avoid having to move the patient for this service. A small darkroom to develop the x-rays also is essential.

Oral hygiene section

In addition to her valuable patient care services, the dental hygienist assists the doctor in gaining the patient's confidence, in maintaining a steady practice through the recall system, and in conducting a program of preventive dental health education. When a full-time dental hygienist is employed, her operatory is furnished with special equipment associated with her particular operations. In those offices that employ a part-time dental hygienist, this room may be furnished the same as the dentist's operatories and used by the dentist in the absence of the dental hygienist.

Operative section

The dentist should have available at least 2 operating rooms, not only for increased productivity, but also to have available an extra room for emergency patients or in case of breakdown of equipment. The number of additional operating rooms he needs will depend upon his work habits and capacity. Each operatory should be equipped in the same manner.

Central dispensary (Fig. 5-3)

An ideal office design should include a separate central dispensary for storage of supplies, sterilization of instruments, assembly and storage of tray preparations, and preparation of materials to reduce clutter and duplication of these items in each operatory. Also, it is useful to have an auxiliary typewriter in this area for use by the dental assistants. In addition, a bulletin board located in this area is useful for the daily appointment schedule and other daily instructions to the staff.

Prosthetic laboratory

The design of a separate room for laboratory procedures will depend upon the type of practice and whether or not the dentist employs a laboratory technician. In those offices in which a laboratory technician is employed, the laboratory should be adequate to accommodate 2 work benches, one for ceramic work and another for other laboratory procedures. Wall cabinets for supplies and waist-high work benches for equipment are needed in this area.

Dental staff

Number

There should be one dental assistant available for each operatory in the office. An additional dental assistant, with bookkeeping and accounting training, also is needed as a receptionist in the business office. Also, it may be desirable to supplement these personnel with a dental assistant trainee. Although each dental assistant is assigned to her particular area, she should be cross-trained to perform all duties in the office, including the business office responsibilities, x-ray work, and chairside assisting. The efficiency of the office and the productivity of the doctor is dependent upon availability of adequate personnel. A dental assistant cannot be developing x-rays, talking on the phone, setting up trays, or draping the patient if she is needed by the dentist for chairside assistance. There must be enough personnel to perform these other duties without interupting chairside assistance.

In order to provide a complete dental care service, the office staff also should include a dental hygienist and a dental laboratory technician.

Training

In order for the dentist to maintain control of all affairs in the office, instruct personnel, make necessary changes, and provide 2-way communications, regular staff meetings should be scheduled at least once a week. As emergency situations arise, additional staff meetings may be called as needed. Every member of the staff should be encouraged to make suggestions for improvement whenever possible. All members of the staff also should be encouraged to attend the regular meetings of their respective professional group, take postgraduate courses, and relay important information from these meetings to the staff.

Reception

Patient relations

The impression a patient receives of the dental office is usually created by the person who first receives the patient. Patients should always be greeted with a pleasant smile and addressed by their proper name. It may be occasionally necessary to be firm, but never rude about financial matters.

Always answer the telephone with a smile on your face; it reflects in your voice. Speak slowly and clearly with sufficient volume for the listener to understand, but not too loud. When answering the telephone, first identify the office and then identify yourself and ask, "May I help you?" Answer all questions if possible without keeping the patient waiting. When making an appointment, state the day, date, and time of the appointment, and repeat this information before closing the conversation.

Chief complaint and vital statistics

On the patient's first visit to the office, obtain and record the following data:

1. Chief complaint
2. Patient's name
3. Home address and phone number
4. Business address and phone number
5. Age
6. Employer
7. Occupation
8. Referred by
9. Physician's name

Tour of office

In the process of getting acquainted and welcoming a new patient, it is desirable to show him through the office, introduce him to the other members of the staff, and briefly explain use of the equipment, sterilization procedures, and routines of the office. Your attitude should be one of pride, enthusiasm, and desire to serve.

I. Business office
  A. Equipment and supplies
    1. Four telephones with 3 outside lines to allow up to 3 incoming or outgoing calls at one time, located at the front desk, the central dispensary, the laboratory, and the doctor's private office. The telephones should be connected from the front desk by a buzzer system.
    2. IBM Selectric typewriter
      a. Changeable balls permitting different typing styles for various purposes.
      b. Absence of movable carriage to save space in tight quarters.
    3. Adding machine with capacity for addition, subtraction, and multiplication to reduce arithmetical errors.
    4. Duplicating machine to make extra copies of office documents as needed.
    5. Horizontal files for folders containing patient's dental charts and x-rays (Fig. 5-4).
    6. Safe and fireproof drawer for active and inactive statement ledger cards and other vital records (Fig. 5-5).
    7. Two comfortable secretary

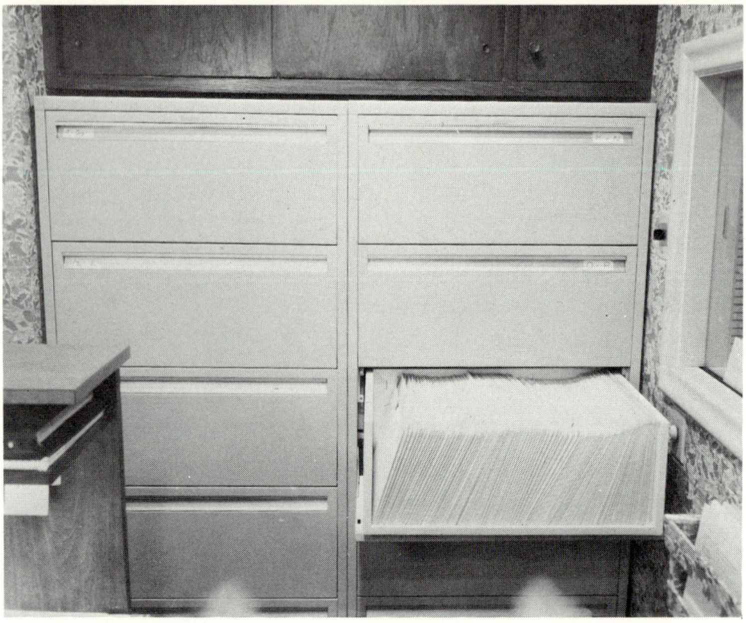

Fig. 5-4. Horizontal files for patients' folders in business office.

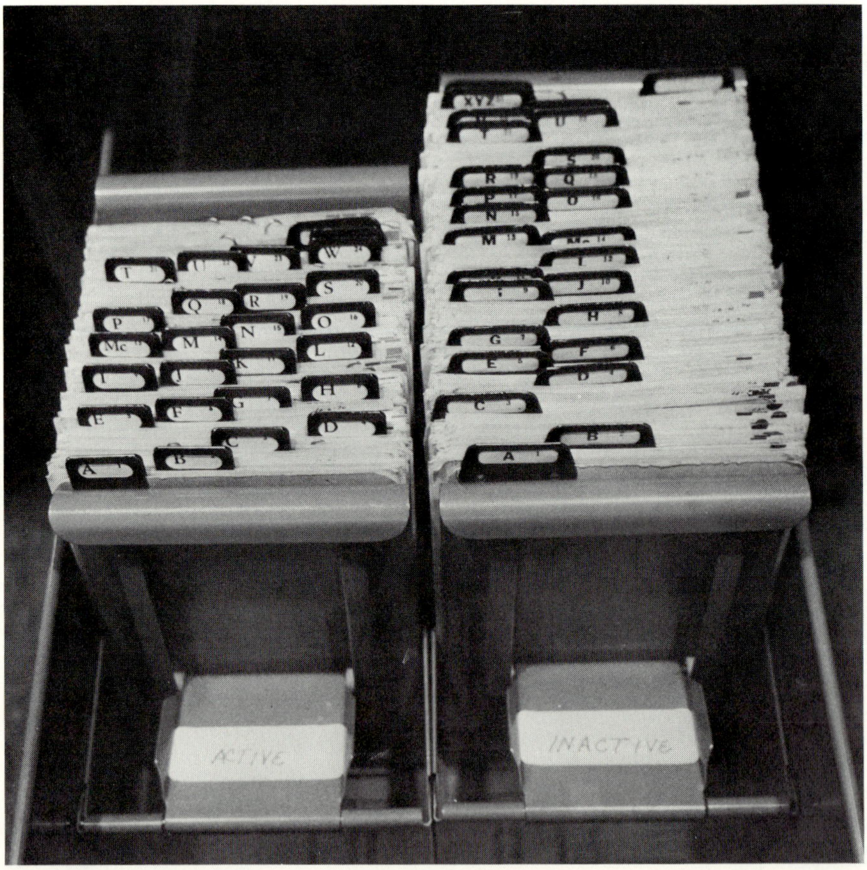

Fig. 5-5. Safe and fireproof drawer for active and inactive statement ledger cards in business office.

chairs to permit prolonged desk work with minimum physical fatigue.

8. Stationery notebook file of business stationery, cards, and forms with letter of shelf or number of drawer where item can be found for reference purposes and for training new employees (Figs. 5-7, 5-9, 5-15, and 5-16).
9. Roladex file for frequently used names, addresses, and telephone numbers of supply companies, repair men and business contacts.
10. Equipment file box (3″ × 5″) containing alphabetical listing of nomenclature, serial number, cost, source, and date of purchase of all items of equipment in the office.
11. Supply file box (3″ × 5″) containing an alphabetical listing of the name of product, source, minimum and maximum stock levels, date ordered, amount ordered, date received, and cost of all supplies stored in the dispensary. A similar supply file box should be maintained for all supply items stored in the laboratory.
12. Supply inventory and locator chart hung on wall in the dispensary, containing an alphabetical listing of all supplies stored in the dispensary followed by a letter or number indicating the cabinet, shelf, or drawer where item is stored. A similar chart should also be developed for all supplies in the laboratory (Fig. 5-6).
13. Metal desk organizer with slots for bills to be paid, letters to be mailed, and so on, to keep desk free of clutter.
14. Desk calender, pencil holders, spindles, scratch pads, staplers, tape dispensers, pencil sharpener.

B. Ordering procedures
   1. When product is needed
      a. When an item of supply reaches the minimum stock level, the card is pulled by the person recognizing the need for ordering.
      b. Card is placed in "TO ORDER" box in the business office.
      c. Ordering should be handled by 1 person, usually the receptionist or senior dental assistant, in consultation with the dentist when indicated.
      d. Order is placed by phone or mail with supply company or detail man to bring the item up to the maximum stock level.
      e. Take advantage of sales or savings by making "bulk purchases" when available, but beware of short shelf-life on some items.
      f. Order some bulk items with long shelf-life in quantities to last a year.
      g. After ordering, place card in the "ORDERED" box.
   2. Back orders
      a. Record date of back order on file card.
      b. Place card in "BACK ORDER" box.
      c. Cancel back order if not delivered in 2 weeks, and replace order with another firm.
      d. Refrain from ordering from firms that constantly put items on back order.
   3. Delivery of supplies
      a. Check and verify items delivered with invoice.

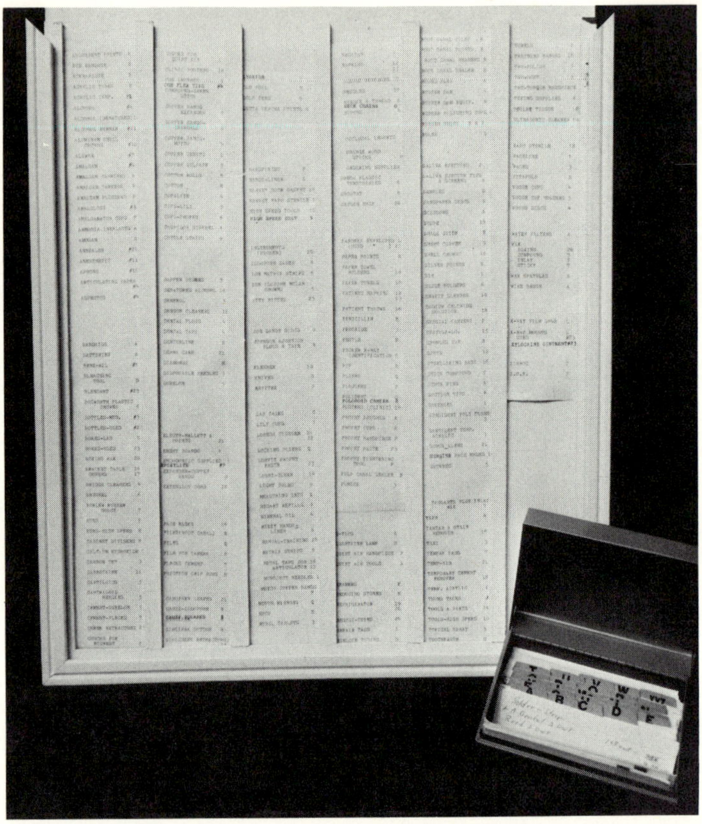

Fig. 5-6. Supply inventory and locator chart and supply file box in central dispensary.

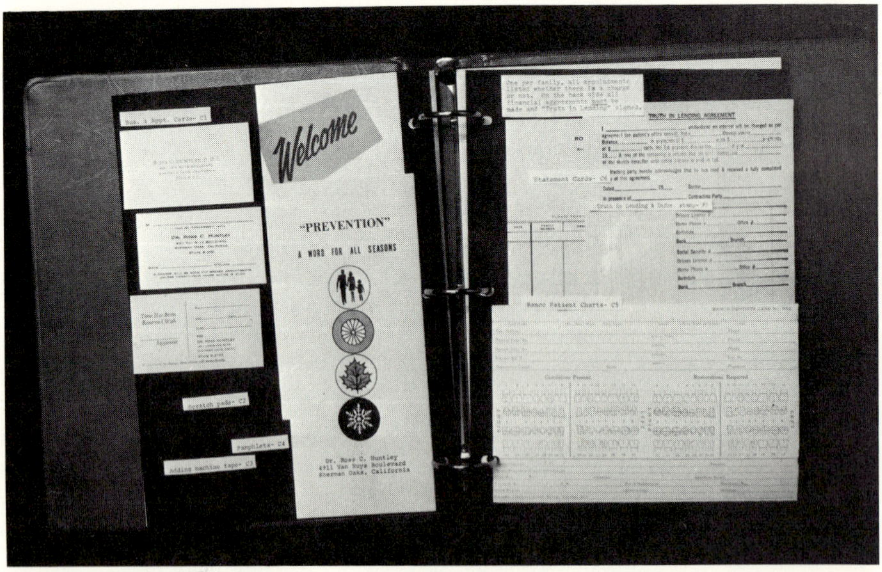

Fig. 5-7. Stationery notebook file. **Right,** statement cards with "Truth in Lending Agreement" on reverse side and patient's dental record; **left,** business cards and patient education handouts.

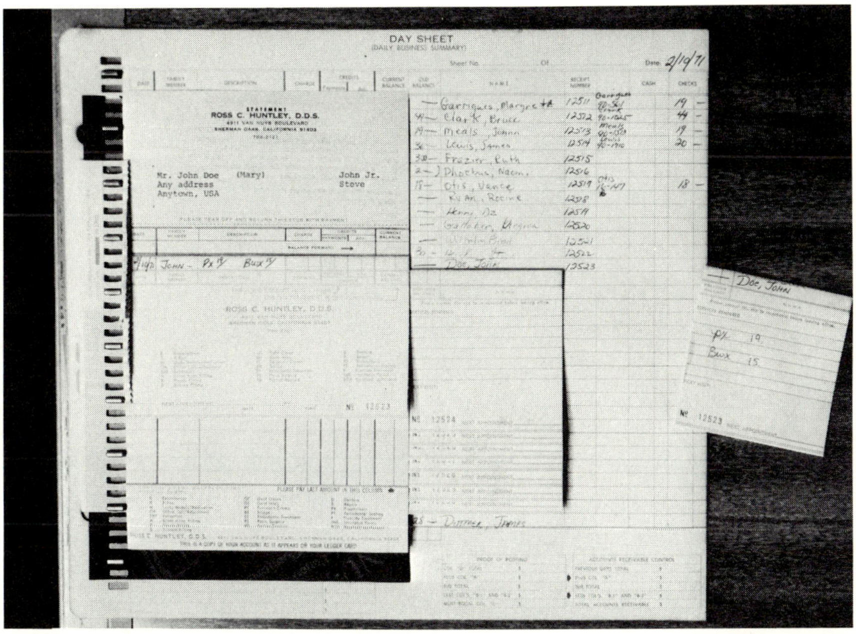

Fig. 5-8. Pegboard bookkeeping system, showing services-rendered slip, receipt slip, statement card, and day sheet.

b. File invoice with bills to bc paid.

c. Replace card in supply file box.

C. Billing procedures

1. Agreements

The method of payment for services to be rendered is agreed upon by the doctor and the patient in the presence of the receptionist at the time of oral examination and case presentation. The agreement is signed by the patient on the reverse side of the dental chart (see Fig. 5-7). Boundaries should be set for credit to patients, depending upon the judgment of the dentist.

2. Payment plans

Several payment plans are offered, depending upon the patient's circumstances and ability to pay. They include the pay-as-you-go plan, payment-by-the-month plan, dental society finance plan, and union insurance plan.

3. Bookkeeping (pegboard system)

This system consists of day sheet, ledger card, statement card, receipt, and services-rendered slip overlaid on pegboard to make several carbon copies of each entry (see Fig. 5-8).

a. After patient is greeted by receptionist, the date and name of family member is entered on the recept and services-rendered slips. These entries are transmitted to the statement card, the ledger card, and the day sheet by means of the carbons. The services-rendered slip is then taken to the dispensary or to the hygienist's operatory, as indicated, and placed on the

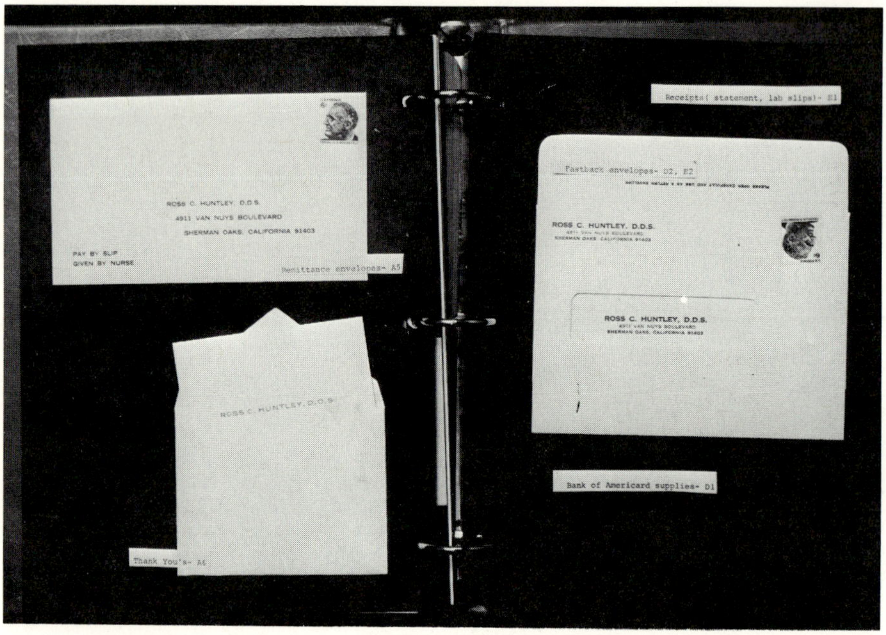

Fig. 5-9. Stationery notebook file. **Right,** fastback envelopes for statements; **left,** remittance envelopes and thank-you cards.

patient's file. This action informs the dental assistant or the hygienist that the patient has arrived and is ready to be seated.

b. When the seating is completed, the dental assistant or hygienist enters the services rendered and the fee on the services-rendered slip and escorts the patient to the business office, where the next appointment is made, fees collected, and appropriate entries made on the pegboard. If payment is made, patient is given the receipt slip. If there is an unpaid balance, the receipt slip (used as an appointment reminder) is given to the patient with a stamped envelope addressed to the office for easy payment (Fig. 5-9). The services-rendered slip showing the date of the next appointment is given to the laboratory technician whenever prosthetic procedures are involved. The laboratory technician attaches this slip to the laboratory pan for identification and planning purposes.

c. The day sheet is balanced daily, and checks received are made ready for deposit by mail.

d. A fee schedule for all types of services rendered in the office should be maintained by the receptionist and should be memorized without hesitancy by all personnel in the office for purposes of clarity and to avoid misunderstanding when asked about fees by the patient.

A

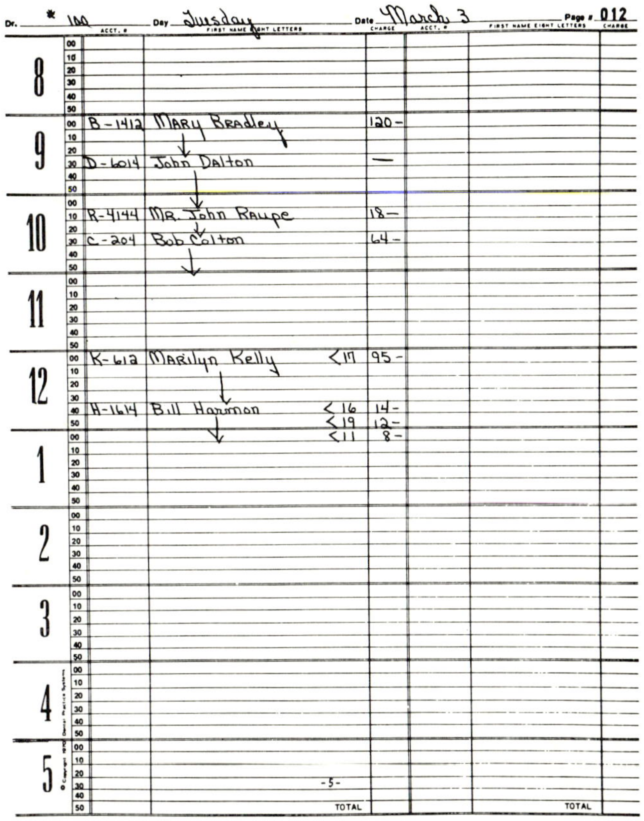

Fig. 5-10. A, Daily appointment sheet, used with computer system as input for charges; **B,** daily control summary, used with computer system as input record of payments, account adjustments, recalls, and messages for the day; **C,** master file form, used to enter all new accounts, changes of address, and deletions into the computer. (Courtesy Dental Practice Systems Corporation, Placentia, California.)

4. Bookkeeping (computer system)

   The use of computerized systems for office accounting procedures remove from the office the time-consuming tasks of handling statements and billing, accounts receivable, accounts aging, appointment control, and recall. These computer systems allow the receptionist to be more productive with appointments and collections and provide the doctor with greater practice information than internal accounting systems.

A typical computer system is comprised of 3 input forms —daily appointment sheet, daily control summary, and master file form (see Fig. 5-10). The daily appointment sheet is used as the input record of charges for professional services rendered. The daily control summary sheet is used as the input record of all payments, account adjustments, recalls, and messages for the day. The master file form is used to enter all new accounts into the system. It also

B

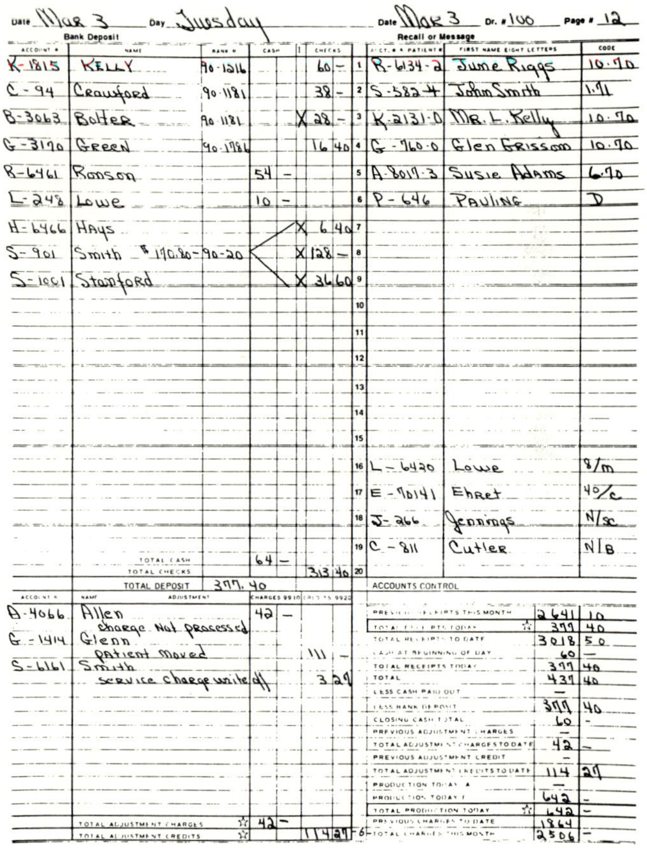

Date Mar 3 Day Tuesday — Bank Deposit

Date Mar 3 Dr. # 100 Page # 12 — Recall or Message

Account #	Name	Bank #	Cash		Checks		Acct. # & Patient #	First name eight letters	Code
K-1815	Kelly	90-1216			60 –	1	R-6134-2	June Riggs	10.70
C-94	Crawford	90-1181			38 –	2	S-582-4	John Smith	1.71
B-3063	Botter	90-1181		X	28 –	3	K-2131-0	Mr. L. Kelly	10.70
G-3170	Green	90-1786			16 40	4	G-760-0	Glen Grissom	10.70
R-6461	Ronson		54 –			5	A-8017-3	Susie Adams	6.70
L-248	Lowe		10 –			6	P-646	Pauling	D
H-6466	Hays			X	6 40	7			
S-901	Smith $170.80	90-20		X	128 –	8			
S-1001	Stanford			X	36 60	9			
						10			
						11			
						12			
						13			
						14			
						15			
						16	L-6420	Lowe	8/m
						17	E-70141	Ehret	40/c
						18	J-266	Jennings	N/sc
	Total cash		64 –			19	C-811	Cutler	N/B
	Total checks				313 40	20			
	Total deposit	377.40							

Account #	Name / Adjustment	Charges 9910	Credits 9920
A-4066	Allen — charge not processed	42 –	
G-1414	Glenn — patient moved		111 –
S-6161	Smith — service charge write off		3 29
	Total adjustment charges ☆	42 –	
	Total adjustment credits ☆		114 29

Accounts control

Previous receipts this month	2641	10
Total receipts today ☆	377	40
Total receipts to date	3018	50
Cash at beginning of day	60	–
Total receipts today	377	40
Total	437	40
Less cash paid out	–	
Less bank deposit	377	40
Closing cash total	60	–
Previous adjustment charges	–	
Total adjustment charges to date	42	–
Previous adjustment credit	–	
Total adjustment credits to date	114	29
Production today A	–	
Production today F	642	–
Total production today ☆	642	–
Previous charges to date	1864	
Total charges this month	2506	–

Fig. 5-10, cont'd. For legend see p. 47.

is the method by which change of address information or deletion of an account is entered into the system. These sheets, prepared by the dental office, are sent weekly to the computer company.

Typical output information is provided the doctor by the computer company.

a. Statement including postage and double-window return envelope is sent to patient.
b. Monthly recall reminder is sent to patient.
c. Monthly recall register is sent to the doctor.
d. Patient billing and aged accounts receivable ledger are sent monthly to the doctor (see Fig. 5-11).

5. Delinquent accounts

These are handled immediately by telephone or personal contact with the patient. The agreements reached by this contact are recorded on the patient's billing record. At the next billing period a duplicate copy of this billing record is sent to the patient. Depending upon the circumstances involved, if the account remains delinquent for a period of 90 days, a copy of the billing record with previous agreements

C

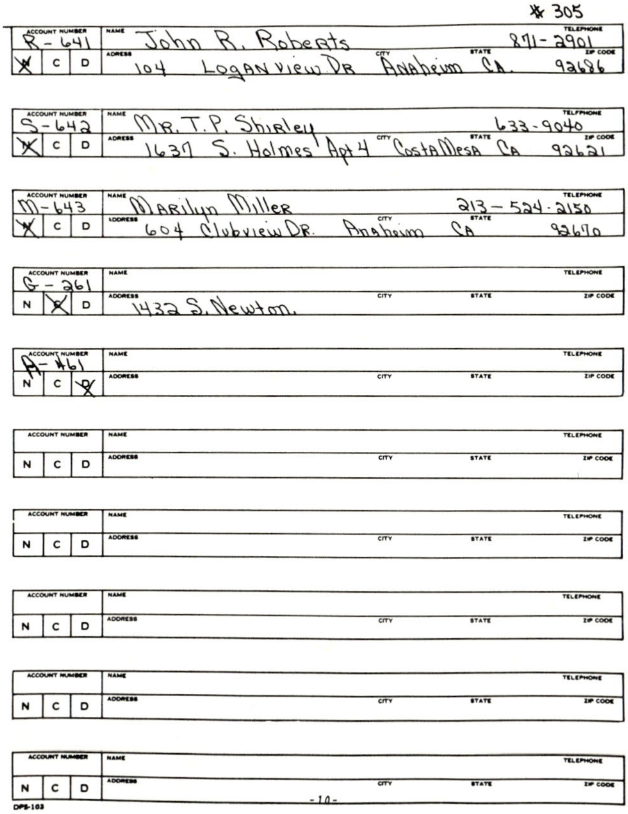

Fig. 5-10, cont'd. For legend see p. 47.

recorded may be sent to the patient with the statement attached that the account has been referred to a collection agency.

6. Dental society finance plans

When a patient is unable to afford the cost of complete dental care, he may be referred to a bank to arrange a loan sufficient to pay for the cost of the treatment anticipated. Many local dental societies have arranged finance plans with banks in the community to help such patients budget the cost of dental treatment over a period of time. After the patient's loan has been approved, the bank notifies the doctor, and treatment can be started (see Fig. 5-12).

7. Union insurance plans

A notebook should be kept to record actions taken in behalf of patients eligible for union insurance benefits (Fig. 5-13). Authorization for payment of these benefits should be obtained from the insurance company prior to starting treatment. The file of these patients should be labeled by colored stickers for easy identification. It should be explained to all insurance patients at the time of case pre-

A

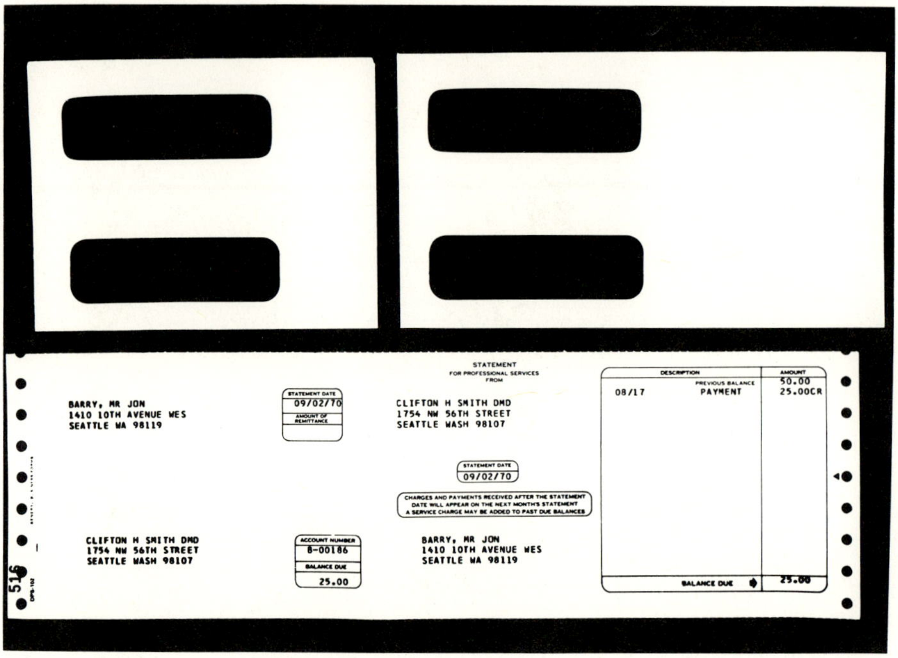

B

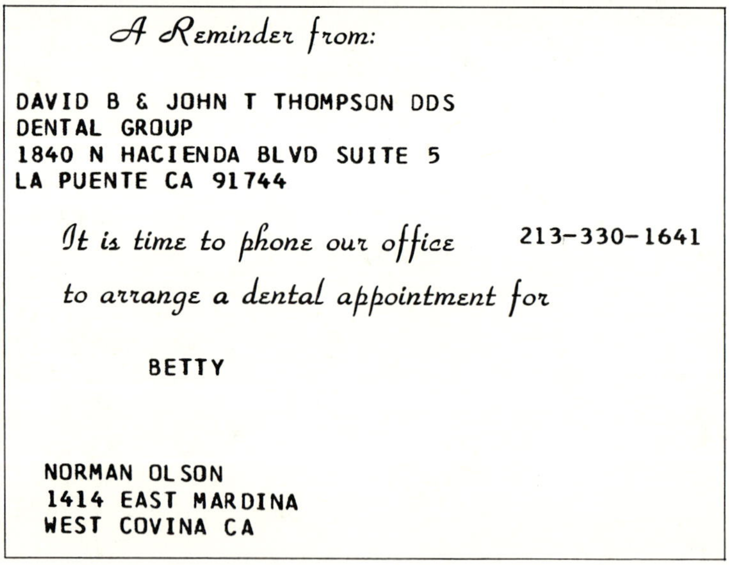

A Reminder from:

DAVID B & JOHN T THOMPSON DDS
DENTAL GROUP
1840 N HACIENDA BLVD SUITE 5
LA PUENTE CA 91744

It is time to phone our office 213-330-1641
to arrange a dental appointment for

BETTY

NORMAN OLSON
1414 EAST MARDINA
WEST COVINA CA

Fig. 5-11. A, Statements, including postage and double return envelope, sent to patient by computer company; **B,** monthly recall reminder, sent to patient by computer company; **C,** monthly recall register, sent to doctor by computer company; **D,** patient billing and aged accounts receivable ledger, sent monthly to the doctor by the computer company. (Courtesy Dental Practice Systems Corporation, Placentia, California.)

C

RECALL REGISTER

PATIENT NUMBER	PATIENT	NAME	DATE	PATIENT NUMBER	PATIENT	NAME	DATE
A-3048	A J ANSTETT 2427 BUCKINGHAM ANAHEIM CALIF - 528-7010	MR. KATHY	70-03*	B-0310	MR E BASURTO 8591 JOYZELLE DR GARDEN GROVE CALIF - 529-9010	MRS	70-03*
A-3129	ALEXANDER ALMOIAN 4381 NOGAL AVE YORBA LINDA CALIF	ALEX	70-03*	B-0319	MR C BLACKWOOD P O BOX 417 YORBA LINDA CALIF - 528-3769	JANICE CARI BETH	70-03*
A-3151	EDWARD ALSKY 5262 LIVERPOOL YORBA LINDA CALIF - 528-6010	MR. MRS.	70-03*	B-0322	MR E BONETA 4731 LIBRA PL YORBA LINDA CALIF - 528-6404	MRS	70-03*
B-0008	MR L BARTON 18911 CAMINO VERDE YORBA LINDA CALIF - 529-2431	SUSAN	70-03*	B-1083	MR ROBERT BUSH 17651 BROOKLYN AVE YORBA LINDA CALIF	ROBERT RICHARD	70-03*
B-0009	MR J GORDON BOTTS 397 TOLBERT ST. BREA CALIF - 637-0437	LARRY TOM MRS	70-03*	B-2567	HARLAN BERGDALE 17421 CALGARY YORBA LINDA CALIF - 526-4599	DIANE	70-03*
B-0019	MR W. BERNSTEN 18041 AVOLINDA DR. YORBA LINDA CALIF 213 524-6486	MRS.	70-03*	B-2736	BEN BAKER 18602 AVOLINDA DR YORBA LINDA CALIF 213 528-7071	MRS	70-03*
B-0305	MR LARRY BOUCHEY 4852 PROSPECT YORBA LINDA CALIF 213 633-1505	MR.	70-03*	B-2737	HAROLD L. BAYS 5091 STONE CANYON YORBA LINDA CALIF - 528-9001	MR MRS	70-03*
B-0308	MRS EVELYN BRIGGS 1140 S BELBURY DR WALNUT CALIF 772-1014	MR EVELYN DEAN	70-03*	B-2776	PETER A. BROCNIK 914 APPLING PLACENTIA CALIF 213 999-6007	PETER	70-03*

D

PATIENT BILLING AND [illegible]GED ACCOUNTS RECEIVABLE

DOCTOR C0560 PHILIP D WHITENER,D.D.S. DATE 12-31-69 PAGE 36

	PATIENT NUMBER	PATIENT NAME — DESCRIPTION	DATE MO.	DATE DAY	DATE YR.	PRIOR BALANCE	CURRENT PRODUCTION	CURRENT PAYMENTS	CURRENT ADJUSTMENTS	OVER 30 DAYS	OVER 60 DAYS	OVER 90 DAYS	ENDING BALANCE
	Y-0281	MR FAY YOUNG											
		18001 AVOLINDA DR											
		YORBA LINDA CALIF				.00							
		- - FANNIE	12	15	69		18.00						
							18.00*						18.00 *
	Y-2921	MICHAEL R YOUNG											
		5075 MANOR VIEW											
		YORBA LINDA CALIF											
		- -				6.00							
		LAST PAYMENT 25.00	10	15	69							6.00	6.00 *
	Z-0285	MR L J ZIMMERMAN											
		P O BOX 497											
		YORBA LINDA CALIF				.00							
		- - L	12	10	69		30.00						
		HELEN	12	23	69	.	18.00						
							48.00*						48.00 *
	9-9999	TRANSCIENT ACCT											
		- -				20.00CR							
			12	01	69			6.00					
			12	05	69		6.00						
			12	05	59		6.00						
			12	05	69		10.00						
			12	15	69			12.00					
			12	15	69			6.00					
			12	15	69			40.00					
			12	18	69			10.00					
			12	29	69		40.00						
			12	29	69		12.00						
		LAST PAYMENT 10.00	12	19	69		74.00*	74.00*					20.00CR*
00560						18342.04*	6360.00*	7474.18*	92.00CR*	3916.90	2973.50	7434.58	17,135.86*

Fig. 5-11, cont'd. For legend see opposite page.

To Bank of America NATIONAL TRUST AND SAVINGS ASSOCIATION

DENTAL SOCIETY PAYMENT PLAN

No.______

and Dr.______, ______, 19__

APPLICANT'S STATEMENT

Name In Full______ Age______ First Name of Spouse______ Number of Dependents______

Home Address______ City______ How Long______ Phone______

Former Address______ City______ Soc. Sec. Number______ Operator's License No.______

Employer______ Address______ Business Phone______

Position______ How Long______ Monthly Salary $______ Amt. Other Income $______ Source______

Spouse's Employer______ Address______

Do You Own An Automobile?______ Make______ Year______ Legal Owner______ Balance Due $______ Mo. Paym't. $______

Name and Address of Mortgage Holder or Landlord______ Monthly Mortgage or Rental Paym't. $______

Name of Nearest Relative Not Living with You______ Complete Address______ Relationship______

Bank Account Carried at______ Branch Address______ Checking ☐ Savings ☐ BankAmericard No.______

Credit references (banks, stores, credit unions, finance companies, etc.) Attach additional sheet if necessary. INCLUDE ALL DEBTS NOW OWING.	PRESENT UNPAID BALANCE	AMOUNT OF MONTHLY PAYMENT

Bill Amt. $______

I prefer to make my payments on the 1st, 5th, 10th, 15th, 20th, 25th, day of each month. (Circle date selected.)

Signature______

INSTALMENT NOTE
(DENTAL SOCIETY PAYMENT PLAN)

No.______

$______ ______ California ______, 19__

For Value Received, I promise to pay to the order of Dr.______ at the Bank of America in this city______ dollars in instalments as follows:______ dollars ($______) on______ and______ equal successive______ monthly instalments of______ dollars ($______), beginning ______, 19__ together with a delinquency charge on each instalment in default for 10 days in an amount equal to 5% of such instalment, but not less than $1.00.

If default be made in the payment when due of any part or instalment of principal or interest, then the whole sum of principal and interest shall become immediately due and payable at the option of the holder of this note, without notice.

In the event of suit to enforce payment of this note, I agree to pay such additional sum as attorney's fees as the Court may adjudge reasonable.

Signature______
BORROWER

Signature______
WIFE OR HUSBAND OF BORROWER

TPL-359Y 11-66 (REV.)

Fig. 5-12. Dental society finance plan application form.

sentation that the amount of insurance benefit is determined by a schedule of allowances agreed upon by the insurance company and the buyer of the contract. The patient should understand that the fees charged by the dentist may not be the same as the schedule of allowances. Financial agreements made with such patients should include the following signed statement on the reverse side of the dental chart: "I, ______, understand I am financially responsible for balance of bill not taken care of by my insurance benefit." Additional financial arrangements, including the amount to be paid per month, also should be made as previously explained.

D. Office expenditures (pegboard system)

A check-writing and posting system to record all expenditures of the office is shown in Fig. 5-14. It consists of a series of blank checks overlaid on a ledger sheet showing the breakdown of expenses by payee, date, amount, and purpose. This system reduces check-writing and posting to 1 step by means of carbons on the underside of each check.

E. Recall procedures

1. Prophylaxis recall appointments are made 3, 6, or 12 months in

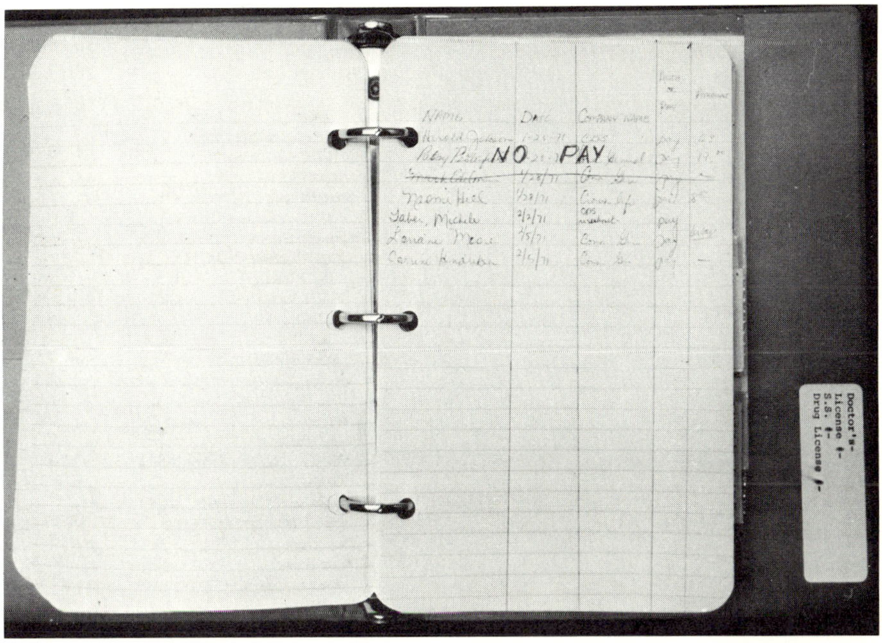

Fig. 5-13. Notebook record of insurance plan authorizations and payments.

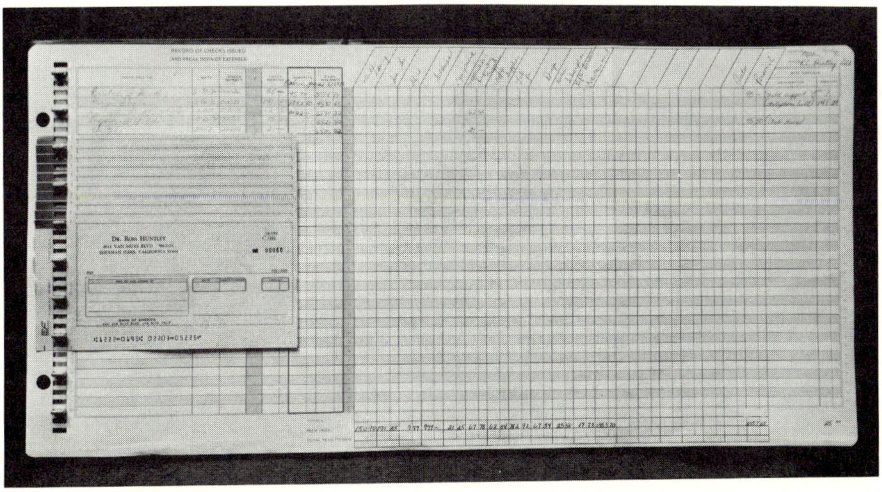

Fig. 5-14. Pegboard checkwriting system, used to record checks issued and breakdown of expenses.

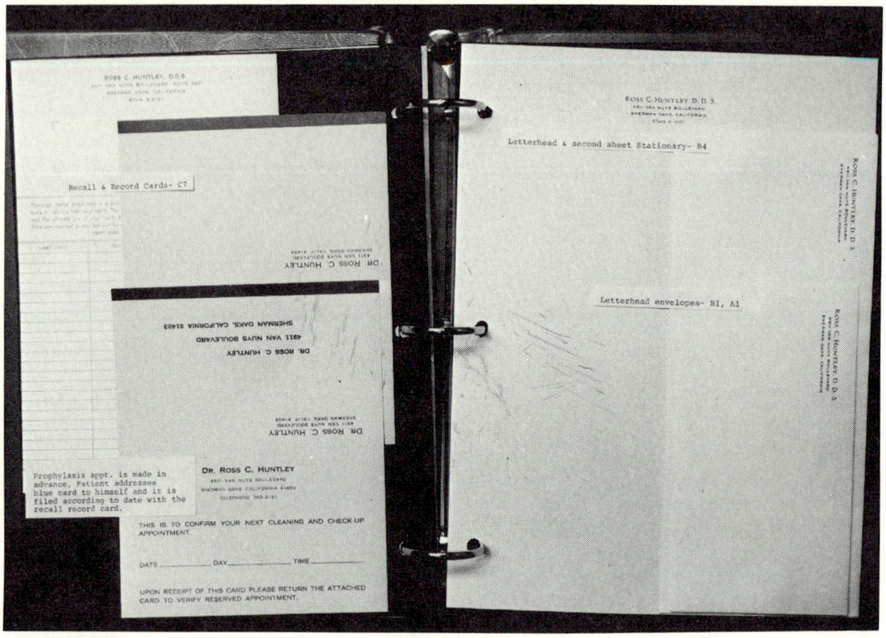

Fig. 5-15. Stationery notebook file. **Right,** letterhead stationery and envelopes; **left,** recall cards and recall record cards.

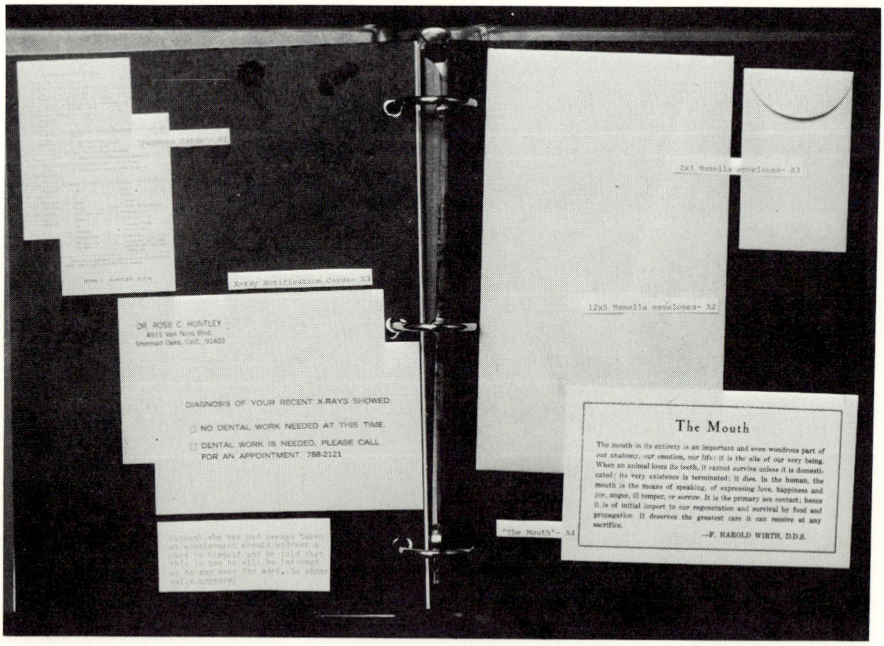

Fig. 5-16. Stationery notebook file. **Right,** manila envelopes and patient education handouts; **left,** patient education handouts and x-ray notification cards.

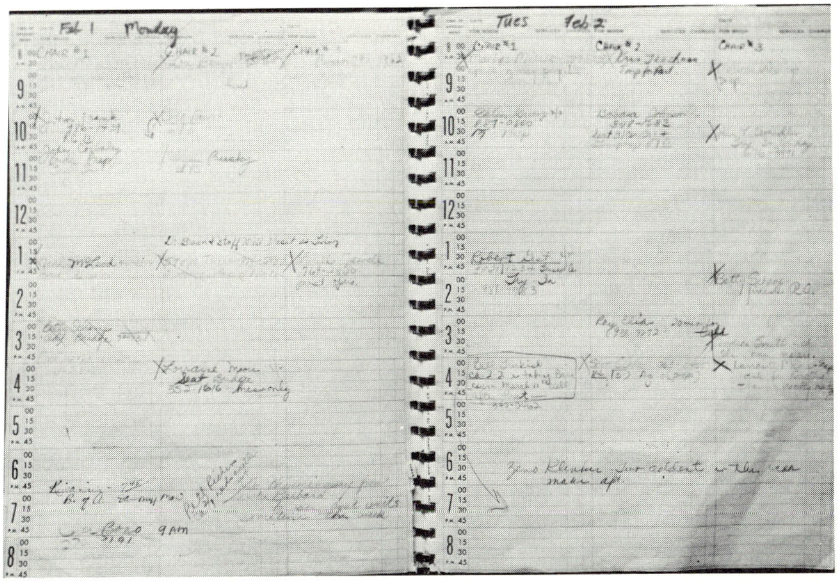

Fig. 5-17. Doctor's appointment book. Note separate columns for each chair.

advance at the time of the last prophylaxis visit. The patient addresses a blue recall card to himself; this card is filed chronologically with the recall record card. Two weeks prior to the appointment, the blue recall card is sent to the patient. Upon receipt of this card, the patient returns the attached card to confirm or cancel the appointment. A patient who does not return his card is contacted by telephone 1 or 2 days in advance of the reserved appointment to confirm or cancel the appointment (see Fig. 5-15).

2. Those patients not on prophylaxis recall are annually sent reminders to make an appointment for reexamination and x-rays, if needed.
3. Another type of recall is initiated by any additional x-rays taken by the dental hygienist at the time of the prophylaxis appointment. After these x-rays are developed and viewed by the doctor, those patients needing additional treatment are notified to call the office for an appointment (see Fig. 5-16).

F. Appointment scheduling
   1. One patient should be scheduled for each operatory at the beginning of the morning and the afternoon (see Fig. 5-17). Subsequent appointments for each operatory should be scheduled on a time allowance basis for each operation, as follows:
      a. Preps
         Gold inlays and crowns—45 minutes for one, 15 minutes extra for each additional prep.
      b. Seating
         Gold inlays, crowns, and bridges—30 minutes per inlay or crown; 15 minutes extra

for each additional inlay or crown.

c. Try-ins
Forty-five minutes.

d. Amalgams
One surface—20 minutes; two or more surfaces—45 minutes.

e. Resins
First tooth—45 minutes; ten minutes for each additional tooth.

f. Endodontics
Pulpectomy—30 minutes.
Root canal enlargement—15 minutes.
Obturation—45 minutes.

g. Periodontal surgery
Twenty minutes per tooth.
Thirty minutes per quadrant.

2. Several copies of the dentist's and dental hygienist's appointment schedule are typed for the following day, indicating time of appointment, patient's name, and treatment scheduled to be done. One copy is for the business office, one for each operatory, one for the doctor's private office, and one for the dispensary.

3. The receptionist pulls the patients' folders for the following day and places them in sequence in a holder in the dispensary. The x-ray and chart of the patients are placed on end to facilitate easy access from the folder. The following morning all tray preparations for the morning patients are set out on the counter with the patients' folders on top. All tray preparations and folders for the afternoon patients are similarly set out at noon (see Fig. 5-3).

II. X-ray section

A. Equipment and supplies

1. Panoramic x-ray machine located in a separate room (Fig. 5-18).
2. Conventional x-ray machine, wall mounted, located in each operatory (Fig. 5-20).
3. Panoramic x-ray film and cassettes stored in dark room.
4. Bite-wing and periapical film stored in lead box in each operatory.
5. X-ray mounts stored in dispensary.
6. X-ray viewers located in each operatory, the dispensary, and the doctor's private office.

B. Personnel

Each dental assistant should be trained to take all types of x-rays, including panoramic, bite-wings, and periapicals. She also should be trained to distinguish landmarks and abnormalities, to be able to mount them correctly, and to be able to identify them if they get mixed-up during developing. However, she should not attempt to make a diagnosis from the x-rays or discuss them with the patient.

C. Types of x-rays and when x-rays are taken

1. Panoramic x-rays
   a. Taken by dental assistant on all new patients.
   b. Taken by hygienist on all recall patients every 3 years, or as indicated by dentist.
   c. Taken by hygienist on all patients with periodontal and periapical disease every 1 to 2 years.
2. Bite-wings and anterior periapicals
   a. Taken every year at recall by the dental hygienist.
3. Miscellaneous periapicals
   a. Taken by dental hygienist at recall, when indicated.

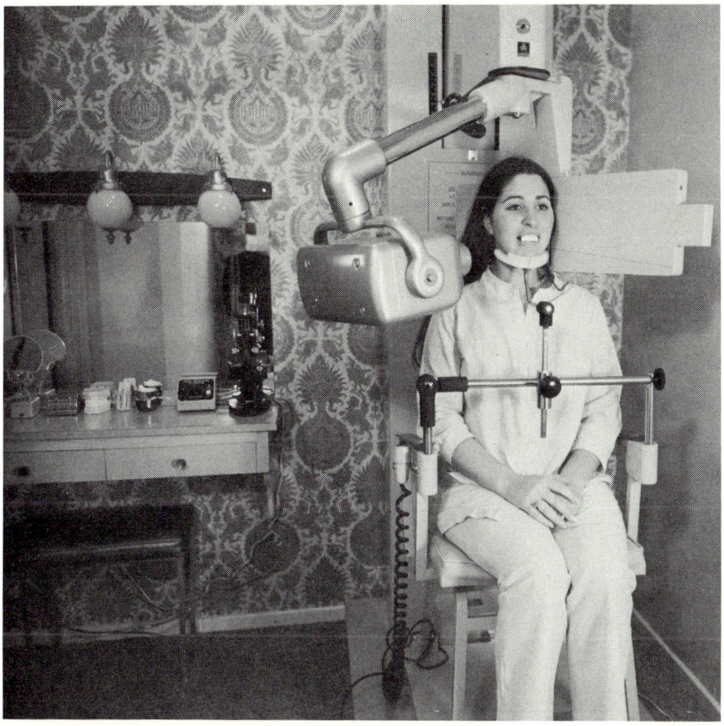

Fig. 5-18. Panoramic x-ray machine in dressing room. Note dressing table with phase microscope for patient education on left.

b. Taken by dental assistant during and after endodontic treatment, as indicated by doctor.

c. Special third molar examinations taken by dental assistant, as indicated by doctor.

D. Routines

1. Patient's name and type of x-ray are listed on the daily appointment schedule.
2. If panoramic x-ray is to be taken, a label with name and date is typed in advance by the receptionist for imprinting on the film.
3. X-rays are developed by the person who takes them while the patient waits to be certain x-ray is satisfactory.
4. Patient is dismissed after development of x-ray, unless he has an appointment to see the dentist.
5. X-rays are mounted promptly next morning in the dispensary by the person who took them.
6. X-rays are identified by patient's name, date taken, and initials of person who took them. Notation is made if x-rays are to be referred to another doctor.
7. All mounted and identified x-rays are then placed on the doctor's desk for diagnosis.
8. Dentist attaches notations to each x-ray and returns them to the business office where appointments are made for patients needing treatment. Patients not needing treatment also are notified.

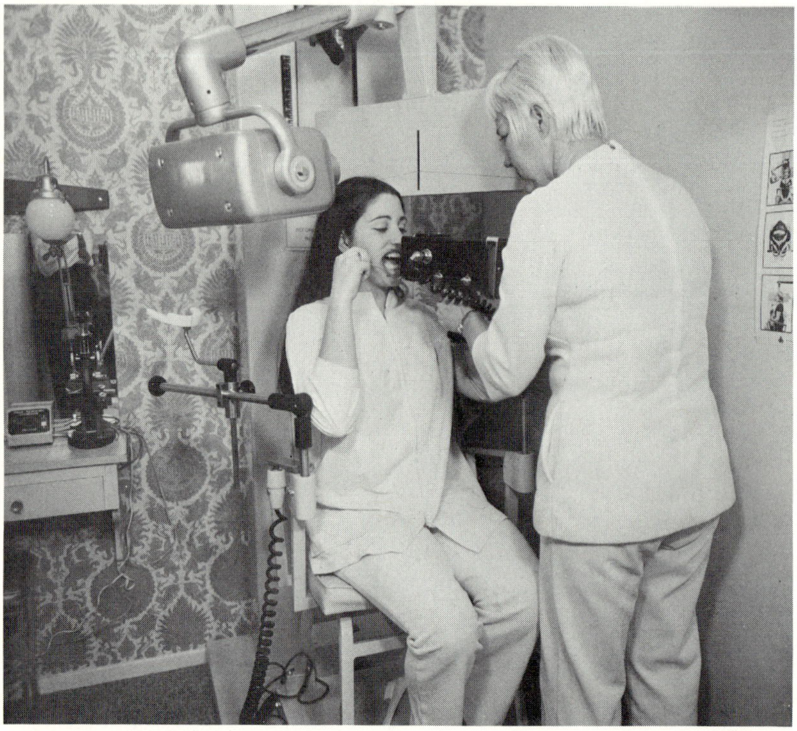

Fig. 5-19. Preoperative photography taken of all new patients.

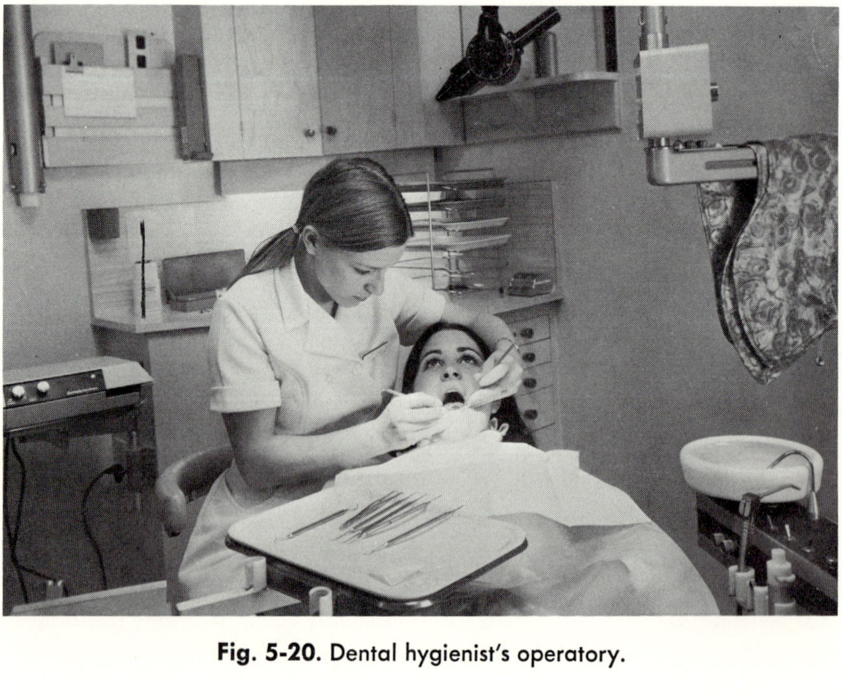

Fig. 5-20. Dental hygienist's operatory.

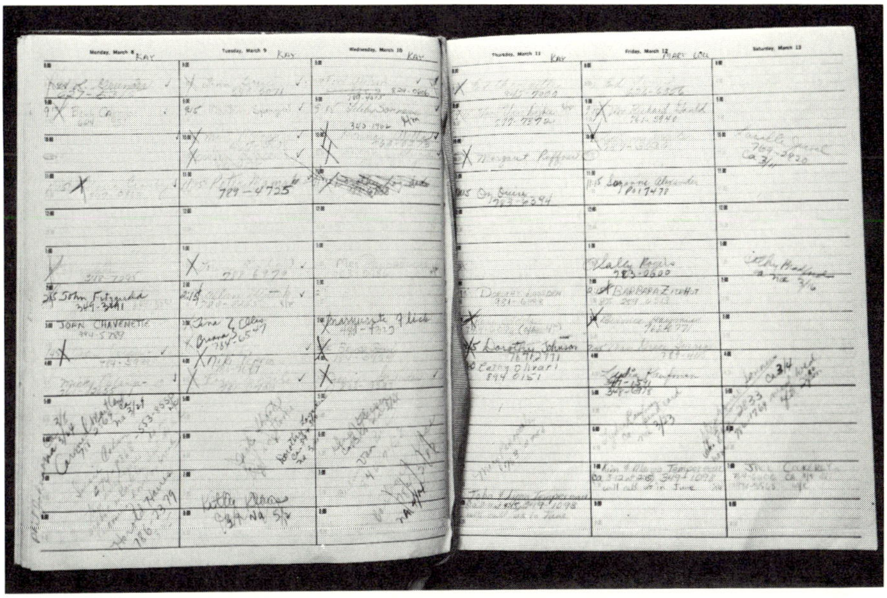

Fig. 5-21. Dental hygienist's appointment book.

9. X-rays are *not* filed in patient's folder until the patient is notified.

E. Photographs
1. Preoperative intraoral photographs of all new patients are taken with Polaroid camera by the dental assistant who takes the panoramic x-ray (Fig. 5-19).
2. Postoperative photographs are also taken by the dental assistant of all patients receiving major restorative or periodontal treatment.

III. Oral hygiene section (see Fig. 5-20)

A. Equipment
1. Contour dental chair for patient
2. Right side
   a. Mobile operating stool
   b. Mobile unit containing one contra-angle handpiece with swing-away bracket tray
   c. X-ray viewer recessed in wall
   d. Dental folder rack on wall with clip for dental chart
   e. Ultrasonic unit on swing-away bracket arm
3. Left side
   a. Mobile, swing-away unit attached to dental chair containing air, water, suction, and cuspidor
   b. X-ray machine
   c. Lead apron
4. Corner cabinet
   a. Shelves, drawers, sink, and counter top
   b. Draping materials, auxiliary supplies
   c. Alcohol and gauze sponges in containers on counter top
   d. Tray rack on counter top for tray preparations

B. Routines

The oral hygiene section operates as nearly as possible on its own. A separate appointment book is kept for the dental hygienist, and fees are listed separately on the day sheet. Appointments are usually made at 45-minute intervals (see Fig. 5-21). The dental hygienist utilizes time-tested recall methods (see p. 52). The hygienist's appointments are made to coincide with the doctor's schedule, so that he will be available for consultation and/or treatment when needed. If the dentist is unable to see the patient when the dental hygienist has completed her treatment, notes are made on the patient's chart for the dentist's attention at the next appointment.

C. Charting

During prophylaxis the oral hygienist notes all findings, such as cavities, pockets, or inflammation, on the dental chart. On the back of the chart, she writes the date and findings; she then checks with the doctor to see if any operative work indicated can be done that same day. The dental hygienist may also make personal notes of interest about the patient on the chart.

D. X-rays

As mentioned previously, panoramic, bite-wing, and periapical x-rays are taken by the dental hygienist for diagnosis by the dentist. In addition, the dental hygienist may take bite-wing x-rays after scaling to check for remaining calculus prior to dismissal.

E. Tray set-ups

At the end of the day, 10 trays are prepared in advance for the following day. Contaminated instruments from the day's operations are washed in running water and placed in an ultrasonic cleaner. At this point, the instruments are assembled in sets and placed in sealed paper packets for autoclaving. After autoclaving, 1 packet of instruments is placed on each tray with sterile dappen dishes, polishing cups, brushes, and napkins. The trays are stored on racks shown in Fig. 5-20. The handpieces are cleaned and oiled, supplies replenished, and the room vacuumed and dusted.

F. Sharpening instruments

The dental hygienist uses several varieties of stones for sharpening sickles and curets (see Chapter 11). Separate drawers are maintained for sharpened and nonsharpened instruments.

G. Patient education

In conducting a program of preventive dental health education adapted to the needs of each patient in the practice, the dental hygienist may perform the following functions:

1. Give instruction in tooth brushing, flossing, and interdental stimulation.
2. Demonstrate use of disclosing tablets.
3. Give each new patient a toothbrush of proper design.
4. Demonstrate diseased conditions in his mouth by means of illustrations and models.
5. Use dietary analysis sheets and give dietary instruction when indicated.
6. Demonstrate microbes in the patient's mouth using a phase microscope before and after treatment.
7. Schedule group presentations to patients to reinforce issues presented by means of cartridge sound films.

IV. Operative section

A. Equipment and supplies (Fig. 5-22)

1. Contour dental chair for patient
2. At doctor's side
   a. Mobile operating stool
   b. Mobile unit containing 1

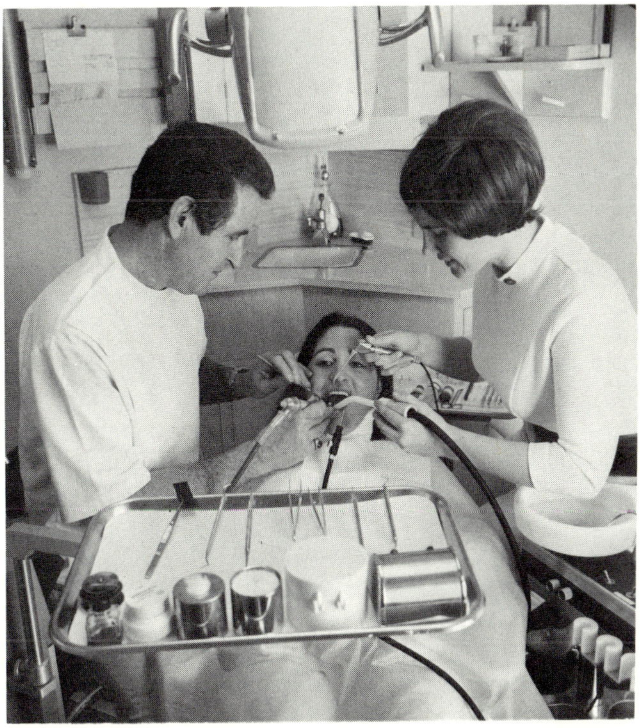

Fig. 5-22. Doctor's operatory. (Each operatory is equipped the same.)

contra-angle and 2 high-speed handpieces with swing-away bracket tray
c. Portable electrosurgery unit
d. X-ray viewer recessed in wall
e. Dental folder rack on wall with clip for dental chart
3. At dental assistant's side
a. Mobile operating stool
b. Moble swing-away unit attached to dental chair containing air, water, suction, and cuspidor
c. A low swing-away bracket tray attached to the wall
d. X-ray machine
e. Lead apron
4. In corner cabinet
a. Shelves, drawers, sink, and counter top
b. Draping materials stored on shelves
c. Temporizing materials and auxiliary supplies stored in drawers
d. Corner cabinet above sink containing impression materials
e. Syringes in bactericidal solution recessed in counter top
f. Anesthetic cartridges, needles, alcohol gauze sponges stored in separate containers on counter top
g. Lead box for film on counter top
h. An inventory list kept in each cabinet or drawer for reference purposes in replenishing supplies
B. Seating patient
1. The services-rendered slip, placed on the chart in the dispensary by the receptionist,

signifies that the patient has arrived.

2. Check for vacant operatory, and make certain that it is spotlessly clean. Do not leave patient in waiting room when a vacant operatory is available.
3. Go to waiting room, greet patient by name, and invite him in.
4. Take patient's wraps, and seat him in dental chair.
5. Bring in tray and folder from dispensary.
6. Place tray on low bracket arm at the rear left side of the patient.
7. Place x-rays on viewer, and clip dental chart to wall rack.
8. Drape patient with folded towel wrapped around the neck and plastic apron overlaid with paper napkin.
9. Transfer basic instruments consisting of mirror, explorers, and cotton pliers to the bracket arm on the doctor's side.
10. Place indicated burs, stones, and discs in handpieces.
11. Doctor is informed that the patient is ready.

C. Operative routines
1. One dental assistant is responsible for each operatory.
2. Step-by-step procedure cards for each operation should be prepared by the dentist and memorized by the dental assistant. (For hints in preparing the procedure cards see Chapter 6.) These cards are very useful for reference purposes and for training a new assistant.
3. Allow no interruption until a stopping point is reached once the operation is started.
4. The same assistant who starts the operation stays with the doctor until it is completed.
5. Never leave the dentist alone with the patient.
6. The doctor concerns himself only with irreversible procedures in the field of operation.
7. Keep your eyes upon the field of operation.
8. Maintain field of operation visible and free of debris by controlling the lights, air, suction, and water.
9. Deliver and receive instruments and materials at chin level as needed.
10. Always be 1 step ahead of the dentist.
11. A second, or roving, assistant triturates filling materials and prepares impression materials in the central dispensary as needed.
12. Perform all other reversible procedures permitted within the limits of the State Dental Practice Act (see also Chapter 4).

D. Dismissal and reappointment
1. Enter the following type of information on the services-rendered slip upon completion of the operation:
   a. #13 MOD inlay prep
   b. Fee
   c. Next visit: #13 MOD seat inlay (see Fig. 5-8).
2. Similar information is entered on the patient's dental chart.
3. Offer patient facial tissues and water for rinsing.
4. Undrape patient, hand him services-rendered slip, and direct him to the business office where the next appointment is made and fees collected as indicated by the receptionist. Be

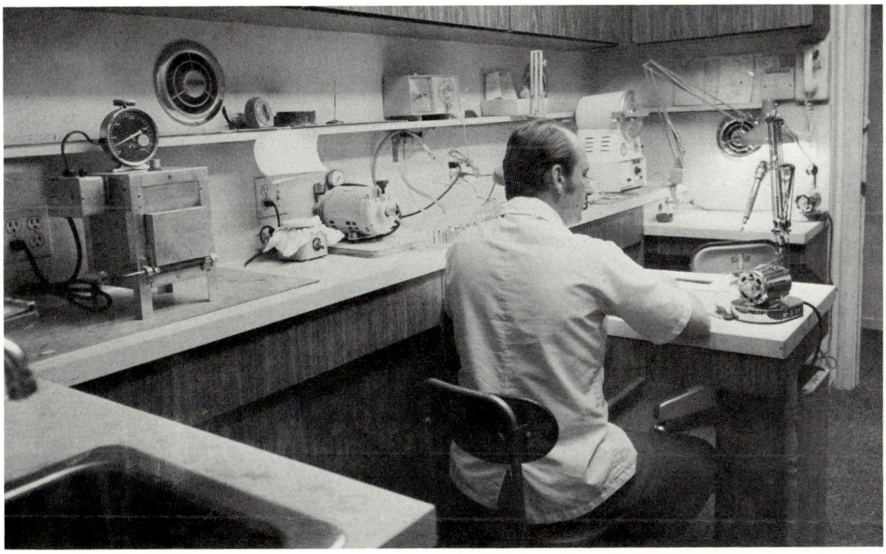

Fig. 5-23. Prosthetic laboratory. Note separate work bench for ceramic work.

sure patient has his wraps and other personal belongings.

E. Clean up and sterilization of instruments
   1. Clean operatory, wipe handpieces, syringes, and bracket arm with alcohol sponges, and return tray and contaminated instruments to the dispensary.
   2. Immerse contaminated instruments in ultrasonic cleaner 5 to 10 minutes before transferring them to the autoclave or chemical sterilizer.
   3. Replenish tray with instruments, burs, and stones from the drawers and bur blocks containing sterile instruments. Replace prepared tray in cabinet (see Fig. 5-3).
   4. Upon completion of the sterilization cycles, replace sterilized instruments in appropriate storage drawers and bur blocks in the dispensary.
   5. At the end of the day, sweep and vacuum all operatories, check cabinets, and replenish supplies.

V. Prosthetic laboratory section
   A. Equipment (see Fig. 5-23)
      1. Model trimmer
      2. Casting machine
      3. Burnout oven
      4. Sandblaster
      5. Ultrasonic cleaner
      6. Vacuum mixers for stone and investment
      7. Vacuum porcelain furnace located at separate bench for ceramic work
      8. Polishing lathe with dust collector
      9. Bench lamps with color-correct light
      10. Bench engines with handpieces
      11. Safe for gold
      12. Vibrator
   B. Routines
      1. Before starting any prosthetic operation, the laboratory technician is called to meet the pa-

tient and to take the shade, if necessary.

2. Preliminary impressions for study models and photographs may be taken at this time.
3. The laboratory technician is called to observe completed tooth preparations prior to final impressions to improve his understanding of the case.
4. Notation of the shade and special instructions are entered on the services-rendered slip, which is given to the patient at the completion of the appointment. This slip is retained by the receptionist, who enters the next appointment date and gives the slip to the laboratory technician for attachment to the laboratory pan.
5. In making appointments for prosthetic cases, the receptionist allows 1 week for inlays, 2 weeks for ceramic work, 1 week for try-ins, and 1 week for finish. Should the need arise for expediting the case, the technician should be consulted before an earlier appointment is made.

CHAPTER 6 TRAY PREPARATIONS AND CHAIRSIDE PROCEDURES

CHARLES M. BELTING, B.A., M.S., D.D.S.

The same essential skills of chairside assistance are required whether a dental operation is upon the hard or the soft tissues of the oral cavity. These include preparing the armamentarium, passing and cleaning instruments and materials, and maintaining the operating field visible and free of debris. A dental assistant cannot perform these tasks intelligently unless she has some understanding of the purpose of the operation and knows the names, the order of use, and the functions of the wide variety of instruments and materials used. It is the purpose of this chapter to explain these functions, so that she might better understand her role as chairside assistant during each type of treatment procedure commonly performed in the general practice of dentistry.

Preparing the armamentarium on trays in advance of scheduled appointments saves chairtime and avoids repeated contamination of instrument drawers and drawer handles during the course of the operation. One or more separate trays are prepared for each common operation performed in the office and are stored in an appropriate cabinet (Fig. 6-1). Until the dental assistant has learned the order of use and the purposes of all instruments and materials required for each operation, she will find it helpful to refer to photographs or lists of items to be placed on the tray. Since every dentist has his own personal preferences for the instruments and materials to be used for each operation, it is advisable for every office to develop its own manual of tray preparations for training and reference purposes. Such a manual can easily be prepared from photographs blown up to 8 × 11 inches and mounted on cardboard (Fig. 6-2).

A wide variety of dental instruments are used in dental practice, and the "tray system" requires several duplicates of each instrument. Colored plastic bands that fit over the instrument handles can be used to identify different classes of instruments or to identify instruments that are stored in different drawers. By this means, paired instruments also can be distinguished from one another by a second color added to the handle of one instrument of the pair, and so on. The plastic bands withstand both heat and chemical methods of sterilization (Fig. 6-3).

The order of arrangement of the tray preparations shown in this chapter follows the usual sequence of performing dental treatment for a patient in general practice, starting with oral examination and progressing through periodontics, oral surgery, en-

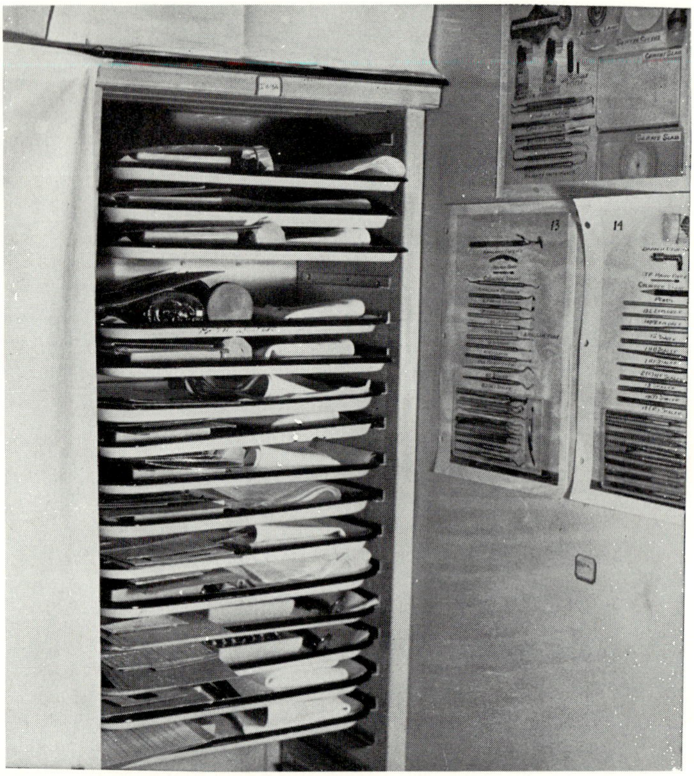

Fig. 6-1. Cabinet of prepared trays. (From Jackson, G. I.: Dent. Radiogr. Photogr. **28:** 69-71, 1955.)

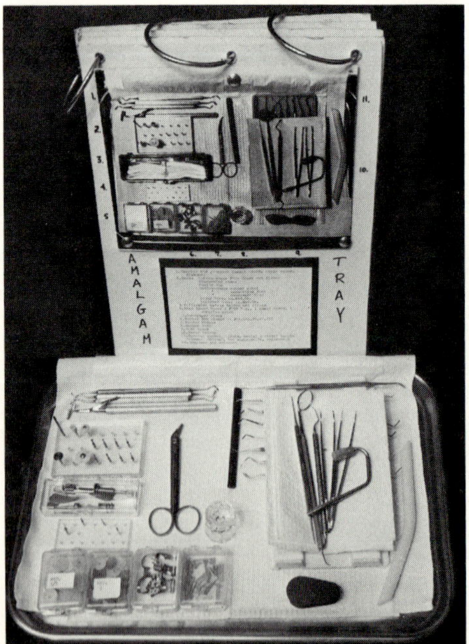

Fig. 6-2. Manual of tray preparations for reference and training purposes. Note prepared tray in front.

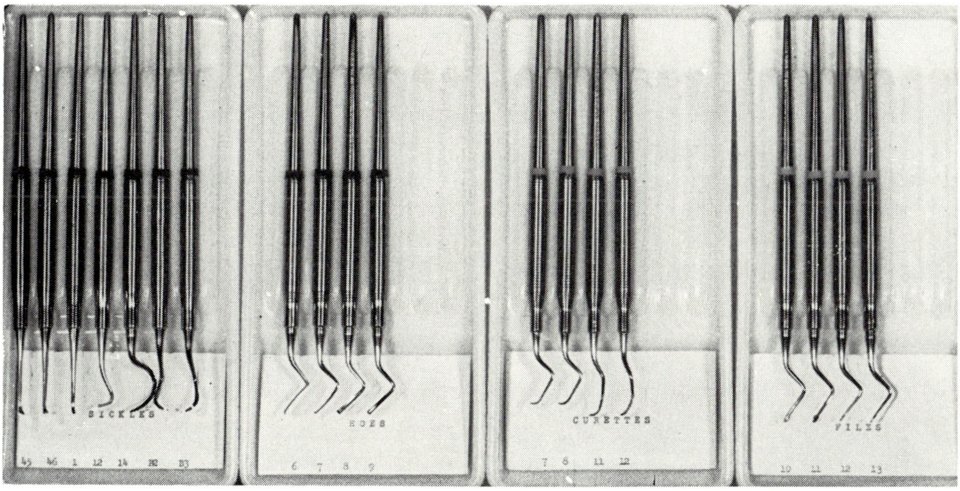

Fig. 6-3. Colored plastic identification bands on instruments.

dodontics, operative dentistry, crowns and bridges, partial dentures, and complete denture aspects of dental treatment. The instruments and materials shown for each tray are identified by numbers, starting with number one in the lower left-hand corner of the illustration and ending with the highest number in the upper right-hand corner. By this method of identification, an attempt has been made to indicate the sequence in which the items shown are used, as well as their location on the tray. The numbers also serve as a key to the nomenclature given in the legend accompanying each photograph.

ORAL EXAMINATION

It is necessary for a dentist to make a diagnosis, decide upon a plan of treatment, and present this information to the patient before treatment can be started. This procedure involves the appraisal and evaluation of many factors, which are recorded on the dental record by the dental assistant. The importance of completeness and accuracy of the information recorded cannot be overemphasized, since the dental record becomes, in effect, a legal document upon which treatment and fees are based.

Procedure checklist

1. Record vital statistics.
   a. Patient's name
   b. Home address and phone number
   c. Business address and phone number
   d. Age
   e. Employer
   f. Occupation
   g. Person referred by
   h. Physician's name
2. Record chief complaint.
3. Take dental radiographs (panoramic, periapical, and bite-wing), and mount them on illuminator during oral examination.
4. Record medical and dental history (obtained by dentist or by use of oral health questionnaire).
5. Chart oral findings on dental record (dictated by dentist).
   a. Lips and buccal mucosa
   b. Palate
   c. Tongue and floor of mouth
   d. Oral hygiene and calculus
   e. Periodontal status
   f. Occlusion
   g. Fillings or crowns present
   h. Caries and erosion

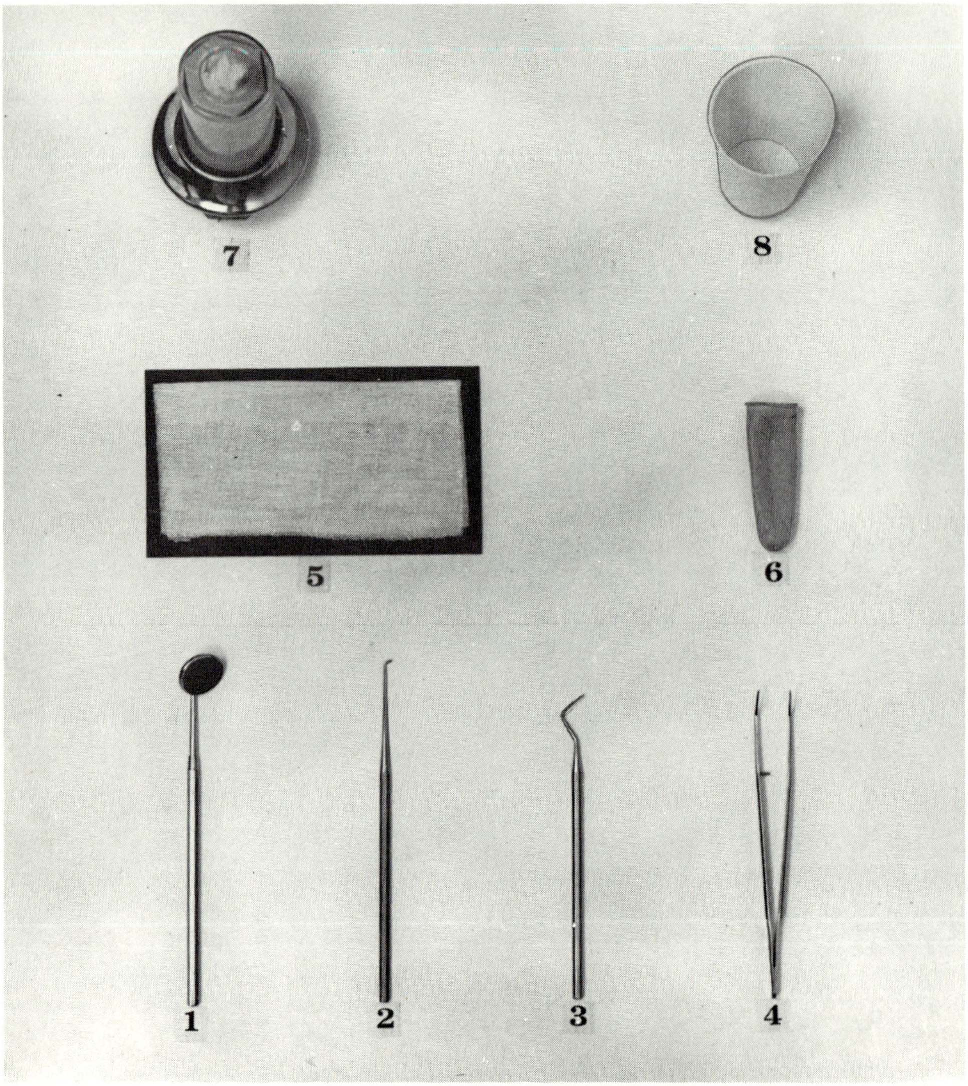

Fig. 6-4. Armamentarium for oral examination.

1. Mirror, mouth, examining, #4.
2. Explorer, #6.
3. Probe, pocket, gauge (Williams).
4. Forceps, dressing, #17.
5. Gauze, dental, napkin, 6 by 6 inches.
6. Cot, finger, rubber.
7. Cotton, absorbent, cylinder (for use in cotton font).
8. Cup, drinking, paper.

i. Missing teeth
j. Devitalized teeth
k. Radiolucencies and radiopacities
l. Alveolar resorption

6. Record study models or photographs taken.
7. Case presentation is made to patient by dentist
   a. Record estimated fees for services needed.
   b. Record method of payment agreed upon by patient.

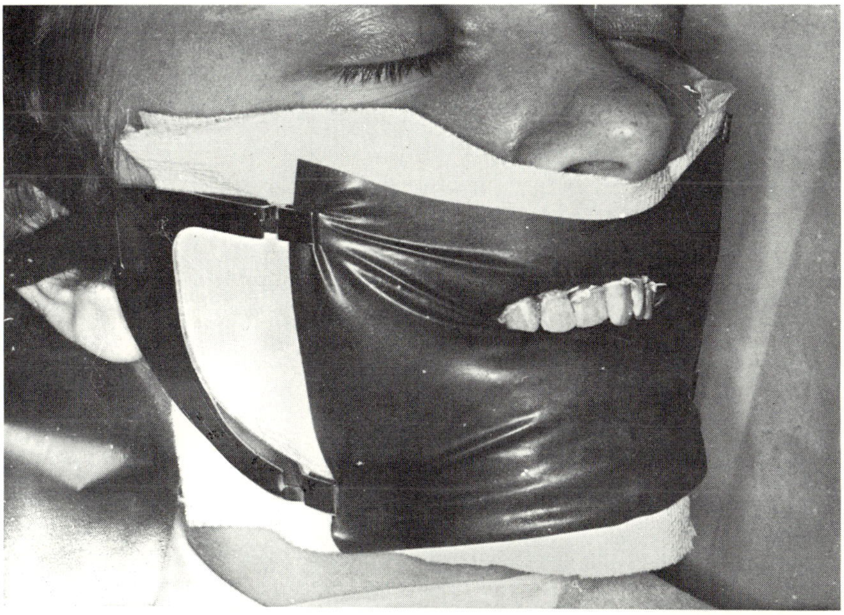

Fig. 6-5. Rubber dam applied to patient. (From Peterson, S., editor: Clinical dental hygiene, ed. 3, St. Louis, 1968, The C. V. Mosby Co.)

For illustration of armamentarium see Fig. 6-4.

SUPPLEMENTAL TRAYS

Rubber dam

A rubber dam is used to isolate one or more teeth for the purpose of keeping the field of operation sterile and/or dry for relatively long periods of time (see Fig. 6-5). A sterile field of operation is required during endodontic procedures, and a dry field of operation is required during the placement of all types of restorations. When dryness is required for shorter periods of time, isolation of the teeth with cotton rolls, skillful chairside assistance, and use of suction and warm air, can be used as a substitute for the rubber dam. The dental assistant who is trained to apply and remove the rubber dam by herself can save the dentist considerable operating time. The armamentarium required for application and removal of a rubber dam is shown in Fig. 6-6.

Procedure checklist
Rubber dam application

1. Punch holes in rubber dam to correspond with the teeth to be isolated. A template may be used to locate the position of the holes.
2. Clear the contact points in the field of operation with dental floss.
3. Lubricate the patient's lips with vaseline or cocoa butter.
4. Attach rubber-dam clamp to the selected posterior tooth with rubber-dam clamp forceps.
5. Apply the rubber dam to the selected teeth, taking care not to tear the rubber as it passes the contact point.
6. Place gauze napkin between cheeks and rubber dam, and attach to holder.
7. Cut hole in appropriate location for insertion of saliva ejector.
8. Adjust the rubber dam by curling the edges of the rubber into the gingival sulci with a beaver-tail burnisher and dental floss.

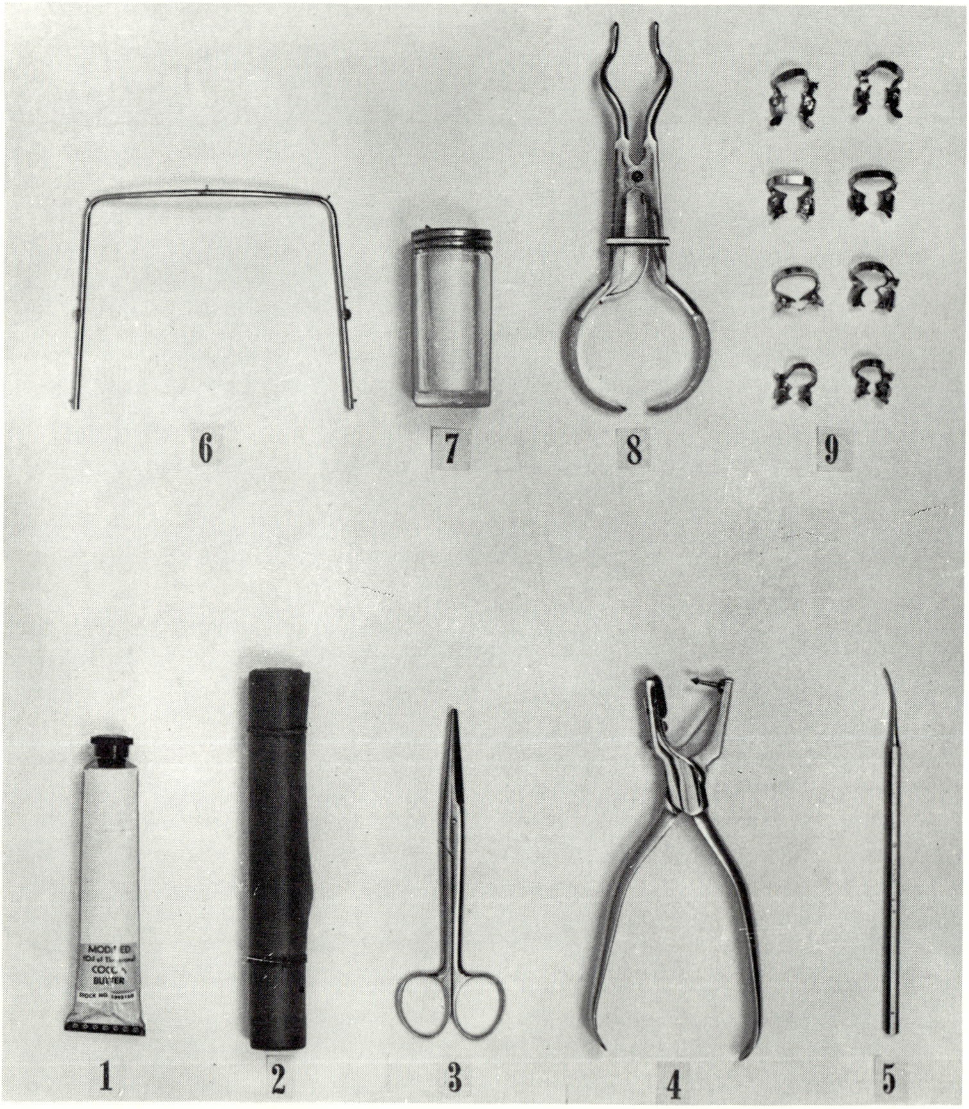

Fig. 6-6. Armamentarium for application of rubber dam.

1. Lubricant, silicate cement (cocoa butter).
2. Rubber dam.
3. Scissors, straight, Mayo, blunt points, 5½-inch.
4. Punch, rubber-dam.
5. Burnisher, #2 (beaver-tail).
6. Holder, rubber-dam.
7. Floss, waxed, dental.
8. Forceps, clamp, rubber-dam.
9. Clamps, rubber-dam (assortment).

9. Tie dental floss ligatures around the teeth where indicated to maintain the seal and to hold the rubber dam in place.

Rubber dam removal

1. Cut and remove dental floss ligatures around the teeth.
2. Stretch the rubber dam away from the teeth, and cut the interproximal rubber septa.
3. Remove clamp with clamp forceps.
4. Detach holder and napkin, and gently remove rubber dam in an occlusal direction.
5. Examine rubber dam for tears and missing pieces of rubber. *Missing pieces of rubber remaining around the teeth must be located and removed at once.*
6. Massage the gingival tissues, and irrigate the mouth.

Finishing and polishing

The final step in the placement of all restorations, including crowns and bridges, consist of the contouring and polishing of all margins and surfaces of the restorations to proper form and function. Frequently, this final step is performed subsequent to the session at which the restoration is placed for the following reasons: (1) in this way several restorations can be finished and polished at the same time; (2) occlusal adjustments frequently are necessary after a trial period in the mouth; and (3) finishing and polishing must await final setting and hardening of the filling material in the case of amalgam and silicate cement restorations. The armamentarium for finishing and polishing is shown in Fig. 6-7.

Procedure checklist

1. Learn to anticipate the dentist's need for each of the materials used in finishing and polishing.
2. Remember that the order of usage of abrasive materials progresses from the coarser to the finer abrasives.
3. The occlusion is first checked by the dentist with articulating paper.
4. Occlusal contours are then perfected with finishing burs and stones.
5. All exposed margins and surfaces are contoured and polished with assorted abrasive paper and Burlew disks.
6. Proximal surfaces and gingival margins are contoured and polished with assorted finishing strips.
7. All exposed surfaces are polished with flour of pumice and whiting.
8. The dental assistant will usually be required to run water on stones as they are rotated on the restoration.
9. Attach abrasive paper disks to the mandrel with the grit "inside" or "outside," according to the directions of the dentist.

Local anesthesia

Local anesthetics are widely employed in the dental office for the purpose of eliminating the pain associated with a great variety of dental operations. Local anesthesia is produced by the injection of an anesthetic solution into the tissues around the nerve or nerves that supply sensation to the part of the mouth to be operated upon. The anesthesia produced when the solution is deposited around a main nerve trunk is called "conduction anesthesia," or a "nerve block." "Mandibular," "zygomatic," "mental," and "infraorbital" are the usual types of intraoral nerve block injections. When the solution is deposited around the terminal branches of a nerve, "infiltration anesthesia" is produced.

The materials used in making the injection include the following: (1) syringe (cartridge type), (2) needle, (3) hub, (4) cartridge (containing anesthetic solution), (5) applicator (cotton-tipped), and (6) germicidal solution.

The plunger end of the cartridge type of syringe opens on a hinge to permit insertion of the glass cartridge containing the anesthetic solution. The plunger on the older type of syringe (Fig. 6-8) has a flat

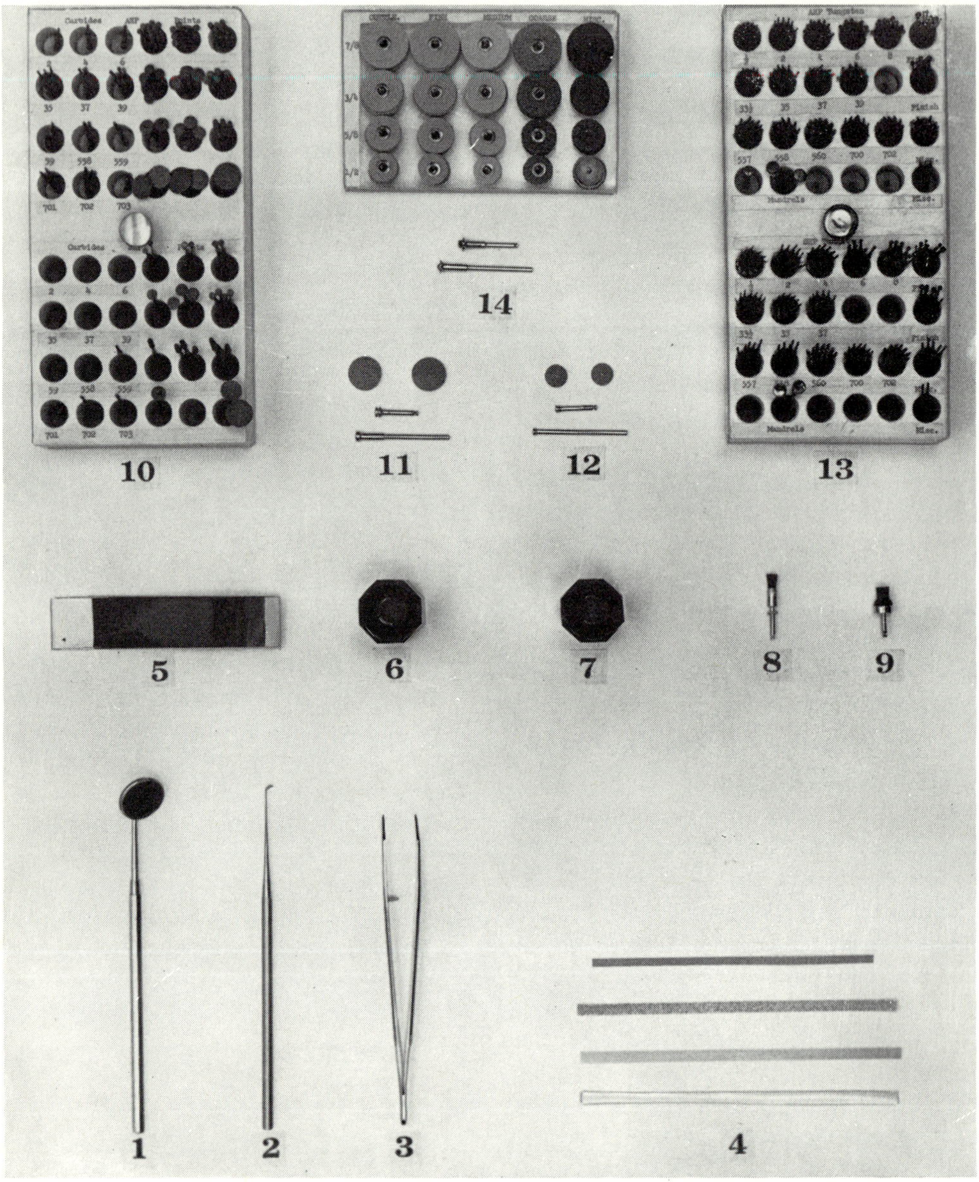

Fig. 6-7. Armamentarium for finishing and polishing.

1. Mirror, mouth, examining, #4.
2. Explorer, #6.
3. Forceps, dressing, #17.
4. Strips, finishing (assortment).
5. Paper, articulating, blue (twelve sheets).
6. Dish, glass, medicament, dappen (for polishing agent).
7. Dish, glass, medicament, dappen (for whiting, calcium carbonate).
8. Brush, tooth-polishing, bristle, AHP.
9. Cup, polishing, rubber, AHP.
10. Points, silicone carbide (assortment).
11. Disk, wheel-shaped, knife-edged, cleaning and polishing, Burlew type (with screwhead mandrels, AHP and SHP #303).
12. Disk, wheel-shaped, knife-edged, sulci, Burlew type (with small screwhead mandrels, AHP and SHP #303½).
13. Burs, excavating, tungsten steel (assortment).
14. Disk set, abrasive paper, with brass center (assortment) and mandrels, Moore type, AHP and SHP.

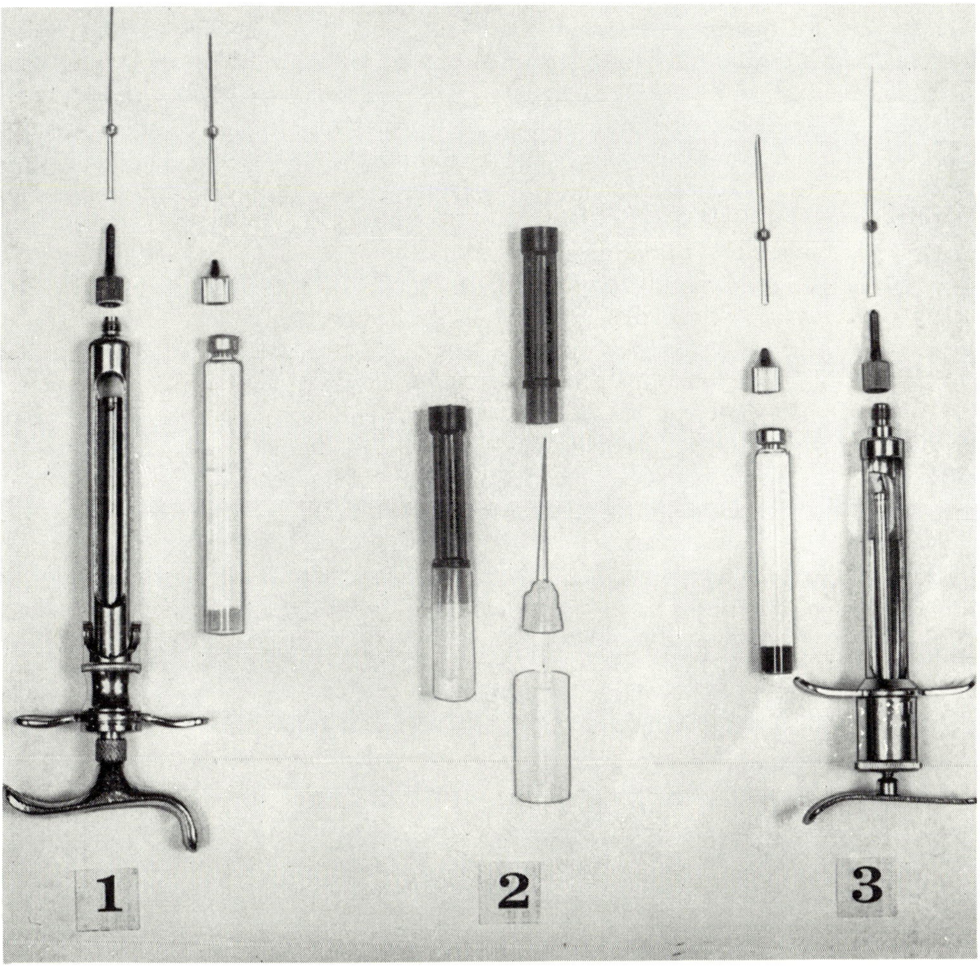

Fig. 6-8. Armamentarium for production of local anesthesia.

1. Syringe, cartridge, with ⅞-inch and ½-inch screw-on hubs; needles, hypodermic, cartridge type, 27-gauge, 1⅝-inch and 1-inch; Novocain 2 percent with Neo-Coberfin 1:20,000, cartridge, 2.2 ml.
2. Needle, hypodermic, cartridge type, 25-gauge, 1½-inch, disposable, with self-threading plastic hub sterilized and sealed in protective polyethylene cartridge.
3. Syringe, cartridge, aspirating, with ⅞-inch and ½-inch screw-on hubs; needles, hypodermic, cartridge type, 27-gauge, 1⅝-inch and 1-inch; Xylocaine hydrochloride 2 percent with epinephrine 1:100,000 cartridge, 1.8 ml.

end, which is pressed against the rubber plunger in the glass cartridge when the injection is made. The plunger on the newer type of syringe (Fig. 6-8) has a hook or screw end, which engages the rubber plunger in the glass cartridge, permitting aspiration as well as injection.

Two lengths of needles, 1-inch and 1⅝-inch, are commonly used for injecting intraoral local anesthetics; which is used depends upon the type of the injection. As a general rule, the 1-inch needle is used for the infiltration type of injection, and the 1⅝-inch needle is used for the nerve block type of injection. However, some dentists prefer to simplify the armamentarium by using the 1⅝-inch needle for both types of injection. The caliber of the needles may be 25, 26, or 27 gauge. The needles have an external end that extends out from the syringe and an internal end that extends into the barrel of the syringe. The needle and hub are assembled by inserting the external end of the needle through the hub. The hub is then screwed onto the end of the syringe. A newer type of sterile, packaged, disposable needle with plastic hub attached (Fig. 6-8) eliminates the problem of washing, sterilizing, and reusing the needles. Disposable needles are a safeguard against dull, inadequately sterilized old needles.

The anesthetic solutions are supplied in rubber-stoppered glass cartridges. The rubber stopper in one end of the cartridge acts as a plunger; the stopper in the other end acts as a cap. When the plunger end of the syringe is opened on its hinge, the cartridge is inserted, cap end first, into the barrel of the syringe and pressed firmly into place until the cap is punctured by the internal end of the needle. The syringe is closed, and it is then ready for use. After a syringe has been used, the needle and hub should be disassembled, and the needle should be soaked in a blood-solvent solution if it is to be resterilized.

An aseptic technique is always used for producing local anesthesia. For this reason, the foregoing items of equipment must be sterilized and kept sterile until ready for use. If resterilized needles are to be used, a convenient method of preparing the syringes is to assemble some with short needles and others with long needles and to place a cotton roll over each needle. The assembled syringes and needles are then autoclaved together. They can be stored in a separate drawer, in which they are laid on a sterile towel and covered with another sterile towel.

Anesthetic cartridges should be stored in a closed container. Before inserting the cartridge into the barrel of the syringe, the cap and plunger ends of the cartridge should be wiped with an alcohol sponge. Do not store anesthetic cartridges in a chemical disinfectant solution because of the possibility of percolation of these solutions through minute flaws in the rubber stoppers.

Procedure checklist

1. When the patient is ready for injection, pass the dentist a sterile cotton-tipped applicator that has been dipped in a germicidal solution.
2. Pass the perpared syringe to the dentist out of sight of the patient.
3. Guard against any sudden reflex movement of the patient's hands during the injection.
4. Be prepared to administer aromatic spirits of ammonia in case the patient shows signs of syncope (fainting).

PERIODONTICS

Coronal debridement (prophylaxis)

Coronal debridement, or prophylaxis, is one of the most common forms of treatment for gingivitis. The operation consists of removing debris, calcareous deposits (calculus), and stains that collect around the teeth coronal to the bottom of the gingival sulcus. Most persons require this type of treatment at 3-, 6-, or 12-month intervals. This particular operation may be performed by a dental hygienist as well as by a dentist. An ultrasonic unit may be used for coronal debridement in addition to armamentarium shown in Fig. 6-9.

Procedure checklist

1. The ultrasonic unit is usually used first, followed by scaling instruments of the sickle type.
2. Sandpaper strips may also be used between the teeth.
3. An astringent may be applied to gingival tissues.

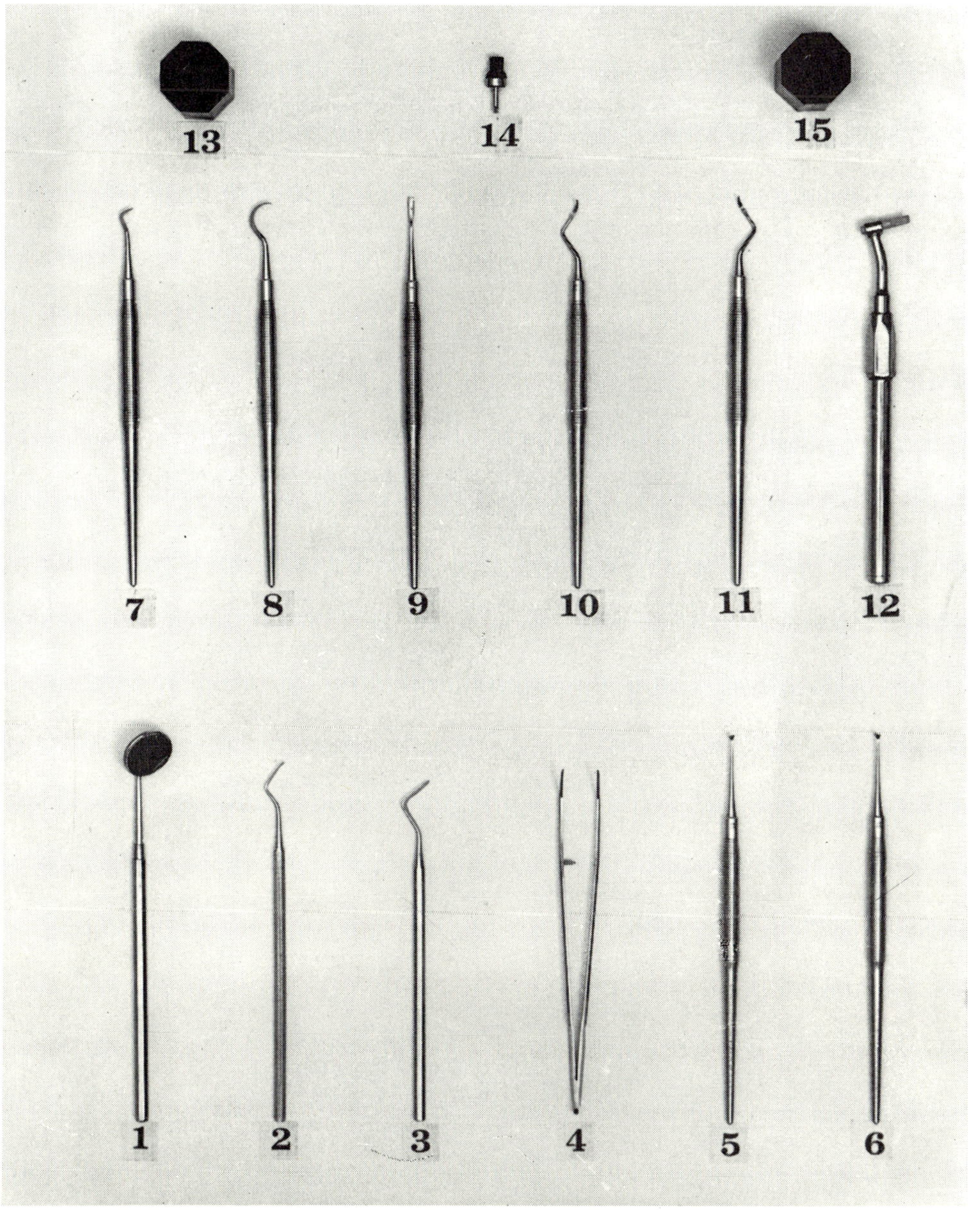

Fig. 6-9. Armamentarium for coronal debridement (prophylaxis).

1. Mirror, mouth, examining, #4.
2. Explorer, #17.
3. Probe, pocket, gauge (Williams).
4. Forceps, dressing, #17.
5. Scaler, wing, #45.
6. Scaler, wing, #46.
7. Scaler, sickle, #5.
8. Scaler, sickle, #14 (Orban).
9. Scaler, push, #1 (McCall).
10. Scaler, sickle, #B2 (Ball).
11. Scaler, sickle, #B3 (Ball).
12. Porte-polisher (with wooden point).
13. Dish, glass, medicament, dappen (for polishing agent).
14. Cup, polishing, rubber, AHP.
15. Dish, glass, medicament, dappen (for astringent).

4. The teeth are polished with a rubber cup and polishing agent.

5. Interproximal spaces are cleared with dental tape.

6. As the scaling instruments are used, the assistant should direct an intermittent steam of air or water on the field of operation to permit better visualization.

7. Wipe the working ends of the instruments with a gauze napkin as they are being used and as they are placed back on the tray.

8. Control the saliva injector to reduce the number of times that the patient must use the cuspidor.

9. Prepare one dappen dish with an astringent and another with a polishing agent.

10. Irrigate the mouth, and clean the patient's face before dismissal.

Subgingival debridement and curettage

Subgingival debridement and curettage commonly are performed as a treatment for periodontal disease. Dental deposits that are not removed from around the teeth at regular intervals by coronal debridement (prophylaxis) extend into and deepen the sulcus that exists between the gingiva and the tooth. A deepened gingival sulcus is called a periodontal pocket. Subgingival debridement, which is an extension of coronal debridement into a periodontal pocket, requires the use of different instruments. The basic armamentarium used for gingival debridement consists of hoes, files, and curets, as shown in Fig. 6-10.

Procedure checklist

1. Since gingival hemorrhage results from subgingival instruments, the assistant must keep the field of operation visible and free of hemorrhage by the alternate use of water and air and by controlling the saliva injector.

2. Wipe instruments with moist napkin as they are used and as they are placed on the bracket table.

3. Prepare cotton pellets or cotton strands for application to the pocket.

4. Prepare one dappen dish with astringent and another with a polishing agent.

5. Irrigate the mouth, and clean the patient's face before dismissal.

Surgical gingival resection

Surgical gingival resection is performed in the treatment of more advanced types of periodontal disease. The operation consists of surgically removing the gingival wall of the periodontal pocket. The armamentarium used for surgical gingival resection is shown in Fig. 6-11.

Procedure checklist

1. Prepare cotton-tipped applicator and syringe for local anesthesia.

2. Keep the field of operation visible and free of hemorrhage with gauze sponges (2×2 inches) and by controlling the suction apparatus.

3. Using a hemostat or tissue forceps, hold one end of the resected tissue while the dentist frees the tissue from around the teeth.

4. Cleanse and pass instruments as granulation tissue and any remaining calculus is removed from around the teeth.

5. Prepare dappen dish with 1:1,000 epinephrine solution.

6. Prepare ¼-inch gauze strips soaked in epinephrine solution for application to the wound surface.

7. Prepare surgical cement dressing to cover and protect the wound surface.

Postoperative treatment

Postoperative treatment after surgical gingival resection is ordinarily scheduled every 5 to 7 days until healing is completed. The armamentarium used for postoperative treatment is shown in Fig. 6-12.

Procedure checklist

1. Dispose of the cement dressing as it is removed by the dentist.

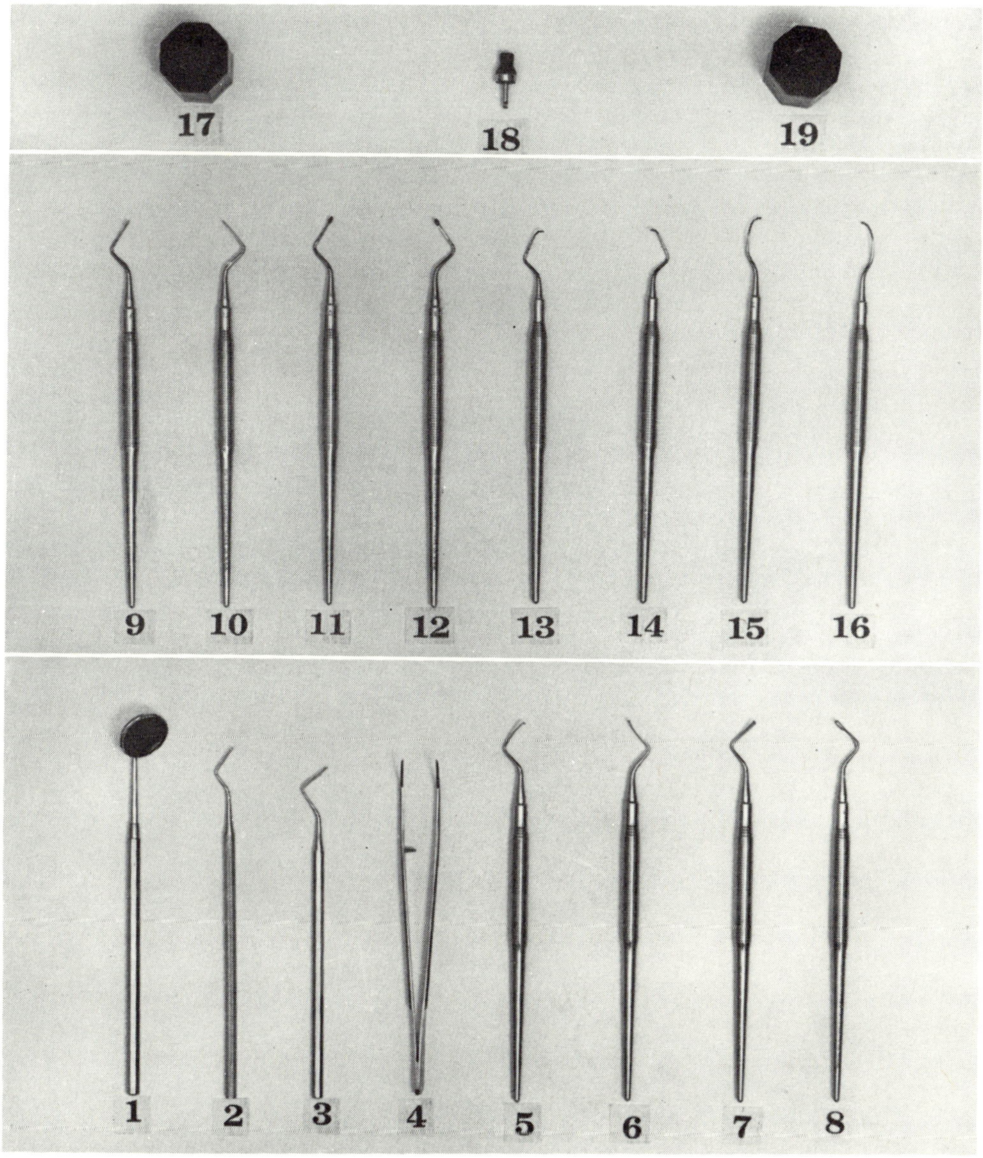

Fig. 6-10. Armamentarium for subgingival debridement and curettage.

1. Mirror, mouth, examining, #4.
2. Explorer, #17.
3. Probe, pocket, gauge (Williams).
4. Forceps, dressing, #17.
5. Scaler, hoe, #7 (Orban).
6. Scaler, hoe, #6 (Orban).
7. Scaler, hoe, #8 (Orban).
8. Scaler, hoe, #9 (Orban).
9. File, #13 (Orban).
10. File, #12 (Orban).
11. File, #10 (Orban).
12. File, #11 (Orban).
13. Curet, #7 (Gracey).
14. Curet, #8 (Gracey).
15. Curet, #11 (Gracey).
16. Curet, #12 (Gracey).
17. Dish, glass, medicament, dappen (for polishing agent).
18. Cup, polishing, rubber, AHP.
19. Dish, glass, medicament, dappen (for astringent).

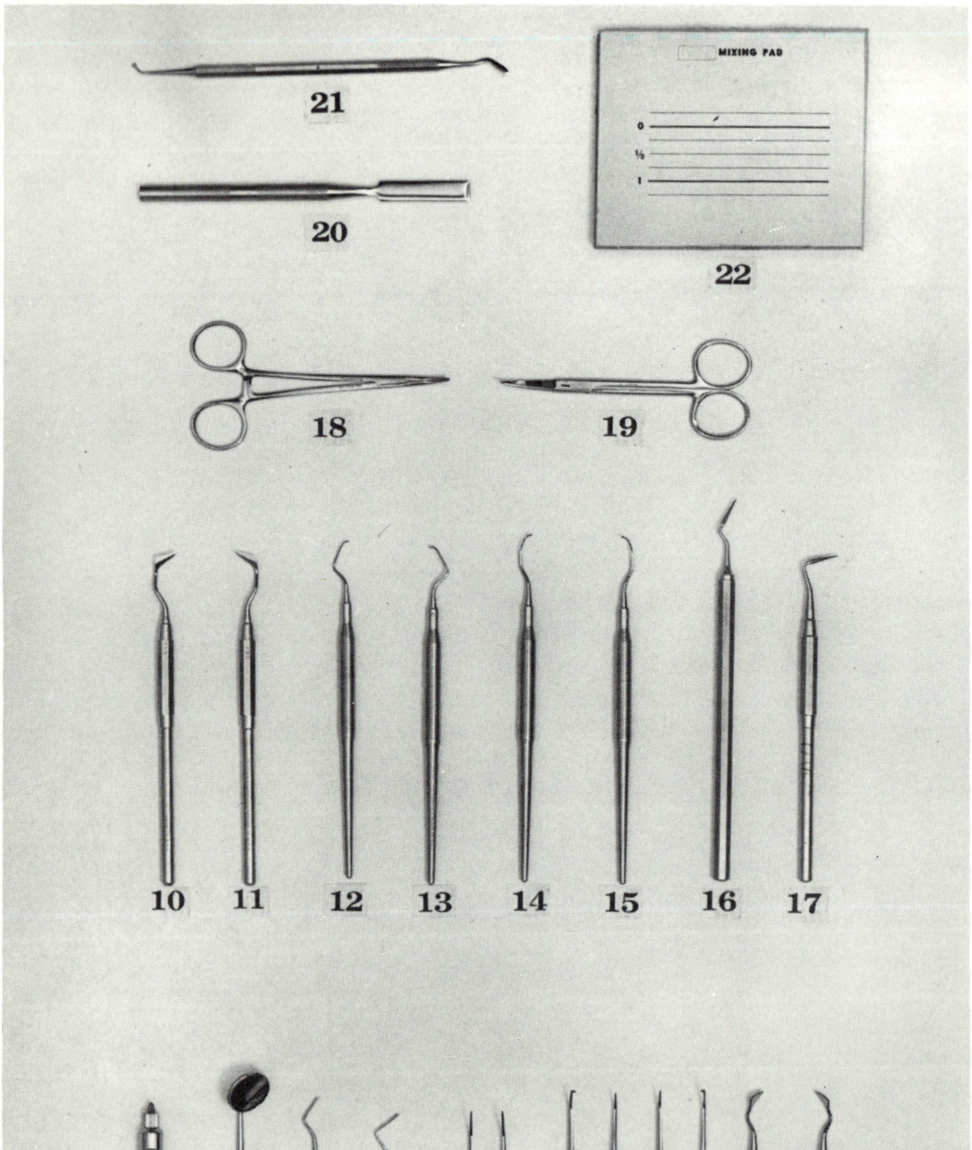

Fig. 6-11. For legend see opposite page.

2. Pass and receive sickle scalers as needed for removal of remaining debris and calculus around the teeth.

3. Gently direct *warm* air on the area being treated (exposed root surfaces are hypersensitive to temperature changes).

4. Prepare wisps of cotton in dappen dish with medicament (trichloracetic acid) for application to the wound surface.

5. Prepare surgical cement dressing for reapplication to the wound surface. (At the last postoperative treatment after the gingival tissues have healed, the teeth are polished, and the cement dressing is not replaced.)

ORAL SURGERY

Oral surgical routine

Preoperative medication

Preoperative medication is commonly indicated prior to oral surgical procedures. A sedative may be routinely prescribed to reduce apprehension before an operation. Preoperative antibiotic therapy frequently is prescribed when infection exists in the area of operation. As soon as the patient arrives in the dental office, the dental assistant should make certain that he has taken the prescribed medications. A kind and reassuring attitude at this time and during the operation is an important factor in obtaining the patient's cooperation, which is essential to the success of the procedure.

Aseptic procedure

Oral surgical operations involve procedures that break the epithelial barrier of the oral mucous membrane and expose the bloodstream and underlying connective tissues to the external environment. For this reason, aseptic procedures must be followed in the preparations for and performance of these operations. All instruments, towels, gauze, and rubber gloves to be used must be sterilized before the operation and maintained under aseptic conditions until needed.

Autoclaving is the most effective method of sterilizing instruments and materials, with the exception of scalpel blades and surgical burs. These latter items are dulled by autoclaving and, therefore, should be sterilized by means of a suitable chemical solution (Fig. 6-13). When surgical burs are to be used, the sleeve of the straight handpiece should also be autoclaved prior to the operation. Sterile instruments and materials are handled *only* with sterile transfer forceps until the hands have been properly prepared (Fig. 6-14).

The assistant scrubs thoroughly and wears rubber gloves, if these are required, in the same manner as the dentist. After

---

Fig. 6-11. Armamentarium for surgical gingival resection.

1. Syringe, cartridge.
2. Mirror, mouth, examining, #4.
3. Explorer, #17.
4. Probe, pocket gauge (Williams).
5. Forceps, dressing, #17.
6. Forceps, periodontal pocket marking, #1 (Goldman-Fox).
7. Forceps, periodontal pocket marking, #2 (Goldman-Fox).
8. Knife, #K15 (Kirkland).
9. Knife, #K16 (Kirkland).
10. Knife, #T19 (Towner).
11. Knife, #T20 (Towner).
12. Curet, #7 (Gracey).
13. Curet, #8 (Gracey).
14. Curet, #11 (Gracey).
15. Curet, #12 (Gracey).
16. File, #00 (Buck).
17. File, #12 (Buck).
18. Forceps, hemostatic, curved, mosquito, 5-inch.
19. Scissors, iris, straight, sharp-pointed, 4¼-inch.
20. Spatula, #2.
21. Plugger, plastic filling, Woodson, double-ended, #2.
22. Pad, waxed surface (for mixing surgical dressing).

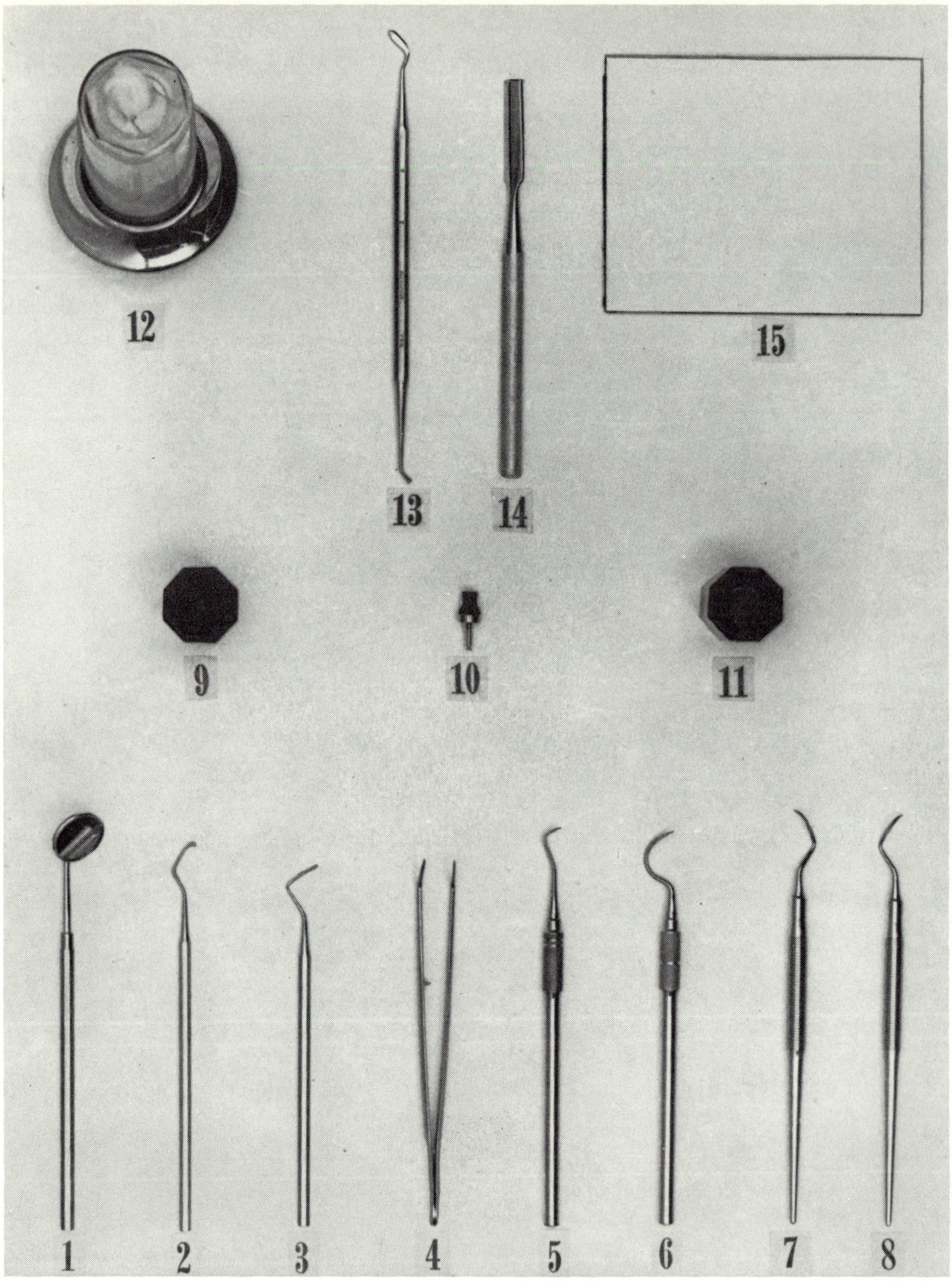

Fig. 6-12. Armamentarium for postoperative treatment.

1. Mirror, mouth, examining, #4.
2. Explorer, #17.
3. Probe, pocket, gauge (Williams).
4. Forceps, dressing, #17.
5. Scaler, sickle, #5.
6. Scaler, sickle, #14 (Orban).
7. Scaler, sickle, #B2 (Ball).
8. Scaler, sickle, #B3 (Ball).
9. Dish, glass, medicament, dappen (for polishing agent).
10. Cup, polishing, rubber, AHP.
11. Dish, glass, medicament, dappen (for caustic).
12. Cotton, absorbent, cylinder (for use in cotton font).
13. Plugger, plastic filling, Woodson, double-ended, #2.
14. Spatula, #2.
15. Pad, waxed surface (for mixing surgical dressing).

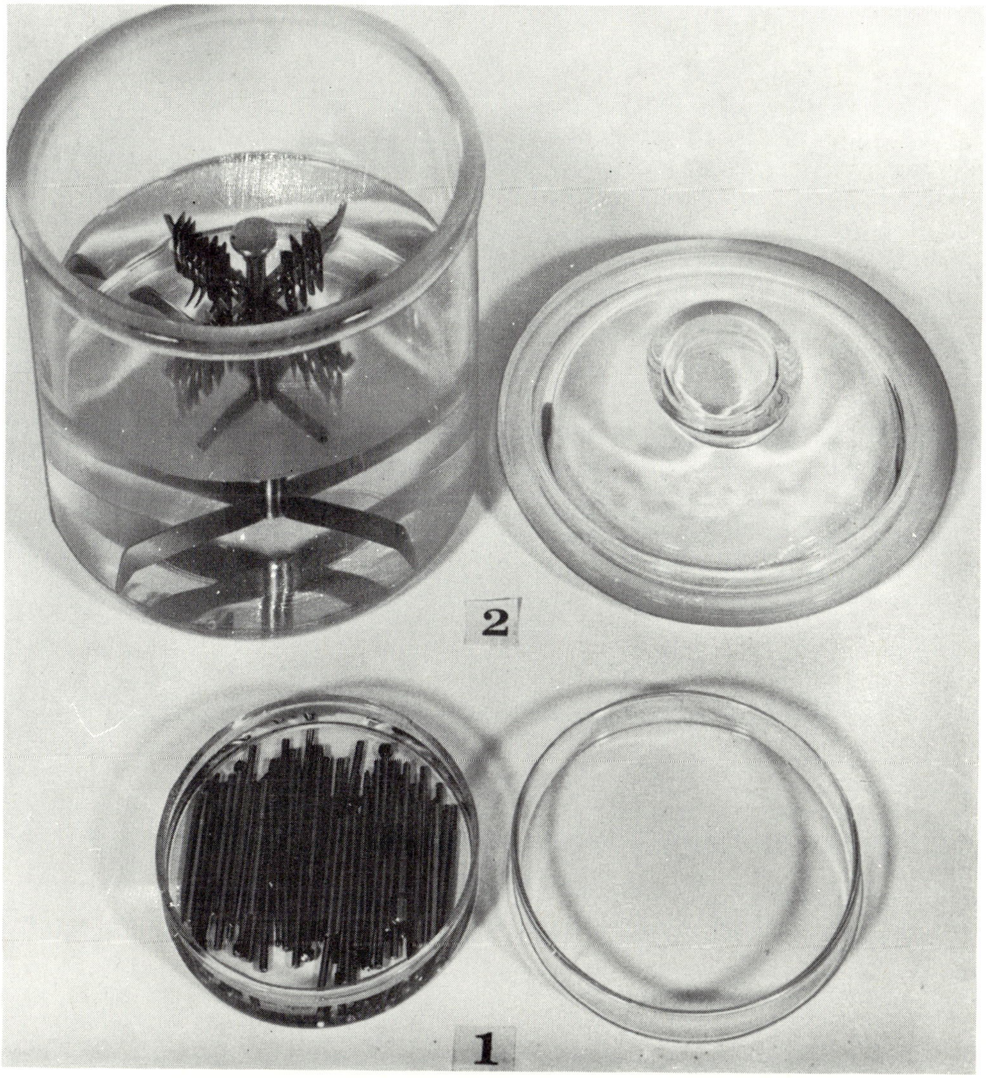

Fig. 6-13. Chemical sterilization of surgical burs and blades.

1. Burs, SHP, surgical, assortment, immersed in benzalkonium chloride solution 1:1000.
2. Blades, surgical, assortment, immersed in benzalkonium chloride solution 1:1000.

the hands are prepared, they should remain free of any contaminants outside the field of operation until the operation is completed. Therefore, when only one assistant is available, it is essential that complete preparation be made before the operation begins. If it should become necessary for the assistant to touch any unsterile article, such as the operating light or dental chair, during the course of the operation, her hands must be reprepared before she handles sterile instruments and materials or enters the field of operation. A second, unscrubbed assistant relieves the operating assistant of the necessity for touching any unsterile article.

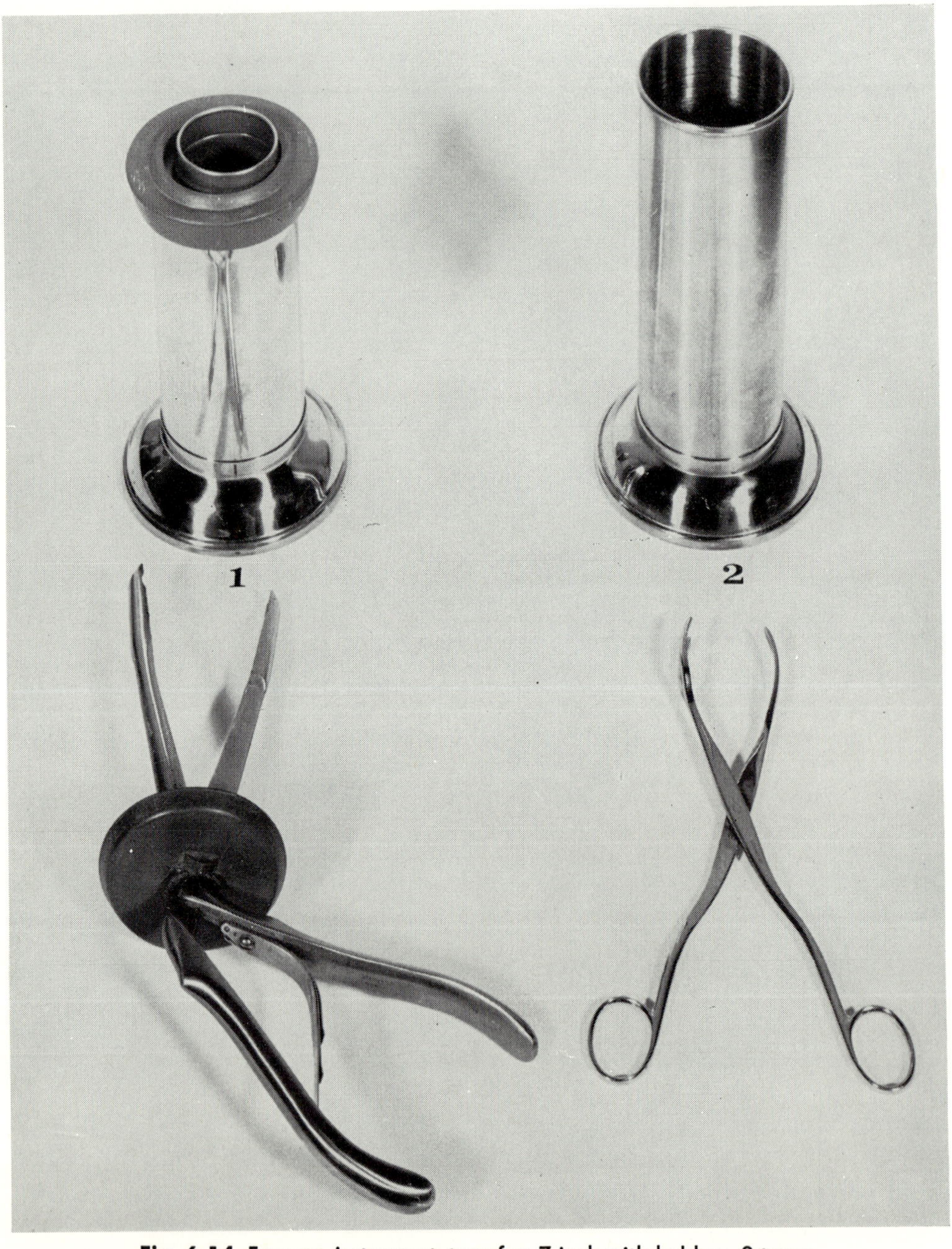

Fig. 6-14. Forceps, instrument, transfer, 7-inch with holders; 2 types.

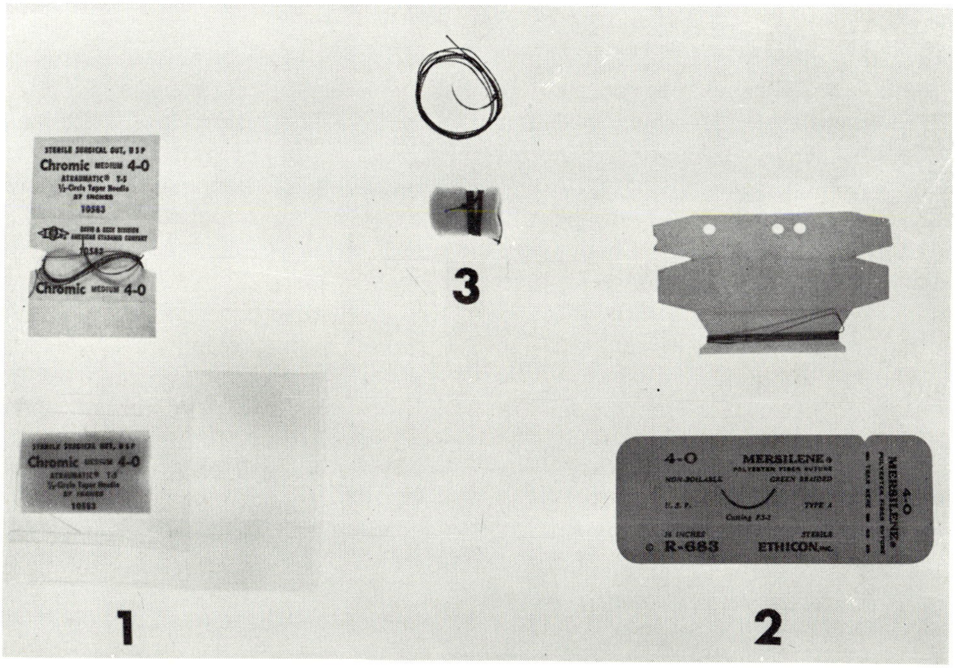

Fig. 6-15. Sutures.

1. Suture, gut, sterile, chromic, medium, size 4-0, 27-inch, with ½-circle taper, eyeless, atraumatic needle.
2. Suture, polyester fiber, sterile, green braided, size 4-0, 18-inch, with ⅜-circle eyeless Atraloc needle.
3. Suture, nylon, size 3-0, threaded on needle, suture, cleft palate, ½-circle, size #2, wrapped on cotton roll, sterilized by immersion in 70-percent alcohol.

The first step in all oral surgical procedures is to scrub the oral tissues in the field of operation with a germicidal solution. Usually it is not possible to sterilize the field of operation in the mouth, but every effort is made to cleanse the area as thoroughly as possible and to avoid introduction of foreign bacteria.

Chairside assistance

The same essential skills of chairside assistance are required for oral surgical operations as for any other type of dental operation. In other words, the assistant passes and cleans instruments and keeps the field of operation visible and free of debris, saliva, and/or hemorrhage. The latter task is accomplished by means of sterile gauze sponges to retract the cheeks, tongue, and tissue flaps and by controlling the suction apparatus.

The assistant should also be alert to early signs of syncope (fainting) manifested by the patient during the course of the operation. These signs, which include marked facial pallor, cold sweat on the forehead, and a vacant stare, should be called to the attention of the dentist, and measures should be taken to counteract them immediately by tipping the dental chair backward so that the patient's head is lower than his feet, by applying a cold damp towel to the forehead, and by holding aromatic spirits of ammonia under the patient's nostrils. Mouth-to-mouth airways or oxygen equipment, if available, also may be used.

Closure of the surgical wound is the final step in all oral surgical operations. Sutures used for this purpose are made of surgical gut, silk, or nylon. They may be obtained in presterilized packages having the thread fused to an eyeless needle (Fig. 6-15), or they may be hand-prepared before the operation using approximately 24 inches of suture threaded around a cotton roll for convenience, and sterilized by immersion in 70-percent alcohol (Fig. 6-15). Surgical gut sutures are eventually absorbed and for that reason are usually used when it is not possible for the patient to return for removal of the suture; silk and nylon sutures will not absorb and must be removed after healing has occurred. As the dentist passes the needle through the tissue, the assistant can help by holding the tissue taut with tissue forceps. After the dentist ties the suture, the assistant should be prepared to cut the loose ends with scissors. When all sutures have been placed, the patient is asked to bite upon a gauze sponge placed over the operative site and to lie down in the recovery room for 15 minutes before being dismissed by the dentist.

Postoperative instructions

In the recovery room the assistant should give the patient written postoperative instructions, such as the following:

1. Do not rinse the mouth for 6 hours after the operation to avoid disturbing the blood clot.
2. Some bleeding normally continues for a short time after the operation. If bleeding has not stopped after a reasonable period of time, call Dr. ________. In the meantime, place a tea bag or a wad of gauze over the wound, and bite firmly for 30 minutes.
3. Some swelling may occur after the operation. Swelling may be reduced by applying an ice bag to the face over the affected area for the first day only.
4. Take ____ tablets every ______ hours as necessary for relief of pain (envelope attached).
5. Avoid coarse foods that can disturb the wound. Select soft foods, soups, and fruit juices for a few days.
6. Cleanse the mouth after each meal. A mouthwash may be used after the first day. Use a gauze-wrapped finger to gently cleanse the teeth and gums in the area of the operation. In all other areas of the mouth, brush the teeth as usual.
7. Promptly report any condition that causes concern.

Biopsy

A biopsy consists of the removal of a piece of tissue from a lesion for the purpose of making a diagnosis. Lesions are biopsied either by excision of the entire lesion or by incision into the edge of the lesion. The excised tissue is *immediately* placed in a small bottle of 10-percent formalin and sent to an oral pathologist for histopathologic examination. The specimen should be accompanied by a report containing the name, age, and sex of the patient; the history, description, and clinical impression of the lesion; and, if possible, a photograph or radiograph taken before the biopsy. The armamentarium used for taking a biopsy is shown in Fig. 6-16 .

Procedure checklist

1. Take photograph of lesion, retracting the cheeks or tongue in such a manner as to provide the best view of the lesion.
2. Remind dentist to record the history, description, and clinical diagnosis of the lesion before taking the biopsy.
3. Prepare cotton-tipped applicator and syringe for local anesthesia.
4. Use suction apparatus and gauze sponges to keep the field of operation free of hemorrhage during biopsy.
5. Immediately place biopsy specimen in a bottle of 10-percent formalin.
6. Assist dentist in the placement of suture to close the wound.

Incision and drainage

Periapical and periodontal infections frequently cause acute abscesses in the oral cavity. The occurrence of such abscesses must be considered a dental emergency. These infections may extend into the tissues of the face and neck and endanger the life of a patient. Extensive abscesses of dental origin are ordinarily treated in a hospital. Less extensive abscesses may be treated in the dental office. Incision and drainage is one phase of the

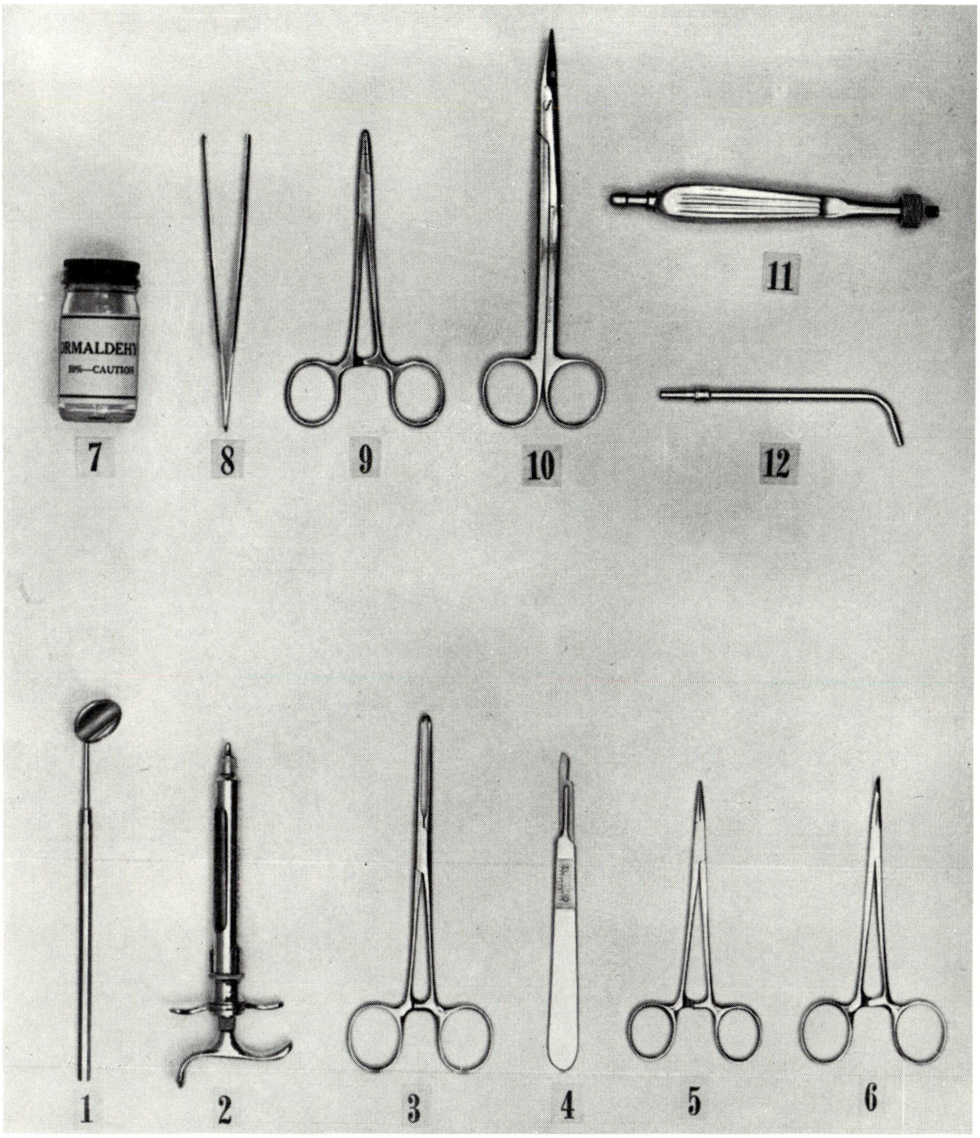

Fig. 6-16. Armamentarium for biopsy procedure.

1. Mirror, mouth, examining, #4.
2. Syringe, cartridge.
3. Forceps, tissue, straight, Allis, 6-inch.
4. Handle, operating knife, #3; blade, #15.
5. Forceps, hemostatic, mosquito, straight, 5-inch (Halstead).
6. Forceps, hemostatic, mosquito, curved, 5-inch (Halstead).
7. Bottle specimen, 1 ounce (for formaldehyde, 10 percent).
8. Forceps, tissue, spring, 5-inch.
9. Holder, needle, 5-inch.
10. Scissors, oral surgery, Dean, 6¾-inch.
11. Handle, suction, vise grip.
12. Tip, tapered, #3, hole $\frac{3}{32}$-inch.

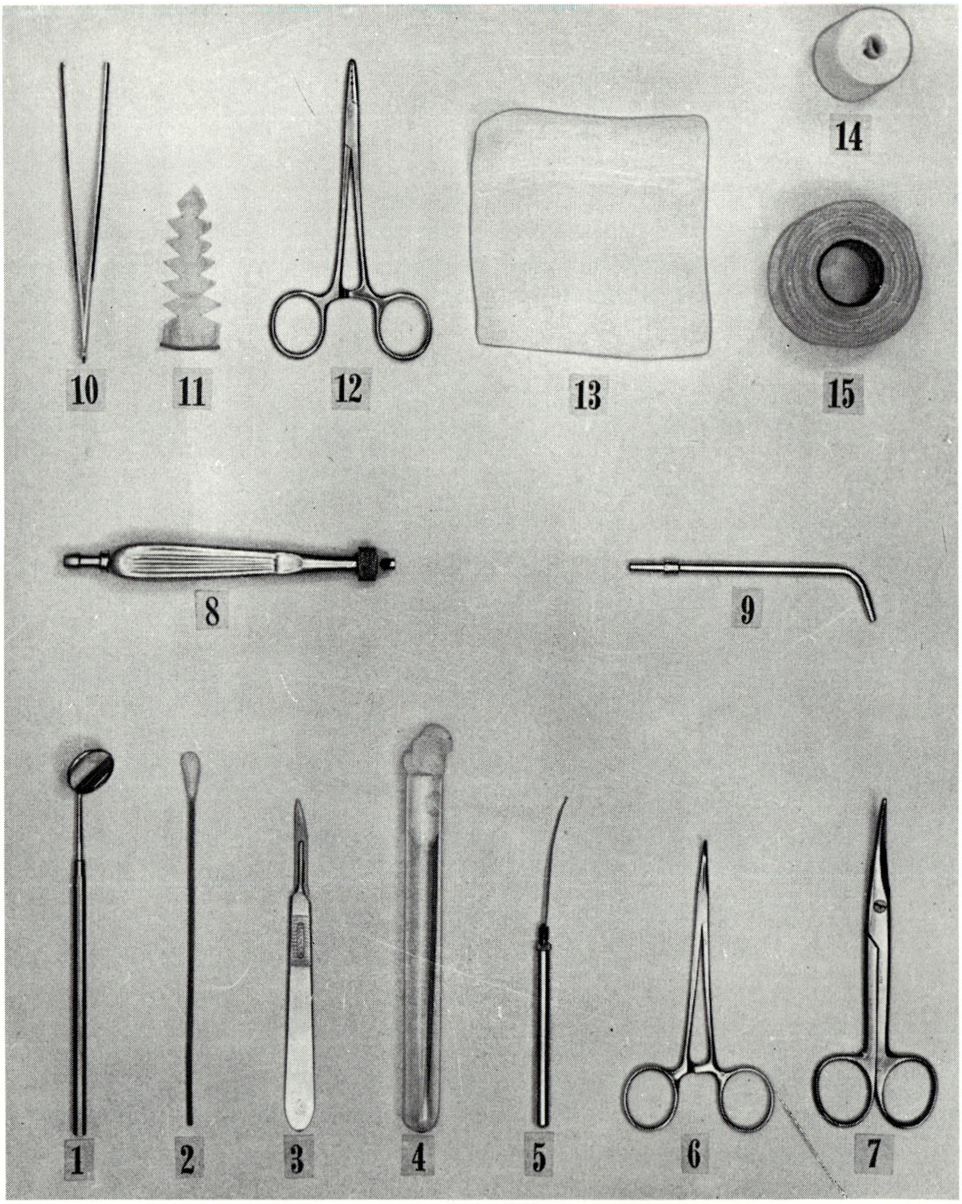

Fig. 6-17. Armamentarium for incision and drainage.

1. Mirror, mouth, examining, #4.
2. Applicator, cotton-tipped, 6⅜-inch.
3. Handle, operating knife, #3; blade, #11.
4. Test tube, culture (with applicator, cotton-tipped).
5. Probe, abscess, silver.
6. Forceps, hemostatic, mosquito, curved, 5-inch (Halstead).
7. Scissors, curved, Mayo (blunt points, 5½-inch).
8. Handle, suction, vise grip.
9. Tip, tapered, #3; hole $\frac{3}{32}$-inch.
10. Forceps, tissue, spring, 5-inch.
11. Drain (cut from cot, finger, rubber).
12. Holder, needle, 5-inch.
13. Sponge, surgical, 4 by 4 inches.
14. Bandage, gauze, roller, 2 inches by 6 yards.
15. Adhesive plaster, surgical, 2 inches by 5 yards.

treatment of such abscesses. This phase is usually followed by antibiotic therapy and removal of the tooth in question or endodontic or periodontal therapy. An intraoral or extraoral incision may be made. The armamentarium used for incision and drainage is shown in Fig. 6-17.

Procedure checklist

1. Take and record patient's temperature before beginning the operation.
2. Prepare cotton-tipped applicator with germicidal solution for scrubbing area of operation.
3. Prepare syringe for local anesthesia.
4. Deliver scalpel for incision into abscess.
5. Have ready a sterile applicator and culture tube for taking bacteriologic cultures of exudate from abscess.
6. Deliver probe and hemostat as needed, and keep field of operation free of hemorrhage by use of gauze sponges and suction apparatus.
7. Prepare rubber drain if needed.
8. Prepare sutures as needed.
9. Prepare gauze bandage if an extraoral incision has been made.
10. Remind dentist of possible need for prescription of antibiotics and sedatives.

Removal of maxillary and mandibular teeth

Teeth may be removed because of advanced caries, advanced periodontal disease, apical cysts, apical granulomas, malposition, and prosthetic or orthodontic reasons. One or several teeth may be scheduled for removal during a given session. Frequently, those teeth to be removed at one time are limited to the maxilla or to the mandible. Therefore, the instruments have been divided into 2 trays—one for removal of teeth in the maxilla and the other for removal of teeth in the mandible (Figs. 6-18 and 6-19). The technique employed for uncomplicated tooth removal is essentially the same whether the tooth is located in the maxilla or in the mandible.

Procedure checklist

1. Prepare cotton-tipped applicator with germicidal solution and syringe for local anesthesia.
2. Help to support the lower jaw during forceful manipulations by the dentist in removing a mandibular tooth.
3. Guard against injury to the patient's lips during manipulations of the forceps by the dentist.
4. Immediately after removal of a tooth, guard against salivary contamination of the tooth socket with sponges and the suction apparatus.
5. *Do not* disturb blood clot in tooth socket unless further examination of the socket is necessary by the dentist.
6. Have a small bottle of 10-percent formalin available in case any tissue is removed from the tooth socket.
7. Prepare and assist in the placement of sutures.
8. Prepare gauze sponge for placement over operative site, and ask patient to bite firmly.
9. Clean patient's face, and ask him to wait in recovery room for 15 minutes or until hemorrhage has stopped.
10. In the recovery room, give patient postoperative instructions and any indicated prescriptions for drugs before dismissal.

Removal of impacted teeth

Teeth that fail to erupt into normal position during growth and development of the jaws are commonly referred to as "impacted or embedded teeth." Those teeth most susceptible to impaction are third molars, canines, premolars, and upper incisors, in that order. Impacted teeth frequently must be removed because of pericoronal infection, root resorption of a adjacent tooth, follicular cysts, and prosthetic requirements. Removal of impacted teeth is a

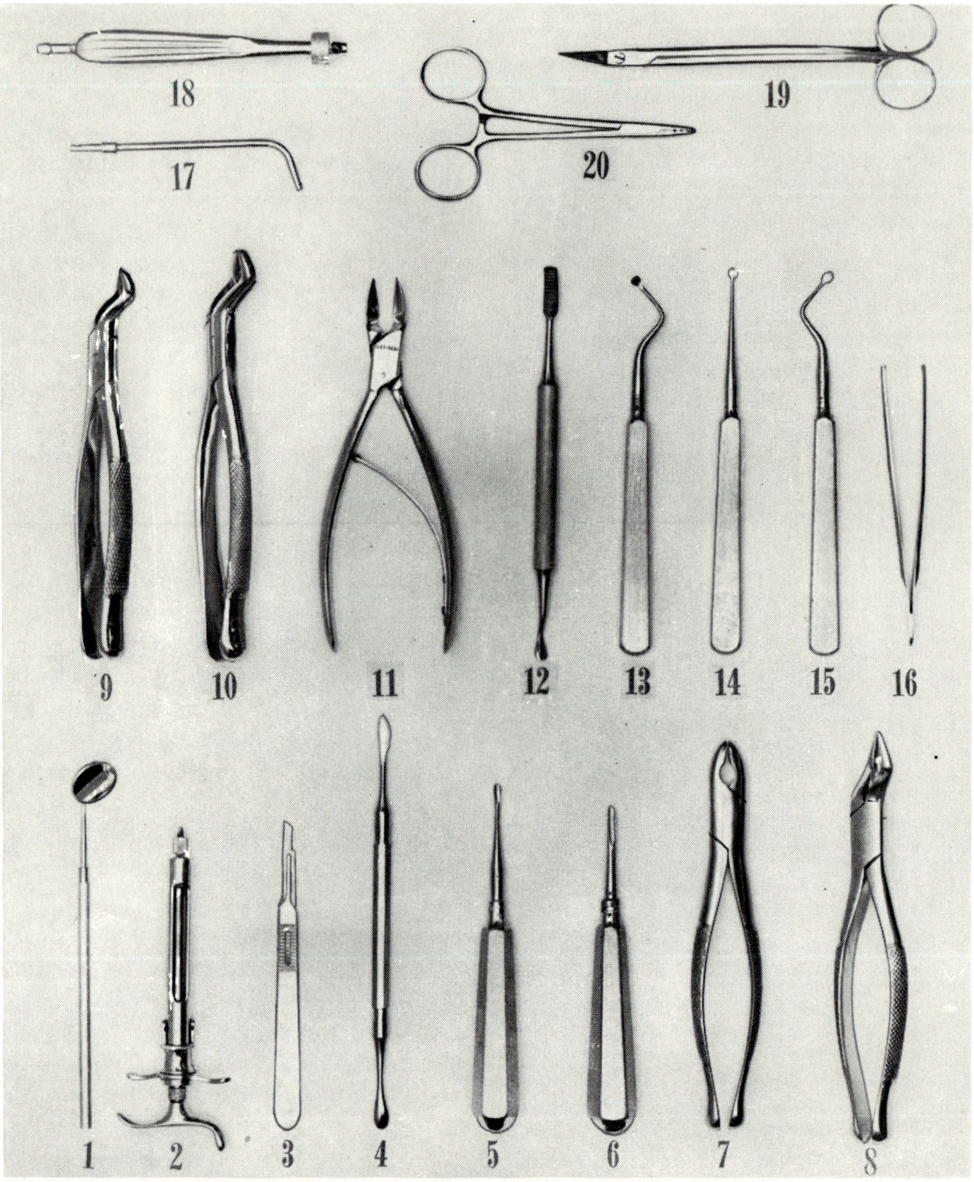

Fig. 6-18. Armamentarium for removal of maxillary teeth.

1. Mirror, mouth, examining, #4.
2. Syringe, cartridge.
3. Handle, operating knife, #3; blade, #15.
4. Periosteotome, #9.
5. Elevator, root, Friedman, #81.
6. Elevator, root, Friedman, #34S.
7. Forceps, tooth extracting, #99C (for upper premolars, canines, and incisors).
8. Forceps, tooth extracting, #286 (for upper anterior teeth, premolars, and roots), bayonet-shaped.
9. Forceps, tooth extracting, #53R (for right upper first and second molars), bayonet-shaped.
10. Forceps, tooth extracting, #53L (for left upper first and second molars), bayonet-shaped.
11. Forceps, bone, rongeur, #5 (side-cutting).
12. File, bone, double-end, #61 and #70 (Friedman).
13. Curet, alveolar, Molt, #9L.
14. Curet, alveolar, Molt, #2.
15. Curet, alveolar, Molt, #10R.
16. Forceps, tissue, spring, 5-inch.
17. Tip, tapered, #3; hole $\frac{3}{32}$-inch.
18. Handle, suction, vise grip.
19. Scissors, oral surgery, Dean, 6¾-inch.
20. Holder, needle, 5-inch.

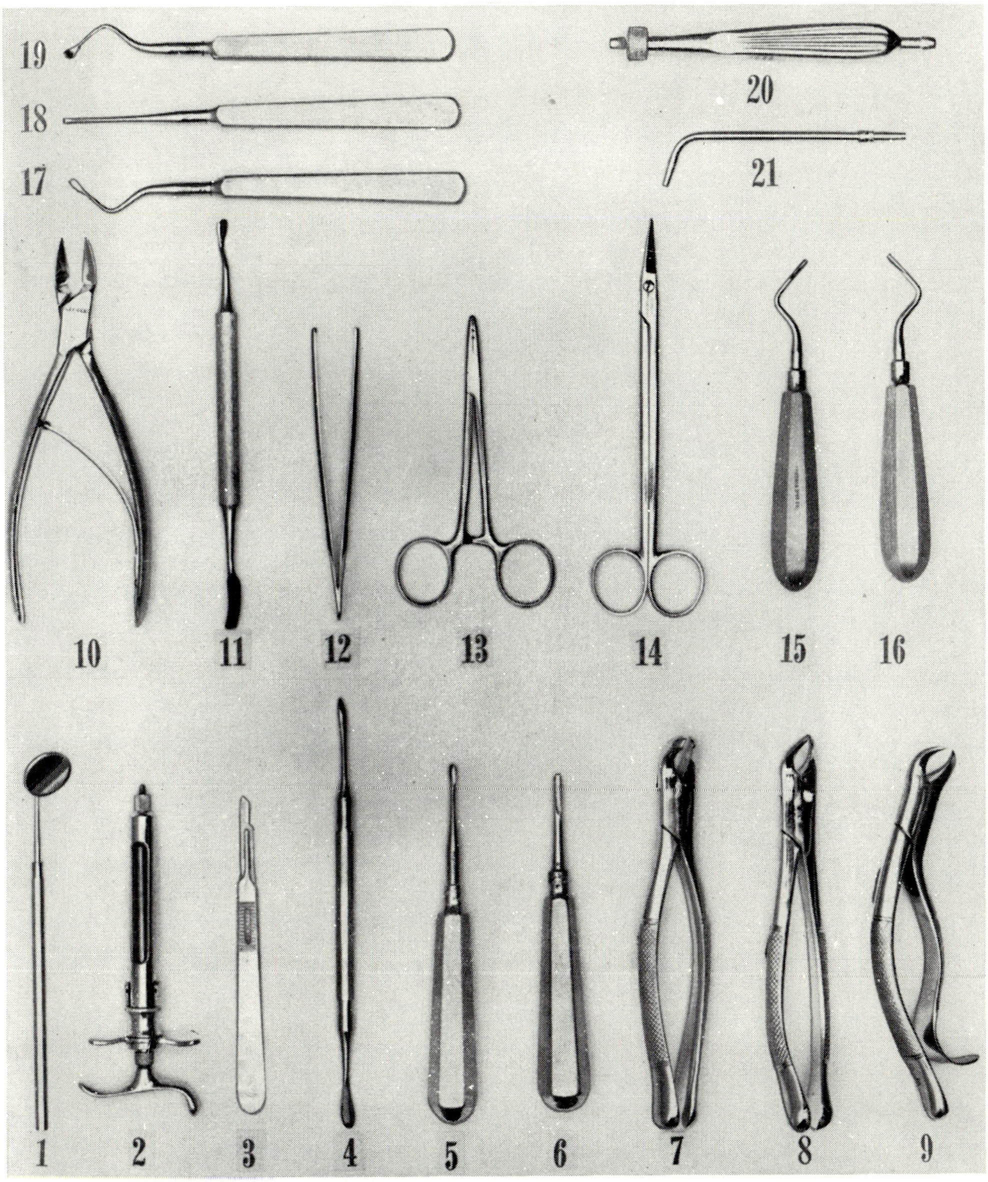

Fig. 6-19. Armamentarium for removal of mandibular teeth.

1. Mirror, mouth, examining, #4.
2. Syringe, cartridge.
3. Handle, operating knife, #3; blade, #15.
4. Periosteotome, #9.
5. Elevator, root, Friedman, #81.
6. Elevator, root, Friedman, #34S.
7. Forceps, tooth extracting, #17 (for lower first and second molars).
8. Forceps, tooth extracting, #151 (for incisors, premolars, and roots).
9. Forceps, tooth extracting, #16, horn-beaked (for lower first and second molars).
10. Forceps, bone, rongeur, #5 (side-cutting).
11. File, bone, double-end, #61 and #70 (Friedman).
12. Forceps, tissue, spring, 5-inch.
13. Holder, needle, 5-inch.
14. Scissors, oral surgery, Dean, 6¾-inch.
15. Elevator, root, Friedman, #90.
16. Elevator, root, Friedman, #91.
17. Curet, alveolar, Molt, #9L.
18. Curet, alveolar, Molt, #2.
19. Curet, alveolar, Molt, #10R.
20. Handle, suction, vise grip.
21. Tip, tapered, #3; hole $\frac{3}{32}$-inch.

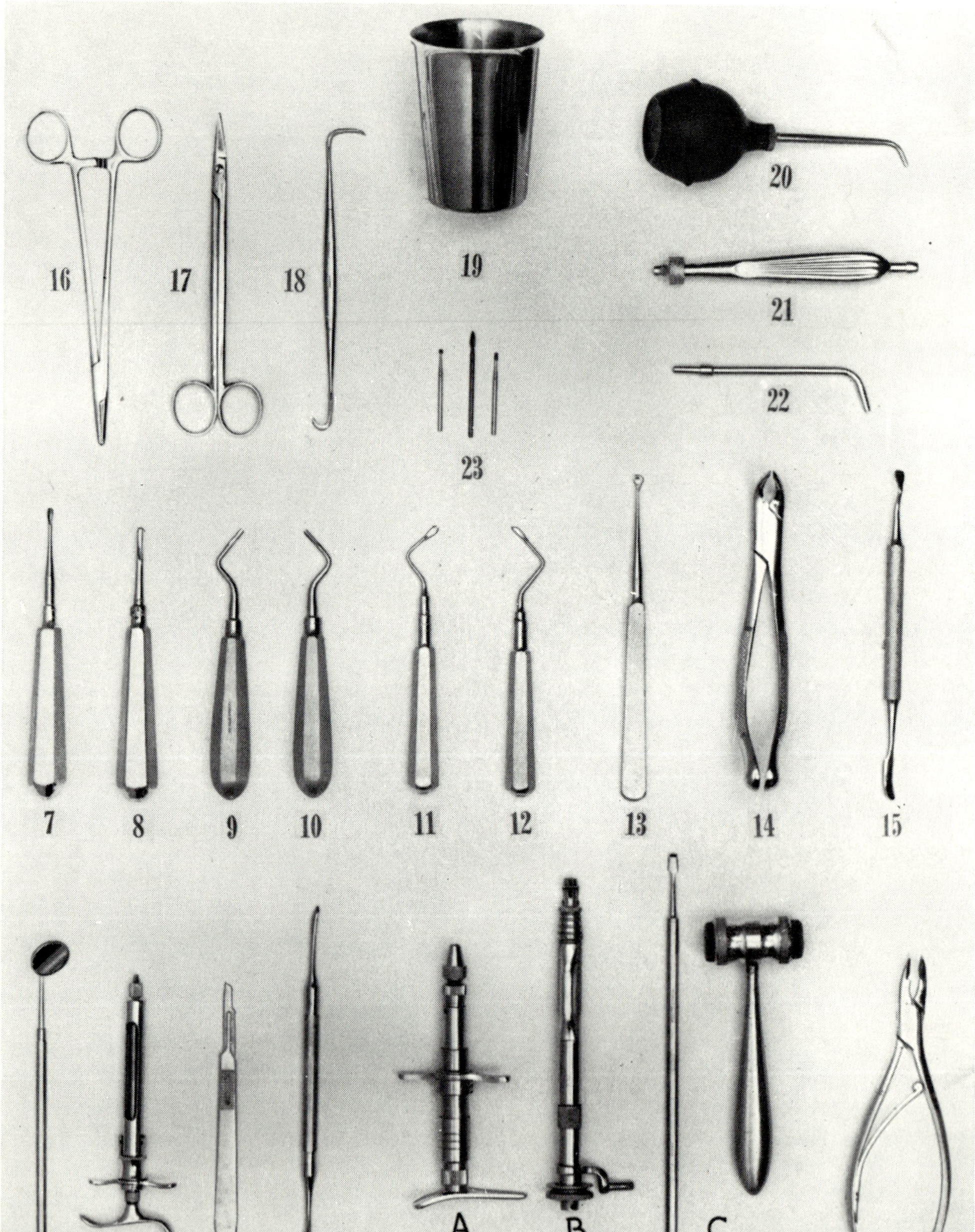

Fig. 6-20. For legend see opposite page.

complicated and difficult surgical procedure. The technique of removal will vary according to the location and position of the impaction. The armamentarium used for the removal of impacted teeth is shown in Fig. 6-20.

Procedure checklist

1. Prepare cotton-tipped applicator with germicidal solution for scrubbing area of operation.
2. Prepare syringe for local anesthetic.
3. Deliver scalpel for incison of mucoperiosteum.
4. Deliver periosteotome to reflect mucoperiosteal flap.
5. Assist with retraction of mucoperiosteal flap using periosteotome or retractor.
6. Continue retraction, and control hemorrhage with sponges and suction while dentist removes bone overlying the impacted tooth. (The dentist may use surgical burs or a chisel and mallet for this purpose.)
7. If a chisel and mallet is used, the assistant will use the mallet while the dentist holds the chisel.
   a. The assistant must learn to judge the force of the blow required in different tissues and different locations.
   b. A stronger blow is required in the dense bone of the mandible than in the softer bone of the maxilla.
   c. A considerably stronger blow is required to split the crown of a tooth.
   d. Manipulate the mallet with wrist-action only.
   e. Use a sharp tap, with immediate recoil of mallet.
   f. Gauge strength of the blow by watching the results at the working end of the chisel.
   g. The dentist usually will nod his head to indicate when to strike each blow.
8. Prepare physiologic saline solution in a cup for irrigation of the operative site with a rubber bulb syringe after removal of impacted tooth.
9. Have gelfoam pack ready for placement in the tooth socket.
10. Assist dentist in placement of sutures to close the wound.
11. Prepare gauze sponge for placement over operative site, and ask patient to bite firmly.
12. Clean patient's face, and ask him to wait in recovery room for 15 minutes or until hemorrhage has stopped.
13. In the recovery room, give patient

Fig. 6-20. Armamentarium for removal of impacted teeth.

1. Mirror, mouth, examining, #4.
2. Syringe, cartridge.
3. Handle, operating knife, #3; blade, #15.
4. Periosteotome, #9.
5. Choice of operator:
   A. Mallet, surgical automatic (Reiter).
   B. Mallet, oral surgery, engine-driven (Dudley).
   C. Chisel, osseous (Stout), #1.
      Mallet, oral surgery, hand-operated (Mead).
6. Forceps, bone, rongeur, #2A (end-cutting).
7. Elevator, root, Friedman, #81.
8. Elevator, root, #34S.
9. Elevator, root, Friedman, #90.
10. Elevator, root, Friedman, #91.
11. Ejector, root, Heidbrink, #98.
12. Ejector, root, Heidbrink, #99.
13. Curet, alveolar, Molt, #1.
14. Forceps, tooth extracting, #151 (for incisors, premolars, and roots).
15. File, bone, double-end, #61 and #70 (Friedman).
16. Holder, needle, 7-inch.
17. Scissors, oral surgery, Dean, 6¾-inch.
18. Retractor, tissue, double-end, three prongs.
19. Cup, stainless steel (for physiologic saline solution).
20. Syringe, irrigating, dental, 1-ounce, rubber bulb.
21. Handle, suction, vise grip.
22. Tip, tapered, #3; hole 3/32-inch.
23. Burs, straight handpiece. Excavating tungsten carbide, spherical, #8; surgery, steel, special, #1; excavating, tungsten carbide, taper fissure, #703.

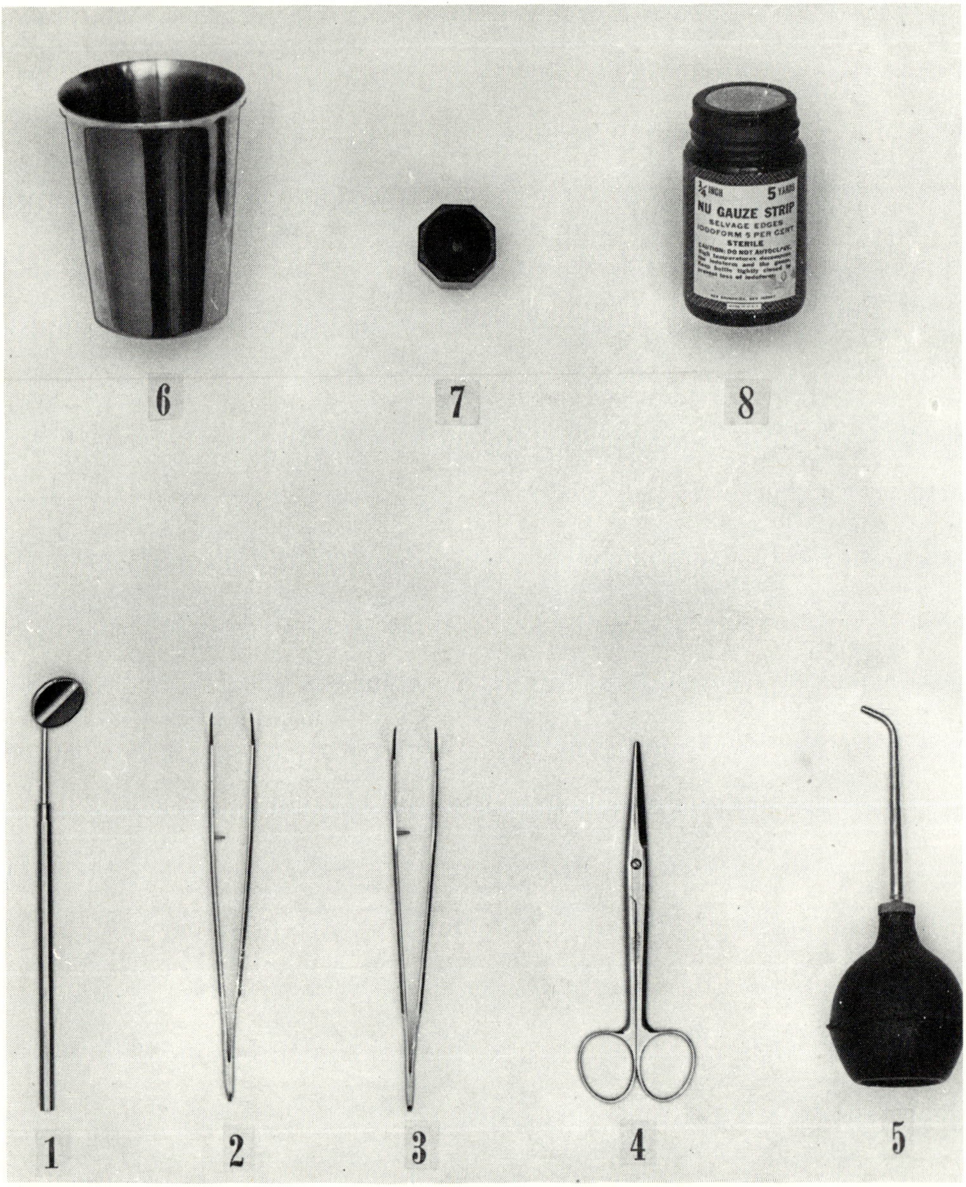

Fig. 6-21. Armamentarium for treatment of infection following removal of tooth (dry socket).

1. Mirror, mouth, examining, #4.
2. Forceps, dressing, #17.
3. Forceps, dressing, #17.
4. Scissors, curved, Mayo (blunt points, 5½-inch).
5. Syringe, irrigating, dental, rubber bulb.
6. Cup, stainless steel (for physiologic saline solution).
7. Dish, glass, medicament, dappen (for topical germicidal and/or obtundent).
8. Gauze, absorbent, iodoform-impregnated, ¼-inch by 5 yards.

postoperative instructions and any indicated prescriptions for drugs before dismissal.

Infection after removal of tooth (dry socket)

A painful infection of the tooth socket, commonly referred to as a "dry socket," occasionally follows removal of a tooth. The pain usually begins on the first or second postoperative day. The condition may be associated with (1) excessive trauma during the operation, (2) the entrance of bacteria-laden saliva into the tooth socket before a blood clot has formed, or (3) the rinsing away of the blood clot by use of a mouthwash too soon after the operation. The armamentarium used for the treatment of infection after removal of a tooth (dry socket) is shown in Fig. 6-21.

Procedure checklist

1. Prepare warm saline solution in a cup for irrigation of the socket with a rubber bulb syringe.
2. Prepare cotton rolls for isolation of the socket, and control saliva ejector.
3. Prepare cotton pellets to dry the socket.
4. Prepare dappen dish with eugenol.
5. Prepare iodoform gauze moistened with eugenol for application to the dry socket.
6. Reschedule patient *daily* for replacement of the iodoform dressing until the pain has subsided.
7. Remind the dentist to prescribe a sedative.

Alveolectomy

Alveolectomy, more properly called alveoloplasty, is the operation performed to shape the alveolar ridges of the maxilla and mandible in preparation for the reception of dentures. Sharp projections of the alveolar process, bulbous tuberosities, and bony undercuts that interfere with proper adaptation of dentures are removed. The operation may be performed immediately following removal of several teeth, or it may be performed subsequently at a separate sitting. The armamentarium used for alveolectomy is shown in Fig. 6-22.

Procedure checklist

1. Prepare cotton-tipped applicator with germicidal solution for scrubbing area of operation.
2. Prepare syringe for local anesthesia.
3. Deliver scalpel for incision of mucoperiosteum.
4. Deliver periosteotome to reflect mucoperiosteal flap.
5. Assist with retraction of mucoperiosteal flap using periosteotome or retractor.
6. Continue retraction, and control hemorrhage with sponges and suction while dentist removes bone with rongeur forceps, bone files, or burs.
7. Remove spicules of bone with sponges and suction apparatus.
8. Assist dentist in placement of sutures to close the wound.
9. Prepare gauze sponge for placement over operative site, and ask patient to bite firmly.
10. Clean patient's face, and ask him to wait in recovery room for 15 minutes or until hemorrhage has stopped.
11. In the recovery room, give patient postoperative instructions and any indicated prescriptions for drugs before dismissal.

Cyst removal

A cyst—a fluid-containing, epithelium-lined cavity—may develop within the jawbone, usually from inflammatory or developmental causes. It starts as a small cavity and tends to become larger and larger, weakening the jawbone as it grows. Cysts are treated either by enucleation or by marsupialization (the so-called Partsch operation). The armamentarium used for cyst removal is shown in Fig. 6-23.

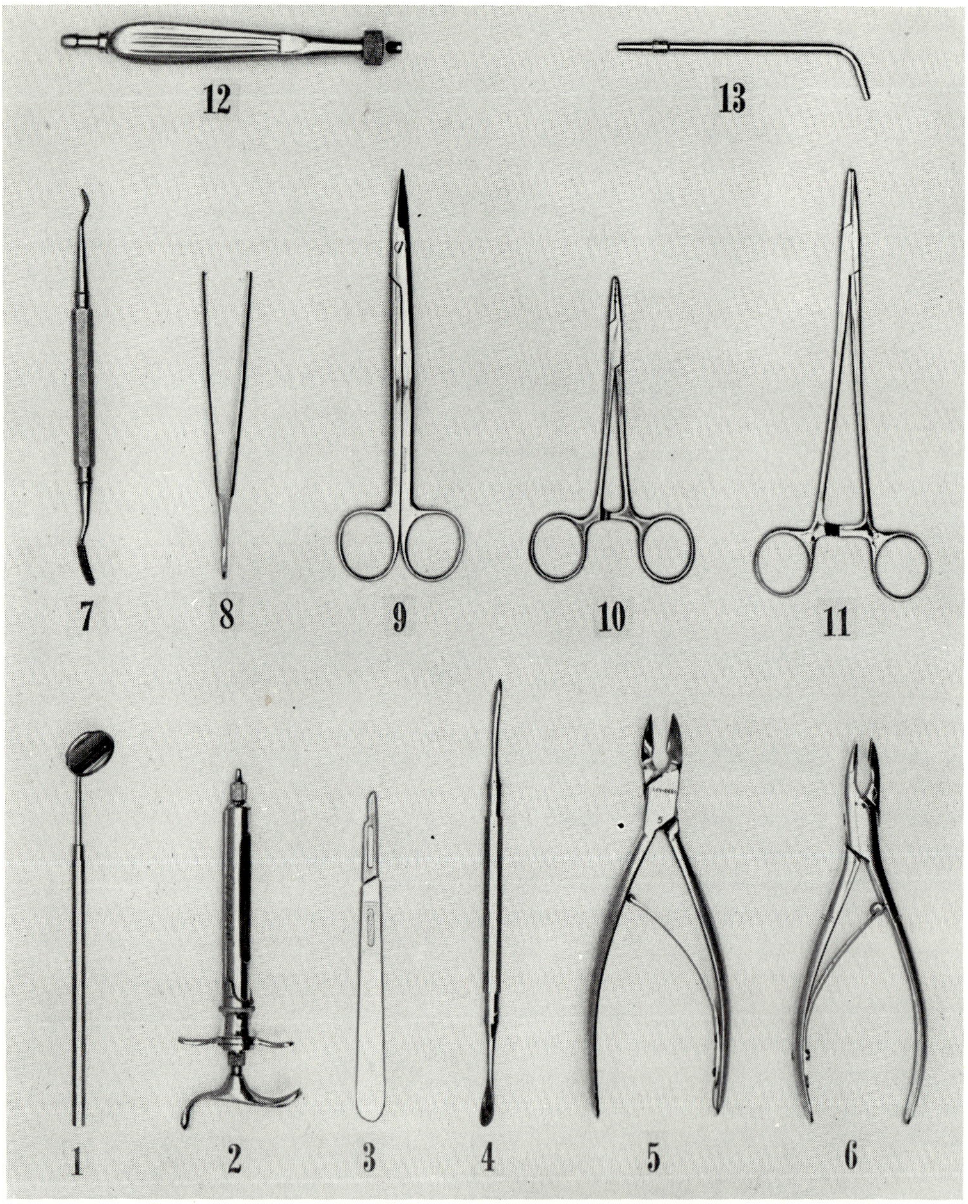

Fig. 6-22. Armamentarium for alveolectomy.

1. Mirror, mouth, examining, #4.
2. Syringe, cartridge.
3. Handle operating knife, #3; blade, #15.
4. Periosteotome, #9.
5. Forceps, bone, rongeur, #5 (side-cutting).
6. Forceps, bone, rongeur, #2A (end-cutting).
7. File, bone, double-end, #61 and #70 (Friedman).
8. Forceps, tissue, spring, 5-inch.
9. Scissors, oral surgery, Dean, 6¾-inch.
10. Holder, needle, 5-inch.
11. Holder, needle, 7-inch.
12. Handle, suction, vise grip.
13. Tip, tapered, #3; hole 3/32-inch.

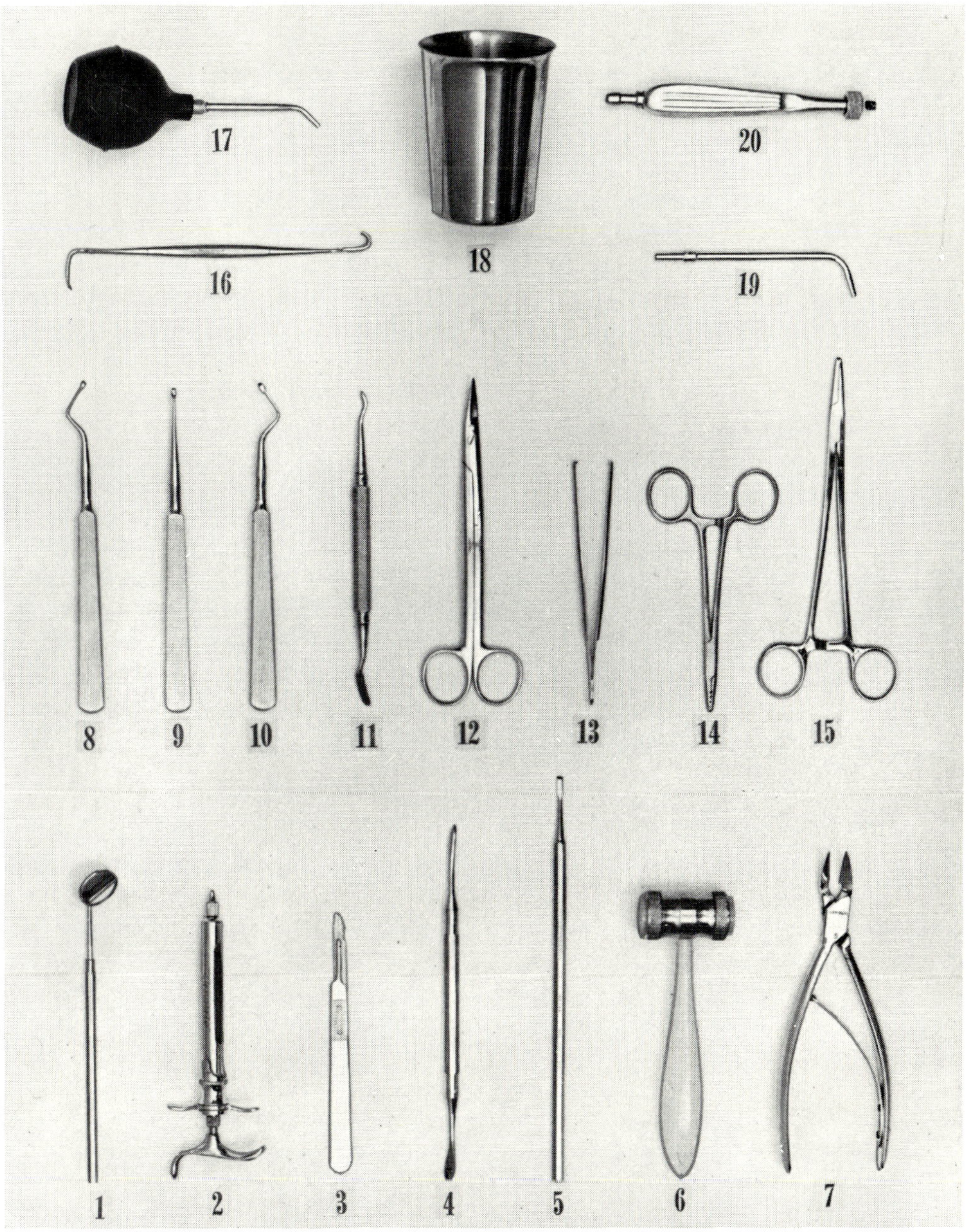

Fig. 6-23. Armamentarium for cyst removal.

1. Mirror, mouth, examining, #4.
2. Syringe, cartridge.
3. Handle, operating knife, #3; blade, #15.
4. Periosteotome, #9.
5. Chisel, osseous, Stout, #1.
6. Mallet, oral surgery, hand-operated (Mead).
7. Forceps, bone, rongeur, #5 (side-cutting).
8. Curet, alveolar, Molt, #5L.
9. Curet, alveolar, Molt, #1.
10. Curet, alveolar, Molt, #6R.
11. File, bone, #61 and #70, double-end (Friedman).
12. Scissors, oral surgery, Dean, 6¾-inch.
13. Forceps, tissue, spring, 5-inch.
14. Holder, needle, 5-inch.
15. Holder, needle, 7-inch.
16. Retractor, tissue, double-end, three prongs.
17. Syringe, irrigating, dental, 1-ounce, rubber bulb.
18. Cup, stainless steel (for physiologic saline solution).
19. Tip, tapered, #3; hole 3/32-inch.
20. Handle, suction, vise grip.

Procedure checklist

1. Prepare cotton-tipped applicator with germicidal solution for scrubbing area of operation.
2. Prepare syringe for local anesthesia.
3. Deliver scalpel for incision of mucoperiosteum.
4. Deliver periosteotome to reflect mucoperiosteal flap.
5. Assist with retraction of mucoperiosteal flap using periosteotome or retractor.
6. Continue retraction, and control hemorrhage with sponges and suction while dentist removes bone overlying the cyst. (Dentist may use surgical burs or chisel and mallet for this purpose.)
7. Assist in the removal of the cyst membrane or sac by using a hemostat and suction.
8. Have bottle of 10-percent formalin ready for fixing the cyst membrane after it is removed.
9. Deliver bone files for smoothing the margins of the bony cavity.
10. Prepare physiologic saline solution in a cup for irrigation of the bony cavity with a rubber bulb syringe.
11. Have gelfoam ready for packing into the bony cavity.
12. Assist dentist in placement of sutures to close the wound. (In the marsupialization, or Partsch operation, the cyst membrane is not removed except over the opening into the cystic cavity. The mucoperiosteal flap is then sutured to the cyst membrane around the periphery of the opening to the cystic cavity.)
13. Clean patient's face, and ask him to wait in recovery room for 15 minutes or until hemorrhage has stopped.
14. In the recovery room, give patient postoperative instructions and any indicated prescriptions for drugs before dismissal.

Jaw fracture

Fractures of the maxilla and mandible frequently result from an external blow, a fall, or an automobile accident. Simple fractures of the mandible may be treated on an outpatient basis in the dental office. Fractures of the maxilla and more complex fractures of the mandible are usually treated in a hospital. The objectives of treatment are (1) reduction and fixation of the fractured jawbone and (2) restoration of the proper maxillomandibular relationship or articulation of the teeth. Many variations in technique are employed to accomplish these objectives, depending upon the type and severity of the fracture. Intermaxillary elastic traction or wiring are methods commonly employed in the treatment of simple mandibular fractures when natural teeth are present. A mental splint or arch bar is wired to the teeth in each jaw to reduce the fracture. The teeth are then brought into proper occlusion and held fixed in the closed position by rubber elastic bands or wires attached to the arch bars in each jaw. The armamentarium used for the treatment of jaw fractures is shown in Fig. 6-24.

Procedure checklist

1. After the dentist has adapted arch bars to the maxilla and mandible, deliver wire ligatures as needed, and hold arch bar in place while he wires the arch bar to the teeth.
2. Cut twisted wire ligatures when indicated by the dentist.
3. Deliver intermaxillary rubber elastics as needed.
4. Give patient printed instructions concerning diet, oral hygiene, and nausea, for example, as follows:
    a. *Diet:* You must remain on a liquid diet while the arch bars are in place. You should have at least 6 servings (8 oz.) per day of a high protein, vitamin enriched food supplement, such as Meritene. This may be supplemented with fruit juices, malted milk, cocoa, eggnog, meat juices and soups, cooked and thin cereal, and puréed baby foods. *Abstain* from any type of alcoholic beverages.

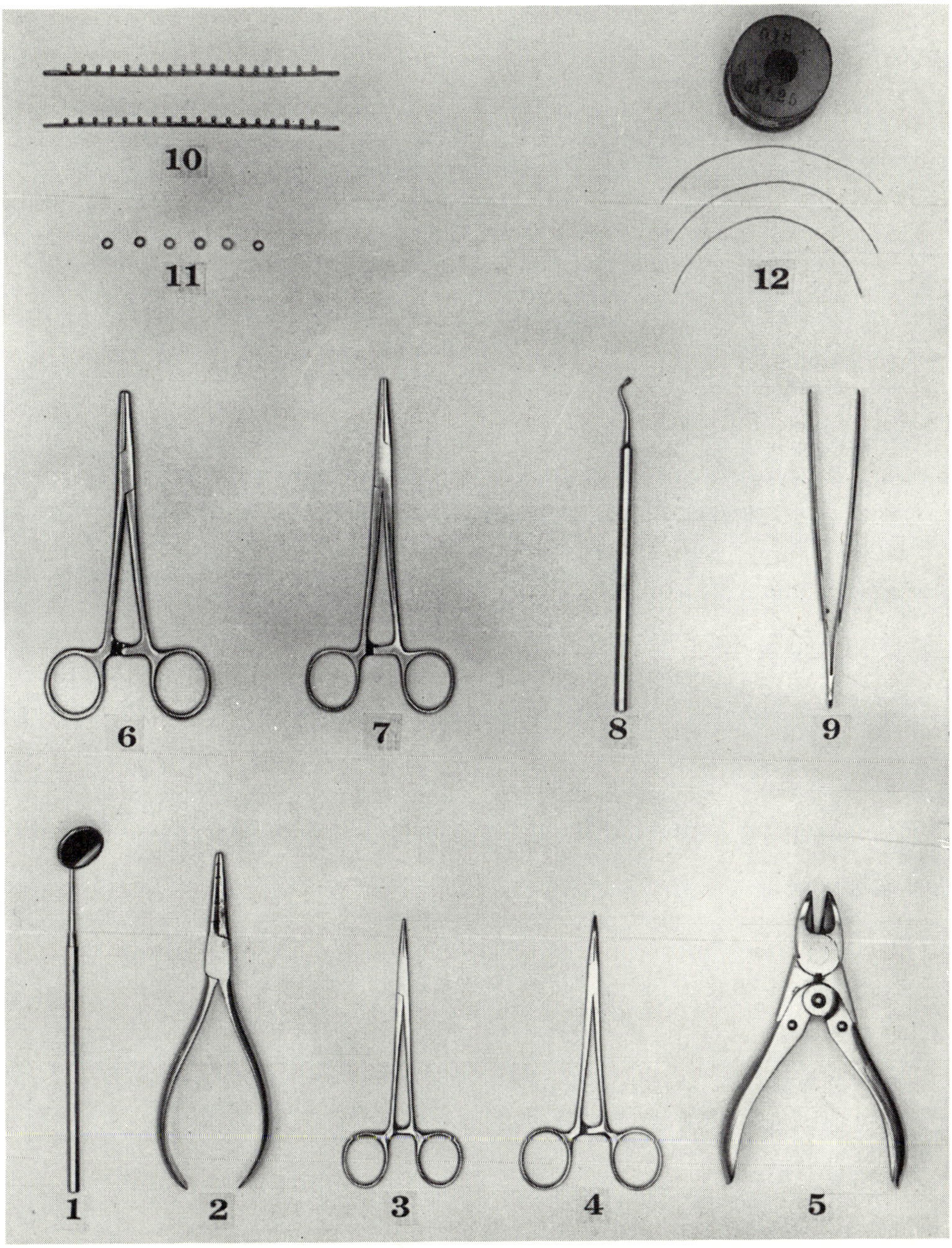

Fig. 6-24. Armamentarium for treatment of jaw fracture.

1. Mirror, mouth, examining, #4.
2. Pliers, clasp-bending, Jelenko.
3. Forceps, hemostatic, mosquito, straight, 5-inch (Halstead).
4. Forceps, hemostatic, mosquito, curved, 5-inch (Halstead).
5. Pliers, wire, diagonal-cutting, 5½-inch.
6. Forceps, Rankin-Kelly, straight, 6¼-inch (tips blunted by grinding).
7. Forceps, Rankin-Kelly, straight, 6¼-inch (tips blunted by grinding).
8. Plugger, amalgam, Black, #2.
9. Forceps, tissue, 5½-inch (serrated tips).
10. Splint, fracture, arch wire, set of two, Jelenko.
11. Ligatures, rubber (cut from tubing, rubber, latex, ⅛-inch, inside diameter, ⅓-inch wall).
12. Wire, stainless steel, 25-gauge.

b. *Oral hygiene:* Brush your teeth after each food serving, using an up and down brushing stroke. Be careful not to break the intermaxillary elastics. Brushing should be supplemented with a water jet appliance.

c. *Nausea:* In the event that you feel like vomiting, *immediately* cut the intermaxillary elastics with a pair of scissors to allow the vomitus to escape.

5. Remind dentist to prescribe any indicated drugs before dismissal.

6. Reschedule patient for *daily* examination and adjustment of arch bars during the first week; reschedule weekly appointments thereafter.

ENDODONTICS

A tooth with a diseased or infected pulp may be retained by endodontic or pulp-canal therapy. The treatment is usually performed in 3 steps—pulpectomy, root-canal enlargement, and root-canal obturation (filling of the pulp canal). Occasionally all 3 steps may be completed in 1 sitting. A separate armamentarium is required for each step. Pulp-canal therapy is a very exacting procedure and must be performed under strict aseptic conditions with the aid of a rubber dam.

In addition to the above steps, endodontic therapy may be supplemented by a surgical operation called "apical curettage" when a diseased pulp has resulted in a periapical cyst or extensive resorption of periapical bone. Apical curettage is also performed to place a retrograde amalgam filling of the pulp canal when it is not practical to open into the pulp chamber through the crown of the tooth.

Pulpectomy

Procedure checklist

1. Prepare cotton-tipped applicator with germicidal solution and syringe for local anesthesia.

2. Deliver rubber-dam tray as shown in Fig. 6-6.

3. Deliver basic endodontic tray as shown in Fig. 6-25.

4. After rubber dam is applied, deliver another cotton-tipped applicator with germicidal solution for scrubbing field of operation.

5. Prepare handpieces with #6 round bur and a #702 fisure bur.

6. Prepare barbed broach for removal of pulp tissue.

7. Prepare tray with indicated medicaments.

a. Sodium hypochlorite

b. Eugenol

Fig. 6-25. Basic endodontic tray.

1. Applicator, cotton-tipped, 6⅜-inch.
2. Mirror, mouth, examining, #4.
3. Explorer, #6.
4. Explorer, #17.
5. Explorer, #23.
6. Forceps, dressing, #17 (two).
7. Chisel, Black, #85, straight.
8. Excavator, Black, #63, spoon.
9. Excavator, Black, #64, spoon.
10. Plugger, amalgam, Black, #2.
11. Plugger, plastic filling, Woodson, double-ended, #3.
12. Burs, excavating, tungsten steel, AHP, spherical, #6; tapered fissure, coarse-cut, cross-cut, #702.
13. Stopping, temporary, dental (gutta-percha).
14. Points, absorbent, pulp canal (assortment).
15. Cup, drinking, paper (for waste).
16. Pellets, cotton (in envelope).
17. Tray, medicament (white opaque glass).
18. Dish, glass, medicament, dappen (for germicide).
19. Dish, glass, medicament, dappen (for physiologic saline solution).
20. Mixing slab, 3 by 6 inches, glass.
21. Spatula, cement, #324.

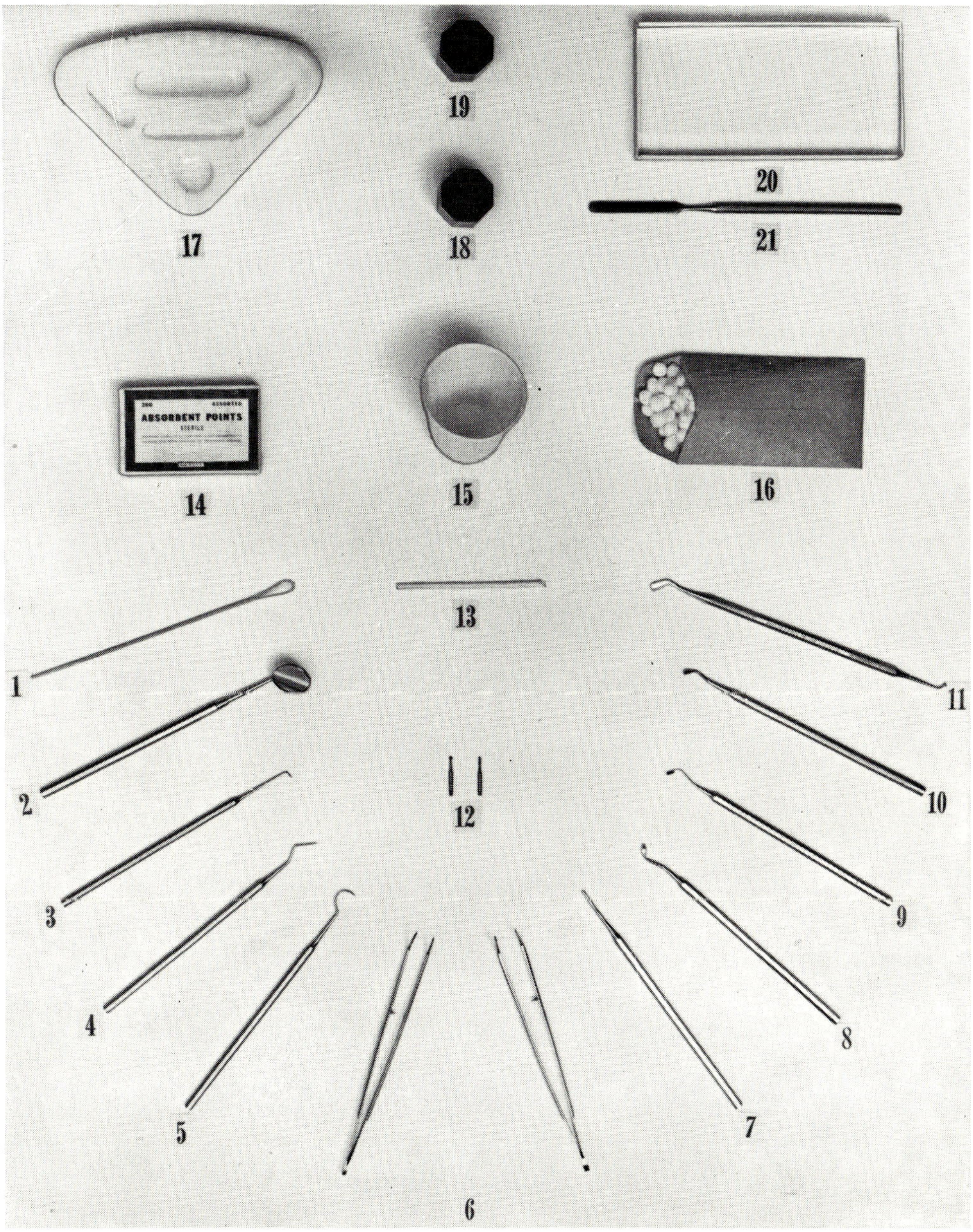

Fig. 6-25. For legend see opposite page.

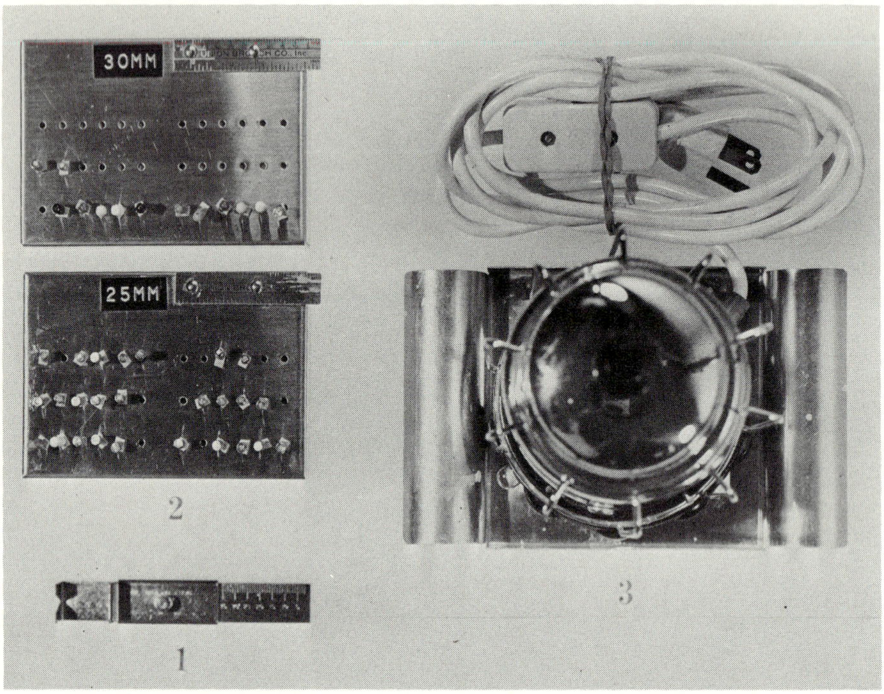

Fig. 6-26. Armamentarium for root canal enlargement.

1. Gauge, measuring, root canal.
2. Steri-boxes with sponge and stainless steel for files and reamers.
3. Sterilizer, glass bead.

c. Formylcresol

d. Camporated monoparachlorophenol (CMPC)

e. Hydrogen peroxide (3-percent)

8. Mix cement for sealing of pulp chamber.

9. Reschedule patient for 1 week after dentist has sealed the pulp chamber and removed the rubber dam.

Root canal enlargement

Procedure checklist

1. Prepare cotton-tipped applicator with germicidal solution and syringe for local anesthesia.

2. Deliver rubber-dam tray as shown in Fig. 6-6.

3. Deliver basic endodontic tray as shown in Fig. 6-25.

4. After rubber dam is applied, deliver another cotton-tipped applicator with germicidal solution for scrubbing field of operation.

5. Prepare tray with indicated medicaments (see previous section on pulpectomy).

6. Deliver root-canal enlargement tray as shown in Fig. 6-26.

7. Take and develop x-ray of tooth with file in pulp canal to establish measurement control.

8. Mix cement for sealing of pulp chamber.

9. Reschedule patient for 1 week after the dentist has sealed the pulp chamber and removed the rubber dam.

Root-canal obturation

Procedure checklist

1. Prepare cotton-tipped applicator with germicidal solution and syringe for local anesthesia.

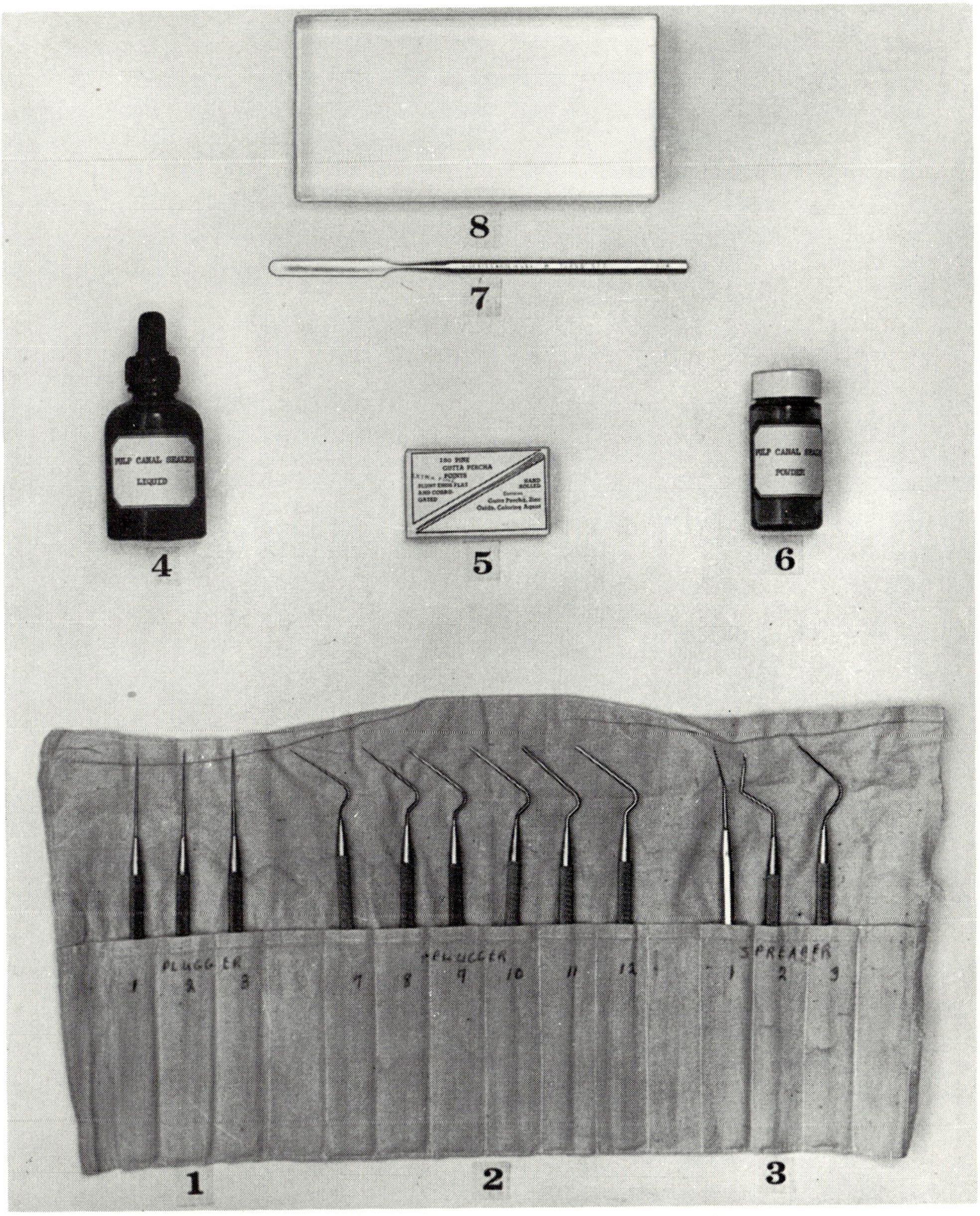

Fig. 6-27. Armamentarium for root canal obturation.

1. Plugger, pulp canal, #1.
   Plugger, pulp canal, #2.
   Plugger, pulp canal, #3.
2. Plugger, pulp canal, #7.
   Plugger, pulp canal, #8.
   Plugger, pulp canal, #9.
   Plugger, pulp canal, #10.
   Plugger, pulp canal, #11.
   Plugger, pulp canal, #12.
3. Spreader, gutta-percha, #1.
   Spreader, gutta-percha, #2.
   Spreader, gutta-percha, #3.
4. Sealer, pulp canal, liquid.
5. Points, pulp canal, gutta-percha (assortment).
6. Sealer, pulp canal, powder.
7. Mixing slab, 3 by 6 inches, glass.
8. Spatula, cement, #324.

2. Deliver rubber-dam tray as shown in Fig. 6-6.

3. Deliver basic endodontic tray as shown in Fig. 6-25.

4. Deliver root-canal obturation tray as shown in Fig. 6-27.

5. After rubber dam is applied, deliver another cotton-tipped applicator with germicidal solution for scrubbing field of operation.

6. Take and develop x-ray of tooth containing primary test cone of gutta-percha.

7. Mix root-canal sealer to thick creamy consistency for placement of primary test cone of gutta-percha.

8. Take and develop final x-ray of tooth.

9. After the dentist has sealed the root canal and pulp chamber, mix indicated filling material (amalgam, resin, or silicate) to restore the cavity in the tooth.

Apical curretage (Fig. 6-28)

Procedure checklist

1. Prepare cotton-tipped applicator with germicidal solution and syringe for local anesthesia.

2. Deliver scalpel for incision of mucoperiosteum.

3. Deliver periosteotome to reflect mucoperiosteal flap.

4. Assist with retraction of mucoperiosteal flap using periosteotome or retractor.

5. Prepare handpiece with #702 bur.

6. Continue retraction, and control hemorrhage with sponges and suction while dentist removes bone overlying the periapical area with the fissure bur.

7. Assist in the removal of the cyst membrane or sac by using a hemostat and suction.

8. Deliver and receive curets as needed.

9. Have bottle of 10-percent formalin ready for fixing tissue removed from the apical area.

10. Have gutta-percha and flame ready for sealing apical end of root canal.

11. Prepare physiologic saline solution in a cup for irrigation of the bony cavity with a rubber bulb syringe.

12. Have gelfoam ready for packing into bony cavity.

13. Assist dentist in placement of sutures to close the wound.

14. Clean the patient's face, and remind dentist to prescribe indicated drugs before dismissal.

15. Reschedule patient for examination and x-ray of tooth 2 days postoperative and again in 1 week for removal of sutures.

OPERATIVE DENTISTRY

"Cavity preparation" is the term applied to the cutting operations performed upon a tooth to remove dental caries and to ensure placement of a restoration that will be strong, resist displacement, and prevent recurrence of caries. Cavities are identified by the surface or combination of surfaces of the tooth on which they occur, as follows:

Occlusal	O	Mesio-occlusal	MO
Incisal	I	Disto-occlusal	DO
Mesial	M	Mesio-occlusodistal	MOD
Distal	D	Mesio-incisal	MI
Facial	F	Disto-incisal	DI
Labial	L	Mesio-incisodistal	MID
Buccal	B	Facio-occlusal	FO
Lingual	L	Linguo-occlusal	LO

Cavities are further classified according to the similarity of instrumentation employed in preparing them (Fig. 6-29):

CLASS I	Cavities in pits and fissures
CLASS II	Cavities on proximal surfaces of premolars and molars
CLASS III	Cavities on proximal surfaces of incisors and canines *not* requiring removal of the incisal angle
CLASS IV	Cavities on proximal surfaces of incisors and canines requiring removal of the incisal angle
CLASS V	Cavities on gingival third of facial and lingual surfaces

The principles of cavity preparation are the same for all teeth. They involve the performance of the following 6 basic steps in sequence: (1) obtaining the outline form, commonly called "extension for prevention of recurrence of caries," (2) obtaining resistance and retention forms, (3)

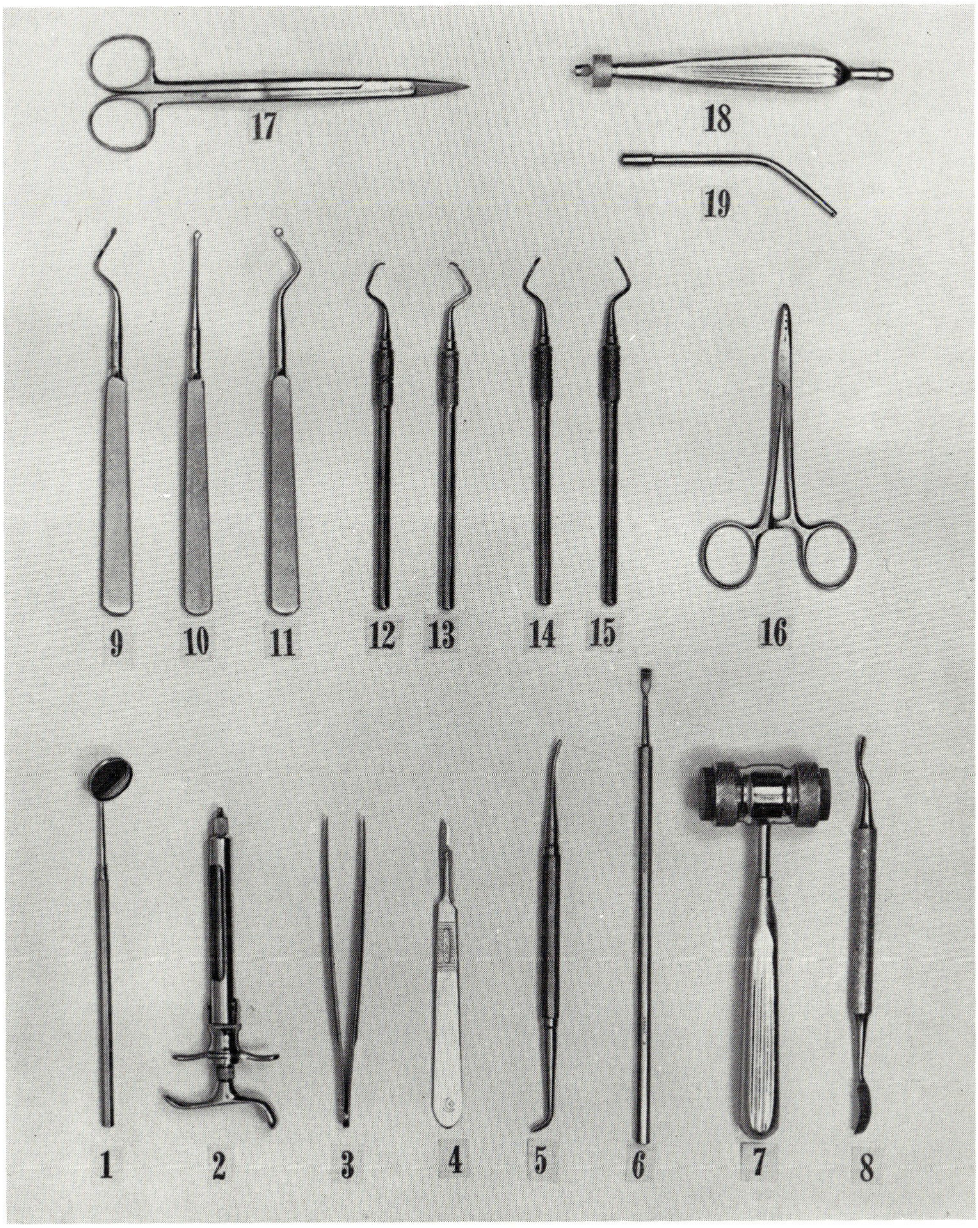

Fig. 6-28. Armamentarium for apical curettage and root resection.

1. Mirror, mouth, examining, #4.
2. Syringe, cartridge.
3. Forceps, tissue, 5½-inch (serrated tips).
4. Handle, operating knife, #3; blade, #15.
5. Periosteotome, #9.
6. Chisel, osseous, Stout, #1.
7. Mallet, oral surgery, hand-operated (Mead).
8. File, bone, #61-70, double-end (Friedman).
9. Curet, alveolar, Molt, #5L.
10. Curet, alveolar, Molt, #1.
11. Curet, alveolar, Molt, #6R.
12. Curet, #15 (Orban).
13. Curet, #16 (Orban).
14. Curet, #17 (Orban).
15. Curet, #18 (Orban).
16. Holder, needle, 5-inch.
17. Scissors, oral surgery, Dean, 6¾-inch.
18. Handle, suction, vise grip.
19. Tip, tapered, #3; hole 3/32-inch.

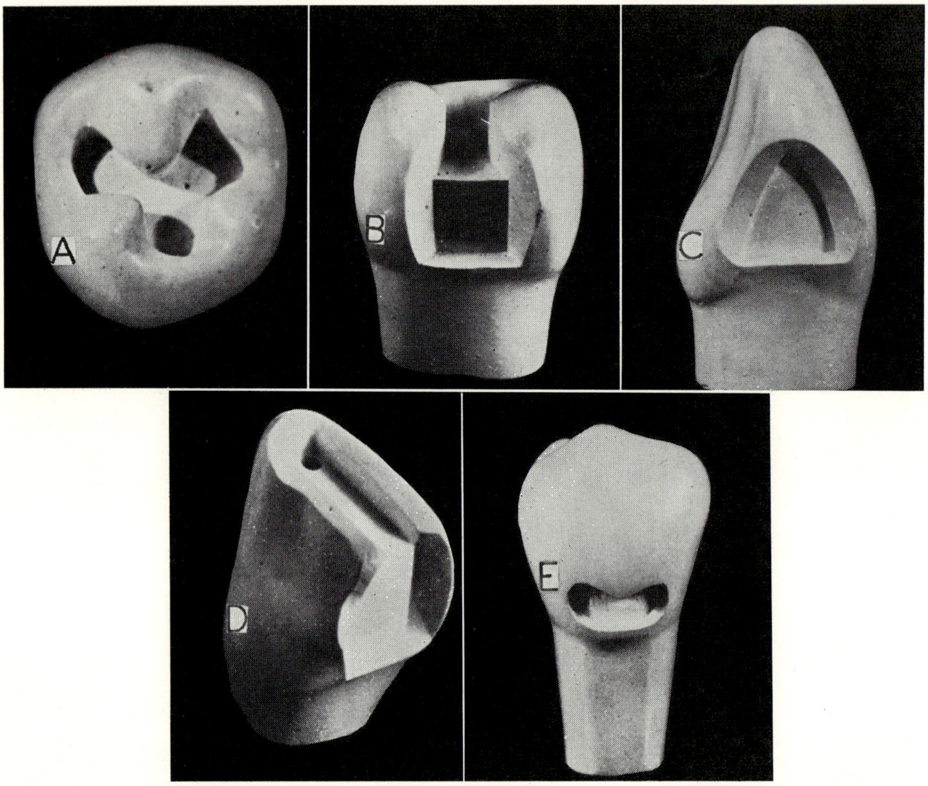

Fig. 6-29. Examples of cavity classification. **A,** Class I; **B,** Class II; **C,** Class III; **D,** Class IV; **E,** Class V. (From Peterson, S., editor: Clinical dental hygiene, ed. 3, St. Louis, 1968, The C. V. Mosby Co.)

removing remaining carious dentine, (4) obtaining the required convenience form, (5) finishing the enamel margins, and (6) cleansing the cavity preparation. The cutting instruments used for cavity preparation will vary according to the location or the type of cavity being prepared. In general, the hand cutting instruments used on anterior teeth are smaller than those of the same type used on posterior teeth. Therefore, 2 trays are shown—one for the preparation of cavities in anterior teeth and another for preparation of cavities in posterior teeth. Each tray includes only the bare essentials. Many additional cutting instruments may be employed.

Two major groups of cutting instruments are used, hand cutting instruments and rotating instruments. The hand cutting instruments are identified as chisels, hatchets, hoes, and spoons. The rotating instruments are identified as burs, Carborundum points or stones, diamond points or stones, and paper disks. These instruments are designed for use in the conventional belt-driven handpiece or in the ultrahigh-speed air-driven handpiece. Convenient methods of storing these instruments are shown in Figs. 6-30 to 6-34.

Rotating instruments used at ultrahigh speeds, as compared with those at slower speeds, greatly simplify cavity preparation, shorten the time required to prepare the cavity, and decrease the discomfort of the patient. Use of ultrahigh-speed equipment is limited, however, to cavity preparations

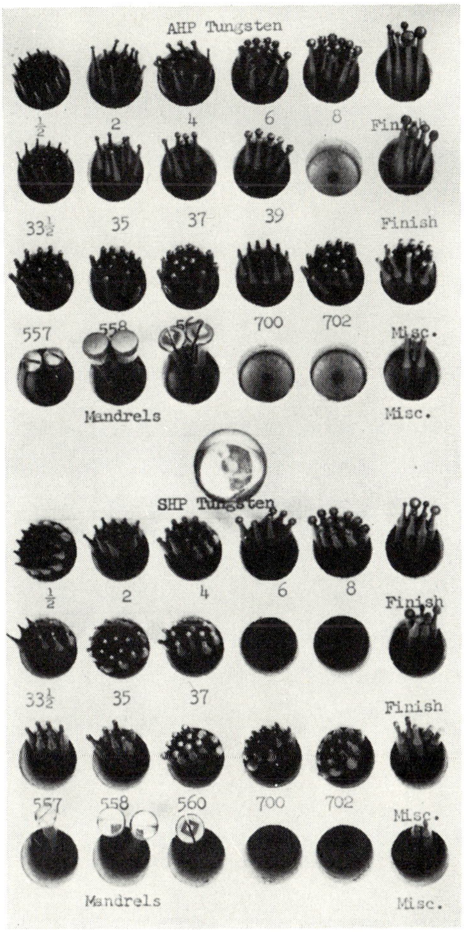

Fig. 6-30. Assortment of tungsten steel burs in wooden block.

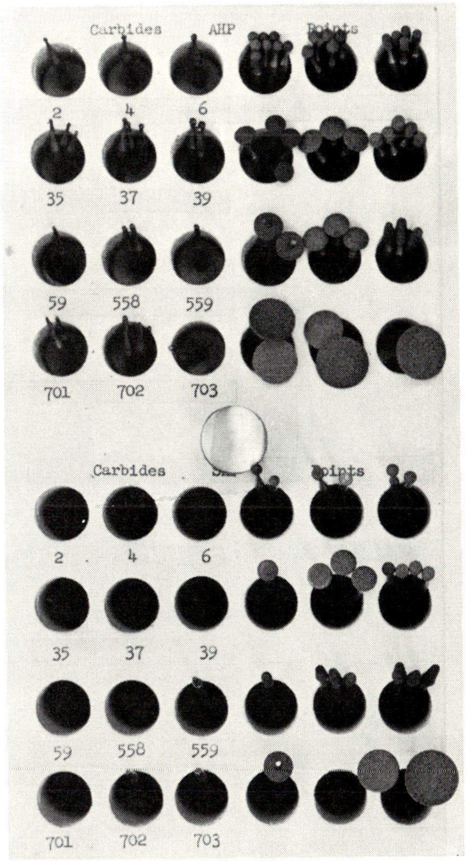

Fig. 6-31. Assortment of tungsten carbide burs and carborundum points in wooden block.

where adequate visibility can be maintained and where relatively large amounts of tooth structure are to be removed. Slower speeds must still be used for cavity preparations where visibility is impaired, tactile sensation is required, or the small amount of tooth structure to be removed requires a slower cutting speed.

The principles of cavity preparation are the same whether hand cutting instruments or rotating instruments are used at slow or ultrahigh speeds. However, the technique employed to accomplish a given objective of treatment will vary according to the preference of the operator. By following his technique, the assistant must learn to anticipate the particular instruments he requires for a given type of cavity preparation. The armamentaria used for anterior and posterior cavity preparations are shown in Figs. 6-35 and 6-36.

Anterior and posterior cavity preparation

Procedure checklist

1. Prepare cotton-tipped applicator with germicidal solution and syringe for local anesthesia.

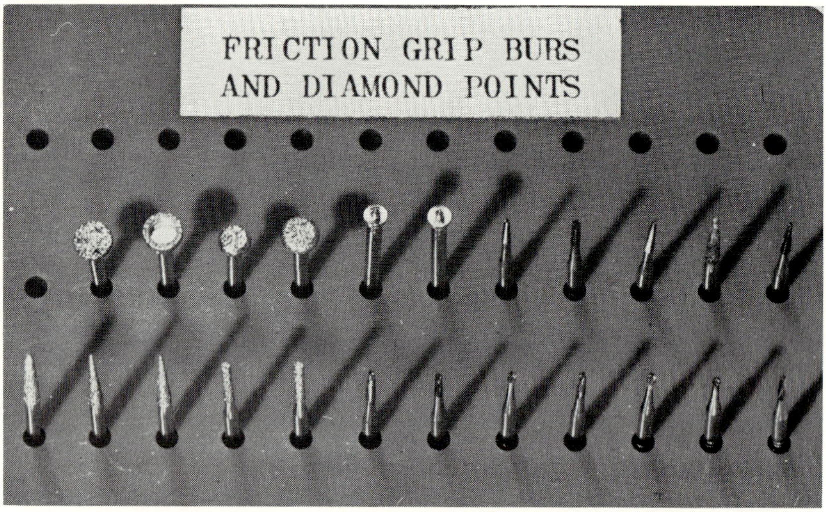

Fig. 6-32. Assortment of friction grip burs and diamond points.

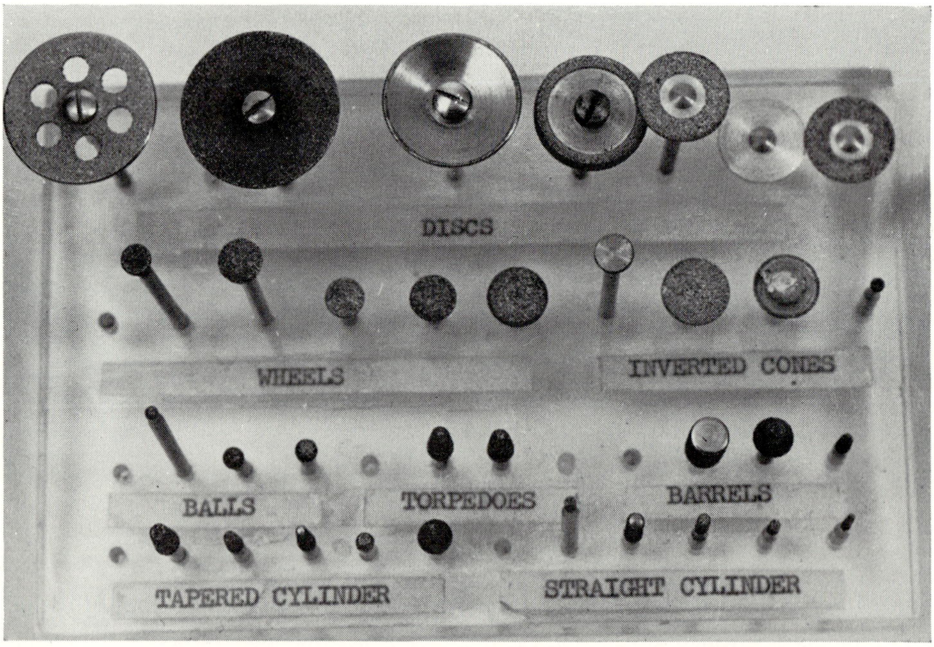

Fig. 6-33. Assortment of diamond points on plastic block.

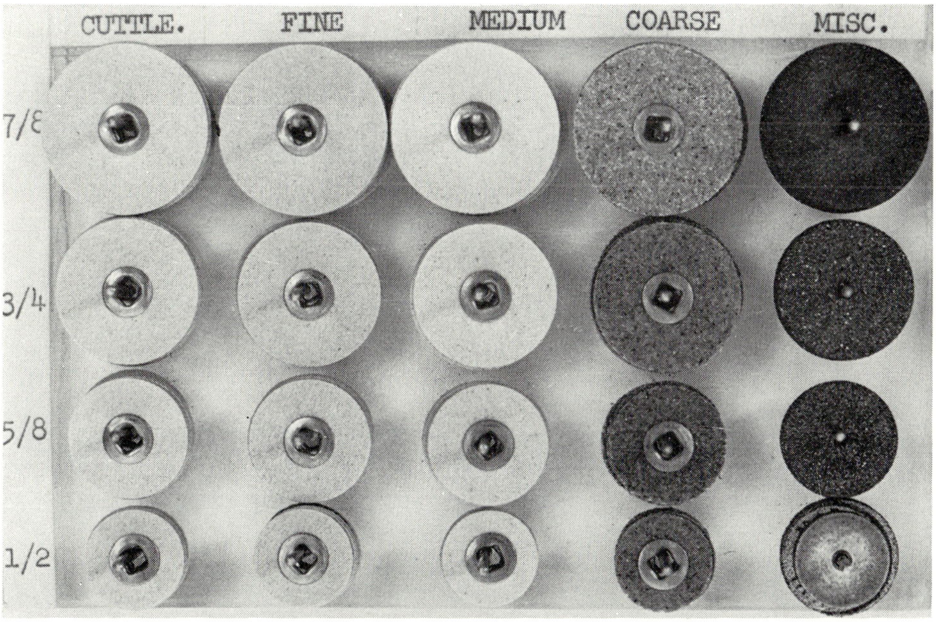

Fig. 6-34. Assortment of abrasive paper disks, carborundum disks, and carborundum wheels on spindles on plastic block.

2. Deliver rubber-dam tray as shown in Fig. 6-6, if rubber dam is to be used.

3. Deliver cavity preparation trays as shown in Figs. 6-35 and 6-36.

4. Prepare high-speed handpieces with friction grip burs #702 and #557.

5. Prepare slow-speed handpiece with #4 round bur, #34 inverted cone bur, or disks as needed.

6. Maintain field of operation visible and free of debris by controlling the lights, saliva ejector, air, water, and suction.

7. Keep your eyes on field of operation.

8. In operations on upper teeth, retract the lips and cheeks with index finger.

9. In operations on lower teeth, retract the tongue with the saliva ejector or a mouth mirror.

10. Deliver, receive, and clean instruments at chin level as needed.

11. Mix temporary or sedative restoration or cement base as needed (Fig. 6-37).

12. When cavity preparation is completed, remove cavity preparation tray, and replace with indicated tray preparation for filling of tooth (amalgam, silicate, resin, or gold foil), or with tray preparation for inlay impression.

Temporary or sedative restoration and cement base

Temporary restorations and protective coverings

Zinc oxide and eugenol cement (Fig. 6-37), in combination with other materials that accelerate the set and give it body, is widely employed as a temporary filling material after cavity preparation. It is also used in aluminum shells as a protective covering after crown preparation on posterior teeth, or in celluloid crown forms after crown preparations on anterior teeth. Silicate cement may be used for cosmetic reasons in place of the zinc oxide and eugenol in the celluloid crown forms. Zinc phosphate cement is used as an outer seal between appointments for endodontic therapy.

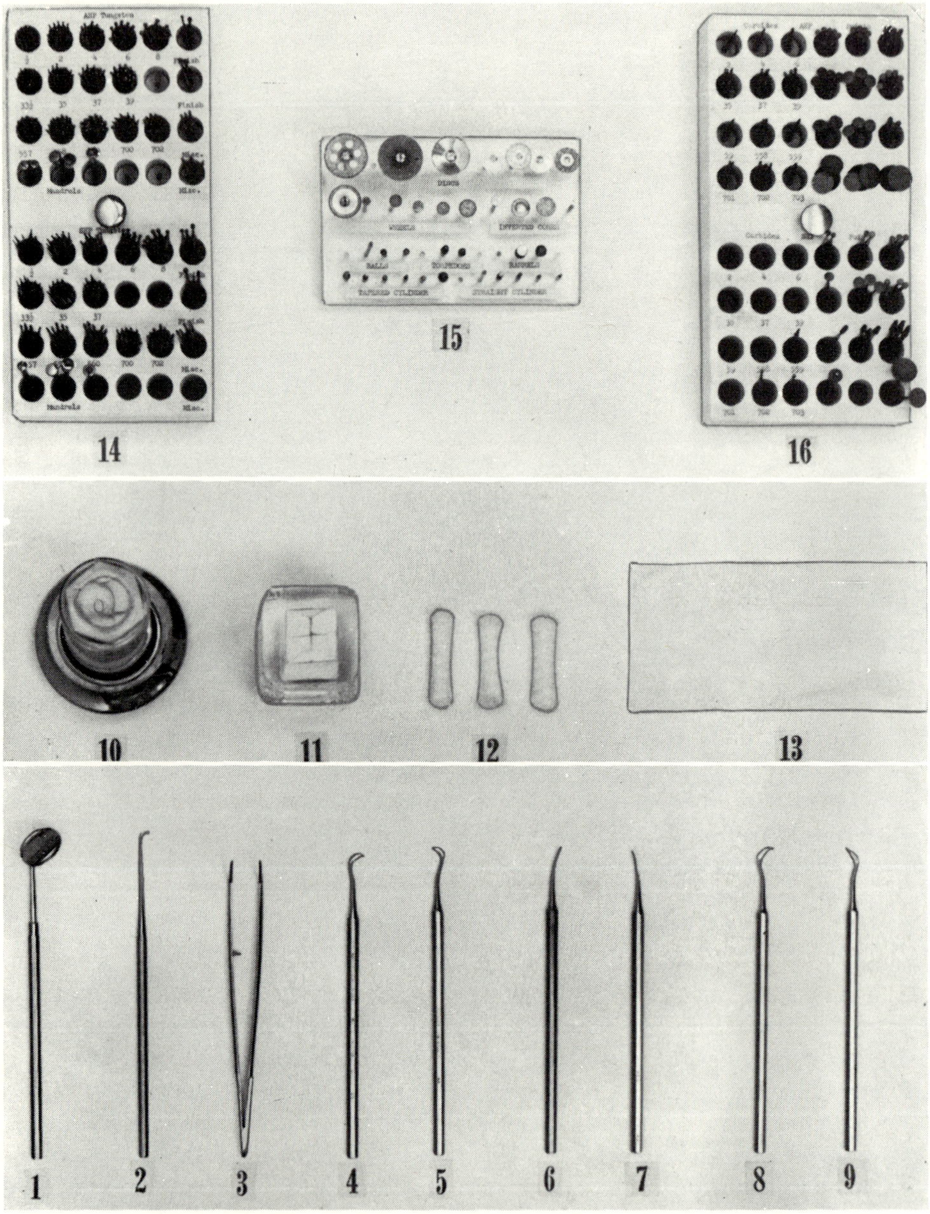

Fig. 6-35. Armamentarium for anterior cavity preparation.

1. Mirror, mouth, examining, #4.
2. Explorer, #6.
3. Forceps, dressing, #17.
4. Excavator, Black, #65 (spoon).
5. Excavator, Black, #66 (spoon).
6. Chisel, Wedelstaedt, #41.
7. Chisel, Wedelstaedt, #42.
8. Excavator, Black, #53 (enamel hatchet).
9. Excavator, Black, #54 (enamel hatchet).
10. Cotton, absorbent, cylinder (for use in cotton font).
11. Waste receptacle.
12. Cotton rolls.
13. Gauze, dental, napkin, 6 by 6 inches.
14. Burs, excavating, tungsten steel (assortment).
15. Points, diamond (assortment).
16. Burs, excavating, tungsten carbide (assortment).

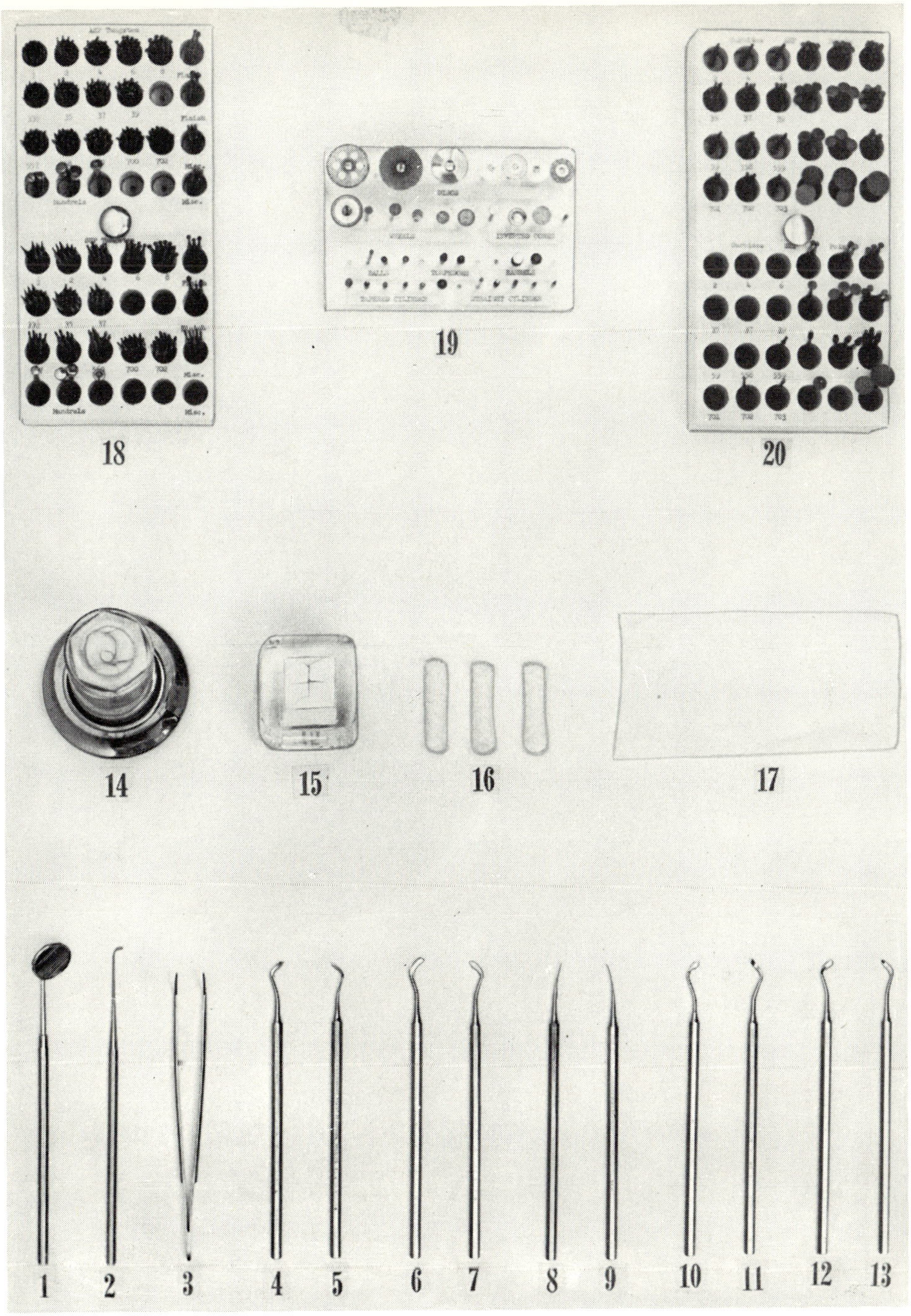

Fig. 6-36. Armamentarium for posterior cavity preparation.

1. Mirror, mouth, examining, #4.
2. Explorer, #6.
3. Forceps, dressing, #17.
4. Excavator, Black, #63 (spoon).
5. Excavator, Black, #64 (spoon).
6. Excavator, Black, #51 (enamel hatchet).
7. Excavator, Black, #52 (enamel hatchet).
8. Chisel, Wedelstaedt, #41.
9. Chisel, Wedelstaedt, #42.
10. Trimmer, gingival margin, Black, #73.
11. Trimmer, gingival margin, Black, #74.
12. Trimmer, gingival margin, Black, #79.
13. Trimmer, gingival margin, Black, #80.
14. Cotton, absorbent, cylinder (for use in cotton font).
15. Waste receptacle.
16. Cotton rolls.
17. Gauze, dental napkin, 6 by 6 inches.
18. Burs, excavating, tungsten steel (assortment).
19. Points, diamond (assortment).
20. Burs, excavating, tungsten carbide (assortment).

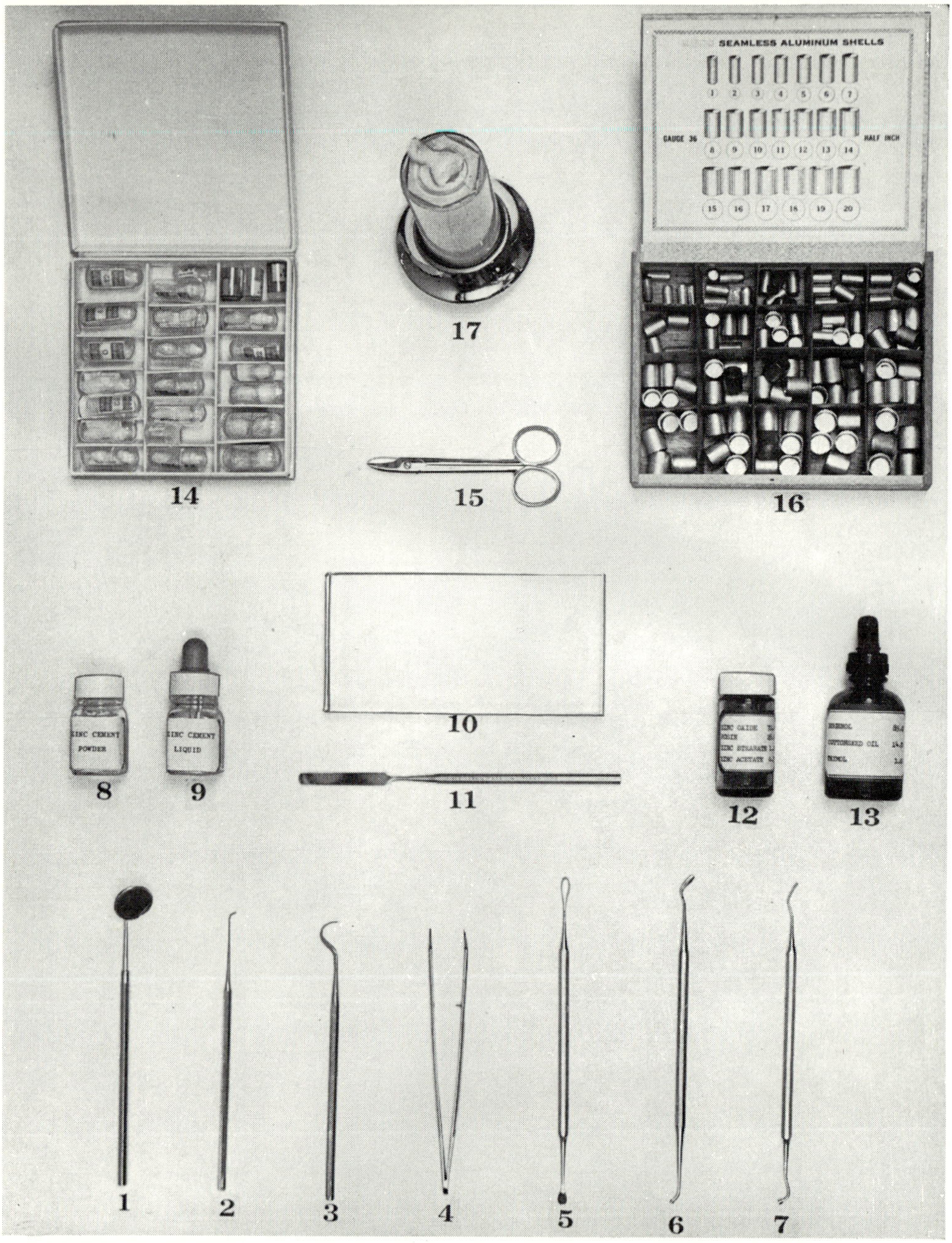

Fig. 6-37. Armamentarium for placement of temporary or sedative restoration and cement base.

1. Mirror, mouth, examining, #4.
2. Explorer, #6.
3. Explorer, #23.
4. Forceps, dressing, #17.
5. Plugger, plastic filling, Woodson, double-ended, #1.
6. Plugger, plastic filling, Woodson, double-ended, #2.
7. Plugger, plastic filling, Woodson, double-ended, #3.
8. Zinc cement powder.
9. Zinc cement liquid.
10. Mixing slab, 3 by 6 inches, glass.
11. Spatula, cement, #324.
12. Zinc oxide.
13. Eugenol.
14. Matrix set, dental, celluloid crown forms (assortment).
15. Shears, crown, curved, Beebe, #11.
16. Shells, aluminum, seamless, 36-gauge, ½-inch (assortment).
17. Cotton, absorbent, cylinder (for use in cotton font).

Sedative restorations

In addition to its other uses, zinc oxide and eugenol cement is widely used as a sedative filling material in cavities of teeth affected with pulpitis (toothache).

Cement base

When caries extends more than halfway through the thickness of the dentine of a tooth, a cavity liner and/or cement base is placed in the deepest portion of the cavity preparation to protect the pulp from chemical and thermal shock. The cavity liners consist of calcium hydroxide suspensions and are supplied as liquids or pastes. These may be covered with a zinc phosphate or carboxylate cement to provide hardness and to build up the resistance form of the cavity preparation. Placement of zinc phosphate cement directly on dentine in deep cavity preparations is contraindicated because of its injurious effect on the pulp.

Because of its unique properties, zinc oxide and eugenol cement is frequently used for the dual purpose of protecting the pulp in deep cavities and acting as a cement base. When zinc oxide and eugenol cement has been used as a temporary filling material in deep cavities, the resistance and retention forms of the cavity are recut within the cement when the patient returns for placement of the permanent restoration. Additional materials and instruments used in the placement of temporary or sedative restorations and cement bases are shown in Fig. 6-37.

Mixing instructions

Zinc oxide and eugenol cement (containing zinc acetate as an accelerator and rosin as a hardener)

1. Powder and 3 or 4 drops of liquid are placed in separate positions on a glass mixing slab.

2. A large amount of powder is incorporated at first with a cement spatula. More powder is incorporated as needed until a sticky, "thick putty" consistency is obtained.

3. The mixing is not critical. The set takes longer than other cements.

Zinc phosphate cement

1. Mixing zinc phosphate cement is a much more critical matter than mixing zinc oxide and eugenol cement.

2. Powder and 3 or 4 drops of liquid are placed in separate positions on a glass mixing slab.

3. The powder is divided into *small equal* parts.

4. The first part of the powder is then incorporated, then the second, third, and so on until a *thick creamy* consistency is obtained. A *thin creamy* consistency is required when the mix is to be used for cementing inlays, crowns, or bridges.

5. If larger amounts of powder are incorporated, the setting time will be accelerated, reducing the working time available.

6. Many dentists prefer to mix the cement themselves while the dental assistant keeps the field of operation dry.

Carboxylate cement

1. For cementing inlays and crowns:
   a. Place 3 drops of liquid from squeeze bottle and 1 measuring spoon of powder in separate locations on mixing slab.
   b. Mix all powder and liquid together simultaneously, and spatulate for 30 seconds to a creamy mix. This creates a mix with a working time of 3 minutes and a setting time in the mouth of an additional 3 minutes.
2. For a cement base:
   a. Place 2 drops of liquid and 1 measure of powder in separate locations on mixing slab.
   b. Mix the powder and liquid together simultaneously, and spatulate for 30 seconds to a *thick* creamy mix. This creates a mix

with a working time of 2 minutes and a setting time in the mouth of an additional 2 minutes. More powder may be added if a thicker mix is desired.

c. Instrument may be dipped in alcohol or powder to facilitate placement of the mix in the cavity preparation.

Amalgam restoration

Dental amalgams are used more widely than any other material for the restoration of lost tooth structure. An amalgam is an alloy, one of the constituents of which is mercury. Dental amalgams contain silver, tin, copper, and zinc, in combination with mercury. The silver-tin-copper-zinc alloy may be supplied as a powder or in preweighed, pressed pellets, to which measured amounts of mercury are added at the time of mixing (Fig. 6-39). If a powder is used, it must be carefully preweighed before the measured amount of mercury is added. The ratio of alloy to mercury recommended by the manufacturer should always be used. The ratio generally used is 5 parts of alloy to 8 parts of mercury by weight. The mixing procedure, called trituration, produces a plastic mass that is condensed into a prepared cavity. Trituration with an amalgamator requires about 10 seconds for 1 measure or pellet of alloy and about 15 seconds for 2 measures or pellets of alloy. Timing of trituration is important, because insufficient trituration results in overexpansion and weakness of the amalgam restoration, and overtrituration results in contraction of the restoration. Each manufacturer supplies instructions for the manipulation of its product, and these instructions should be carefully followed.

The armamentarium used for placement of an amalgam restoration is shown in Fig. 6-38.

Procedure checklist

1. Deliver rubber-dam tray as shown in Fig. 6-6 if rubber dam is to be used.
2. Deliver amalgam tray as shown in Fig. 6-38.
3. Measured amounts of alloy and mercury are placed in the capsule of the amalgamator (1 pellet for a Class I cavity, 2 pellets for a MO or DO cavity, and 3 pellets for a MOD cavity).
4. After the matrix is adapted and the cavity is thoroughly dried, triturate the amalgam on the signal of the dentist.
5. Empty capsule onto a squeeze cloth, and cleanse the capsule and shuttle of wet amalgam.

Fig. 6-38. Armamentarium for placement of amalgam restoration.

1. Mirror, mouth, examining, #4.
2. Explorer, #6.
3. Explorer, #23.
4. Forceps, dressing, #17.
5. Retainer, matrix, #1, and bands (assortment).
6. Retainer, matrix, #9, and bands (assortment).
7. Wedges, ready-cut, Burlew (celluloid).
8. Carrier, amalgam, #10.
9. Choice of operator:
   A. Plugger, amalgam, Black, #1.
   Plugger, amalgam, Black, #2.
   Plugger, amalgam, Black, #3.
   B. "Amal-Pak" with points.
10. Plugger, plastic filling, Woodson, double-ended, #1.
11. Pugger, plastic filling, Woodson double-ended, #2.
12. Plugger, plastic filling, Woodson, double-ended, #3.
13. Plugger, plastic filling, Ladmore, double-ended, #2.
14. Carver, Frahm, #1.
15. Carver, Frahm, #2.
16. Carver, Frahm, #3.
17. Cotton, absorbent, cylinder (for use in cotton font).
18. Cloth, squeeze, dental.
19. Cot, finger, rubber (for mulling amalgam).
20. Strip, finishing, linen; strip, finishing, steel (lightening).
21. Mortar and pestle, glass.
22. Waste receptacle.

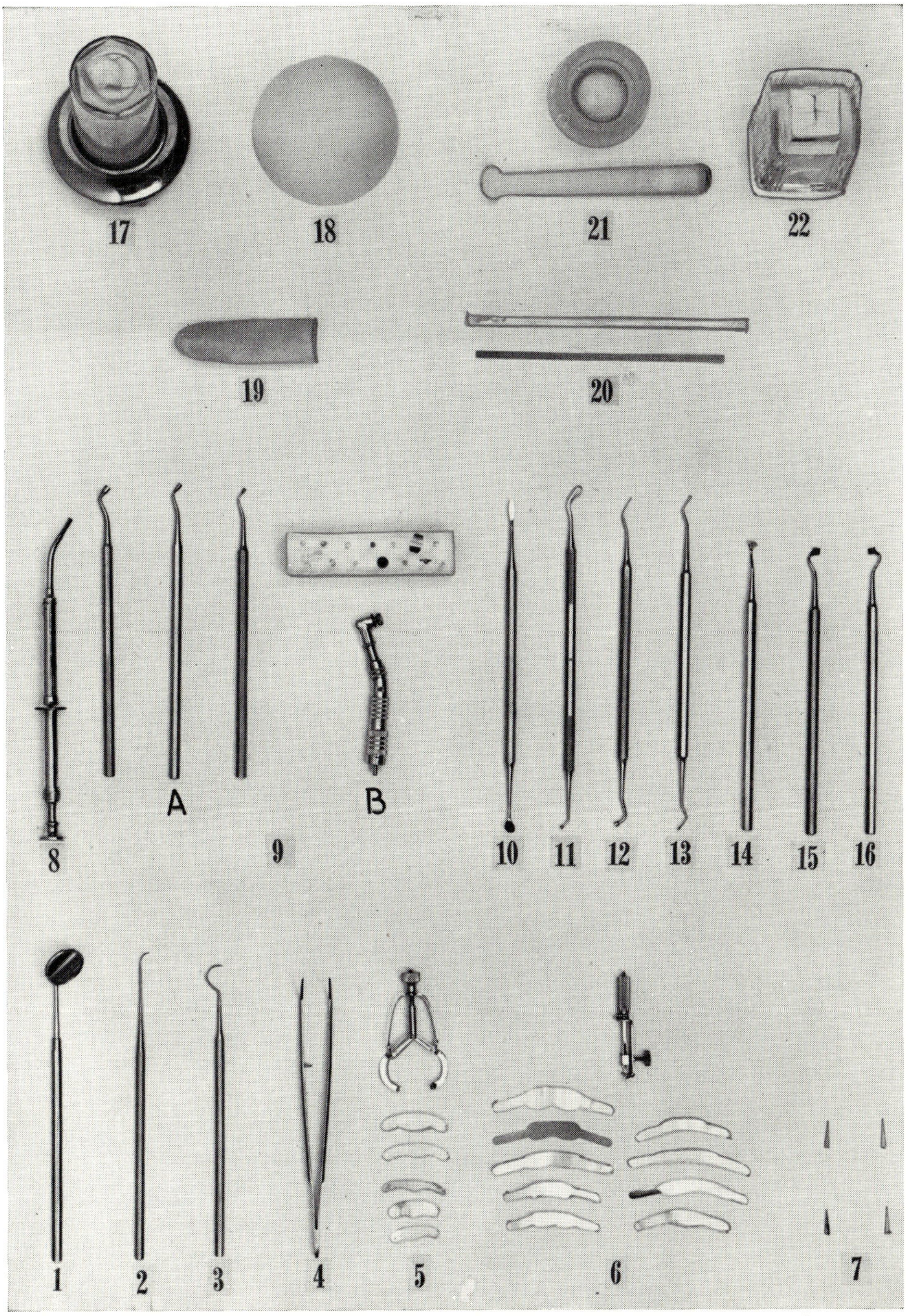

Fig. 6-38. For legend see opposite page.

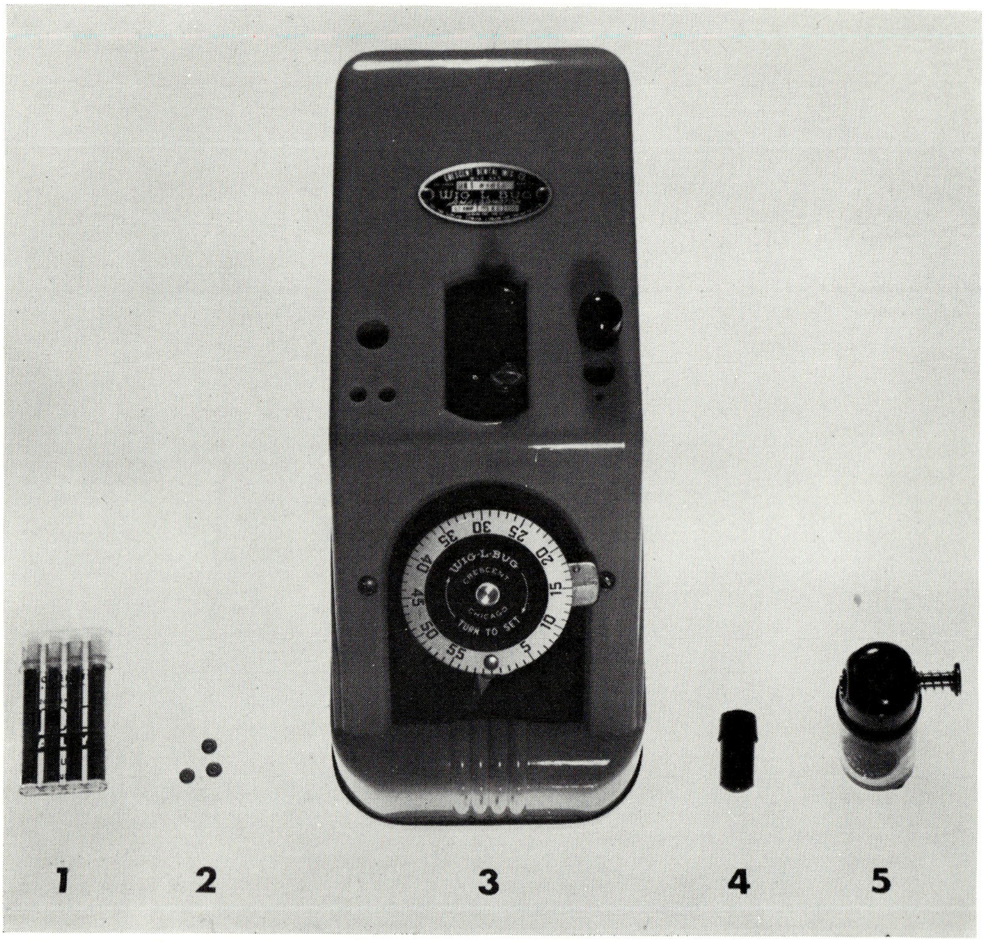

Fig. 6-39. Armamentarium for mixing amalgam.

1. Package containing alloy pellets.
2. Alloy pellets.
3. Amalgamator.
4. Bakelite capsule containing Bakelite shuttle.
5. Mercury dispenser.

6. Mull the amalgam in the squeeze cloth if improvement of consistency is required, taking care that moisture from the fingers does not contaminate the amalgam.

7. Fill amalgam carrier by pressing the end into the amalgam on the squeeze cloth.

8. Eject the amalgam into prepared cavity.

9. Repeat steps 7 and 8 as the dentist continues to condense the amalgam until the cavity is filled.

10. Deliver and receive condensers and carving instruments as needed, maintaining field of operation dry and free of debris with the air syringe.

11. Prepare a cotton pellet for final wiping of the surface of the carved restoration.

12. Assist in removal of the matrix.

13. Before dismissal, give patient a cup of water to rinse away any residual amalgam scrapings.

14. Reschedule patient for finishing and polishing at a later visit.

Silicate cement restoration

Silicate cement may be employed as a semipermanent restorative material. Its chief advantages are harmonious color and ease of manipulation. Its chief disadvantages are solubility in the fluids of the mouth and lack of crushing strength. Silicate cement also has an injurious effect on the dental pulp. For this reason, a liner is always used in the cavity preparation before the restoration is placed. Silicate cement is limited primarily to Class III and Class V cavities in anterior teeth. Silicate cement restorations usually disintegrate over a period of 4 or 5 years and need to to be replaced, although occasionally they may last for a longer period.

Like other cements, silicate cements consist of a powder and a liquid. The powder is supplied in a variety of shades to match the various tooth colors. The liquid consists mainly of phosphoric acid in combination with water and other chemicals. Since the equilibrium of the liquid may change over a period of time, altering the setting time and the quality of the cement, the bottle of liquid should be tightly stoppered when not in use. It should be examined occasionally, and if cloudiness or sediment appears, the liquid should be discarded. The manufacturer's instructions for mixing should be followed, although they should be supplemented with experience and a knowledge of the consistency desired. Silicate cement will not harden properly when contaminated with moisture. Therefore, no moisture must come in contact with the silicate during the mixing or setting processes. The armamentarium used for the placement of a silicate cement restoration is shown in Fig. 6-40.

Procedure checklist

1. Deliver rubber-dam tray as shown in Fig. 6-6 if rubber dam is to be used.
2. Deliver silicate cement tray as shown in Fig. 6-40.
3. After shade has been taken, place silicate cement powder and liquid in separate locations on the mixing slab.
4. Mix calcium hydroxide paste for cavity lining, if indicated.
5. Prepare very small pellet of cotton for application of cavity varnish.
6. Coat celluloid matrix strip with cocoa butter.
7. Mix silicate cement powder and liquid to proper consistency (see following instructions).
8. Hold mixing slab containing freshly mixed silicate cement at chin level, so that the dentist can transfer the cement to the prepared cavity using a stellite instrument.
9. Hold celluloid matrix strip firmly for 3 minutes.
10. Remove matrix strip, and apply coca butter immediately to the restoration.
11. Exclude moisture from the field of operation during the setting process by retracting lips and using cotton rolls, air syringe, and saliva ejector.
12. After 10 minutes, the dentist removes excess silicate with stellite instruments and polishing strips. Further contouring or polishing is done at a subsequent session, at least 48 hours later.

Mixing instructions

1. A cool, clean, dry mixing slab, preferably with a thermometer, is used. Cooling the slab is particularly important on hot, humid days. A cool slab permits incorporation of more powder in the liquid, increases the strength of the restoration, and retards the setting time, thus giving the dentist ample time for manipulation.
2. Powder and liquid should be proportioned as directed. Powder is placed on the slab first and divided into halves. The second half is divided into thirds. The first half of the powder is incorporated; then additional amounts are added, until a mix of *thick putty* consistency is obtained. As much powder should be incorporated as the liquid will absorb and still allow about 2 minutes' working time for insertion.

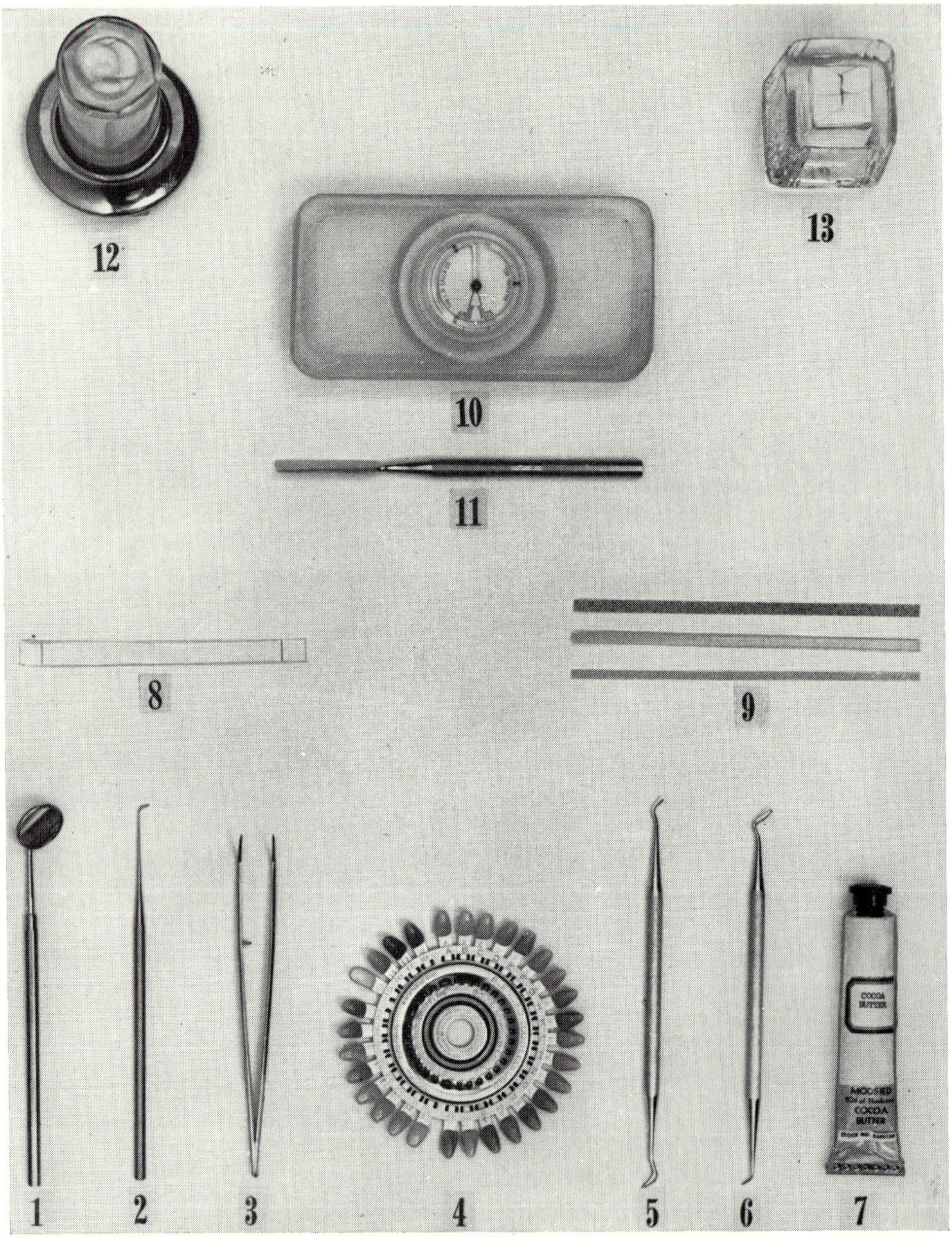

Fig. 6-40. Armamentarium for silicate cement restoration.

1. Mirror, mouth, examining, #4.
2. Explorer, #6.
3. Forceps, dressing, #17.
4. Shade guide, silicate cement.
5. Plugger, plastic filling, stellite, double-ended, #1-2.
6. Plugger, plastic filling, stellite, double-ended, #5-7.
7. Lubricant, silicate cement (cocoa butter).
8. Strips, Mylar, clear.
9. Strips, finishing (assortment).
10. Slab, silicate cement mixing (with thermometer).
11. Spatula, cement, #2 (cobalt-chromium alloy).
12. Cotton, asborbent, cylinder (for use in cotton font).
13. Waste receptacle.

3. The cement is mixed no longer than 1 minute with a stellite spatula. The mixing is done with a rotary motion. A flat, flexible spatula should not be used for silicate cement.

Composite resin restoration

Use of reinforced composite resins in place of silicate cement and unreinforced resins has become widespread for class III, IV, and V restorations. The term "composite" indicates that a reinforcing filler has been added to the acrylic resin matrix. The reinforcing filler, as compared with the unreinforced resin filling materials, increases compressive strength, hardness, and resistance to abrasion, and reduces polymerization shrinkage and thermal expansion. In addition, the nonbrittleness of the composite resins gives them a distinct advantage over the silicate cement restoration. However, pulp response to the resins is similar to silicate cement, and, therefore, the pulp should be protected by a cavity lining. Composite resin filling materials are supplied either in bulk form with a paste and catalyst, which is mixed in proportions indicated by the manufacturer much the same as silicate cement, or in preportioned capsules, which are mixed by vibration in an amalgamator and placed in a syringe for injection of the material into the cavity.

Procedure checklist

1. Deliver rubber-dam tray as shown in Fig. 6-6 if rubber dam is to be used.
2. Deliver composite resin tray as shown in Fig. 6-41.
3. After shade has been taken, place indicated amounts of paste and catalyst in separate locations on paper mixing pad, following manufacturer's instructions.
4. Mix calcium hydroxide paste for cavity lining, if indicated.
5. Prepare very small pellet of cotton for application of cavity varnish.
6. After matrix has been selected and adapted by the dentist, mix the paste and catalyst with wooden spatula for 30 seconds, and use it *at once.*
7. Hold paper mixing pad at chin level, so that the dentist can transfer the composite resin to the cavity using a plastic instrument.
8. Hold celluloid matrix strip firmly for 3 minutes, and then remove the strip.
9. Prepare slow-speed handpiece with diamond stone and disks for finishing restoration.

Gold-foil restoration

Gold foil is the standard to which all other filling material is compared. It possesses most of the qualities of an ideal filling material, including insolubility in the oral fluids, excellent adaptability to the cavity walls, great crushing resistance and edge strength, freedom from dimensional change, and capability of taking and retaining a polished surface. Its only disadvantages are high thermal conductivity, inharmonious color, and difficulty of manipulation. When other factors, such as age, physical condition, color, and prognosis, will permit its use, gold foil is indicated in Classes I, III, V, IV, and II cavities, in that order. The armamentarium used for the placement of a gold-foil restoration is shown in Fig. 6-42.

Gold foil is supplied in the form of cylinders, powdered gold pellets (Goldent), and mat gold. The pieces are placed in the prepared cavity, one at a time, and condensed against the walls of the cavity with a mallet and various types of pluggers. Each succeeding piece becomes welded to the preceding one as the restoration is gradually built up to proper shape and contour. The welding or cohesion will not take place unless the surface of the foil is absolutely free of impurities. Over a period of time, the surface of gold foil tends to become contaminated with a gaseous film. To remove or volatilize the gaseous film the pieces are heated (annealed) over a low flame just prior to use. The pieces are placed on the annealer and picked up with the foil carrier as they are needed.

Procedure checklist

1. Deliver rubber-dam tray as shown in Fig. 6-6.

2. Deliver gold-foil tray as shown in Fig. 6-42.

3. Prepare an annealer over a low flame, or prepare an alcohol lamp, according to the choice of the dentist.

4. Select the type of gold foil to be

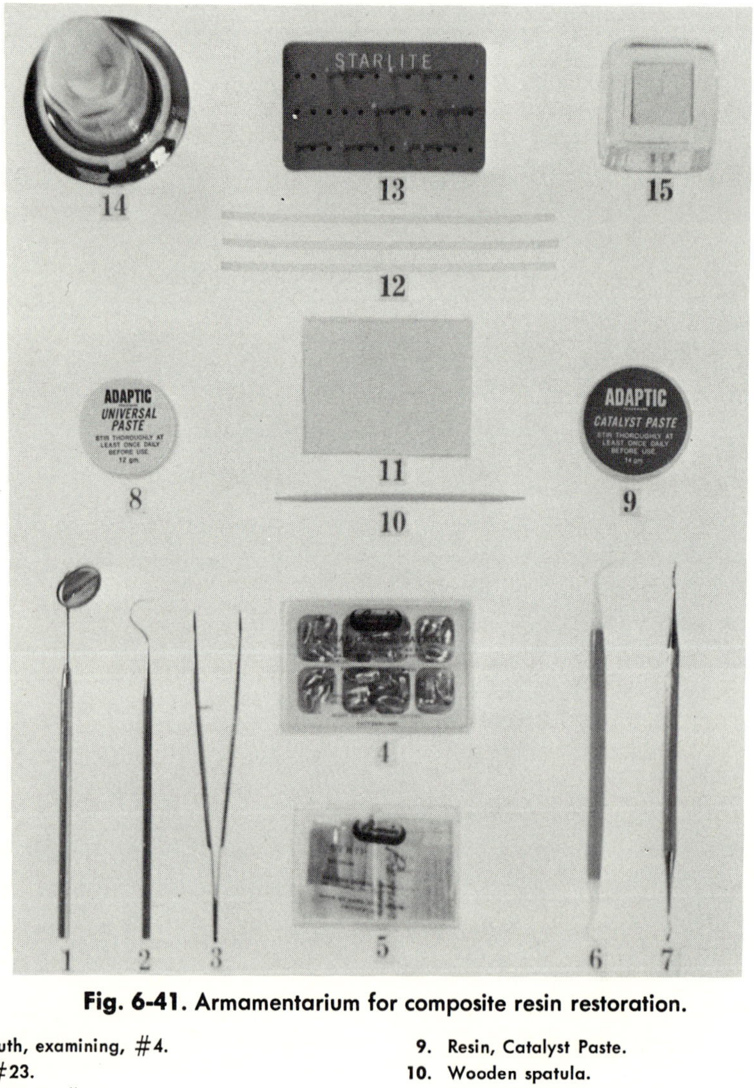

Fig. 6-41. Armamentarium for composite resin restoration.

1. Mirror, mouth, examining, #4.
2. Explorer, #23.
3. Forceps, dressing, #17.
4. Matrices, incisal corner.
5. Strip aids.
6. Temple composite instrument.
7. Plugger, plastic filling, stellite, double-ended, #1-2.
8. Resin, Universal Paste.
9. Resin, Catalyst Paste.
10. Wooden spatula.
11. Mixing pad, paper.
12. Strips, finishing (assortment).
13. Points, diamond (assortment).
14. Cotton, absorbent, cylinder (for use in cotton font).
15. Waste receptacle.

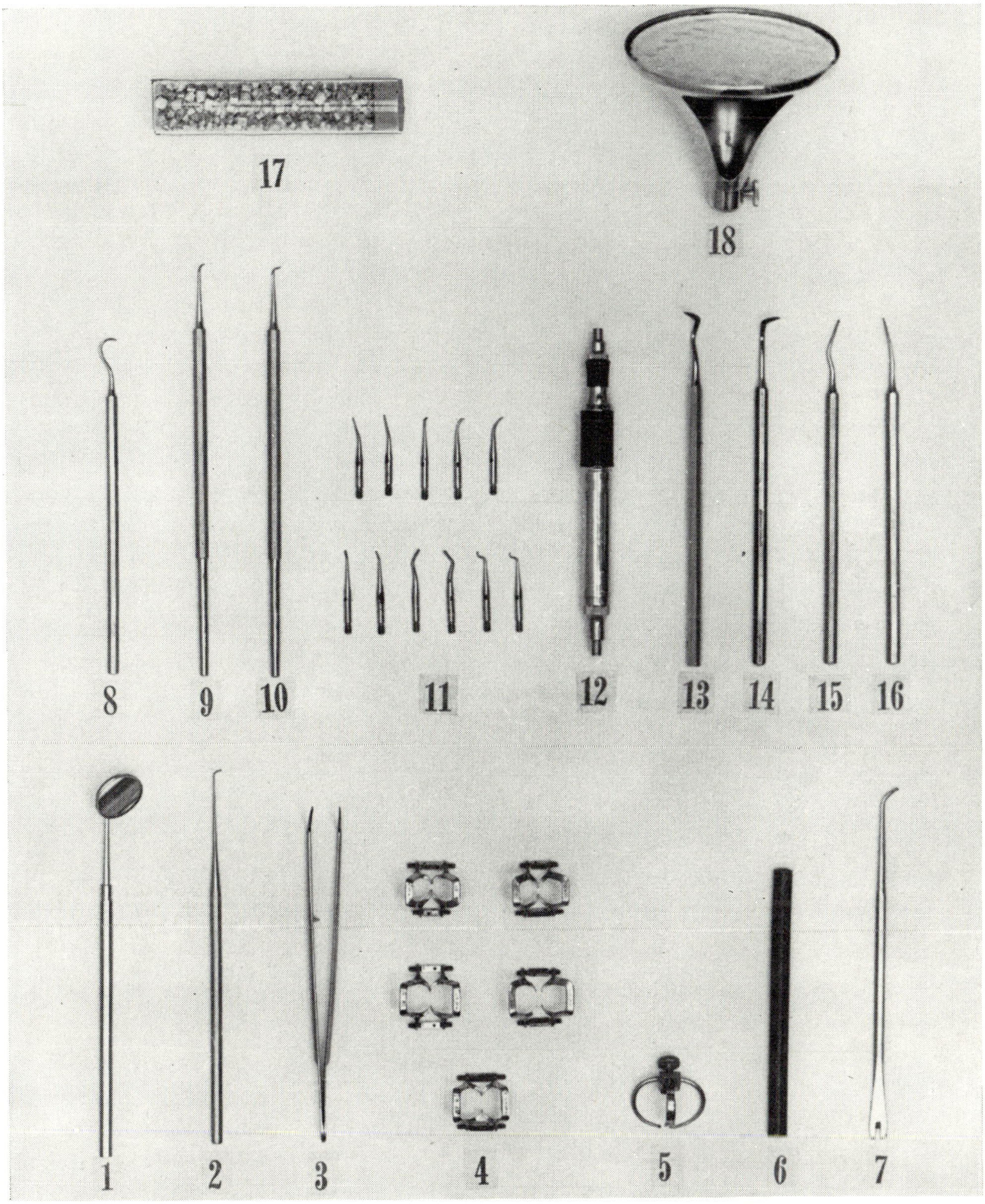

Fig. 6-42. Armamentarium for gold-foil restoration.

1. Mirror, mouth, examining, #4.
2. Explorer, #6.
3. Forceps, dressing, #17.
4. Separators (assortment).
5. Cervical clamp (Hatch).
6. Compound, impression, stick.
7. Wrench (for separators).
8. Instrument, holding, gold-foil.
9. Starter, gold-foil (5-1-23).
10. Starter, gold-foil (5-2-23).
11. Pluggers, gold-foil, black (assortment).
12. Mallet, gold-foil, plugging, automatic.
13. Knife, finishing, Eddy, #1.
14. Knife, finishing, Eddy, #2.
15. File, finishing, #4.
16. File, finishing, #6.
17. Gold, filling, cylinders, cohesive, 1/10-ounce.
18. Annealer, perfection.

used, as indicated by the dentist, and place selected pieces on the annealer.

5. Prepare automatic, pneumatic, or electric mallet, as used by the dentist. ("Round" pluggers are used first for starting the foil, "convex rectangular" pluggers are used next for wedging the foil against the walls of the cavity, and "foot" pluggers are used last for condensing the foil over large open-surfaced areas. The nibs are offset at various angles to permit access to various positions within the cavity.)

6. Transfer pieces of gold foil from the annealer to the cavity using starting instruments as the dentist continues to condense the gold foil within the cavity. (The end of the starter is pressed into the pieces of gold foil on the annealer. Properly annealed gold foil will stick to the end of the starter as the piece is transferred to the cavity. Then press the piece against the previously condensed foil, and continue to hold the instrument in place until the dentist starts to condense it with the mallet. Be careful not to slide the end of the instrument on the gold, since this will burnish the gold and destroy the cohesiveness.)

7. When the cavity is filled, prepare slow-speed handpiece with finishing burs, disks, and polishing cup for finishing and polishing the restoration.

CROWN AND BRIDGE PROSTHESIS

Crown or inlay impression—direct method

Cast-gold inlays or crowns may be used in restoring individual teeth or as retainers in making bridges. In order to fabricate an inlay or crown, the dentist must obtain a wax pattern that fits the prepared tooth exactly the way he wishes the finished restoration to fit. This wax pattern is then used in the laboratory to make a mold into which the gold inlay or crown is cast. When a wax pattern is carved directly on a prepared tooth in the mouth, the technique is called the direct method. This procedure is generally carried out during the same session as the cavity preparation. The armamentarium used for crown or inlay impression by the direct method is shown in Fig. 6-43.

Procedure checklist

1. Deliver crown or inlay impression tray (direct-method) as shown in Fig. 6-43.

2. Light Bunsen flame.

3. After wax has been softened and forced to place by the dentist, insert saliva ejector, and deliver carving instruments.

4. Use short blasts of air to keep the pattern clear of scrapings during the carving procedure.

5. During the final stages of carving, stabilize the wax pattern on the tooth with a finger or a cotton pellet held with forceps as the dentist finishes the carving.

6. Cool the warmed sprue pin with air as the dentist attaches the pin to the wax pattern.

7. As the dentist removes the pattern from the tooth and positions it in the crucible former, remove the crown or inlay impression tray, and deliver instrument tray for placement of a temporary restoration (see Fig. 6-37).

8. Invest wax pattern immediately after dismissal of patient.

Try-in of retainers and bridge impression

Inlays or crowns that support a fixed bridge are called retainers. The teeth to which they are attached are called abutment teeth. When retainers have been made by the direct method, it is necessary to try them on the prepared abutment teeth to check for proper fit. Minor discrepancies are adjusted, and the retainers are seated properly on the teeth before the bridge impression is taken. The bridge impression is used to make a cast on which the retainers are accurately positioned and on which the pontics can be correctly soldered to the retainers. (When retainers have been made

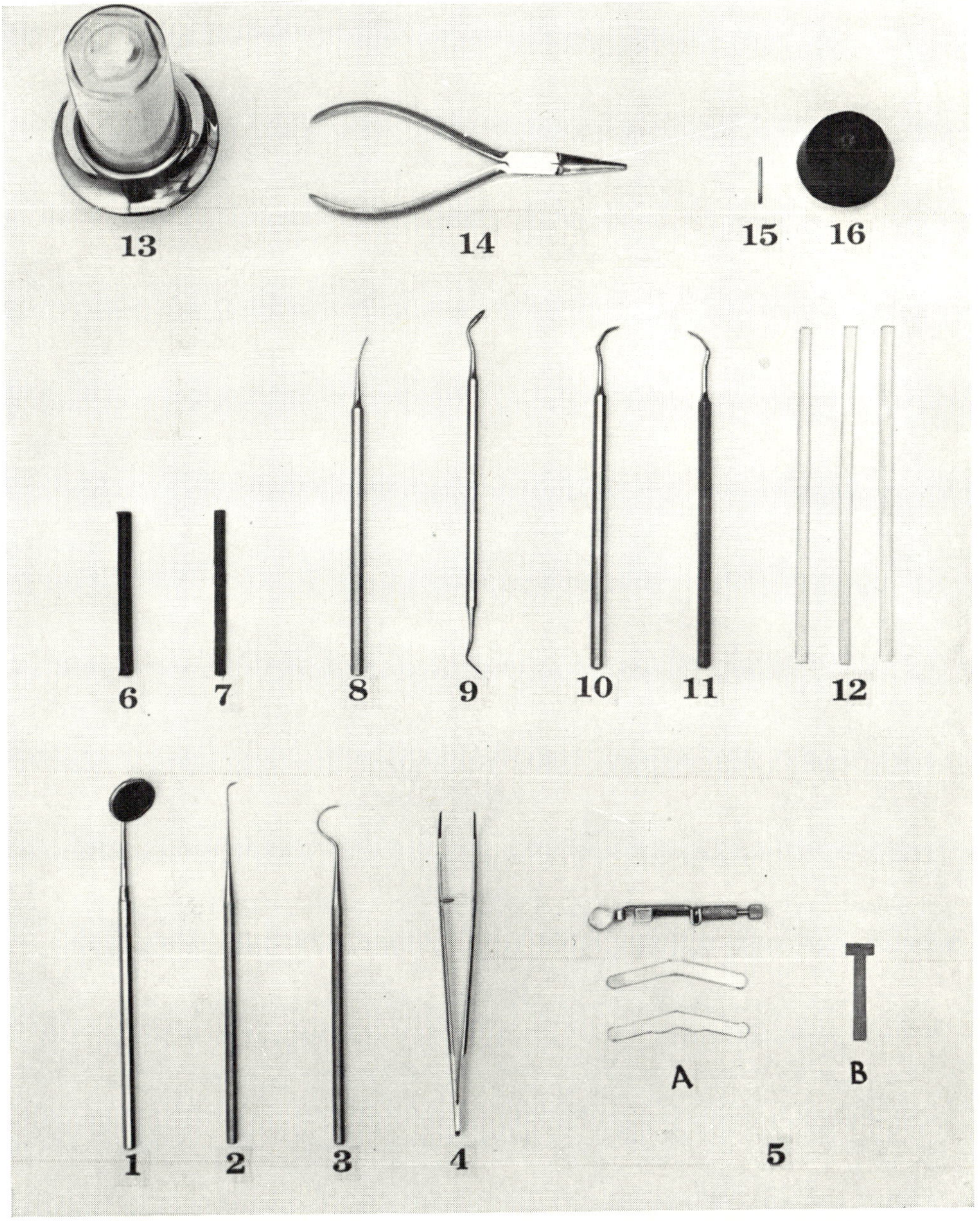

Fig. 6-43. Armamentarium for crown or inlay impression (direct method).

1. Mirror, mouth, examining, #4.
2. Explorer, #6.
3. Explorer, #23.
4. Forceps, dressing, #17.
5. Choice of operator:
   A. Retainer, matrix, Tofflemire (with bands).
   B. T-bands, copper.
6. Wax, casting, inlay, blue.
7. Wax, boxing, stick, red (low-fusing—for correction of wax pattern).
8. Burnisher, #2 (beaver-tail).
9. Carver, wax, Hollenback, #3.
10. Knife, finishing, Eddy, #1.
11. Knife, finishing, Eddy, #2.
12. Strips, finishing, linen.
13. Cotton, absorbent, cylinder (for use in cotton font).
14. Pliers, laboratory and office, #121 (serrated beaks).
15. Pin, sprue.
16. Former, rubber, crucible.

by the indirect method, the try-in appointment may be omitted if the dentist elects to do so.) The armamentarium used for try-in of retainers and bridge impression is shown in Fig. 6-44.

Procedure checklist

1. Deliver tray for try-in of retainers and bridge impression as shown in Fig. 6-44.
2. Deliver spoon excavator and sickle scaler for removal of temporary restorations.
3. Clean and dry abutment preparations by using water, air, and saliva ejector.
4. Deliver retainers for try-in.
5. Assist dentist in seating of retainers by using the mallet while the dentist holds the orangewood stick, if necessary.
6. Deliver articulating paper held by self-locking forceps to check occlusion.
7. Prepare slow-speed handpiece with stones and disks for adjustment of the retainers to the teeth.
8. Select 2 impression trays, one for the bridge impression and one for the opposing arch impression.
9. Prepare impression material for bridge impression according to the dentist's choice, as follows:
   a. Rubber-base impression material.
   b. Hydrocolloid.

(Carefully follow the manufacturer's instructions in the preparation of impression material used.)

10. Fill the impression tray.
11. While the impression material is setting in the mouth, clean the mixing equipment, and get the alginate impression material ready for the opposing arch impression.
12. After bridge impression has been removed, mix alginate impression material for the opposing arch impression, and fill impression tray.
13. While opposing arch impression is setting in the mouth, prepare baseplate wax for the wax occlusal imprint by cutting it to the proper shape and placing it in a bowl of hot water.
14. After wax occlusal imprint has been taken, deliver shade guide, and *record the tooth shade selected.*
15. Remove tray of instruments and materials used, and deliver instrument tray for placement of temporary restorations (see Fig. 6-37).
16. Pour up bridge impression and opposing arch impression with stone *immediately* after dismissal of the patient.

Crown or inlay impression—indirect method

When a wax pattern is carved on a replica or model (commonly called a die) of a prepared tooth instead of directly on the natural tooth, the procedure is referred

Fig. 6-44. Armamentarium for try-in of retainers and bridge impression.

1. Mirror, mouth, examining, #4.
2. Explorer, #6.
3. Forceps, dressing, #17.
4. Stick, orangewood.
5. Mallet, oral surgery, hand-operated (Mead).
6. Paper, articulating, blue (12 sheets).
7. Trays, impression, perforated (maxillary and mandibular—for use with the alginate type of impression material).
8. Choice of operator:
   A. Impression material, accelerator (heavy type). Impression material, rubber-base (heavy type).
   B. Impression material, hydrocolloid, alginate type (2 packages).
9. Spatula, dental, wax, #7, double-ended.
10. Wax baseplate, pink (sheet).
11. Shade guide, tooth.
12. Burs, excavating, tungsten steel (assortment).
13. Disk set, abrasive paper, with brass center (assortment).
14. Points, silicon carbide (assortment).

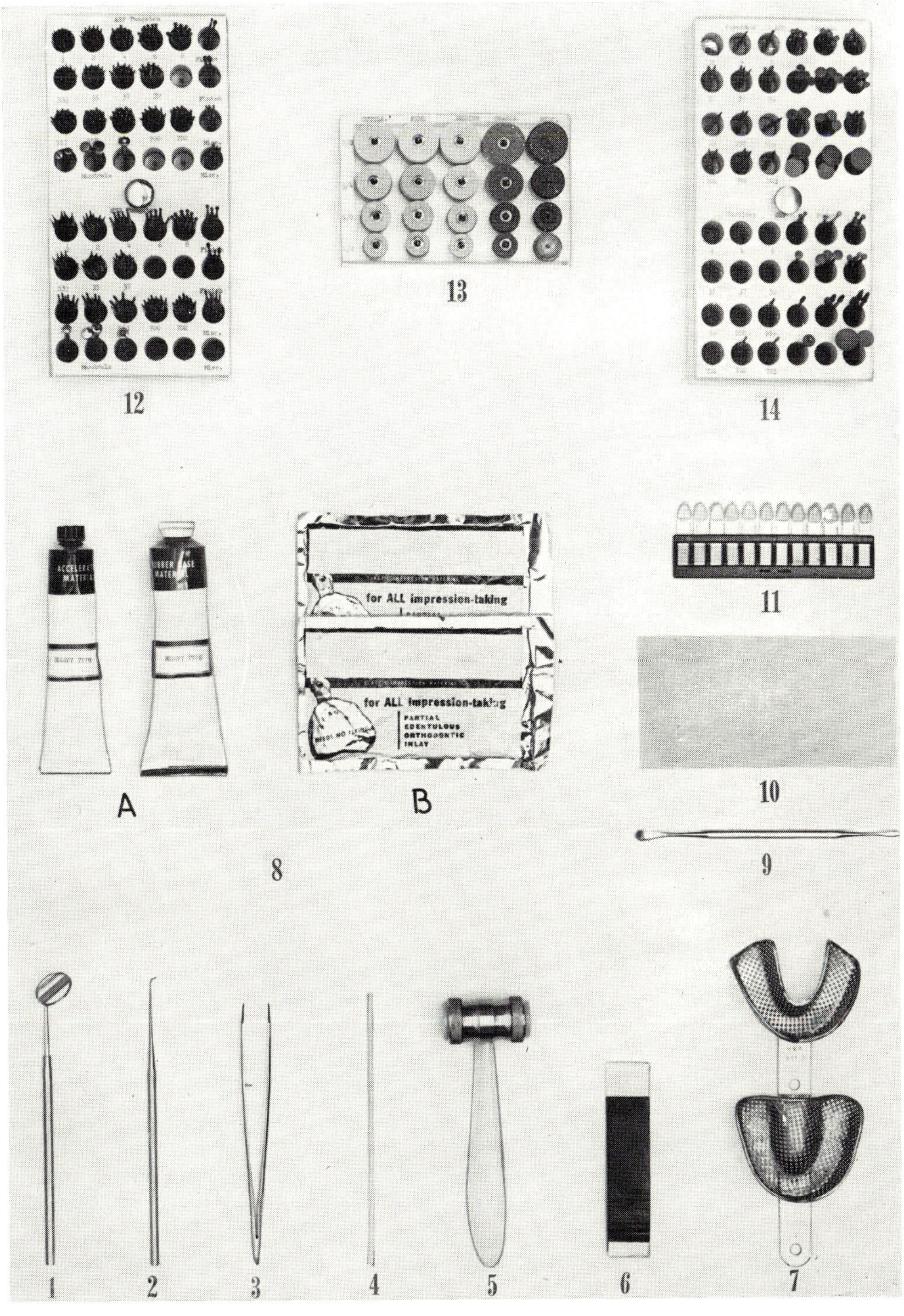

Fig. 6-44. For legend see opposite page.

to as the indirect method of obtaining a wax pattern. Occasionally, a combination of the indirect and direct methods is used; that is, the wax is pattern carved on the die and then tried on the natural tooth to double-check the fit before the pattern is cast into gold. This procedure is called the indirect-direct method of obtaining a wax pattern.

In order to obtain a model of the prepared tooth, it is necessary to first make a negative mold or impression of the tooth. A variety of elastic impression materials may be used, in addition to the synthetic rubber material shown. Detailed instructions for manipulation of each material are provided by the manufacturer. In general, they all require a syringe for injecting part of the material into the cavity preparation and a tray for carrying the bulk of the material into the mouth. The armamentarium used for obtaining a crown or inlay impression by the indirect method is shown in Fig. 6-45.

Procedure checklist

1. Deliver crown or inlay impression tray (indirect-method) as shown in Fig. 6-45.
2. Deliver spoon excavator and sickle scaler for removal of temporary restorations.
3. Clean and dry tooth preparations by using water, air, and saliva ejector, and isolate abutment teeth with cotton rolls.
4. Deliver cotton cord for gingival retraction.
5. Mix impression material of the injection type, fill the syringe, and pass it to the dentist.
6. While the dentist is syringing impression material into the preparations, mix impression material of the heavy type, and fill the custom-made tray coated with tray adhesive. Pass the tray to the dentist, so he can place it in the mouth immediately after he finishes with the syringe. Timing is most important with this procedure.
7. While the impression material is setting in the mouth, clean the mixing equipment, and get the alginate impression material ready for the opposing arch impression.
8. After bridge impression has been removed, mix alginate impression material for the opposing arch impression, fill impression tray, and pass it to the dentist.
9. While opposing arch impression is setting in the mouth, prepare baseplate wax for the wax occlusal imprint by cutting it to the proper shape and placing it in a bowl of hot water.
10. After wax occlusal imprint has been taken, deliver shade guide, and *record the tooth shade selected.*
11. Remove tray of instruments and

Fig. 6-45. Armamentarium for crown or inlay impression (indirect method).

1. Mirror, mouth, examining, #4.
2. Explorer, #6.
3. Forceps, dressing, #17.
4. Plugger, plastic filling, dental stellite, double-ended, #1-2.
5. Cotton cord impregnated with 8:100 racemic epinephrine (Gingi-pak).
6. 8:100 racemic epinephrine (Orostat).
7. Dish, glass, medicament, dappen (for 8:100 racemic epinephrine).
8. Impression material, rubber-base (heavy type).
9. Impression material, accelerator (heavy type).
10. Impression material, rubber-base (injection type).
11. Impression material, accelerator (injection type).
12. Spatula, 3½-inch, steel blade.
13. Pad, mixing, waxed surface.
14. Spatula, 3½-inch, steel blade.
15. Pad, mixing, waxed surface.
16. Tray adhesive.
17. Tray, impression, custom-made (autopolymer resin).
18. Dish, glass, medicament, dappen (for the injection type of impression material).
19. Syringe, injection (for impression material).

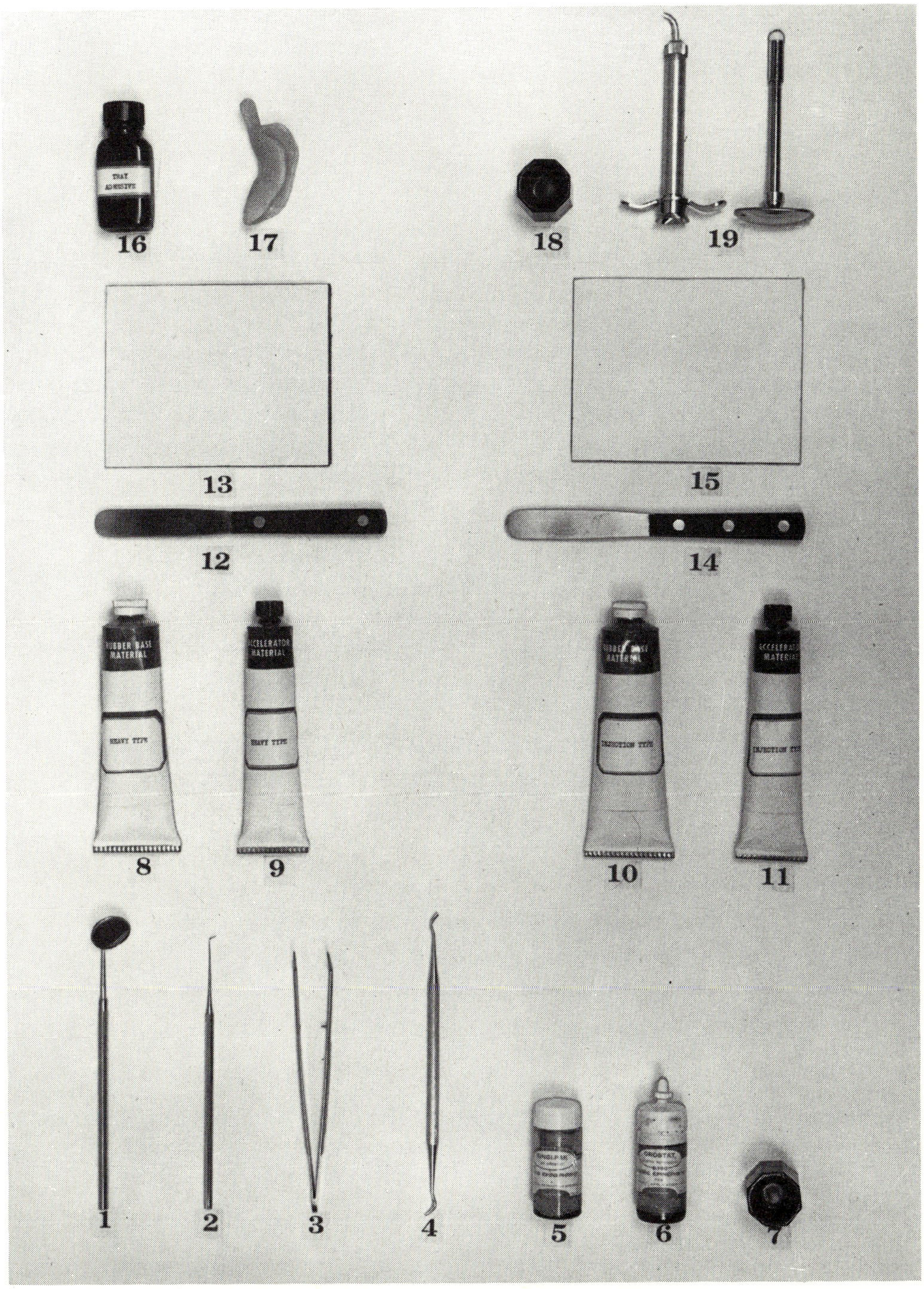

Fig. 6-45. For legend see opposite page.

materials used, and deliver instrument tray for placement of temporary restorations (see Fig. 6-37).

12. Pour up bridge impression and opposing arch impression with stone *immediately* after dismissal of the patient.

Inlay, crown, or bridge cementation

Zinc phosphate or carboxylate cements are used to secure completed inlays, crowns, or bridges to prepare teeth. The procedures employed for cementing these restorations are essentially the same, except that more preparatory adjustments are required in the cementation of a bridge. Porcelain facings must first be adjusted to the pontics of the bridge and to the tissues of the mouth and finally cemented to the pontics outside the mouth before the bridge can be cemented to the abutment teeth. Occasionally, a bridge is seated with temporary cement to allow for minor adjustments of the abutment teeth before permanent cementation of the bridge at a subsequent session. Because of the translucency of the material, the selection of the color of the cement used in cementing porcelain facings and porcelain jacket crowns is more critical than in the cementation of gold castings. The armamentarium used for inlay, crown, or bridge cementation is shown in Fig. 6-46.

Procedure checklist

1. Deliver inlay, crown, or bridge cementation tray as shown in Fig. 6-46.
2. Deliver spoon excavator and sickle scaler for removal of temporary restorations.
3. Clean and dry tooth preparations by using water, air, and saliva injector, and isolate abutment teeth with cotton rolls.
4. If necessary, assist dentist in seating of inlay, crown, or bridge by using the mallet while the dentist holds the orangewood stick.
5. Deliver articulating paper held by self-locking forceps to check occlusion.
6. Prepare slow-speed handpiece with stones and disks for adjustment of the inlay or crowns to the teeth.
7. Remove any remaining scratches on gold by polishing with a buffing lathe.
8. Cement removable porcelain facings to the bridge outside of the mouth.
9. Deliver medicament of the dentist's choice for desensitization of the dentin.
10. Mix cement to a creamy consistency (see mixing instructions for zinc phosphate or carboxylate cements on p. 111).
11. Apply the cement to the inner surface of the inlay or crown while the dentist applies the cement to the tooth preparation. (Timing of this procedure is of utmost importance to permit complete setting of the restoration while the cement still has a creamy consistency. The moment the cement starts to thicken while being applied, the operation should be stopped, and a new mix of cement prepared.)
12. If necessary, assist dentist in seating the inlay, crown, or bridge by using

Fig. 6-46. Armamentarium for inlay, crown, or bridge cementation.

1. Mirror, mouth, examining, #4.
2. Explorer, #6.
3. Explorer, #23.
4. Forceps, dressing, #17.
5. Plugger, plastic filling, Woodson, double-ended, #2 (two).
6. Stick, orangewood.
7. Mallet, oral surgery, hand-operated (Mead).
8. Cotton rolls.
9. Zinc phosphate cement, powder.
10. Zinc phosphate cement, liquid.
11. Mixing slab, dental, glass, 3 by 6 inches.
12. Spatula, cement, #324 (2-inch flat blade).
13. Points, silicon carbide (assortment).
14. Paper, articulating, blue (12 sheets).
15. Disk set, abrasive paper with brass center (assortment).
16. Disks, wheel-shaped, knife-edged, cleaning and polishing, Burlew type.
17. Burs, excavating, tungsten steel (assortment), and mandrels (assortment).
18. Cotton, absorbent, cylinder (for use in cotton font).

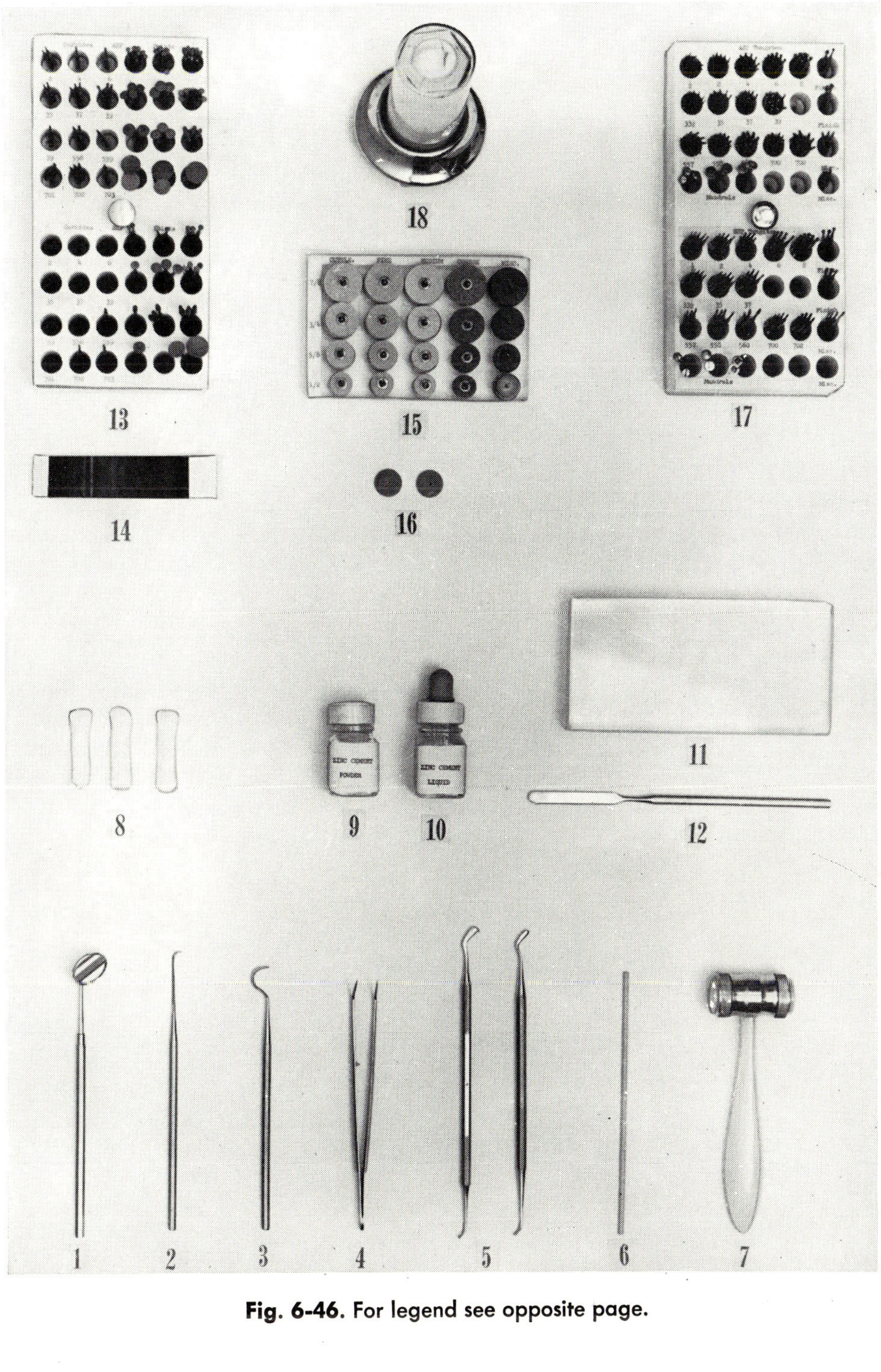

Fig. 6-46. For legend see opposite page.

the mallet while the dentist holds the orangewood stick.

13. Have patient close firmly on cotton roll for 5 minutes.

14. Deliver explorers, sickle scaler, and dental floss for removal of excess cement.

15. Deliver articulating paper held by self-locking forceps for final check of occlusion.

PARTIAL DENTURE PROSTHESIS

Preliminary impression

In anticipation of constructing a removable partial denture prosthesis, preliminary impressions for study models are made of each arch. The study models are mounted on an articulator and analyzed to determine the proper locations for making rest preparations and to evaluate existing contours of teeth. The armamentarium used for obtaining preliminary impressions for partial denture prosthesis is shown in Fig. 6-47.

Procedure checklist

1. Deliver tray for partial denture preliminary impression as shown in Fig. 6-47.
2. Protect patient's clothing with plastic apron, and light Bunsen burner.
3. Lubricate patient's lips with petrolatum.
4. Select maxillary and mandibular impression trays to fit the patient's mouth.
5. After dentist has checked and modified impression trays with boxing wax as needed, give patient a cup of water for thorough rinsing of the mouth.
6. Mix first batch of alginate impression material, fill the tray, and pass it to the dentist.
7. While first impression is setting in the mouth, clean the mixing equipment, and get the alginate material ready for the opposing arch impression.
8. After first impression has been removed, mix second batch of alginate impression material for the opposing arch impression, fill impression tray, and pass it to the dentist.
9. While opposing arch is setting in the mouth, prepare baseplate wax for the wax occlusal imprint by cutting it to the proper shape and placing it in a bowl of hot water.
10. Pour up study models from both impressions with stone *immediately* after dismissal of the patient.

Rest preparation and final impression

The teeth to be clasped and the proper location for making rest preparations are determined from the study models made from the preliminary impressions. The rest preparations are made with stones and disks and are polished before the final impression for the partial denture is taken. The armamentarium used for rest preparation and the final impression for the partial denture prosthesis is shown in Fig. 6-48.

Procedure checklist

1. Deliver tray for partial denture rest preparation and final impression as shown in Fig. 6-48.
2. Protect patient's clothing with plastic apron, and light Bunsen burner.
3. Prepare slow-speed handpiece with stones and disks for making rest preparations.
4. Prepare dappen dish with polishing agent and handpiece with prophylaxis brush and cup for polishing rest preparations, and clasp teeth.
5. Lubricate patient's lips with petrolatum.
6. Select maxillary and mandibular impression trays to fit the patient's mouth.
7. After dentist has checked and modified impression trays with boxing wax and cake compound as needed, give patient a cup of water for thorough rinsing of the mouth.
8. Mix first batch of alginate impression material, fill the tray, and pass it to the dentist.

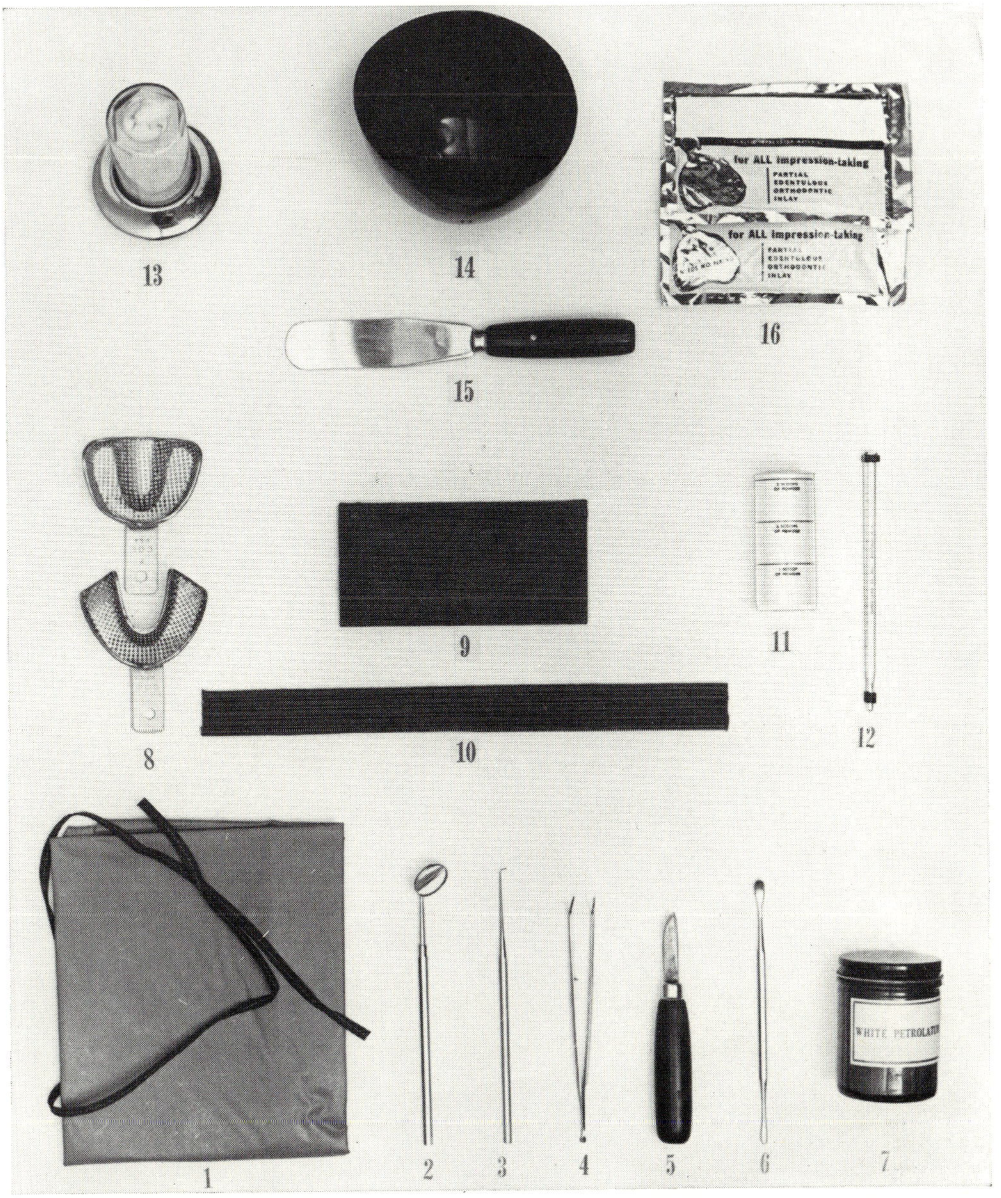

Fig. 6-47. Armamentarium for taking partial denture preliminary impression.

1. Apron, plastic.
2. Mirror, mouth, examining, #4.
3. Explorer, #6.
4. Forceps, dressing, #17 (two).
5. Knife, compound (overall length, 5¼-inch).
6. Spatula, wax, #7, double-ended.
7. Petrolatum, white.
8. Trays, impression, perforated (maxillary and mandibular).
9. Wax, utility, red (sheet).
10. Wax, boxing, sticks, red.
11. Measure, water.
12. Thermometer.
13. Cotton absorbent, cylinder (for use in cotton font).
14. Bowl, mixing, plastic.
15. Spatula, plaster (4½-inch blade, extra stiff).
16. Impression material, hydrocolloid, alginate type (2 (2 packages).

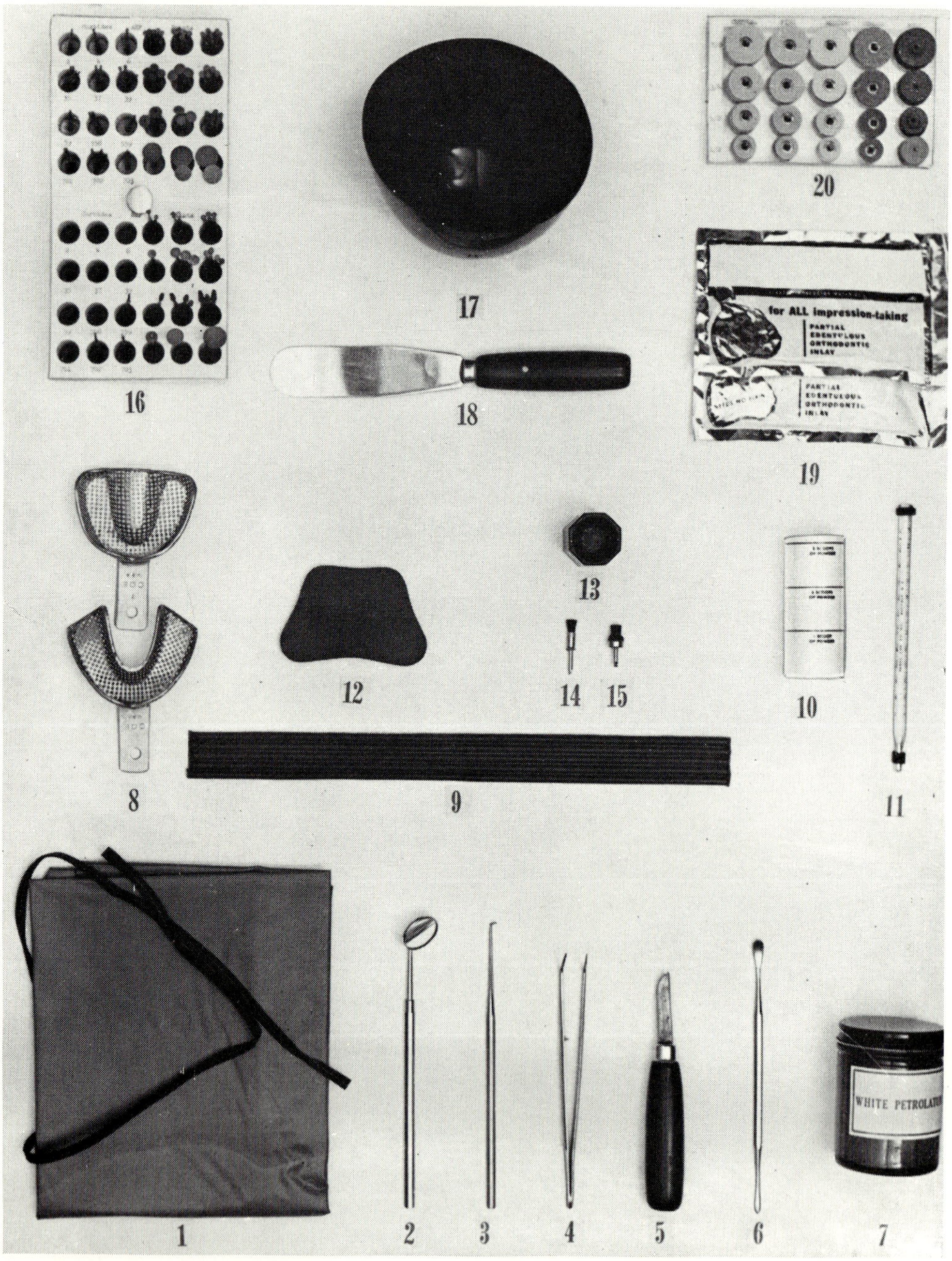

Fig. 6-48. For legend see opposite page.

9. While first impression is setting in the mouth, clean the mixing equipment, and get the alginate material ready for the opposing arch impression if an opposing partial denture is to be constructed. If only 1 partial denture is being constructed, the opposing arch impression may be omitted at this sitting, since the opposing study model made at the previous sitting may be used.

10. The wax occlusal imprint also may be omitted at this sitting if it has been retained from the previous sitting.

11. Pour up master casts from impressions with stone *immediately* after dismissal of the patient.

12. Construct occlusion rims on the stone casts for registration of jaw relations at the next appointment. (If a dental technician is employed in the office, he may construct the occlusion rims.)

Registration of jaw relations

The registration of jaw relations is used to mount the master casts on an articulator in correct positional relationship. The registration involves recording the relation of the jaws when the remaining teeth are in functional occlusal position. The method of recording this relation will vary according to the number and position of the remaining teeth. If occlusal contact is made between teeth in the anterior, right posterior, and left posterior areas of the jaws so that casts can be articulated accurately and with stability, no other occlusal record is required. If occlusal contact is absent in any one or more of these 3 areas, occlusion rims are used to register the positional relation of the jaws and to stabilize the mounting of the casts on the articulator. The armamentarium used for registration of jaw relations with occlusion rims for partial denture prosthesis is shown in Fig. 6-49.

Procedure checklist

1. Deliver tray for registration of jaw relations for partial dentures as shown in Fig. 6-49.
2. Protect patient's clothing with plastic apron.
3. Light Bunsen burner for the dentist's use in adjusting wax occlusion rims to the proper vertical dimension and occlusal position.
4. Deliver shade and mold guides, and *record the mold and shade selected.*

Prior to the next appointment, the dentist or the dental technician will construct the metal framework for the partial dentures, mount the master casts on the articulator, and set up the artificial teeth in wax for a try-in of the trial partial dentures.

Try-in of trial partial dentures

Trial partial dentures consist of the metal framework and wax setup of the

Fig. 6-48. Armamentarium for partial denture rest preparation and final impression.

1. Apron, plastic.
2. Mirror, mouth, examining, #4.
3. Explorer, #6.
4. Forceps, dressing, #17.
5. Knife, compound (overall length, 5¼-inch).
6. Spatula, wax, CRS, #7, double-ended.
7. Petrolatum, white.
8. Trays, impression, perforated (maxillary and mandibular).
9. Wax, boxing, sticks, red.
10. Measure, water.
11. Thermometer.
12. Compound, impression tray, cake.
13. Dish, glass, medicament, dappen (for polishing agent).
14. Brush, tooth-polishing, bristle, AHP.
15. Cup, polishing, rubber, AHP.
16. Points, silicon carbide (assortment).
17. Bowl, mixing, plastic.
18. Spatula, plaster (4½-inch blade, extra stiff).
19. Impression material, hydrocolloid alginate type (2 packages).
20. Disk set, abrasive, paper, with brass center (assortment).

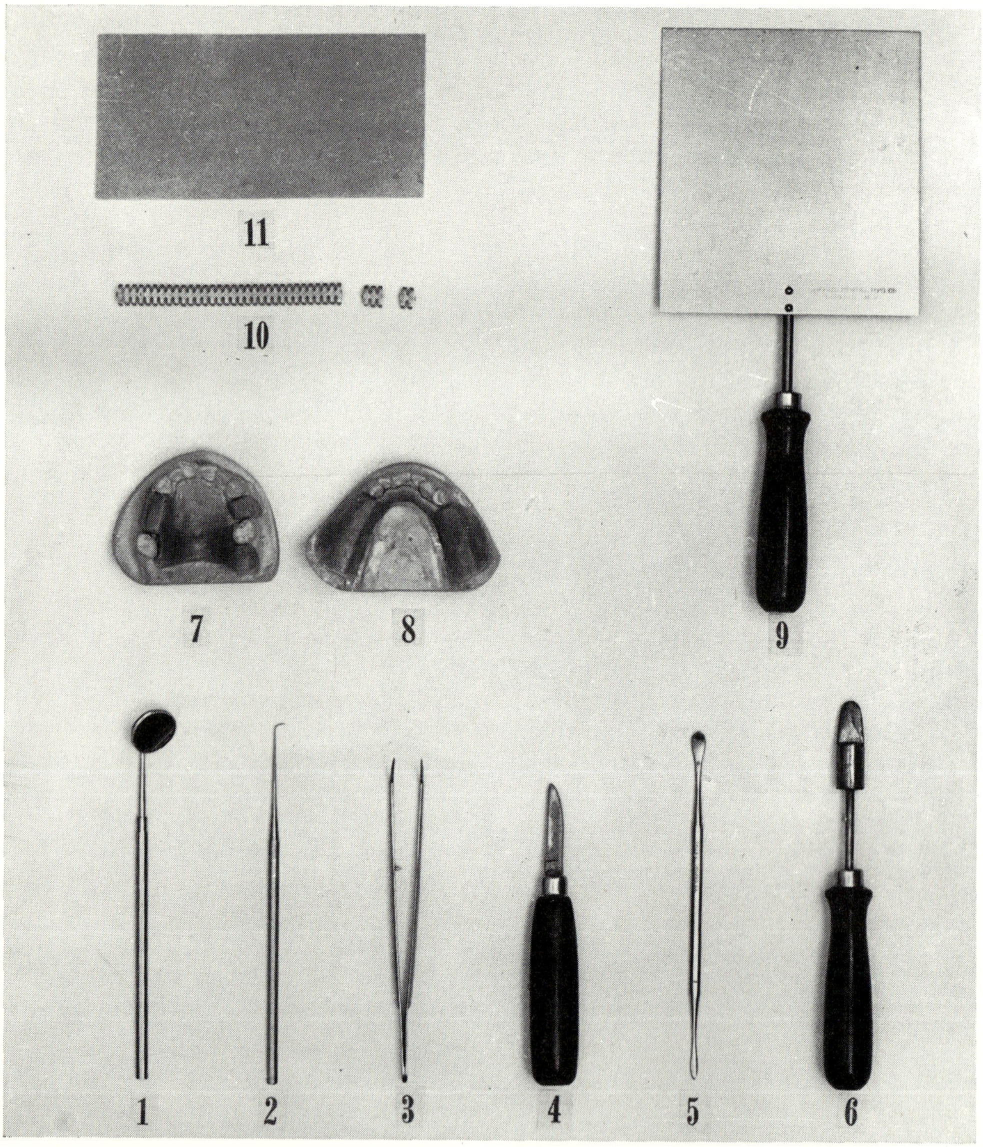

Fig. 6-49. Armamentarium for partial denture registration of jaw relations.

1. Mirror, mouth, examining, #4.
2. Explorer, #6.
3. Forceps, dressing, #17.
4. Knife, compound (overall length, 5¼-inch).
5. Spatula, wax, CRS, #7, double-ended.
6. Spatula, pooling, flat copper blade (for softening wax bite rims).
7. Cast, maxillary, with wax occlusal rim.
8. Cast, mandibular, with wax occlusal rim.
9. Hot plate, aluminum, 5 by 4½ inches (for melting, shaping, and trimming wax bite rims).
10. Staples, steel, automatic, $\frac{3}{16}$-inch legs (for cleating wax bite rims).
11. Wax, baseplate, pink (sheet).

artificial teeth that have been constructed in the laboratory. Trial dentures are tried in the mouth so that any discrepancies in the framework and setup of the teeth can be detected and adjusted before the partial denture is processed to completion. The armamentarium used for a try-in of trial partial dentures is shown in Fig. 6-50.

Procedure checklist

1. Deliver tray for try-in of trial partial dentures as shown in Fig. 6-50.
2. Protect patient's clothing with plastic apron, and light Bunsen burner.
3. Deliver articulating paper held by self-locking forceps to check occlusion.
4. Prepare slow-speed handpiece with stones as indicated.
5. Light Bunsen burner to heat wax spatula for any indicated adjustment of artificial teeth.
6. Deliver hand mirror for patient to examine the arrangement and appearance of the artificial teeth.

After this appointment, the dental technician processes the trial dentures to completion in the laboratory.

Insertion or postinsertion adjustment

Prior to insertion, a completed partial denture should be kept immersed in water to prevent distortion. At the time of insertion, minor occlusal adjustments of the denture teeth are usually required as a result of slight changes that have occurred during processing of the denture. If porcelain facings are used on the partial denture, they should not be cemented to the pontics until they have been adjusted to the tissues of the mouth by the dentist. The armamentarium used for insertion or postinsertion adjustment of partial dentures is the same as for complete dentures (Fig. 6-58).

Procedure checklist

1. Deliver tray for insertion of partial and complete dentures as shown in Fig. 6-58.
2. Scrub partial denture with soap and *cold* water in the presence of the patient.
3. Deliver partial denture to dentist for insertion.
4. Prepare slow-speed handpiece with stones for adjustment of denture as needed.
5. Deliver clasp-bending pliers for adjustment of clasps as needed.
6. Deliver articulating paper held by self-locking forceps to check occlusion.
7. Cement porcelain facings to the partial denture outside of the mouth.
8. Deliver hand mirror for patient to examine the appearance of the partial denture.
9. Be sure patient knows how to remove the partial denture, and reinforce dentist's instructions on care of the partial denture as follows:
    a. "Remove partial denture, and brush your natural teeth after each meal."
    b. "Brush partial denture with soap under *cold* running water after each meal."
    c. "Immerse partial denture in a cup of *cold* water when not being worn."
10. Schedule patient for postinsertion adjustment within 24 hours.

COMPLETE DENTURE PROSTHESIS

Preliminary impression

The objective of impression-taking in complete denture prosthesis is to secure an undistorted imprint of the tissues of the mouth over the denture-bearing area. This is a difficult and exacting operation to perform, since these tissues are easily displaced by the pressure used in taking the impression. Therefore, a preliminary impression of the edentulous arch is first taken to make a stone cast on which a custom-made tray for the final impression is constructed. The armamentarium used for obtaining preliminary impressions for complete denture prosthesis is shown in Fig. 6-51.

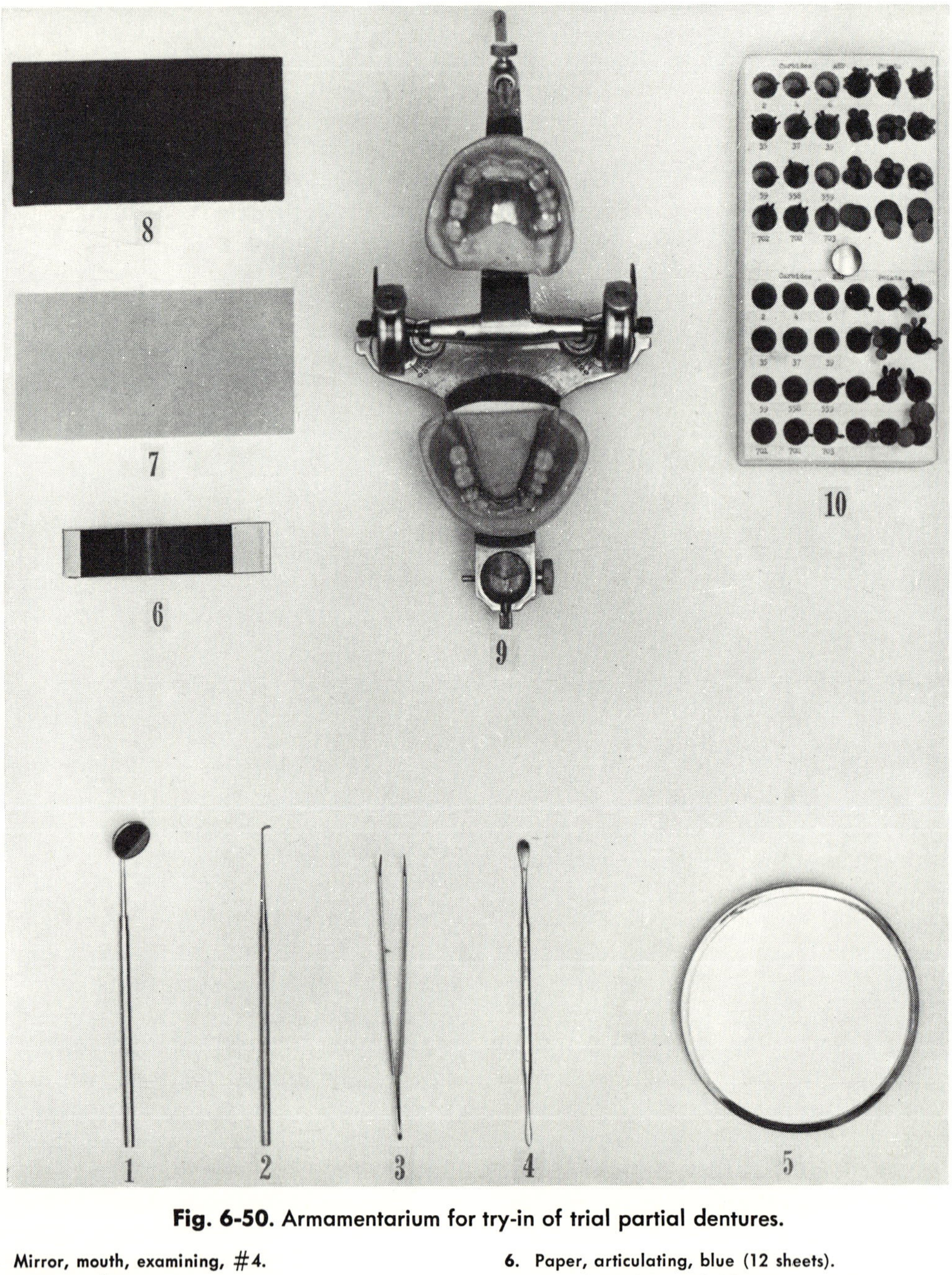

Fig. 6-50. Armamentarium for try-in of trial partial dentures.

1. Mirror, mouth, examining, #4.
2. Explorer, #6.
3. Forceps, dressing, #17.
4. Spatula, wax, CRS, #7, double-ended.
5. Mirror, hand (diameter 5-inch).
6. Paper, articulating, blue (12 sheets).
7. Wax, baseplate, pink (sheet).
8. Wax, utility, red (sheet).
9. Trial partial dentures on articulator.
10. Points, silicon carbide (assortment).

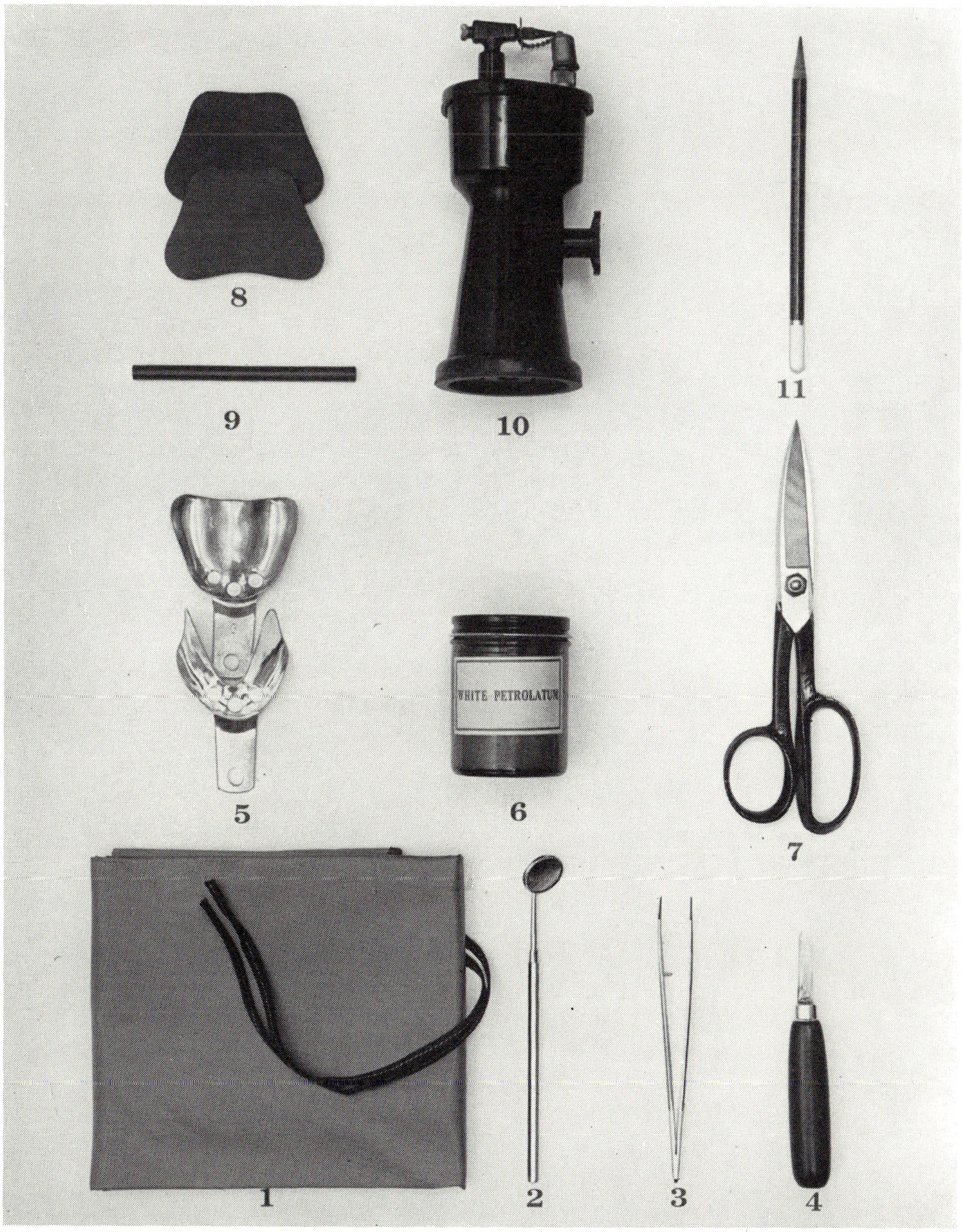

Fig. 6-51. Armamentarium for complete denture preliminary impression.

1. Apron, plastic.
2. Mirror, mouth, examining, #4.
3. Forceps, dressing, #17.
4. Knife, compound (overall length, 5¼-inch).
5. Trays, impression, edentulous (maxillary and mandibular).
6. Petrolatum, white.
7. Shears, metal-cutting, hand, straight, 7¾-inch.
8. Compound, impression tray, cakes.
9. Compound, green, impression, stick.
10. Blowtorch, alcohol.
11. Pencil, lead, indelible.

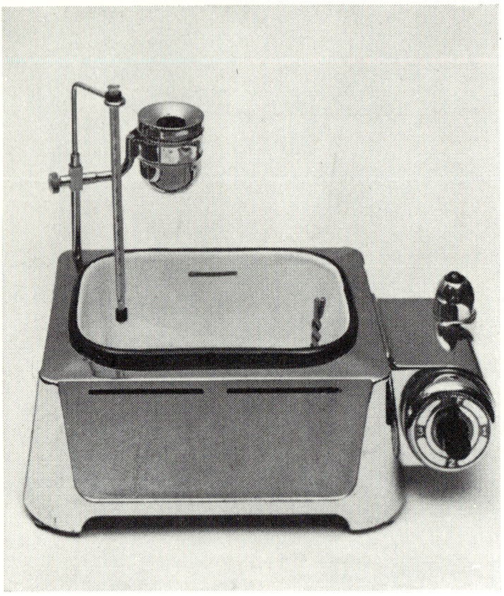

Fig. 6-52. Heater, water bath, dental impression compound, thermostatically controlled, complete with wax melting cup and thermometer.

Procedure checklist

1. Deliver tray for complete denture preliminary impression as shown in Fig. 6-51.
2. Protect patient's clothing with plastic apron, and light Bunsen burner.
3. Fill water bath heater with hot water, and set control switch at position #2 (medium) (Fig. 6-52).
4. Place 3 cakes of modeling compound in the basin of the heater, and maintain temperature of the water at 132 degrees F. (Compound heated to a higher temperature may burn the oral tissues, and compound at a lower temperature will lack the proper degree of plasticity.)
5. Lubricate patient's lips with petrolatum.
6. Select maxillary and mandibular impression trays to fit the patient's mouth.
7. After dentist has checked and modified impression trays as needed, give patient a cup of water for thorough rinsing of the mouth.
8. Fill maxillary impression tray with 1½ cakes of modeling compound, and pass to the dentist.
9. After the impression is seated, chill the tray in the mouth with a stream of cold water.
10. After the dentist has removed and muscle-trimmed the impression with low-fusing, greenstick compound, the same procedure is repeated for the mandibular impression.
11. Pour up study models from both impressions with stone *immediately* after dismissal of the patient. (Custom-made plastic trays are made on the study models prior to the next appointment.)

NOTE: *Alginate impression material, instead of modeling compound, may be preferred by the dentist for obtaining the preliminary impression. If so, the above procedures and armamentarium would need to be modified accordingly.*

Final impression

The final maxillary and mandibular impressions are used to make master casts, on which the complete dentures will eventually be processed. The custom-made plastic trays used for taking the final impressions are constructed in the laboratory prior to this appointment on study models made from the preliminary impressions. The armamentarium used for final impressions for complete denture prosthesis is shown in Fig. 6-53.

Procedure checklist

1. Deliver tray for complete denture final impression as shown in Fig. 6-53.
2. Protect patient's clothing with plastic apron, light Bunsen burner, and fill water bath heater with hot water and set control switch at position #3 (low).
3. Lubricate patient's lips with petrolatum.
4. Scrub custom-made plastic trays with soap and *cold* water in the presence of the patient, and deliver them to the dentist.

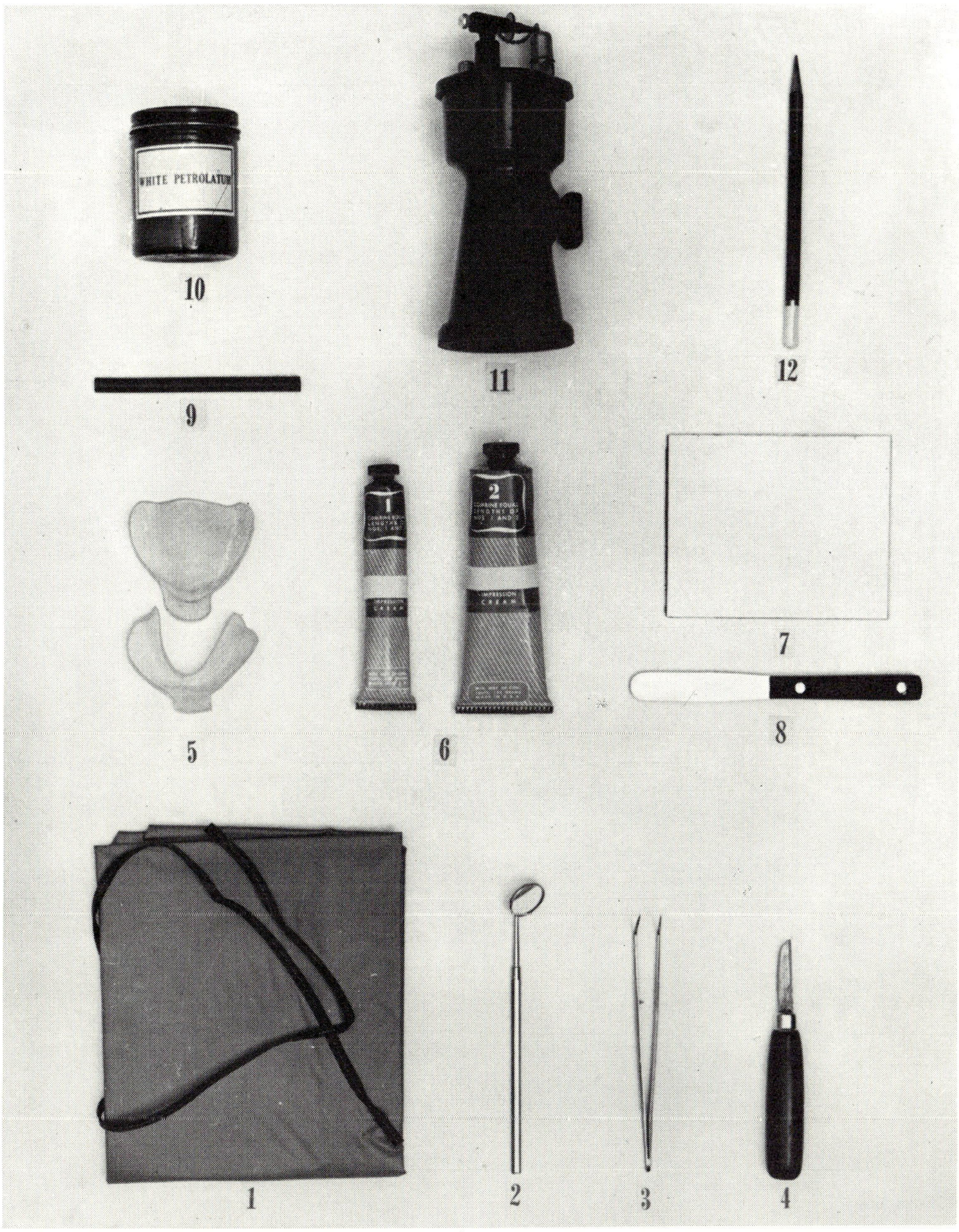

Fig. 6-53. Armamentarium for complete denture final impression.

1. Apron, plastic.
2. Mirror, mouth, examining, #4.
3. Forceps, dressing, #17.
4. Knife, compound (overall length, 5¼-inch).
5. Trays, impression, custommade (autopolymer resin).
6. Paste, impression, zinc oxide–eugenol (tubes 1 and 2).
7. Pad, mixing, waxed surface.
8. Spatula, 3½-inch, steel blade.
9. Compound, green, impression, stick.
10. Petrolatum, white.
11. Blowtorch, alcohol.
12. Pencil, lead, indelible.

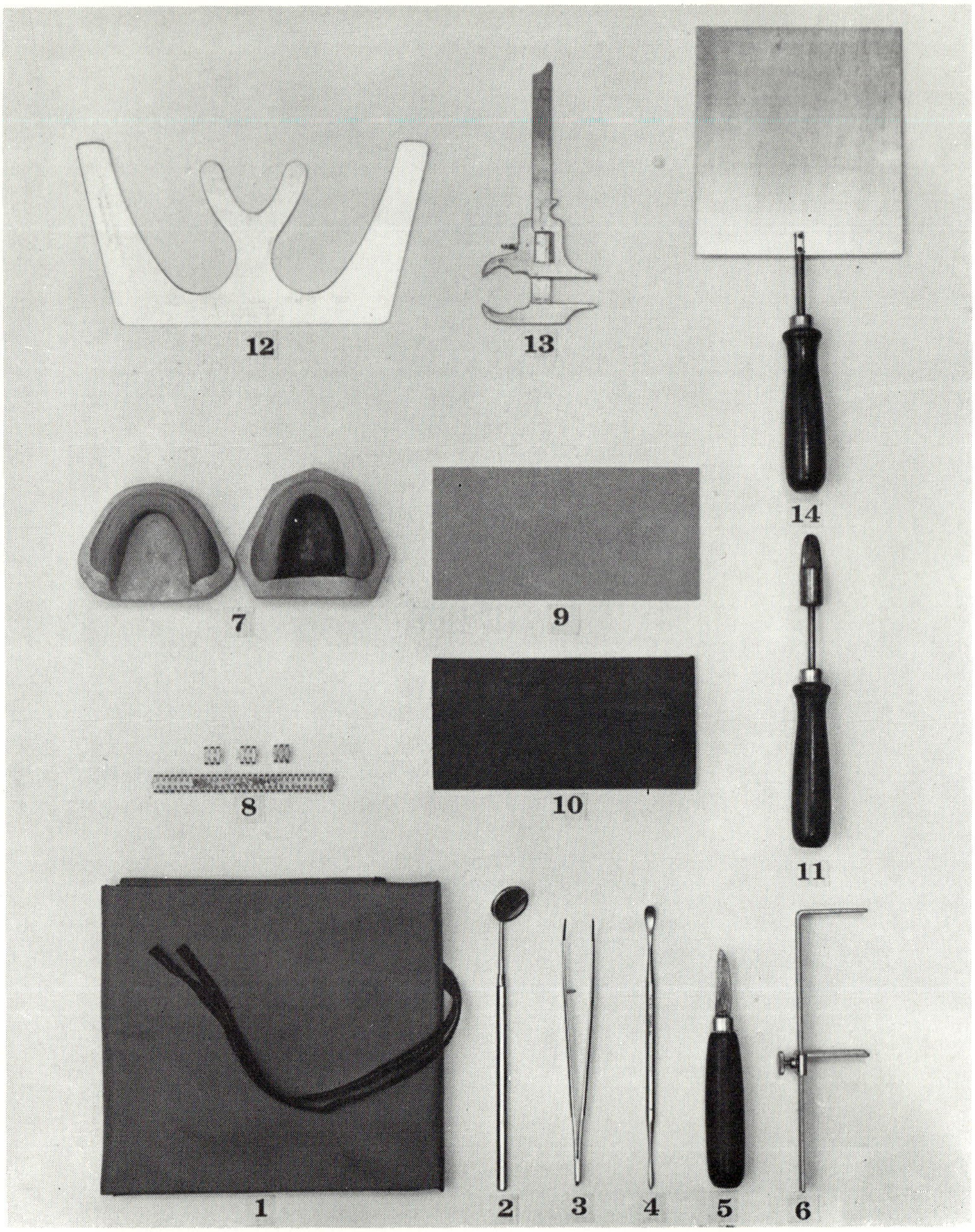

Fig. 6-54. Armamentarium for complete denture registration of jaw relations.

1. Apron, plastic.
2. Mirror, mouth, examining, #4.
3. Forceps, dressing, #17.
4. Spatula, wax, #7, double-ended.
5. Knife, compound (overall length, 5¼-inch).
6. Gauge, bite, Willis (for measuring vertical dimension).
7. Casts (maxillary and mandibular, with wax occlusal rim).
8. Staples, steel, automatic, $\frac{3}{16}$-inch legs (for cleating wax bite rims).
9. Wax, baseplate, pink (sheet).
10. Wax, utility, red (sheet).
11. Spatula, pooling, flat copper blade (for softening wax bite rims).
12. Guide, occlusal plane, aluminum (Fox).
13. Caliper, vernier (Boley).
14. Hot plate, aluminum, 5 by 4¼ inches (for melting, shaping, and trimming wax bite rims).

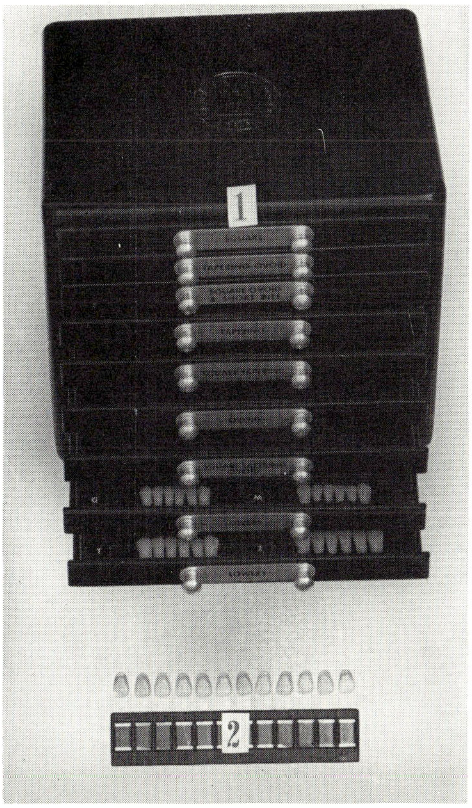

Fig. 6-55.

1. Mold guide, tooth (Bioform).
2. Shade guide, tooth (Bioform).

5. Prepare slow-speed handpiece with denture stone for trimming trays as needed.

6. After dentist has modified and muscle-trimmed custom-made trays with greenstick compound, give patient a cup of water for thorough rinsing of the mouth.

7. Mix impression material of the operator's choice for the maxillary impression. Zinc oxide–eugenol paste (Fig. 6-53) is commonly used, but synthetic rubber or impression plaster may also be used. (The dentist will usually prefer to fill the impression tray himself. In this way, he is better able to judge the quantity and consistency of the impression material in the tray.)

8. Box and pour up master casts from the final impressions with stone *immediately* after dismissal of the patient. (Occlusion rims are constructed on the master casts to be used in the registration of jaw relations at the next appointment.)

Registration of jaw relations

Complete absence of natural teeth results in a loss of the occlusal relationship of the jaws. The purpose of registration of jaw relations is to reestablish that lost relationship with artificial teeth. This is done by making 5 jaw registrations, as follows: (1) rest vertical dimension, (2) occlusal vertical dimension, (3) centric relation, (4) protrusive relation, and (5) face-bow registration.

Rest vertical dimension is the vertical measurement between the jaws when the mandible is in physiologic rest position. Physiologic rest position is used as a position of reference for the subsequent recording of occlusal vertical dimension.

Occlusal vertical dimension is the vertical measurement between the jaws when the teeth are in occlusal contact (2 to 4 mm. less than the rest vertical dimension).

Centric relation is the most retruded, unstrained relation of the mandible to the maxilla from which lateral movement can be made at any given degree of jaw separation. It may be recorded by one of 2 methods, the interocclusal method or the Gothic arch tracing method. The record is used to mount the mandibular cast on the articulator.

Protrusive relation is the relation of the mandible to the maxilla when the lower jaw is in a forward position. The registration of this relationship is used to set the inclination of the condylar guidance on the articulator. Similar registrations of the relationship of the mandible to the maxilla when the lower jaw is in right and left lateral positions are occasionally made for the purpose of setting the lateral condylar inclination on the articulator.

The face-bow registration is a record of the relationship of the maxilla to the tempo-

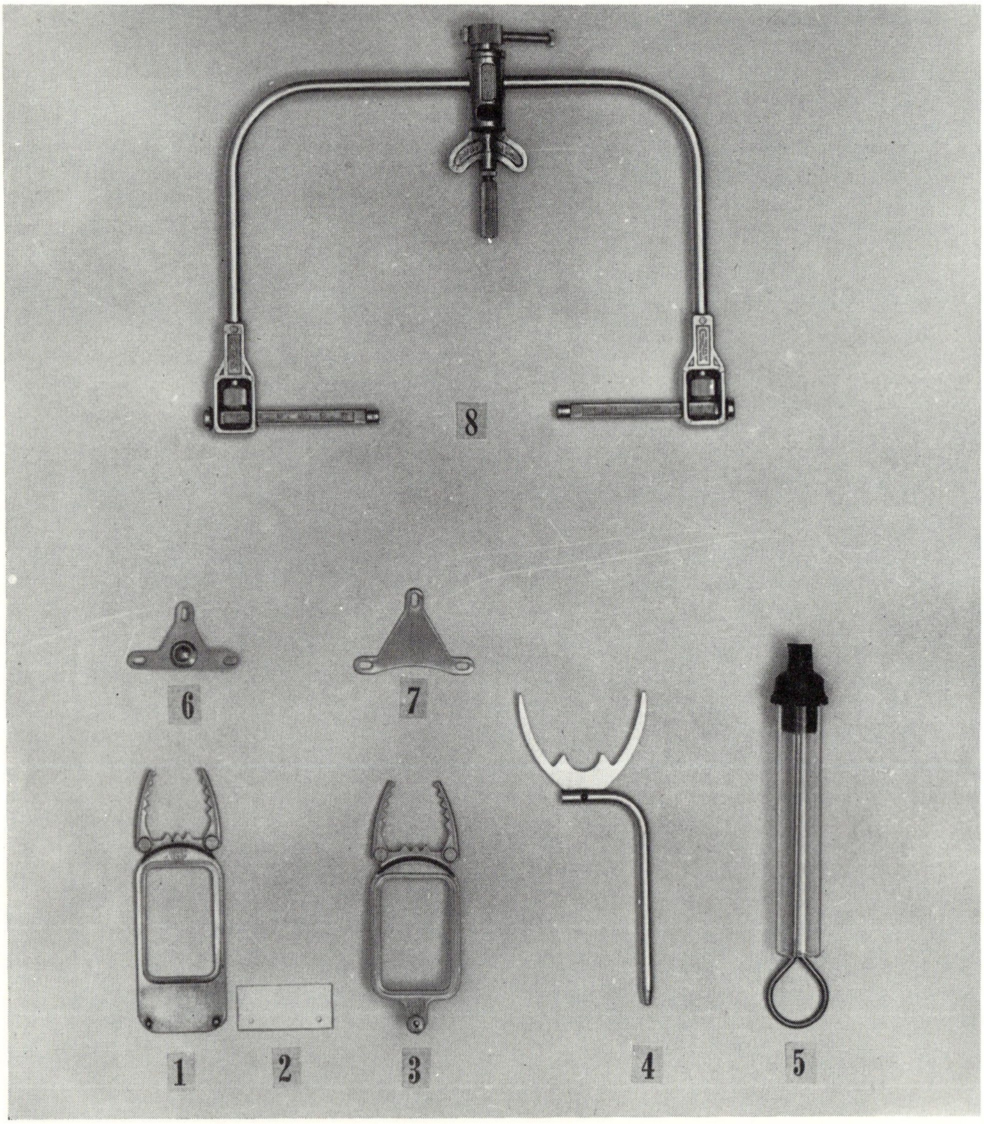

Fig. 6-56. Accessories for registration of jaw relations.

1. Tracer, Hight (tracing table for attachment to mandibular baseplate).
2. Plastic plate (for fixing centric position, attached to tracing table).
3. Tracer, Hight (tracing stylus for attachment to maxillary baseplate).
4. Bitefork, face-bow.
5. Syringe, plaster.
6. Central bearing plate with stud (for attachment to mandibular baseplate).
7. Central bearing plate (for attachment to maxillary baseplate).
8. Face-bow (Hanau).

romandibular joints. It is used for mounting the maxillary cast on the articulator in that same relationship.

Procedure checklist

1. Deliver tray for complete denture registration of jaw relations as shown in Fig. 6-54.
2. Seat patient in an upright position.
3. Protect patient's clothing with a plastic apron, and light Bunsen burner.
4. Lubricate patient's lips with petrolatum.
5. Scrub occlusion rims with soap and *cold* water in the presence of the patient, and deliver them to the dentist.
6. After dentist has obtained rest vertical dimension, occlusal vertical dimension, and centric relation, assist in the attachment of the face-bow to the bite fork (see Fig. 6-56).
7. Deliver mold and shade guides, and *record the mold and shade selected* (see Fig. 6-55).
8. At this point, the patient may be dismissed, unless Gothic arch tracings are to be made. In that case, mount maxillary and mandibular casts on the articulator, and deliver the additional accessories shown in Fig. 6-56.

Prior to the next appointment, the dental technician will set up the artificial teeth for try-in of the trial dentures.

Try-in of trial complete denture

Trial dentures for a complete denture prosthesis consist of a wax setup of the artificial teeth on the baseplates used for registration of jaw relations. The trial dentures are tried in the mouth, so that any discrepancies in arch form, occlusion, balance, phonetics, and appearance may be detected and adjusted before the dentures are processed to completion. Only minor adjustments will be required if the registration of jaw relations, the mounting of casts on the articulator, and the arrangement of teeth have been made correctly. Occasionally, ments will be required, if the registration of jaw relations. Such errors make it necessary to take new interocclusal centric and protrusive records, remount the mandibular cast, and reset the mandibular teeth. The armamentarium used for try-in of trial dentures for complete denture prosthesis is shown in Fig. 6-57.

Procedure checklist

1. Deliver tray for try-in of trial complete dentures as shown in Fig. 6-57.
2. Protect patient's clothing with plastic apron, and light Bunsen burner.
3. Deliver articulating paper held by self-locking forceps to check occlusion.
4. Prepare slow-speed handpiece with stones as indicated.
5. After the arch form, occlusion, position of the teeth, and phonetic ability of the patient have been checked and adjustments made by the dentist, deliver a hand mirror or, preferably, have the patient stand in front of a wall mirror to see the appearance of the trial dentures.
6. After any further needed adjustments are made, the patient may be dismissed.

After this appointment the trial dentures are processed to completion in the laboratory.

Insertion or postinsertion adjustment

Finished dentures should be kept immersed in water prior to insertion to prevent distortion. At the time of insertion, preliminary adjustments of the frenal notches, occlusion, and balance of the dentures are made. Final adjustments are deferred until the patient has worn the dentures for a period of 24 hours. The armamentarium used for insertion or postinsertion adjustment of complete dentures, as well as partial dentures, is shown in Fig. 6-58.

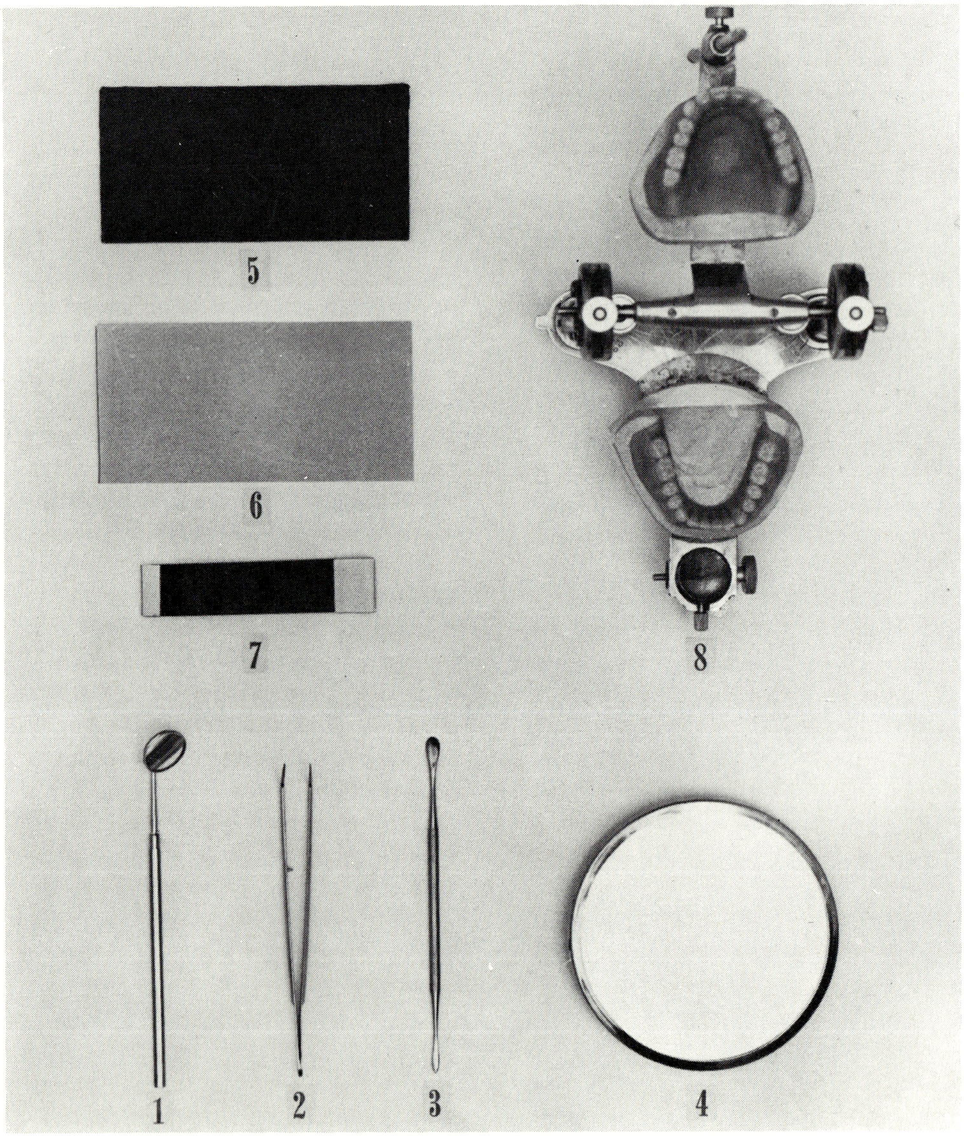

Fig. 6-57. Armamentarium for try-in of trial complete dentures.

1. Mirror, mouth, examining, #4.
2. Forceps, dressing, #17.
3. Spatula, wax, #7, double-ended.
4. Mirror, hand (diameter, 5-inch).
5. Wax, utility, red (sheet).
6. Wax, baseplate, pink, (sheet).
7. Paper, articulating, blue (12 sheets).
8. Trial complete dentures on articulator.

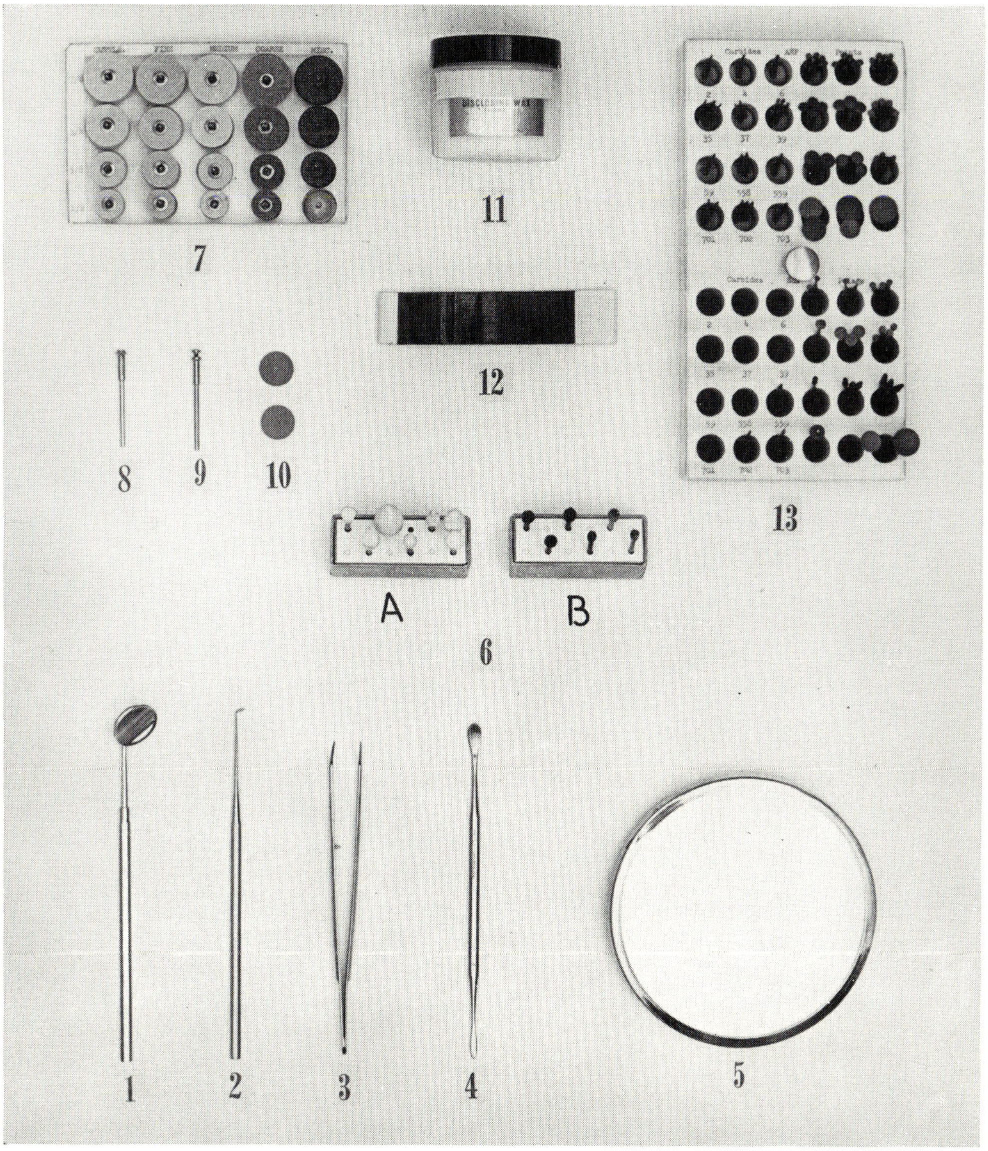

Fig. 6-58. Armamentarium for insertion or postinsertion adjustment of partial and complete dentures.

1. Mirror, mouth, examining, #4.
2. Explorer, #6.
3. Forceps, dressing, #17.
4. Spatula, wax, CRS, #7, double-ended.
5. Mirror, hand (diameter, 5-inch).
6. Choice of operator (for trimming and finishing plastic denture material):
   - **A.** Points, abrasive, "Faskut" (assortment).
   - **B.** Burs, denture, tungsten steel, SHP (assortment).
7. Disk set, abrasive paper, with brass center (assortment).
8. Mandrel, Moore type, SHP.
9. Mandrel, SHP, screwhead, #303.
10. Disks, rubber, wheel-shaped, knife-edged, cleaning and polishing, Burlew type.
11. Wax, disclosing (for locating areas of excessive pressure on tissue side of denture).
12. Paper, articulating (12 sheets).
13. Points, silicon carbide (assortment).

Procedure checklist

1. Deliver tray for insertion of partial and complete dentures as shown in Fig. 6-58.

2. Scrub dentures with soap and *cold* water in the presence of the patient.

3. Deliver dentures to dentist for insertion.

4. Deliver articulating paper held by self-locking forceps to check occlusion.

5. Prepare slow-speed handpiece with stones for adjustment of dentures as needed.

6. When all adjustments have been completed, deliver hand mirror or, preferably, have the patient stand in front of a wall mirror to see the appearance of the dentures. Compliment the patient discreetly, but sincerely, on the appearance of the dentures.

7. Deliver written instructions on care of the dentures as follows, for example:

Cleaning

1. Use a soft brush and soap and water to clean your dentures after every meal and before going to sleep. Rinse your mouth at these times also.

2. If you can't brush after a meal, at least wash the dentures under cold running water, and rinse your mouth.

3. Take your dentures out of your mouth before going to sleep. Clean them, and put them in a cup of cool water.

Eating

1. Begin with soft foods that require little chewing. After several days, start eating more solid food.

2. Cut any solid food in small pieces, and place it on the lower back teeth on *both sides*. Chew on both sides at the same time; this will help to seat the dentures. (If you chew on one side only, the other side tends to wobble.)

3. Take your time when eating—*chew slowly*.

Miscellaneous

1. Let your tongue lay forward so that it just touches the lower front teeth when you are not eating or speaking. The lower denture may jump if the tongue is not in this position.

2. Yawning, coughing, or sneezing will loosen the dentures.

3. You will have a lot of saliva in your mouth the first few days. It will gradually return to normal.

4. At first it may be difficult to speak with your new dentures; practice reading aloud until you can do this properly.

INSTRUMENT SHARPENING

All cutting instruments become dull and lose their effectiveness after repeated use. Dull instruments make cutting harder, decrease the quality of results, prolong operating time, and cause considerably more pain than sharp instruments. Thus, cutting instruments must be resharpened as they become dull. The little time spent in sharpening instruments is more than compensated for by increased speed and precision. With a little instruction and practice, the dental assistant can easily learn to perform this important service. For detailed description on the sharpening of instruments and suggestions on how these instruments can be cared for, see Chapter 11.

CHAPTER 7 PUTTING FOUR HANDS TO WORK

LOIS K. KRYGER,* C.D.A.

In the past 5 years, the words "four-handed dentistry" have been used so extensively in dental literature that they have become part of the vocabulary in a relatively short time. The four hands are those of the dentist and dental assistant, working together while treating patients in the operatory. Since the concept has been accepted by dental educators, dental assisting students and employed dental assistants should prepare themselves to perform competently at the chairside. They should be able to apply basic principles to the methods of procedure that the individual practitioner has adopted.

While the purpose of this book is to provide the dentist and his assistant with material and information to help them to work effectively and efficiently in the office, the purpose of this chapter is to describe and to teach the dentist and his assistant to put their *four hands to work efficiently* while working together at the chair.

It is impossible in one chapter to give examples of all of the different ways in which these four hands are put to work. However, the dentist and his assistant who already work together in the passing of instruments as they work on the patient will have an opportunity to see some examples of how other people go about this task. Those who do not now work with a dental assistant at the chair will undoubtedly receive some ideas as to how this is done in some offices and schools, and these ideas and suggestions will be a challenge to try. However, there are many ways of saving time and motion, and no doubt many dentists and their assistants will discover new and better ways of putting their four hands to work efficiently and effectively.

Dentistry and dental education are changing every year. As new instruments, equipment, materials, and techniques and utilization of new auxiliary personnel are changing the practice of dentistry, so must future developments change and improve the utilization of the four hands. The dentist today is not content to make use of the same methods that he learned in dental school. Neither the dentist nor his assistant are content to be limited and restricted by what they have been doing; thus, we can expect dental office teams to develop and invent new and better ideas for improving dental practice for the future. In other words, this chapter should serve to make one more aware of how the dentist and his assistant are putting their four hands to work efficiently at the present time. Furthermore, it is an effort to help dental as-

*This chapter was contributed by Miss Lois Kryger in her private capacity. No official support or endorsement by the Public Health Service is intended or should be inferred.

sistants become more effective in management of instruments at the chairside, thus helping to increase the productivity of dentistry.

Studies have shown that the dentist and his assistant can provide as much as 60 percent more treatment on patients when they are working effectively as a team than the dentist could working by himself. This is apparent as one examines the teamwork approach described in this chapter. The illustrations will show how the dental assistant is saving the dentist valuable time by having instruments ready for him, thereby eliminating the need to detract his attention from the patient.

One of the factors that has influenced the emphasis upon the full-time use of the dental assistant at the chairside was the 5-year Richmond Study,* in which the individual activities of the dentist and his assistant were catalogued and identified. When all of these activities were analyzed, it was found that the dental assistants actually performed more of the items than the dentist alone, thereby dramatically showing the time saved in the total operation by having the dental assistant lend her two hands to the joint teamwork approach.

Including the seating of the patient, anesthetization, cavity preparation, the restoring of 3 teeth with amalgam, carving the restorations, and dismissal of the patient, the number of activities recorded in the Richmond Study were as follows: dentist, 33; chairside assistant, 57; coordinating assistant, 39. Because twenty-two of the activities of the chairside assistant and the dentist were synonymous (passing and receiving instruments, for example), this figure was reduced to 35 separate and distinct activities performed by the chairside assistant. These tasks could not have been accomplished had the chairside assistant not been constantly at the chairside.* The chairside assistant can be effective only if she is continually at the chairside during treatment and knows all aspects of the treatment involved.

*Public Health Reports, U. S. Department of Health, Education, and Welfare, Public Health Service 67:393, 1962.

*Public Health Reports, U. S. Department of Health, Education, and Welfare, Public Health Service 67:393, 1962.

PRINCIPLES OF CHAIRSIDE ASSISTING

Although the major objective of this chapter is to introduce the basic principles of instrument management, there are a number of factors that contribute to the effectiveness of the dental assistant at the chairside. These factors are the use of prearranged instrument trays; the use and arrangement of equipment that is compatible with "four-handed sit-down dentistry" (see Chapter 8); correct seating of the patient, assistant, and operator; effective delivery of instruments and materials; and basic knowledge by the assistant of steps common to each procedure and the techniques employed by the operator.

Prearranged trays

Stainless steel or plastic instrument trays are often used. The average size of a tray is 12½ by 9½ inches. Instruments required for the preparation and completion of an amalgam restoration can be placed upon a tray of this size. (For discussion of tray preparations for specific procedures see Chapter 6.)

A grooved instrument divider is a strip of metal, plastic, or disposable corrugated paper, 2½ inches wide and the exact length of the tray. The divider helps to keep the instruments in place, and with it they are more easily picked up for delivery. With the narrow side of the tray facing the assistant, the divider should be placed inside of the tray about 3 inches from the left side. If the divider is placed too close to the inside edge, instruments are more difficult to pick up for delivery. Placing the divider in the center creates waste space needed for accessory items, such as burs, matrices, and cotton goods.

Instruments should be placed in sequential order. The end of the instrument used for delivery (the end opposite the working end) should be placed so the junction of the shaft and shank is about one inch away from the left side of the divider, as instruments are picked up at this point. In addition, the instruments should be positioned in relation to the manner they are used by the operator. For example, for an initial oral inspection, the mouth mirror should be delivered to the operator's left hand, and the explorer to his right (assuming the operator is right-handed). Therefore, the mirror is placed upon the tray first, and the handle is to the right of the assistant. The end of the explorer that will be used for delivery is to the left. The mirror will be delivered with the right hand, and the explorer with the left—both at the same time. The left hand of the assistant more conveniently serves the right hand of the operator, and vice versa (see Figs. 7-1 and 7-2).

In most cases, the end of the instrument first used should be placed to the right on the tray, as most hand cutting, condensing, and carving instruments will be picked up with the left hand. The prearranged tray and all required items for the treatment procedure should be placed in the operatory prior to seating the patient.

Seating the patient

Seating the patient comfortably and positioning his head for good visibility and access to the operating field are among the first considerations in the preparation for treatment. This instruction is based on the assumption that a contour or lounge chair is used. This type of chair is comfortable for the patient, and it has the features that permit the assistant and operator to work from seated positions.

Before inviting the patient into the operatory, the assistant should be certain that the prearranged tray and all other materials required are complete and in order. The drape should be folded over the chairback, which has been placed upright. The chair should be lowered to a level that permits the patient to be seated normally.

As the patient is seated and draped, the assistant should inform him that he will be placed in a reclining position for his comfort. The chairback is then slowly lowered, using the appropriate chair switch for this purpose. For treating the mandibular quadrants, the chairback should be lowered until it reaches a 25- to 30-degree angle. For treatment of maxillary quadrants, the chairback is lowered until it is horizontal, or parallel to the floor. The cushion- or cradle-type headrest should be placed near the operator's side of the chair and in a position so the top of the patient's head is as close as possible to the upper edge of the chairback.

The height of the chair is adjusted after the operator is seated. However, the chair should be elevated sufficiently to permit the operator to be seated without it being priorly elevated. When the treatment plan for the appointment is completed, the assistant should elevate the chairback slowly to an upright position. Do not elevate the chairback too quickly.

Operating position for the assistant

In discussing seated operating positions for the assistant and dentist, "the clock" is often used as a point of reference. For purposes of this chapter, the mouth of the patient is the center of the clock. Looking at the face of the patient, the top of his head is referred to as 12 o'clock, and the area beneath the chin is 6 o'clock. The area at the left side of the patient is described as between 1 and 6 o'clock, and the area to the patient's right is 6 to 12 o'clock. An imaginary line drawn from the eyes of the operator or the assistant to the mouth of the patient forms the hands of the clock.

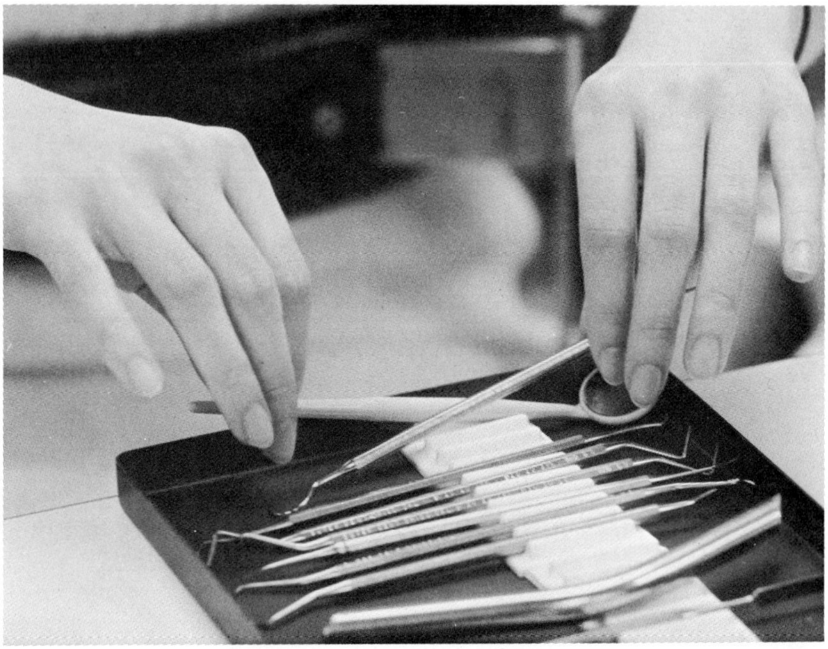

Fig. 7-1. The position of the mouth mirror, explorer, and other instruments on the tray for effective delivery to the operator for initial inspection. The handle of the mirror has been placed for pick-up and immediate delivery to the left hand of the operator. The explorer is placed for delivery to the operator's right hand. A modified pen grasp is used to pick up the instruments from the tray. (Courtesy University of Maryland School of Dentistry.)

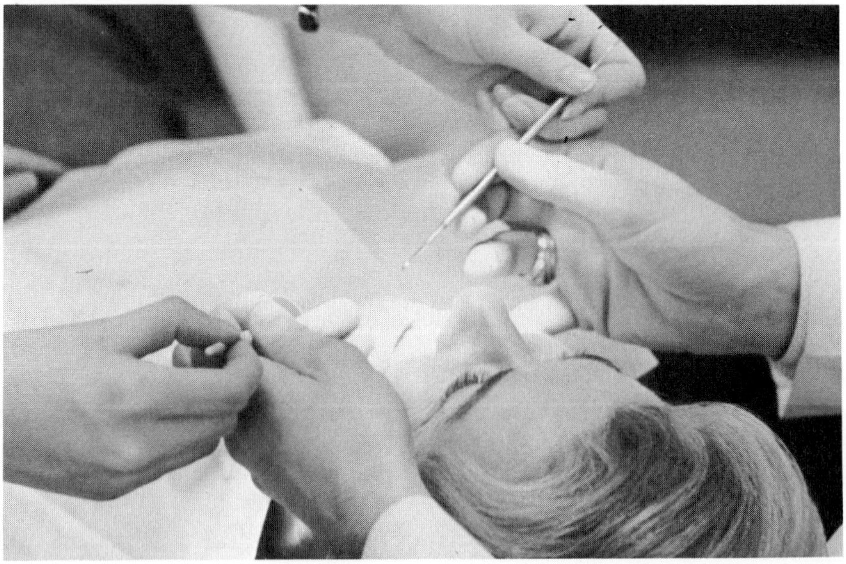

Fig. 7-2. The mirror and explorer are placed firmly between the thumb and index fingers of the operator's left and right hands, respectively. The working end of the explorer is directed upward for inspection of maxillary teeth. The modified pen grasp is adjusted to pen grasp for delivery. (Courtesy University of Maryland School of Dentistry.)

For the operator, the "time" will always be between 6 and 12 o'clock, and for the assistant, 1 to 6 o'clock. (This discussion has described procedure for a right-handed dentist and assistant.)

The assistant's seated position should be at the left of the chair, between 3 and 4 o'clock. Even if the operator varies his seated position, good visibility can be achieved from this position. The left femur (thigh) should be nearly parallel with the left side of the chairback. The body-support arm of the assistant's operating stool should be brought around from the left side and adjusted to a position just below the rib cage.

The assistant should then pull the mobile cabinet (with sliding top), instrument stand, or cart forward. A position similar to that used for typewriting should be assumed.

The operating light and height of the assistant's chair are adjusted after the operator is seated.

Operating position for the dentist

The operator's chair is adjusted so that when he is seated, his thighs are parallel to the floor. If the operator works by the "indirect" method (using a mirror), he will usually sit at the 11 o'clock position. The 8 to 9 o'clock position is used for working by the "direct" method. After the desired operating position is selected, the operator should lower the dental chair so the chairback nearly touches his knees. This places the patient in desirable operating position.

The assistant then directs the operating light to the patient's mouth and makes the required adjustment of the operating stool. The assistant's eye level should be about 4 inches above that of the operator. This height permits the assistant to see the operation and to quickly observe the signals of the operator (see Fig. 7-3).

Instrument grasp

To properly deliver instruments to the hand of dentist, the assistant should know the instrument grasps. Operators use 5 principal instrument grasps. They are described as follows:

1. Pen grasp. Held like a pen, the instrument is grasped with the thumb and first and second fingers at the junction of the shaft and shank; some operators may wish to grasp the instrument higher on the shaft. This grasp is most often used for instruments having an angled shank, blade, or nib. Some operators use the pen grasp on straight-shanked instruments as well. Dental assistants should be aware that these variations in technique exist among operators.
2. Reverse pen grasp. This grasp is identical to the pen grasp, except the working point is toward, rather than away from, the operator.
3. Palm grasp. This grasp is done by grasping the handle of the instrument in the palm of the hand. It is used with surgery and other types of forceps.
4. Palm-thumb grasp. In this grasp, often called the "whittling" grasp, the handle is placed in the palm of the hand and grasped by 4 fingers. The thumb is used as a rest or is placed at the junction of the shaft and shank. This grasp is used with instruments having a straight shank and blade, such as the straight or Wedelstaedt chisels.
5. Palm-thrust grasp. Similar to the palm grasp, in this grasp the end of the large handle is held in the center of the palm. No rest is utilized. This grasp is not often used.

Rests and guards

The dentist will often place the third or fourth finger of the hand grasping the instrument on an adjacent tooth. Called rests, these actions help control and steady the action of the instrument.

Guards are used by applying the thumb and first finger of the opposite hand around the site of operation. Guards protect the operating field from accidental slipping of

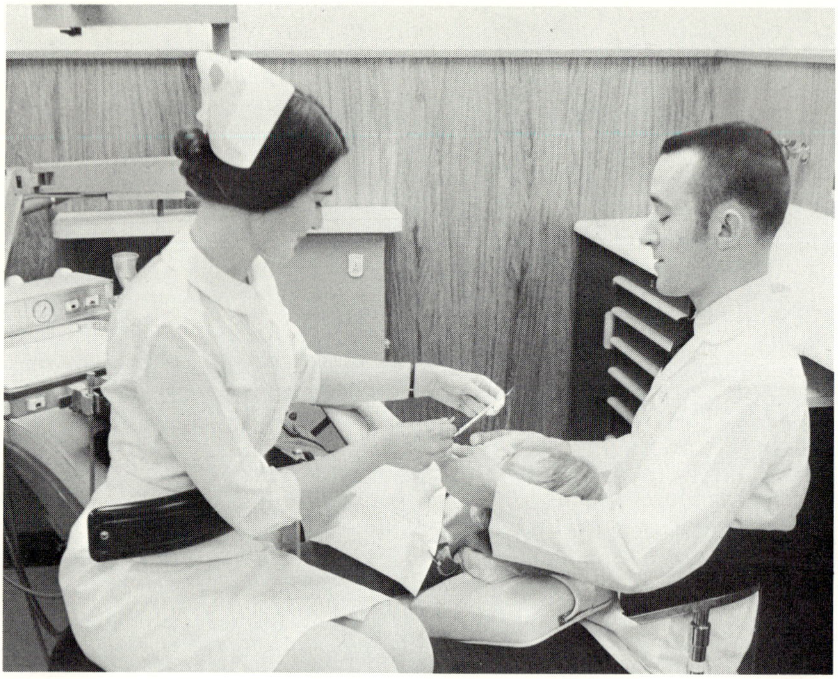

Fig. 7-3. The relative positions of the patient, operator, and assistant. The operator utilizes the "indirect method" for treating mandibular quadrants. The operator is seated at approximately the 11 o'clock position. The assistant is seated at about the 3:30 o'clock position. Both operator and assistant achieve maximum visibility seated in these positions. (Courtesy University of Maryland School of Dentistry.)

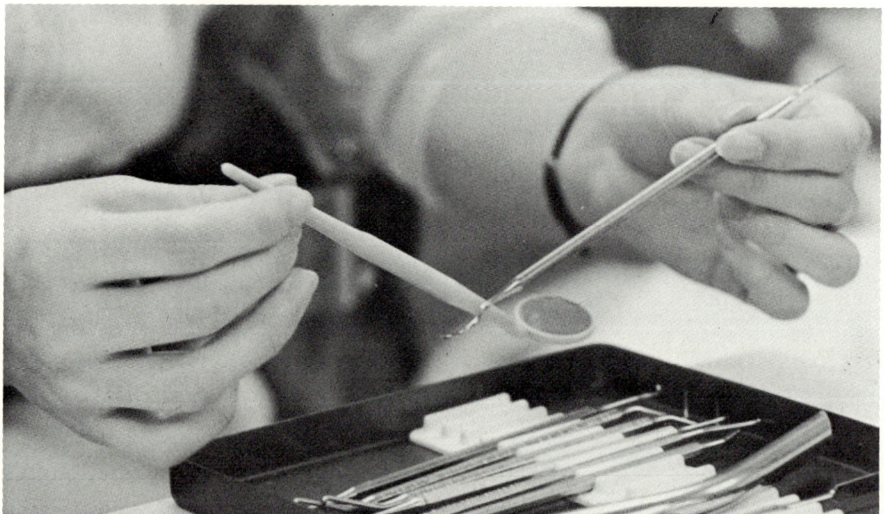

Fig. 7-4. The modified pen grasp is used for picking up instruments from the tray. By slightly relaxing the grasp, the instrument can be placed in pen grasp position for delivery, as shown in Fig. 7-1. (Courtesy University of Maryland School of Dentistry.)

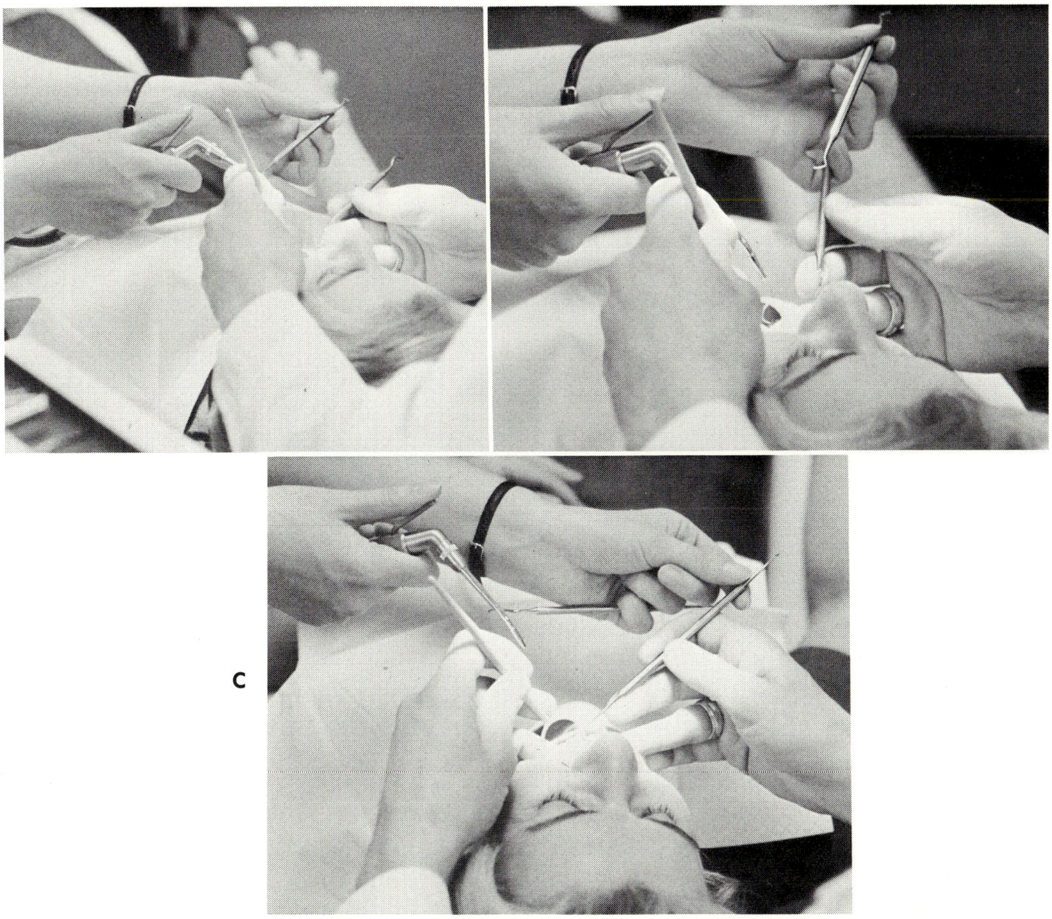

Fig. 7-5. **A,** The instrument is held in the left hand, using a reverse modified pen grasp, paralled to the instrument to be received from the operator; **B,** the instrument is retrieved from the operator by grasping the free end with the small finger of the left hand; **C,** the retrieved instrument is carried away from the operating zone by closing the middle, third, and small fingers toward the thumb. The new instrument is delivered to operating position. (Courtesy University of Maryland School of Dentistry.)

an instrument and possible injury to the patient.

The dental assistant should be aware of the rests and guards used by the operator, so that when assisting, she does not interfere with this part of the operating procedure.

Instrument exchange

A zone of exchange, sometimes called "transfer zone," should be established between the operator and assistant. This zone should be relatively close to the operating field and should involve only a minimum of forearm movements by the operator.

Delivery of pen-grasp instruments

The assistant uses a modified pen grasp for picking up most instruments from the tray (see Fig. 7-4). A point on the shaft, just below the junction of the shaft and shank of the end opposite the working end

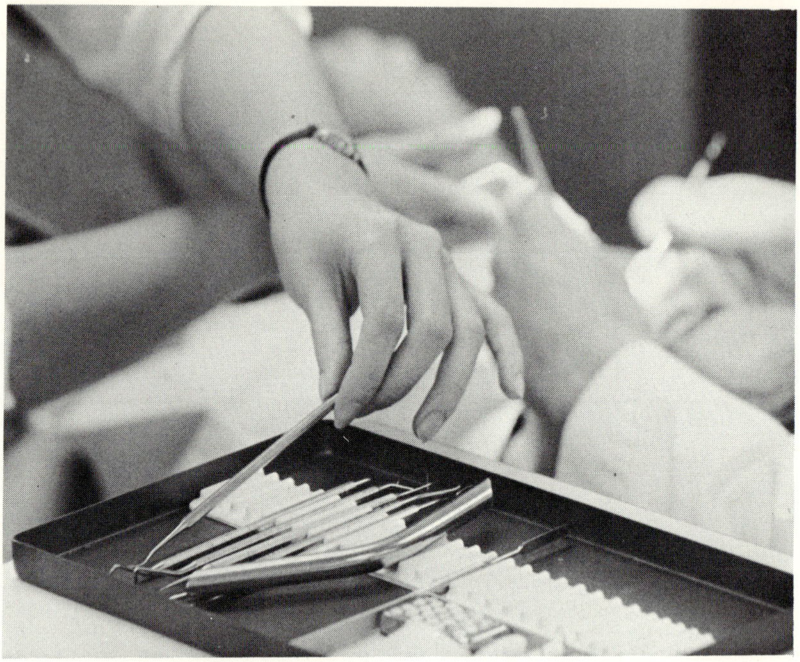

Fig. 7-6. Instruments are returned to the tray in the same relative position. (Courtesy University of Maryland School of Dentistry.)

A

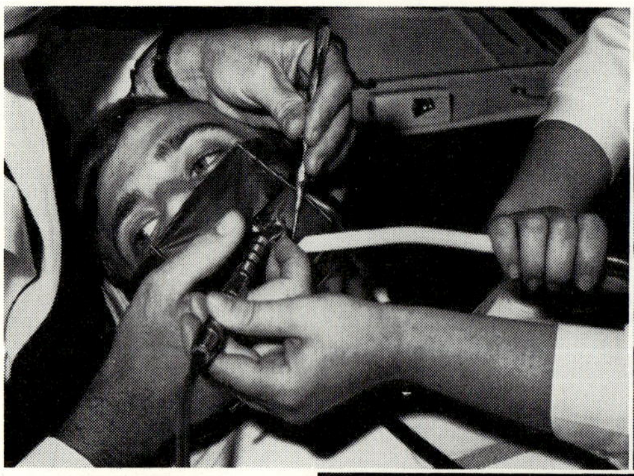

B

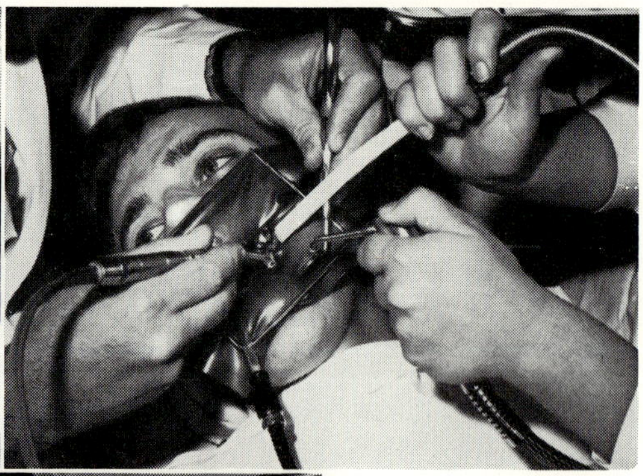

C

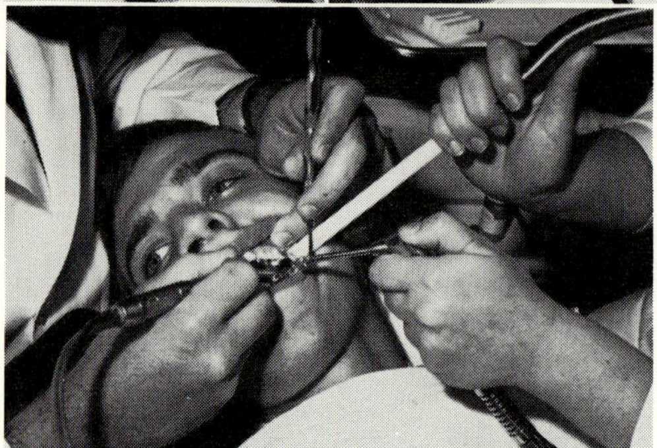

Fig. 7-7. Cavity preparation. **A,** Dentist receives air-turbine handpiece from assistant, who holds oral evacuator in right hand with palm-thumb grasp; **B,** four-handed dentistry in correct position for cutting procedure—with rubber dam in place; **C,** four hands at work for cavity preparation without a rubber dam. (Courtesy University of Tennessee College of Dentistry.)

A

B

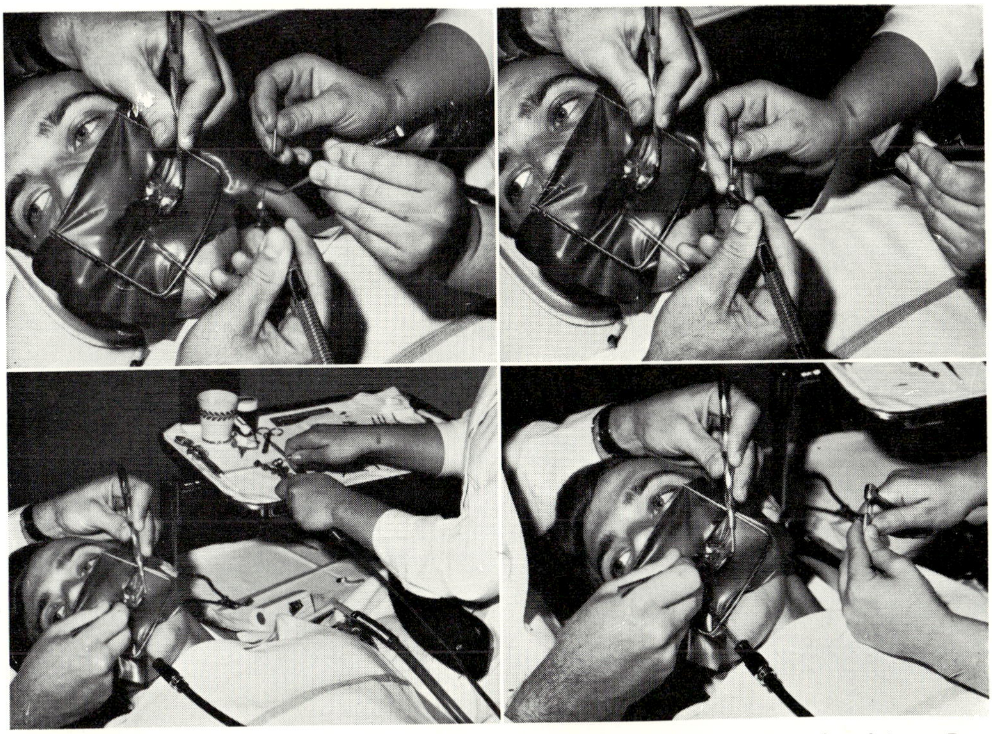

C

D

Fig. 7-8. Bur change. A, Assistant removing bur from conventional type handpiece; B, assistant placing bur in conventional type handpiece; C, assistant removing bur from air-turbine handpiece; D, assistant placing bur in air-turbine handpiece. (Courtesy University of Tennessee College of Dentistry.)

of hand cutting, condensing, and carving instruments, is recommended for delivery of pen-grasp instruments. Deliver pen-grasp instruments with the blade or nib facing downward for treating mandibular teeth. Place the instrument between the operator's thumb and index finger near the junction of the shaft and shank, wherever he has identified as his preference (see Fig. 7-5, A).

Delivery for the reverse pen grasp is made exactly the same as the pen grasp, except that the blade or nib is directed upward.

Release the instrument as soon as it is firmly grasped by the operator.

Delivery of palm-thumb-grasp instruments

Palm-thumb-grasp instruments should be picked up with the thumb and forefinger of the left hand on the shank, about one-fourth of the way from the blade. The instrument should be in the operator's palm so his thumb will contact the junction of the shaft and shank of the instrument.

Delivery of palm and palm-thrust instruments

These instruments should be picked up with the left hand about one-fourth of the way from the working end. Place the instrument in the palm of the operator's hand. The working point should be directed toward the site of operation. If a lower tooth is involved, the working point is directed downward; for upper teeth, the working point is upward.

Delivery of palm-grasp instruments

These instruments, mainly forceps, should be delivered into the operator's open

A B C D E F G H

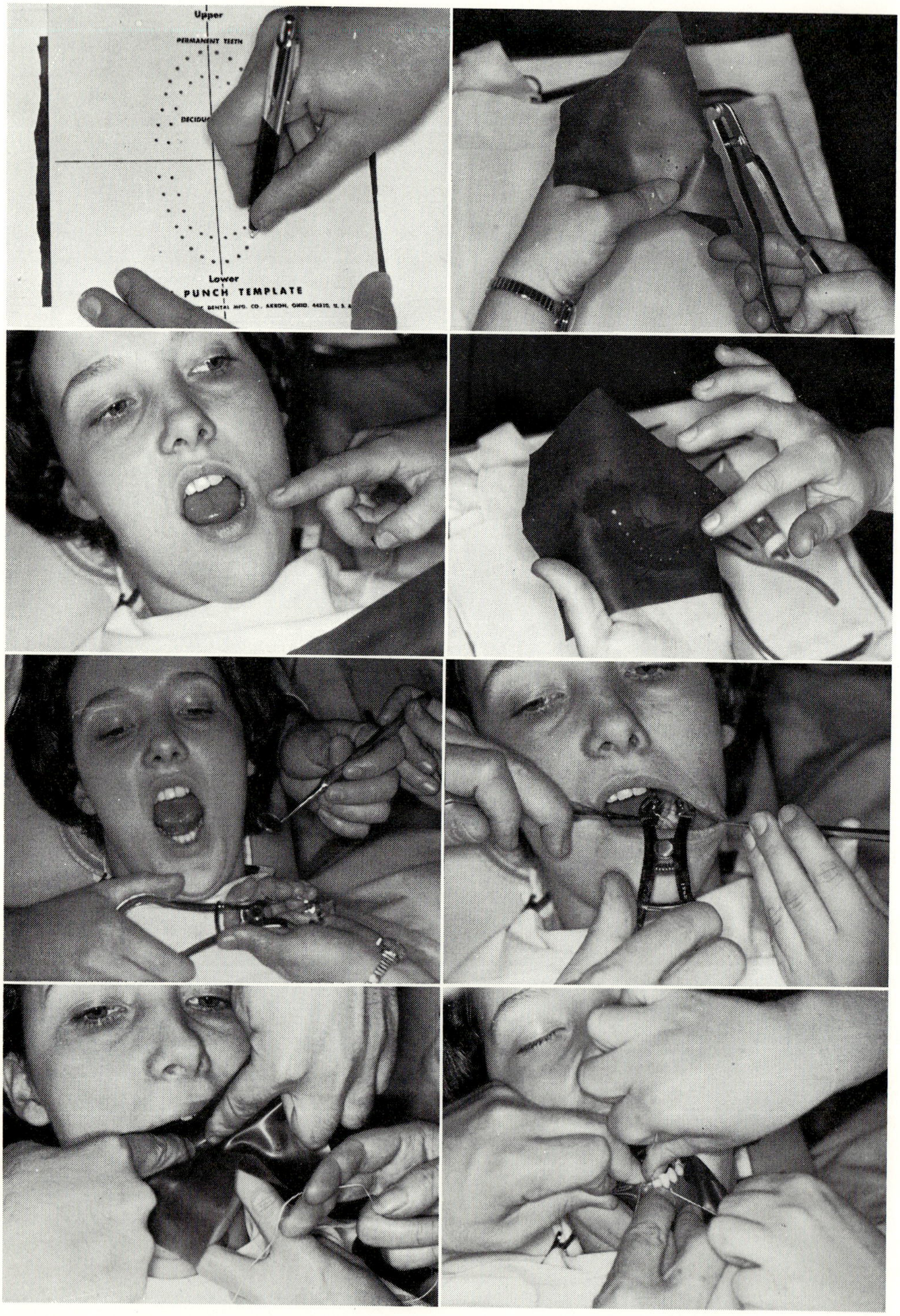

Fig. 7-9. For legend see opposite page.

I J

K L

M

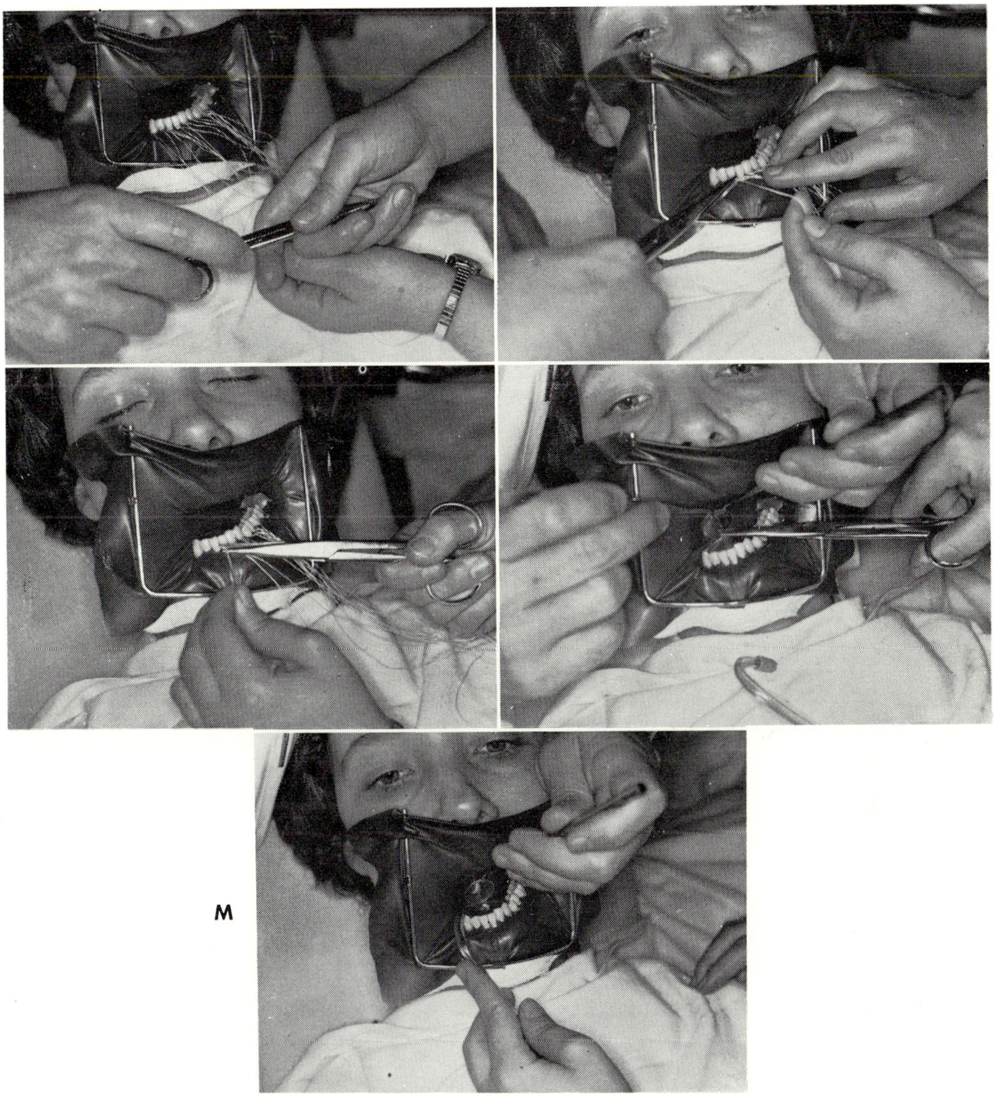

Fig. 7-9. Utilizing the dental assistant in application of the rubber dam. **A,** Use of template to mark dam; **B,** assistant using rubber-dam punch; **C,** assistant lubricates patient's lips; **D,** assistant lubricates dam; **E,** assistant passes clamp holder with clamp to dentist and receives mouth mirror; **F,** dentist places rubber dam on second molar while assistant retracts cheek; **G,** dentist places dam while assistant holds floss in ready position; **H,** assistant passes floss through contacts as dentist positions dam; **I,** assistant passes scissors to dentist to cut ligature; **J,** assistant holds ligature while dentist cuts ligature; **K,** assistant cuts ligature; **L,** dentist holds dam with cotton pliers and assistant cuts small aperture in dam for positioning of saliva ejector; **M,** assistant positions saliva ejector. (Courtesy University of Tennessee College of Dentistry.)

A B C D E F G H

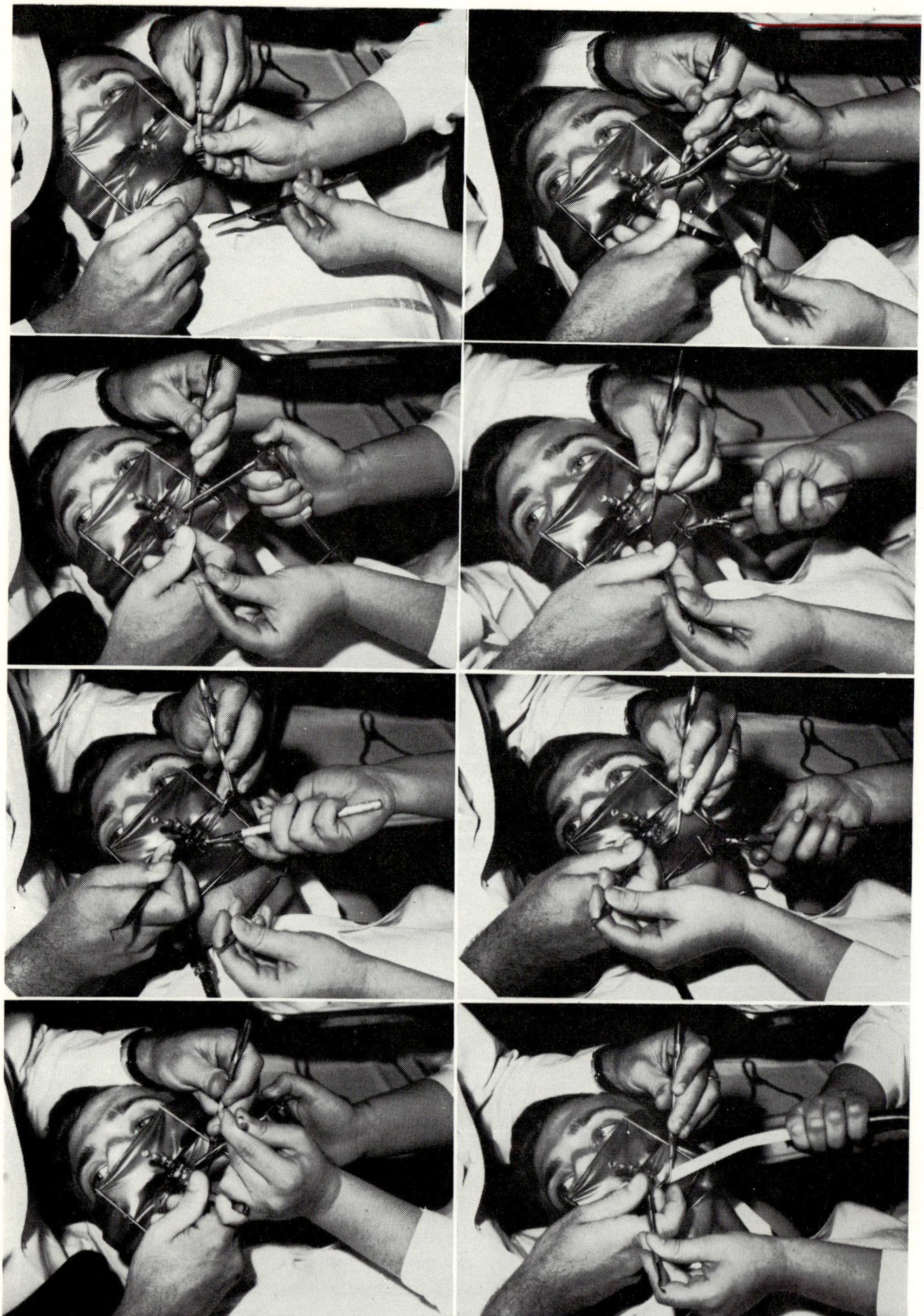

Fig. 7-10. For legend see opposite page.

palm facing upward and with the beaks of the instrument directed upward for use on maxillary teeth. Delivery for use on mandibular teeth is made into the operator's open palm facing downward and with the beaks also directed downward, or toward the position in which the instrument will be used.

Scissors and hemostats should be picked up at the blades or beaks. The loops on the handles are delivered toward the thumb and index or third finger of the operator. These instruments are retrieved as they are delivered—grasped at the blade or beak. Receiving them in the palm creates the need for repositioning for correct placement on the tray.

Receiving instruments from the operator

Unless the operator expects a new instrument immediately, the used instrument may be received in the left hand of the assistant, using a modified pen grasp.

If a new instrument is immediately required, it is held in a modified pen grasp, parallel to the instrument to be replaced. The small finger is extended, and the instrument is retrieved by grasping it an inch or so below the junction of the shaft and shank, opposite the working end just used. When the assistant has firmly grasped the instrument in the crook of the small finger, the operator releases the instrument. The assistant then guides the instrument back toward the palm of the hand, away from the zone of exchange. At the same time, the new instrument is delivered (see Fig. 7-5, *A* to *C*). This method frees the right hand for retracting, evacuating, and other chairside tasks.

All instruments should be returned to the tray to the same space from which they were taken. If instruments are needed a second time, a search will not be required, and an orderly tray can be maintained.

Fig. 7-10. Passing of instruments in amalgam restoration utilizing a rubber dam. **A,** Dentist receives matrix retainer from assistant, who also holds cotton tweezers with wedge in left hand at ready position (inverted pen grasp); **B,** dentist places wedge while assistant holds matrix burnisher with pen grasp for instrument exchange and utilizes her right hand to operate syringe; **C,** assistant places matrix burnisher in hand of dentist, who uses pen grasp; **D,** dentist receives condenser in pen grasp position from assistant also utilizing a pen grasp; assistant with right hand is using modified palm grasp to place amalgam in cavity preparation; **E,** assistant places amalgam in cavity preparation with right hand while holding second condenser as the dentist uses #1-0 condenser in left hand; **F,** Dentist receives #2-0 condenser in pen grasp position from assistant, who has received #1-0 condenser with little finger of left hand; assistant's right hand holds amalgam carrier ready for placement insertion; **G,** dentist receives instruments from assistant for removal of wedges and matrix retainer; **H,** dentist receives amalgam carver from assistant in pen grasp position, after assistant has removed #2-0 condenser from dentist with little finger of the left hand; assistant's right hand holds evacuator in palm-thumb grasp to clear field of operation. (Courtesy University of Tennessee College of Dentistry.)

CHAPTER 8 SELECTING SUITABLE OFFICE EQUIPMENT

CHARLES O. CRANFORD, D.D.S.

SHAILER PETERSON, B.A., M.A., Ph.D.

Every dental student looks forward to the time when he will own his first dental office. Every dental assistant looks forward to the time when she can help in the selection of the equipment she will use and in its arrangement in the office. Today the dentist and his dental assistant can select equipment and gadgetry from a large number of different manufacturers and suppliers. They can choose from a variety of sizes, designs, colors, and shapes, and create a customized and personalized office that will suit their needs and wishes.

Many of today's dentists will not remember that it was only about ten years ago that there were just a few manufacturers of dental chairs and dental units, and that the available equipment that one could choose was all very similar. The different models may as well have all been poured out of the same mold, for they all looked and performed pretty much alike. It used to be that the dentist chose his equipment much like he selected his household refrigerator or his television set. He could choose between different manufacturers and the reputations that they had earned, but basically all refrigerators had about the same selection of sizes and shapes, and all performed the same task with the same speed and reliability. Similarly, all television sets looked a lot alike, used interchangeable tubes, and had the same number and kind of adjustments and controls.

In the last 10 years, dentists have begun to insist that the manufacturers provide equipment that is designed for the comfort and efficiency of the dentist and his chairside assistant. The dentist now wants to choose his equipment like he plans and designs the den or office in the home he is building, selects his favorite hunting or fishing equipment, and selects the color and design of the clothes he wears.

About 1957, dental schools began to teach the dental student to work efficiently and thereby increase the amount of dental service he could deliver. The student was taught that he must be assisted at the dental chair by a competent chairside assistant who could provide him with an extra pair of hands. He was taught that he could operate in a seated position and, not only perform more work each day, but he could finish the day less fatigued. The school experience taught him that the more jumping up and down he did while practicing and the more movement that was required of his whole body, the more fatigued he would become during the day, and the shorter his life span was likely to be.

The dental assistant was taught that

her extra pair of hands at the chair could be her contribution to the success of the dental office. She learned that equipment was now available that could be adapted to the teamwork that she and her doctor has worked out. She learned that she could select equipment that could be adapted to her needs and to those of her dentist, and that it was not necessary for her to be a slave to the equipment and machinery.

The dental assistant observed that she and the dentist had become accustomed to operate at the chair differently than the dentist and his assistant in the neighboring office. They had developed individuality in their approach to the patient. She observed that a personalized office for a dentist and his team employs equipment that had been selected with their particular needs in mind, and an office design that suits one team may be awkward for another. This meant that the dentist and his assistant needed to analyze how they could best work cooperatively in the office, what kinds of equipment could best serve their methods, and how this equipment could be arranged and located in the office so that it was within easy reach.

When there was little selection available, many dentists became inventors and designers of their own customized equipment. Now the manufacturers have also made a study of the preferences and needs of the dentist and his chairside assistant. Companies have been guided by the dental schools that have been teaching dental students to function as a four-handed team. Therefore, today a dentist and his assistant can select from many kinds and styles of equipment.

The photographs in Fig. 8-1 show dentists and their assistants walking through the aisles of exhibits by commercial manufacturers at 2 annual sessions of the American Dental Association. There are many occasions when the manufacturers exhibit and demonstrate their equipment, such as at the Chicago midwinter meeting in February, the Greater New York meeting in December, and the annual American Dental Association session in October. In addition, many of the dental supply houses in the larger cities will maintain show rooms and displays of some of the equipment which they sell, and they have catalogs and illustrations of all of the available equipment. About 26,000 dentists and their auxiliary personnel attend a typical annual American Dental Association session; about 350 different manufacturers, importers, and suppliers exhibit and demonstrate their equipment at such an annual session. Just as a dentist goes to a boat show or to an automobile show, he and his dental assistant need to attend these exhibits of dental manufacturers and suppliers, so that they can keep their dental office practices efficient and up-to-date.

There are many reasons why a dental assistant and her dentist should be encouraged to examine all new pieces of equipment that are available through the local dealers or at the various regional and national meetings. Some of these reasons are as follows:

1. To learn about the function and use of the instrument or equipment.
2. To learn what factors need to be considered in selecting equipment.
3. To learn how different pieces of equipment relate to one another.
4. To learn how other members of the dental health team make use of the equipment.

The level of proficiency of the dental health team can be at its best only if the following conditions are met:

1. The equipment is properly designed.
2. The operator learns how to use the equipment correctly and efficiently.
3. The equipment is compatible with the other associated or related equipment.
4. The equipment is adjusted to operate in the manner the manufacturer intended.

A

B

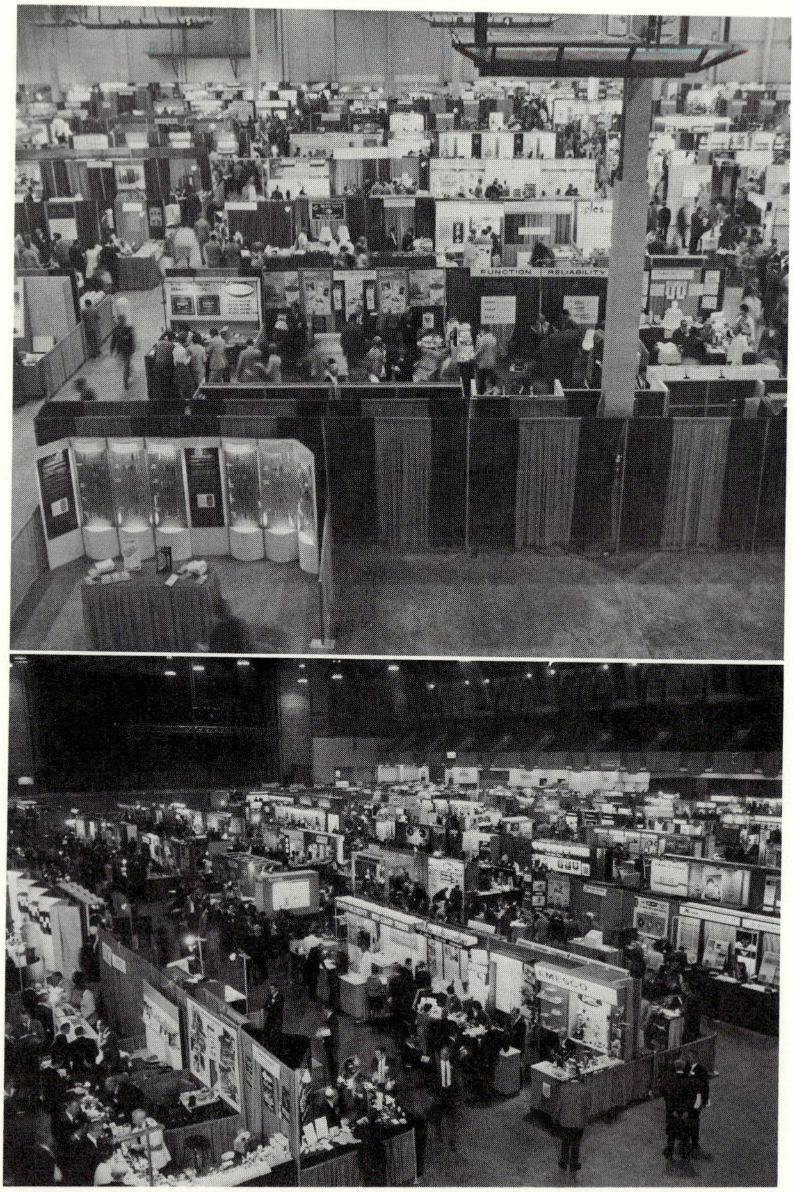

Fig. 8-1. American Dental Association conventions. **A,** 1968 Miami Beach convention; **B,** 1963 Atlantic City convention.

5. The equipment is properly cared for through a preventive maintenance program.
6. The equipment is placed or positioned so that it is convenient for the operator or operators to use.

BASIC OPERATORY EQUIPMENT

The dental unit

Dental units vary a great deal, from traditional to modern design. For many years, they were manufactured with essentially the same basic design, but within the

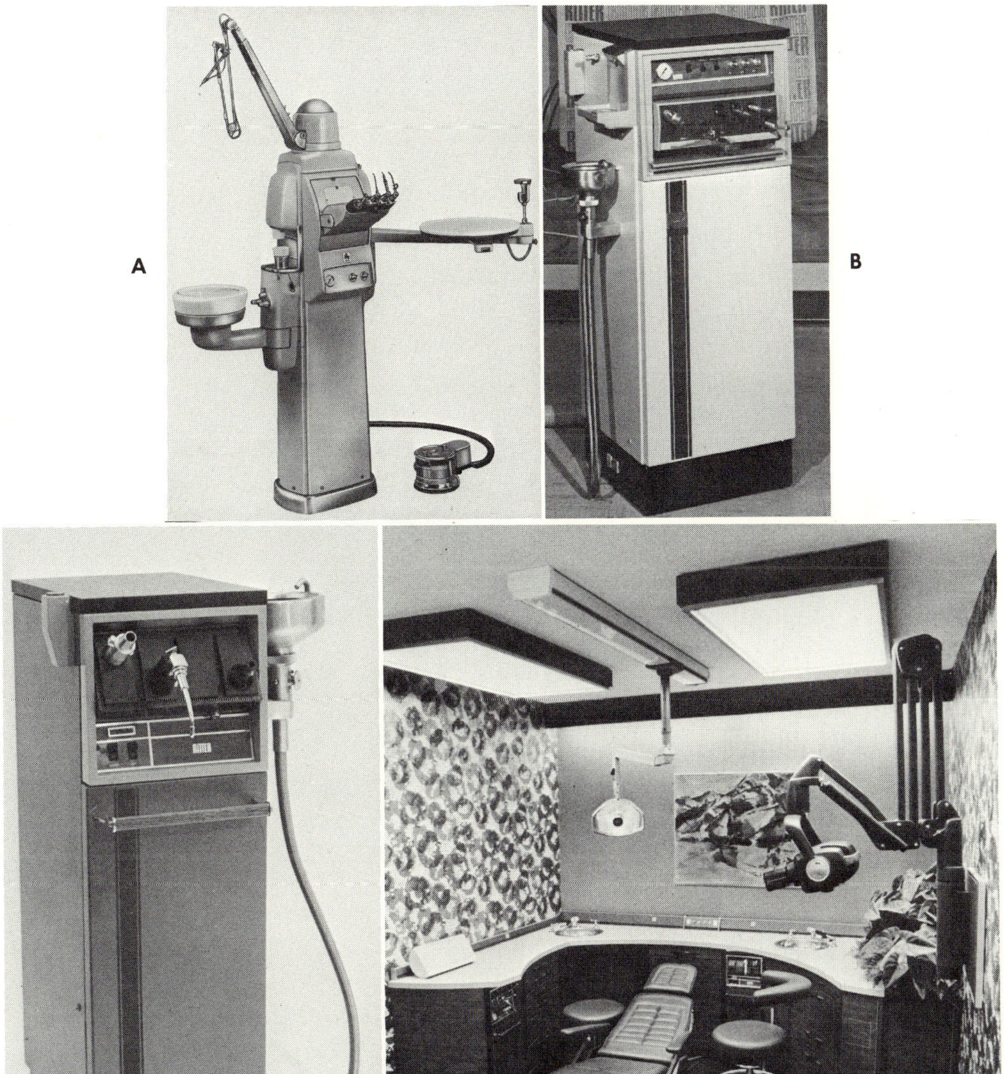

Fig. 8-2. Dental units. **A,** Ritter J2A Unit; **B,** Ritter Orbiter Unit I; **C,** Ritter Orbiter Unit II; **D,** Ritter Sigma Modular Unit; **E,** Pelton & Crane Executive Unit; **F,** A-dec Mobile Unit; **G,** A-dec Chair-Mounted Unit; **H,** Valtronic King-Air I, *left,* and Queen-Air I Mobile, *right,* Dental Units; **I,** Valtronic Total I ("closed") Modular Dental Unit; **J,** Coastal Chair-Mounted Dental Unit; **K,** Weber Unit; **L,** Weber Unit; **M,** Dentsply Spectrum I and II; **N,** Dentsply Spectrum Console; **O,** Dentsply Trimodular Control System. (H and I Courtesy The Valtronic Corp.)

E F G H

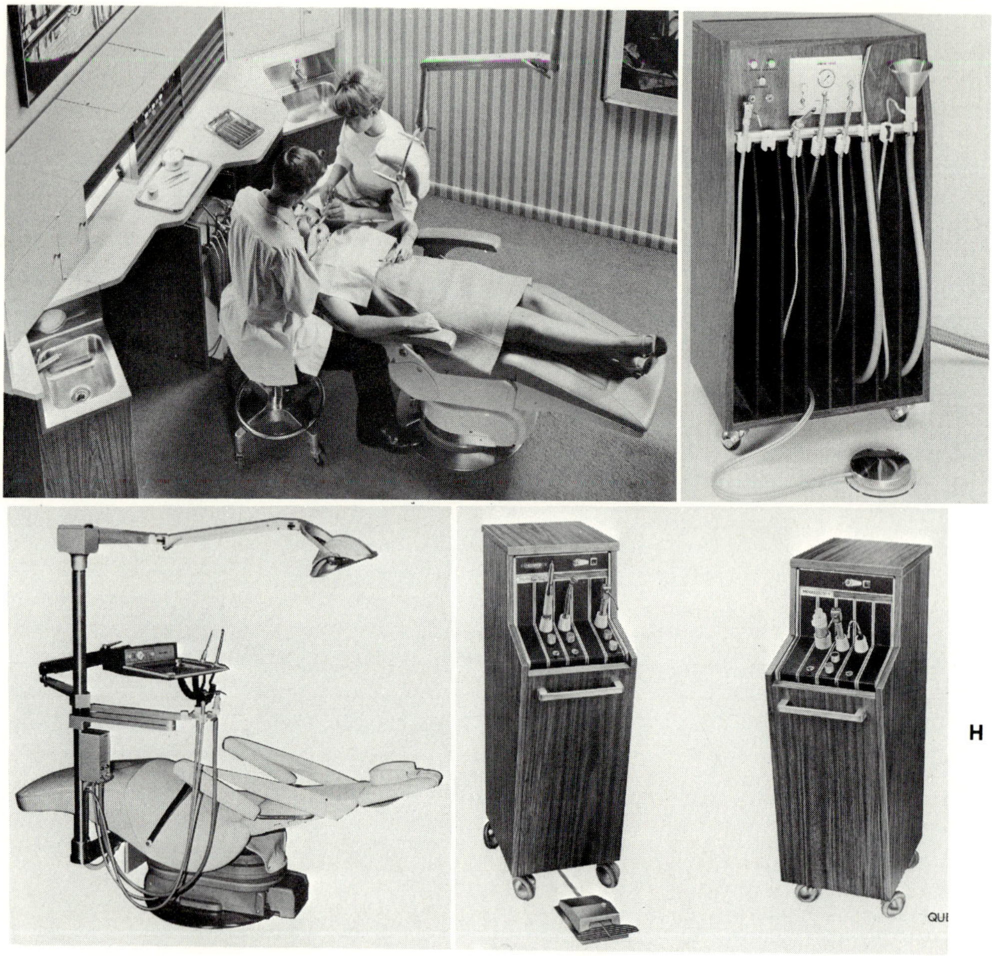

Fig. 8-2, cont'd. For legend see p. 161.

last few years, there have been many innovations in the style of the dental unit. Until recently, the dental operatory was designed around a stationary, or "fixed," dental unit, and the unit was considered by many to be the center or core of operation within the operatory. Now this concept is giving way to one in which the patient is the core of operation. This new concept requires that all elements of the operatory be designed to deliver essential equipment to a working zone around the patient's mouth.

There is a variety of dental units to choose from, as illustrated in Fig. 8-2. They may be fixed or mobile, attached to the dental chair or concealed in a cabinet, and containing fully retractable hoses and cords or featuring simple, free-hanging cord and hose-attached instruments. Despite these differences in design, they generally have one common feature; they are smaller and more compact than the old stationary and more traditional dental unit. Even though there is a variety of styles of modern dental units, most units can be classified in one of the following general categories, based on the relationship of the unit to the operating zone:

I

J

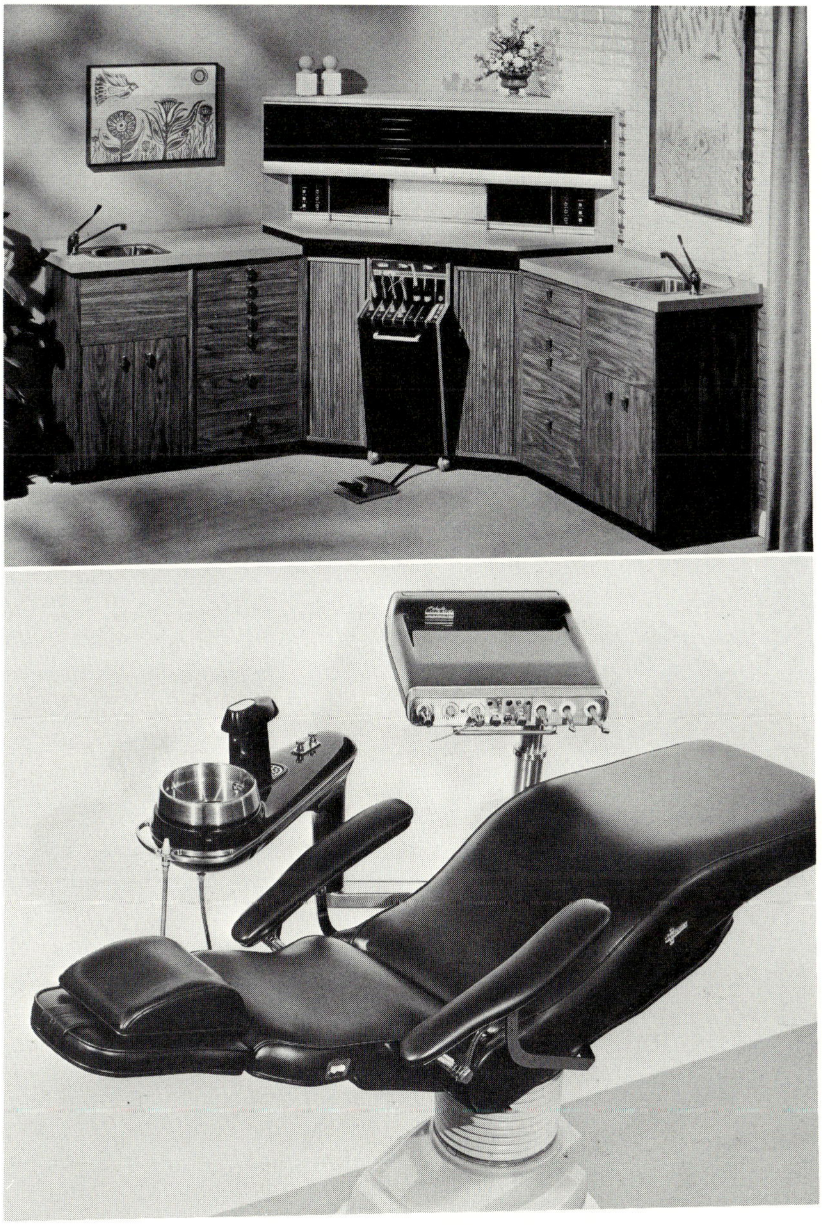

Fig. 8-2, cont'd. For legend see p. 161.

1. Posterior presentation, fixed.
2. Posterior presentation, mobile.
3. Side presentation, fixed.
4. Side presentation, mobile.
5. Frontal presentation.

The dental chair

The dental chair has a dual purpose to perform. It provides support for the patient and positions the patient in a manner to facilitate the performance of den-

K

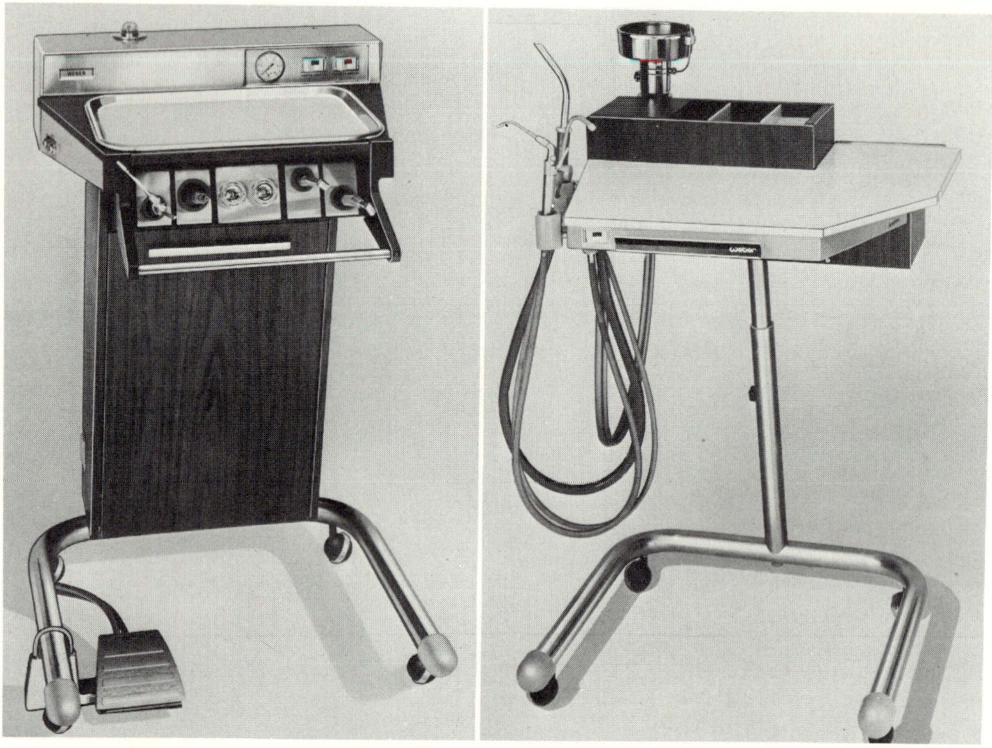

L

Fig. 8-2, cont'd. For legend see p. 161.

tal procedures. The chair may be motor-driven, manually operated, or a combination of the two.

Modern practice methods have spurred development of the so-called contour chair. As the name implies, this chair is intended to fit the contour of the patient's body and provide the optimum of comfort to the patient, while positioning him for the dentist's convenience. This style of chair is rapidly being accepted by the dental profession. In spite of this acceptance, because the contour chair was only developed in the past 10 years, many conventional chairs will still be found in dental offices. The conventional chair may be completely manually operated. This means that the adjustments on the chair are all done by hand, and the chair is raised and lowered by means of a foot-operated hydraulic pump. Other conventional chairs will have been improved by adding an electric motor to raise and lower the chair, thus eliminating the foot-pump operation. A large number of the latter type are still in use in dental offices.

Several special features may be found on contour chairs. These features include:

1. A floor track system for backward and forward movement of the chair.
2. An air-glide base, on which the chair can be moved on a cushion of air, permitting free movement in any direction.
3. Special cushions for the head or adjustable head supports.
4. A sideways-tilting chair for enhancing access during certain operations.

Earlier models of conventional chairs were sparsely padded and usually featured leather-covered cushions. By contrast, today's modern contour chair is well padded and

M

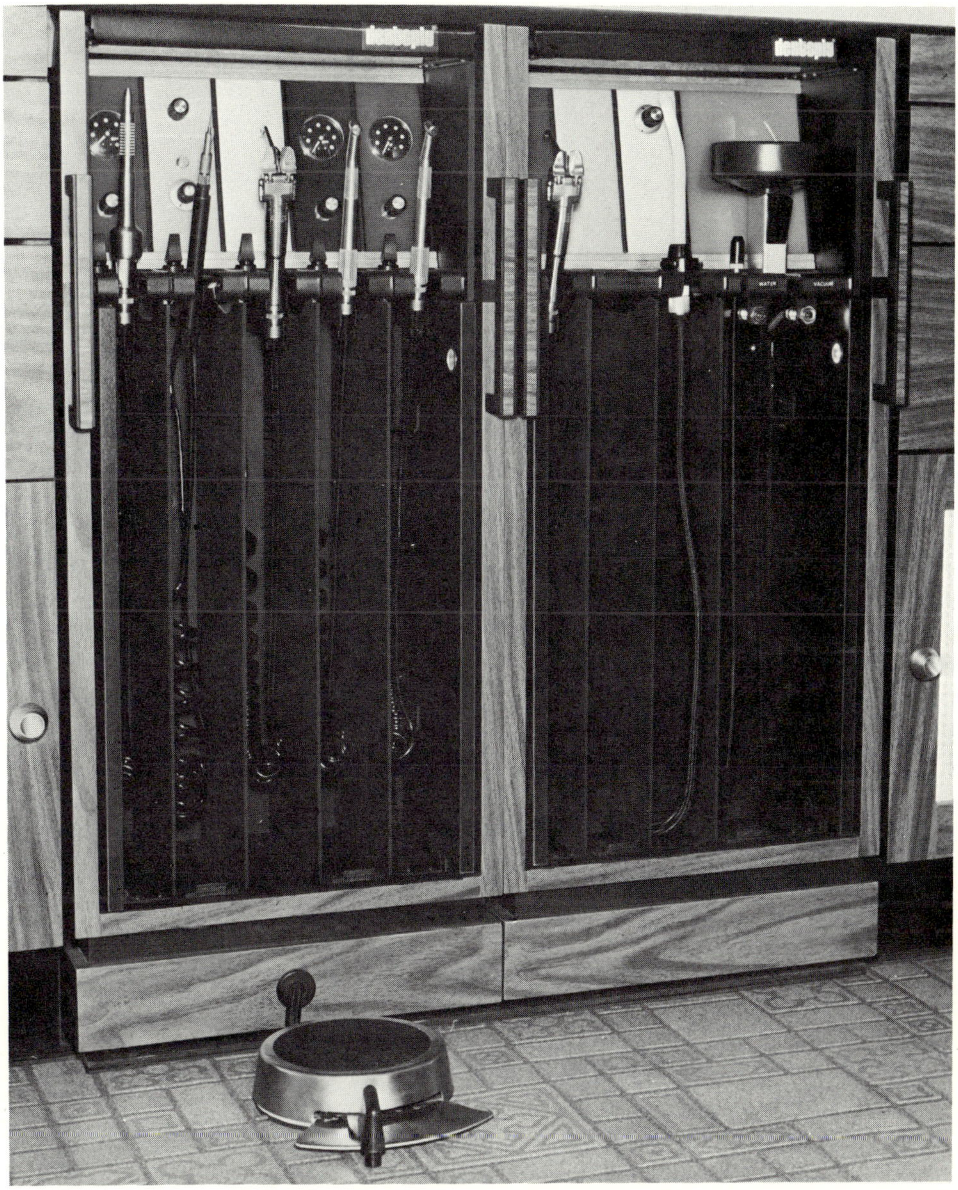

Fig. 8-2, cont'd. For legend see p. 161.

usually covered with vinyl or a combination of nylon and vinyl. Several examples of dental chairs are presented in Fig. 8-3.

The operatory stool

It is generally accepted that the use of stools by the dentist and the assistant will reduce physical fatigue during the day. Moreover, it is believed to add years to the productive life of the dental team. Several kinds of stools are found in the dental office. They include the nonmobile pedestal stool, the semimobile stool attached to the dental chair base, the standard secretarial

N

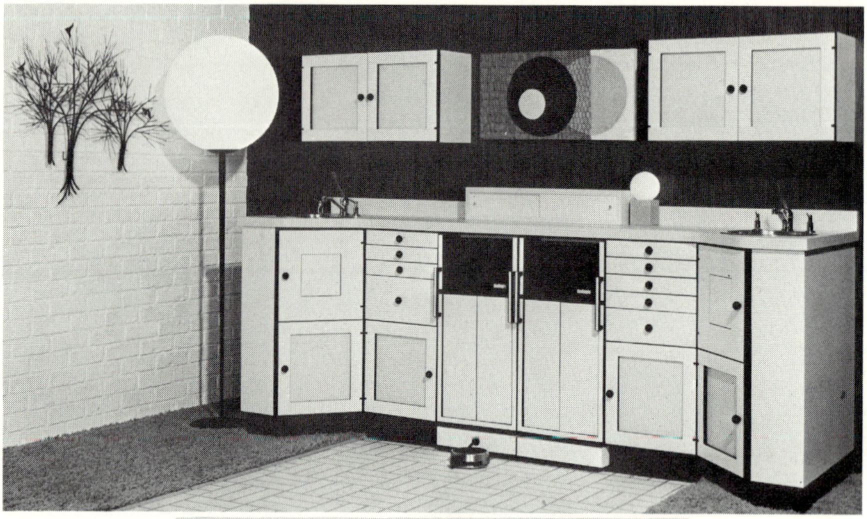

O

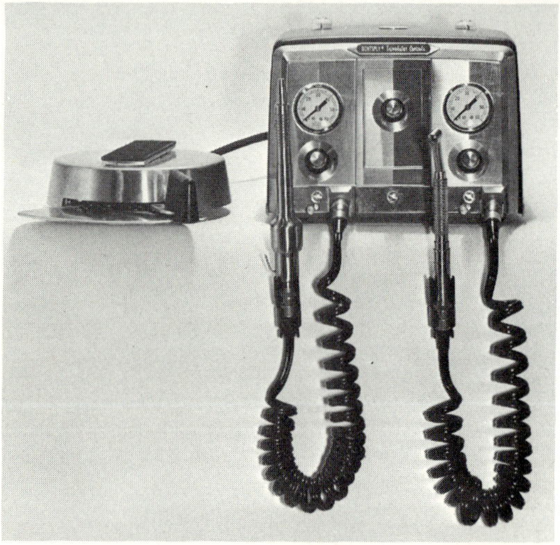

Fig. 8-2, cont'd. For legend see p. 161.

stool, and the mobile, fully adjustable, contoured stool. The nonmobile pedestal stool is mounted on a weighted fixed base, and limited movement of the seat is obtained by rotation of a ball-and-socket joint between the base and the seat pedestal. The semimobile stool, secured by the base of the dental chair, may be single or dual and can be moved around the chair through a combination of arms, posts, and joints. The fully adjustable mobile stool moves on 3, 4, or 5 swivel casters; its height is adjustable, and it is the most versatile of the stools mentioned. Examples of dental stools are presented in Fig. 8-4.

The oral evacuation unit

The introduction of the high-speed handpiece and use of water to cool the tooth while operating demanded the development of an efficient oral evacuating system. Up until that time, the saliva ejector found on the basic traditional dental unit was quite adequate. The use of high-speed

Text continued on p. 172.

A

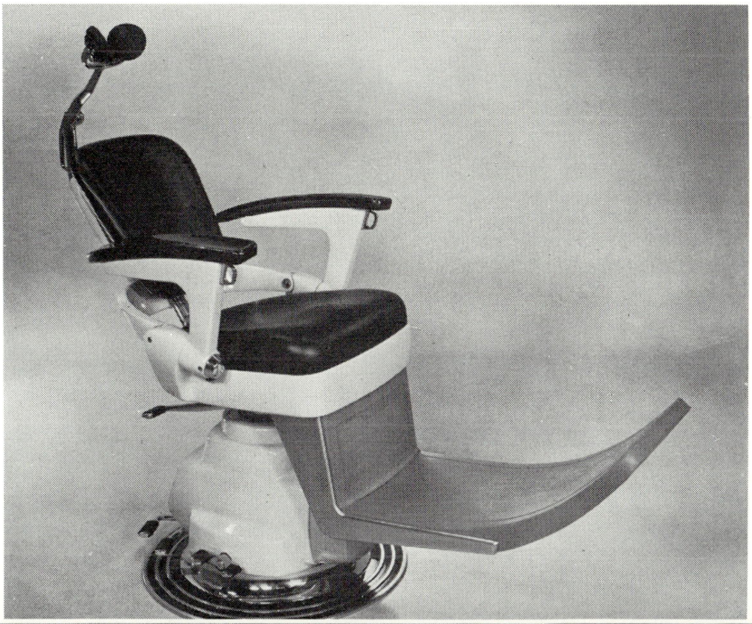

B

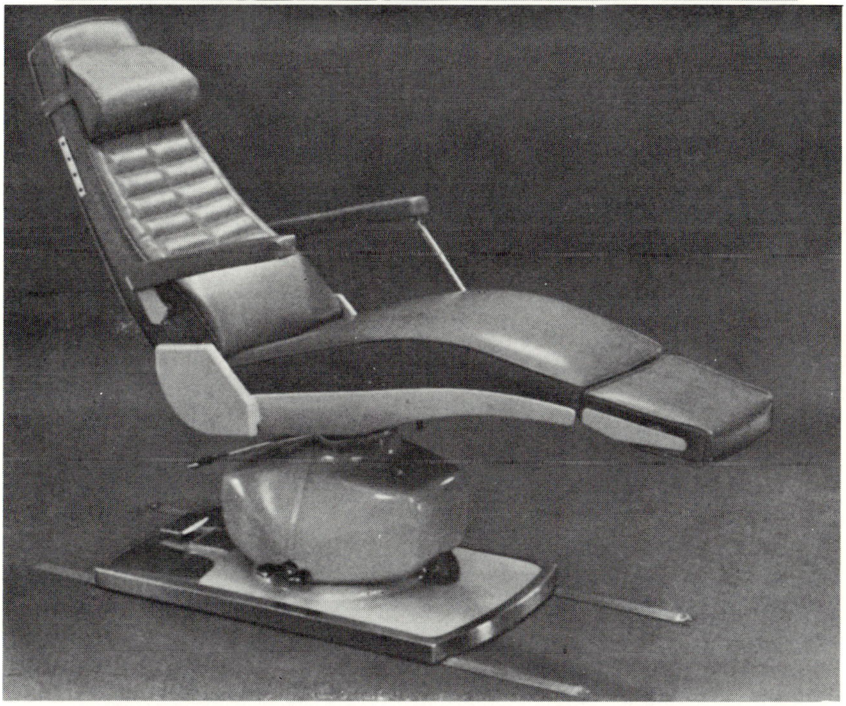

Fig. 8-3. Dental chairs. **A,** Ritter Conventional Dental Chair with motor-driven base; **B,** Ritter Lounge Chair with track on base; **C,** Ritter Lounge Chair with adjustable back and air-glide base; **D,** Den-tal-ez Contour Chair; **E,** Coastal Medallion Dental Chair; **F,** Weber Chair.

C

D

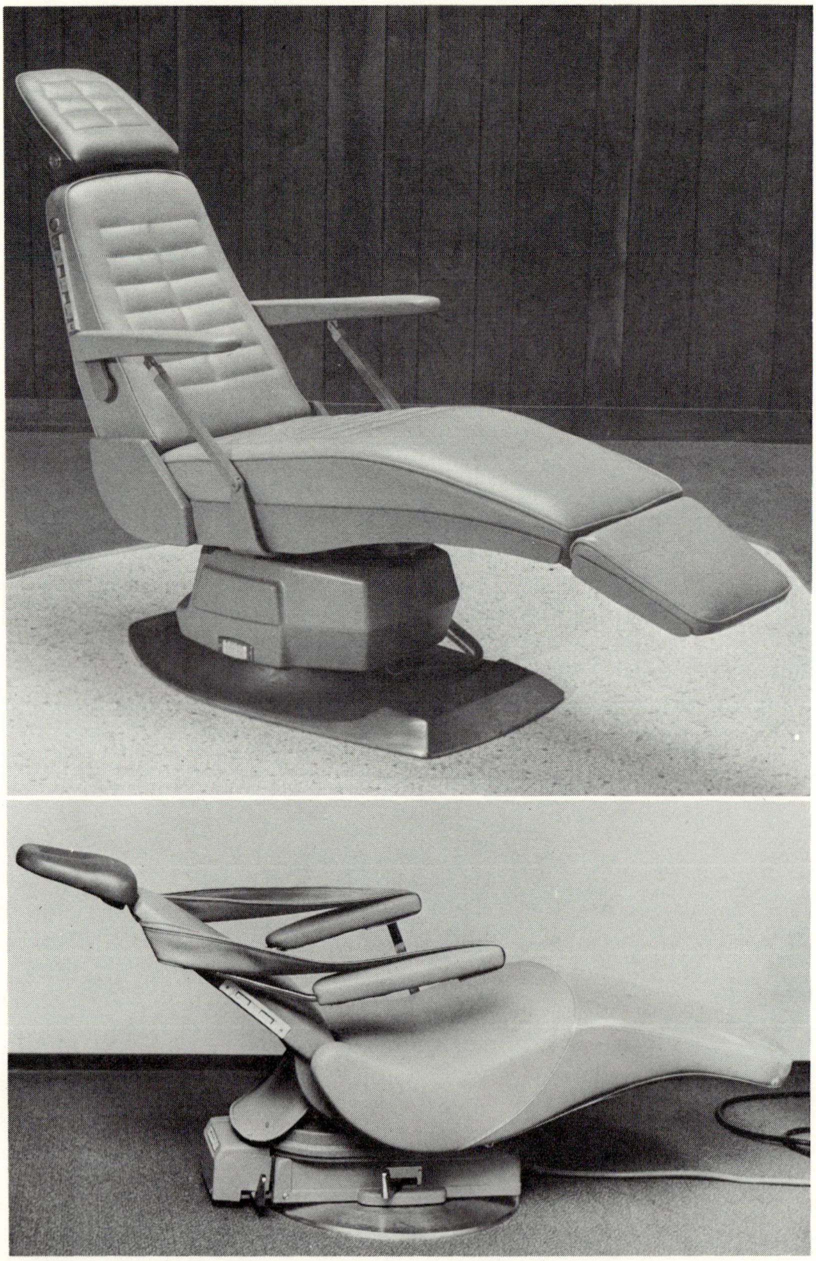

Fig. 8-3, cont'd. For legend see p. 167.

E

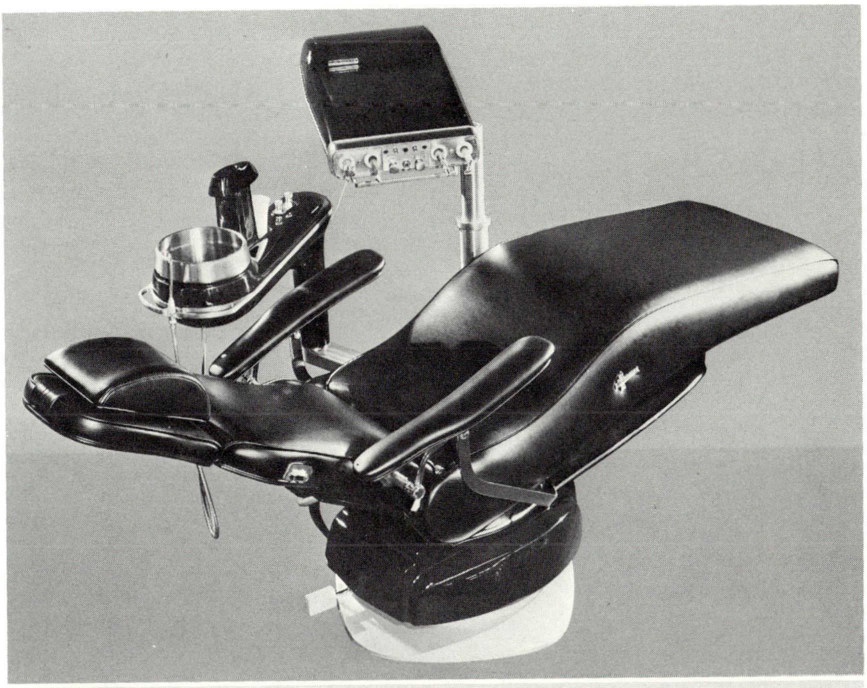

F

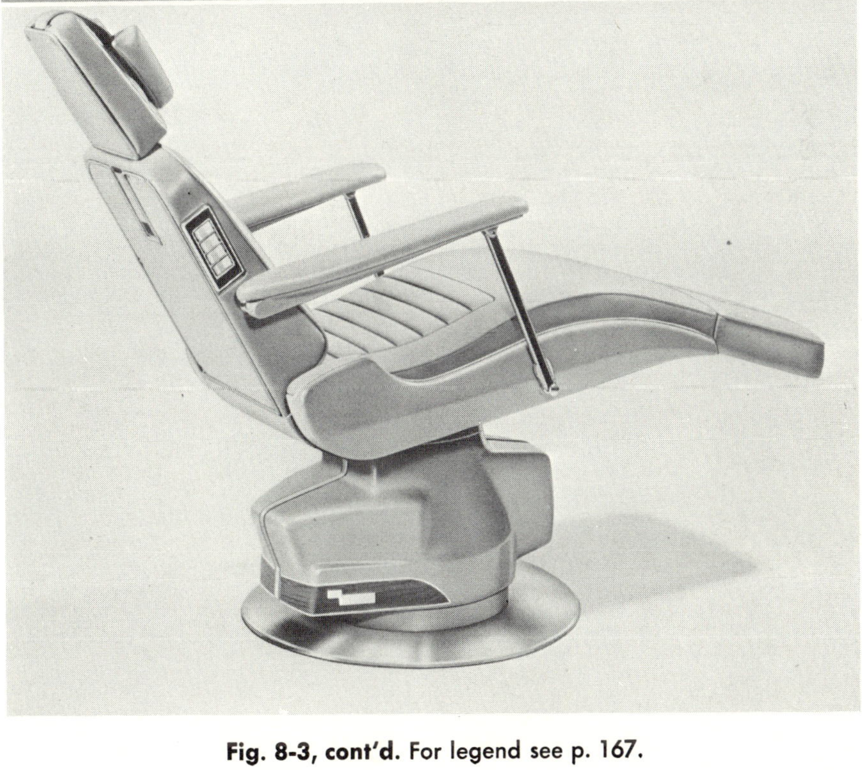

Fig. 8-3, cont'd. For legend see p. 167.

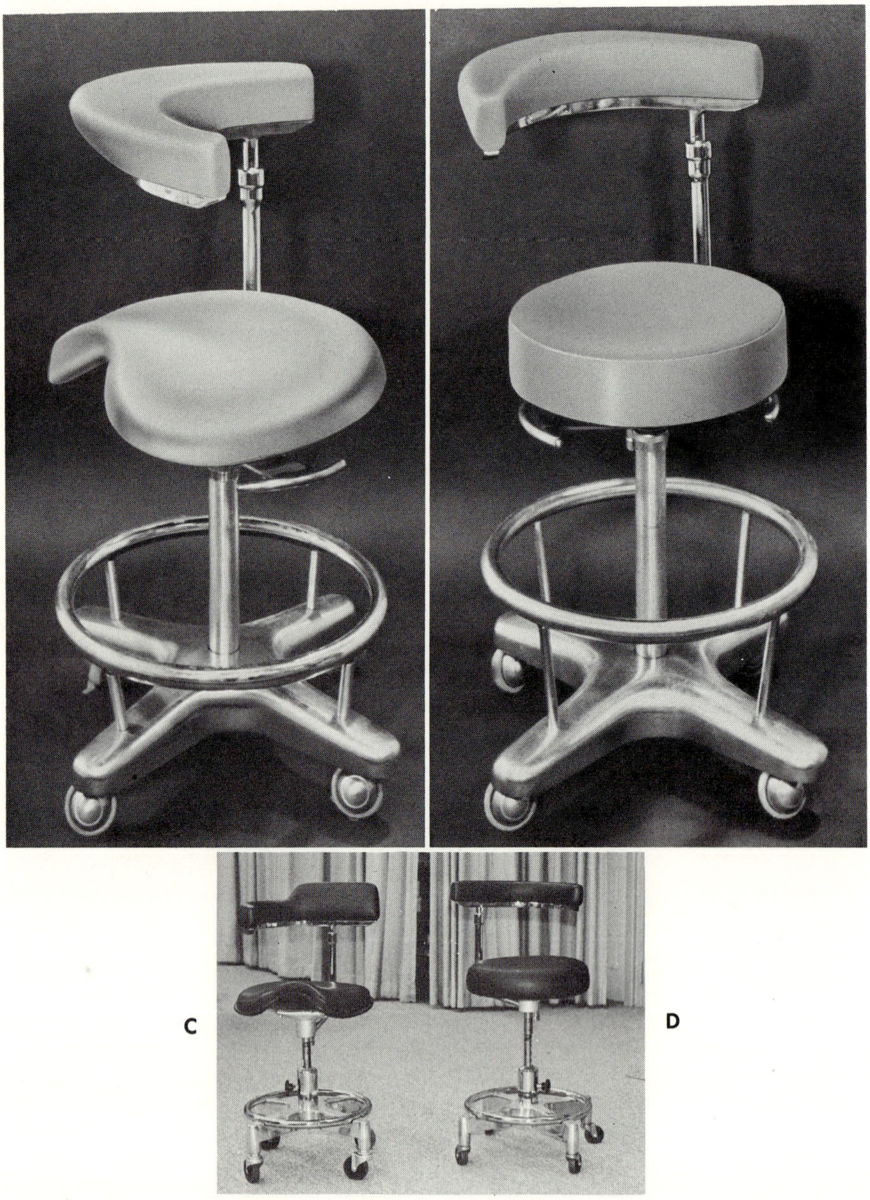

A B C D

Fig. 8-4. Dental operating stools. **A,** Ritter Dentist Stool; **B,** Ritter Assistant Stool; **C,** Den-tal-ez Dentist Stool; **D,** Den-tal-ez Assistant Stool; **E,** Ritter Chair, with dual attached stools; **F,** Dentsply.

E

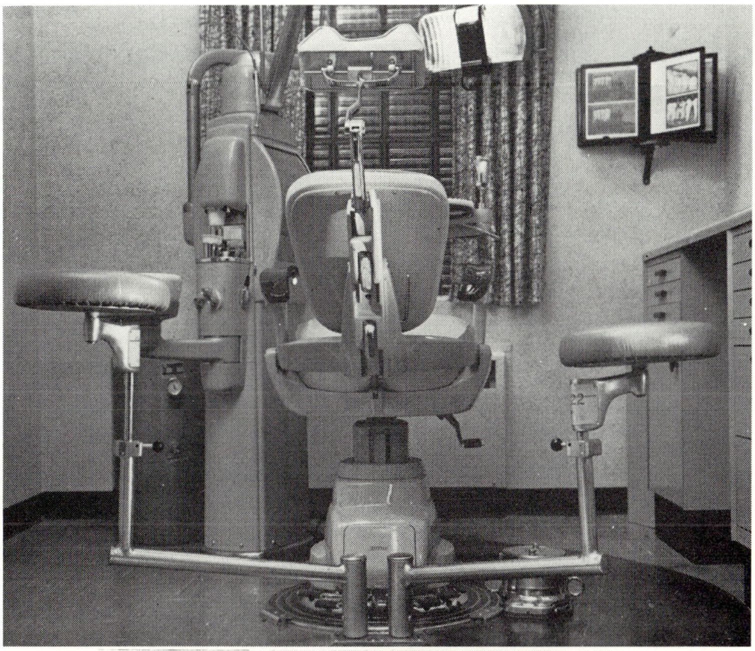

F

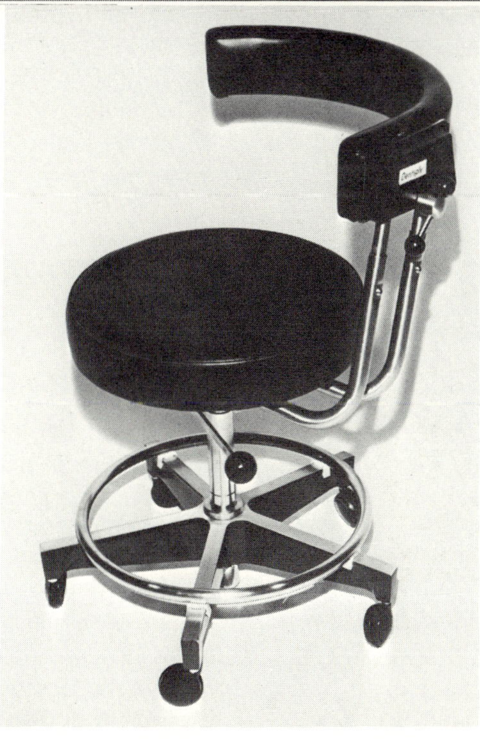

Fig. 8-4, cont'd. For legend see opposite page.

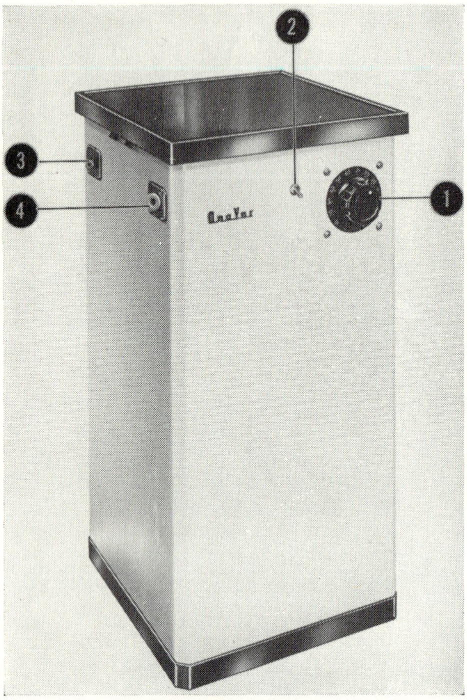

Fig. 8-5. Mobile oral evacuating machine. **1,** Variable power controller; **2,** on-off switch; **3,** retractable tube for saliva ejector or surgical tip; **4,** retractable evacuation tube. (Courtesy Torit Manufacturing Company.)

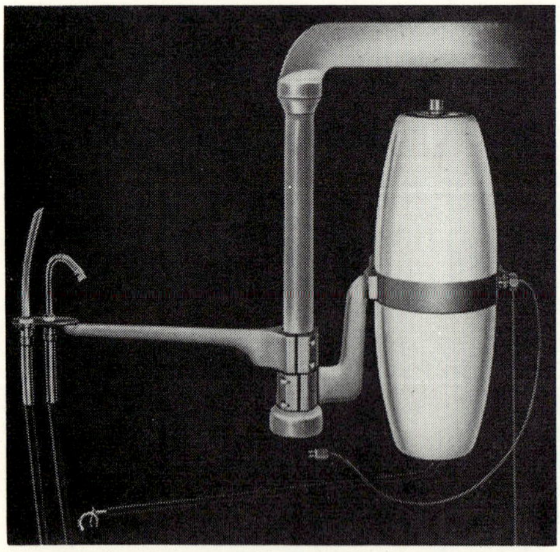

Fig. 8-6. Evacuating machine of the type that is attached to the dental unit. Notice the drainage tube, which is placed in the unit cuspidor. (Courtesy Pelton and Crane Company.)

equipment, with its constant water spray, requires that large volumes of water be removed from the mouth during even routine dental operations. Thus, the oral evacuation unit was developed. This unit is capable of removing water, debris, saliva, and blood from the operating field quickly and efficiently by means of a vacuum air flow that is powerful, yet gentle to the oral tissues. Oral evacuating units are manufactured as a component of a fixed or mobile dental unit, or as a completely separate mobile or fixed unit. The separate unit is usually compact and self-contained, with a motor, a debris separator, and a collection cannister for solid wastes. This self-contained unit may be enclosed in a mobile cabinet or housed in a cannister attached either to the wall, the cabinet, or the support arm of the operating light. Oral evacuation units are illustrated in Figs. 8-5 and 8-6.

The dental cabinet

Dental operating cabinets are available in various sizes and designs. The needs of the dentist will dictate the type of cabinet to be used in the office. Likewise, the mode of operation and the type of practice will influence the positioning of the cabinet. The recent trend is placement of the cabinet behind the patient. The variety of available sizes, styles, and colors makes the modern dental cabinet attractive and serviceable, as shown in Fig. 8-7.

Standard cabinet

The standard type of dental operating cabinet seen in many offices is available in several sizes. Depending upon their size, these cabinets may be mobile, so that they can be positioned for efficiency in various operations. The larger type is usually positioned in the location most convenient for all procedures. All these cabinets are fitted, to a certain extent, to receive the usual assortment of dental instruments and materials. The assistant should not hesitate,

A

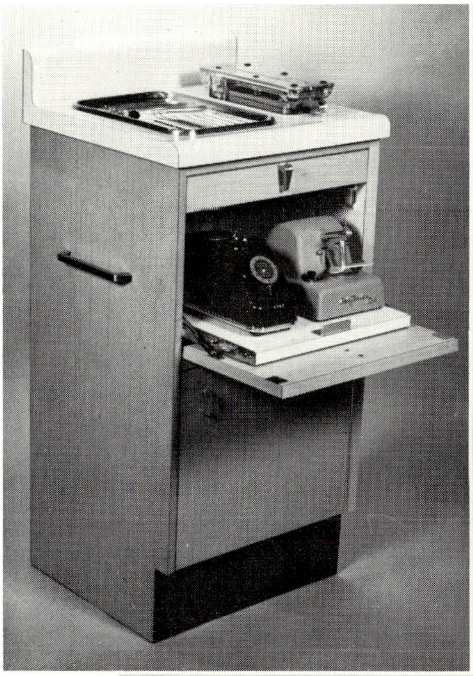

B

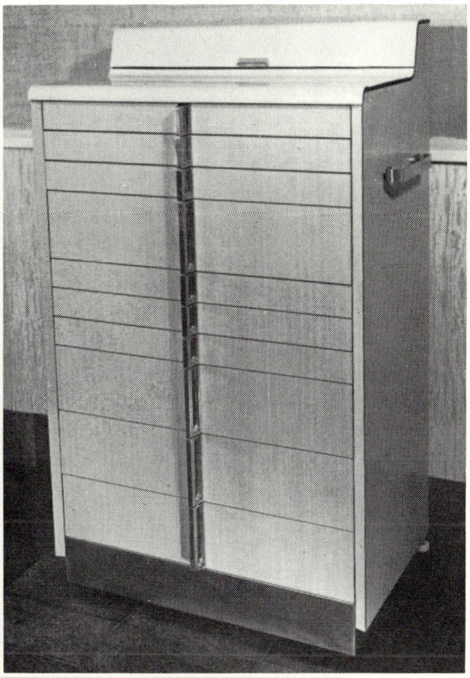

C

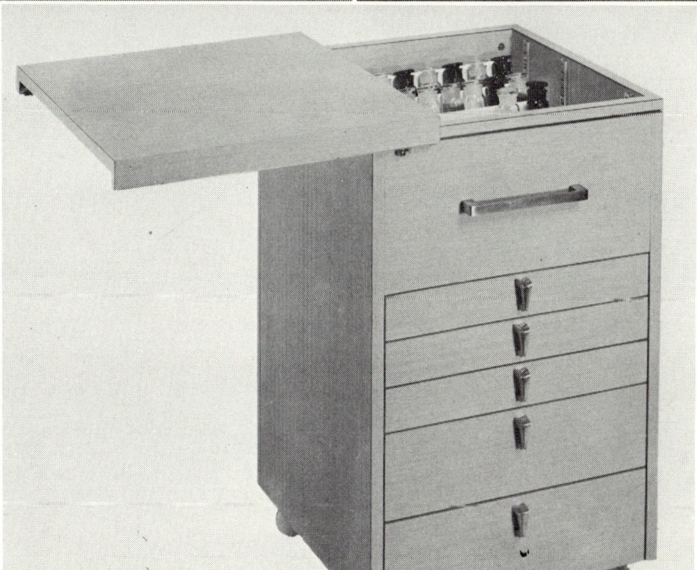

Fig. 8-7. Dental cabinets. **A,** Mobile cabinet with special top and drawer design to accommodate tray setup technique and provide space for amalgamator and spot welder; **B,** mobile dental cabinet. This type of cabinet can be positioned near the chair for the convenience of the dentist and the assistant. (Courtesy Hamilton Manufacturing Company.) **C,** Valtronic Mobile Cabinet with sliding top; MSFL-UAL; **D,** Valtronic Modular Cabinets—Total II Standard. (Courtesy The Valtronic Corp.) **E,** Dentsply Spectrum Console, Heritage Style. (Courtesy Dentsply International.)

D

E

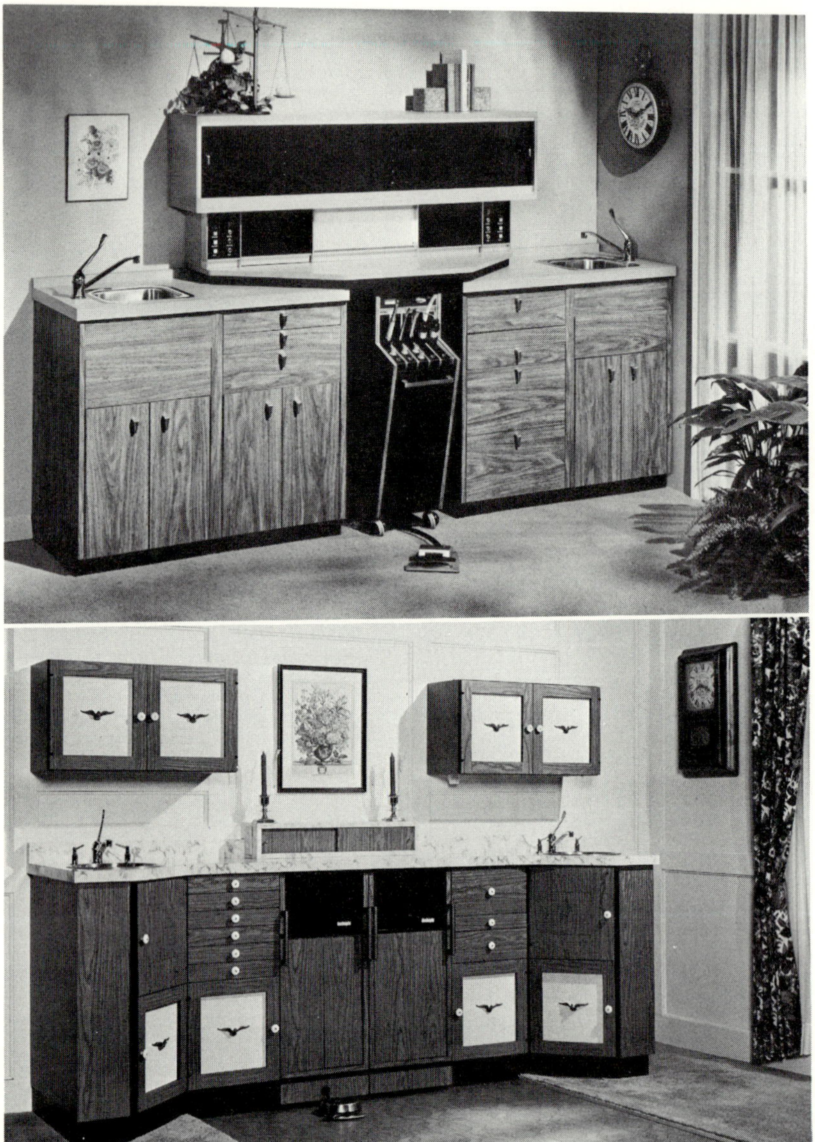

Fig. 8-7, cont'd. For legend see p. 173.

however, to make original innovations for storing special items.

Modular cabinet

The built-in, or modular, cabinets are convenient and compact, and they give the dentist a wider selection in arrangement and fitting of drawers. Convenient storage and fitting are also available for accessory equipment, such as the oral evacuating equipment, mechanical amalgamator, hydrocolloid unit, and instrument sharpener. In some instances, the use of this cabinet system gives more storage space and makes possible more convenient placement of cabinets in the available office space.

The dental operating light

The traditional dental unit is designed to accept a post to which a movable arm is attached. At the end of this movable arm is mounted a dental operating light. This light is adjustable in relation to the field of operation. With the advent of dental units that are positioned in other than the traditional location, it became necessary to find another way of locating and stabilizing the operating light. Several approaches have been developed. The first is by means of a lamppost, either attached to or stabilized by the dental chair base. Attached to this lamppost is a movable arm and operating light, which is similar to the light usually found on the traditional dental unit. Some lamps are mounted on arms that are fastened to the seat portion of the chair. Use of an arm that fastened to the foot of the chair was tried, but this never proved very satisfactory. Another approach is a light system mounted in the ceiling, and even a wall mounting can be used in some locations. In this latter lighting system, one or more operating lights, backed up by a panel of fluorescent lamps, may be used. Frequently, the operating light(s) may be attached to a sliding track to create greater utility.

Dental operatory lighting offers a wide variety of options. Manufacturers and their representatives should be consulted regarding the best light combinations and the correct number of foot-candles required for dental procedures. The assistant should keep in mind the need for correctly balanced light in the dental operatory to help reduce eye fatigue and to aid in the selecting and blending of restorative materials. A foot-candle is the amount or intensity of light falling on an object that is 1 foot from a standard-sized candle. It is usually considered necessary that the dental operatory be so well lighted that the intensity of light falling on any table or working surface is 150 foot-candles. It is further believed that the dentist needs about 10 times that intensity of light for working at the oral cavity, or about 1,500 foot-candles of intensity are required at his point of operation.

It should also be pointed out that not all light is the same tint or color. Ordinary light bulbs usually produce a high proportion of red. Bulbs with colored glass filter out undesirable rays and colors and can produce a more natural appearing illumination. In fluorescent lamps, the color of the glass, as well as the gaseous chemicals in the bulb control the tint that is produced. Most lighting experts try to combine bulbs and light sources to simulate natural light coming from the Northern sky in bright daylight.

The color or tint of the lighting not only affects the eye comfort of the persons working under these conditions, but there are some shades or tints that also help one discern detail in the object being studied. Women are conscious of the fact that different shades of cosmetics appear very different under various kinds of lighting. Similarly, the color of tissues and the coloring in teeth appear different under various lighting conditions. When the dentist selects a shade of silicate filling, he attempts to match the shade of the teeth being filled, and he wants to match it under the same lighting conditions in which the teeth will normally be viewed.

The dental handpiece

Handpieces are classified in several different ways. The fundamental classification is based on speed, or revolutions per minute. In this classification are the conventional, or low-speed, high-speed, and ultrahigh-speed handpieces. Perhaps one should not classify the low-speed handpiece as conventional, because the high-speed instruments are becoming more common and have actually replaced many of the older, low-speed instruments. The term "conventional" basically refers to the belt-driven handpiece, which was the forerunner of

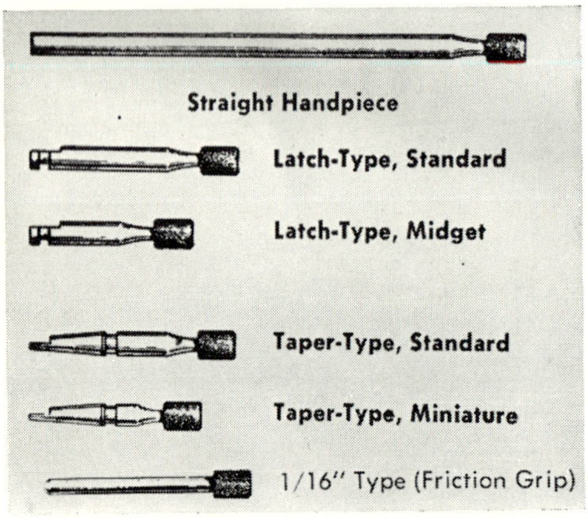

Fig. 8-8. Mounted stones showing various types of shank adaptable to different handpieces. (Courtesy Densco, Inc.)

the various turbine models. Handpieces may also be classified according to the type of propellant that drives them—belts, air, or water. Contra-angles are usually classified by the type of bur shank that they receive, such as taper, latch, friction-grip, or special (Fig. 8-8).

Conventional handpiece

The conventional type of handpiece and angle are driven by the engine on the dental unit and the cord arm belt. The speed of this type of handpiece ranges to a maximum of 9,000 r.p.m. (Fig. 8-9, *A*). The contra-angle, the prophylactic angle, and the condensing angle are placed on the end of the handpiece (Fig. 8-9, *B*).

Gear-driven handpiece

The high-speed handpiece may be run by gears or by a belt. Those operated by gears and ball bearings can assume speeds of over 50,000 r.p.m. The high-speed contra-angles used with this type of handpiece are known as "sleeve" angles (Fig. 8-10). When teeth are cut at high speeds, a coolant must be used to avoid injury to the tissue and to preserve the efficiency of the burs and stones.

Belt-driven handpiece

The belt-driven high-speed handpieces will run at speeds up to 150,000 r.p.m.

A

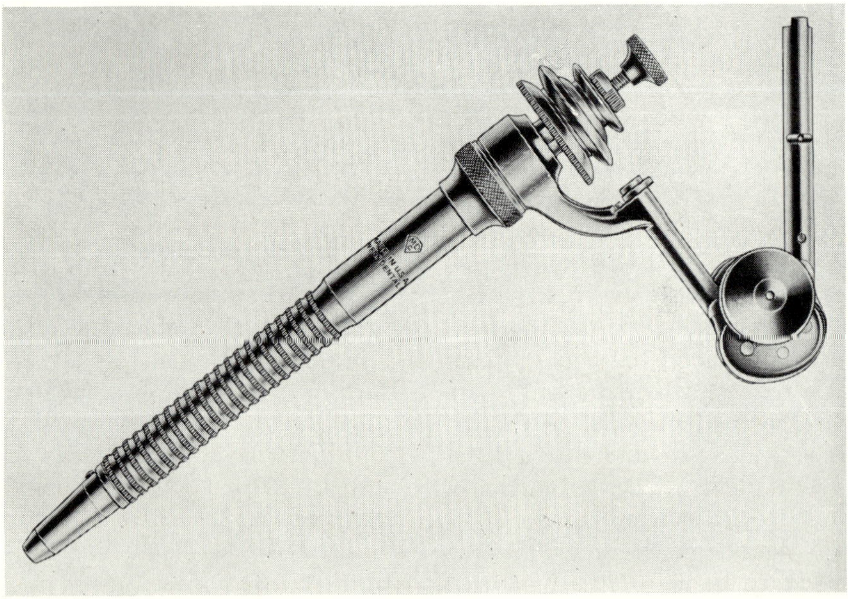

Fig. 8-9. A, Conventional straight handpiece, which is also termed a sleeve-bearing handpiece. This type of handpiece is often used with the dental engine in the laboratory; **B,** prophylactic angle *(below)* and shortsleeve contra-angle *(above)* for use with the conventional straight handpiece. (Courtesy Midwest Dental Manufacturing Company.)

B

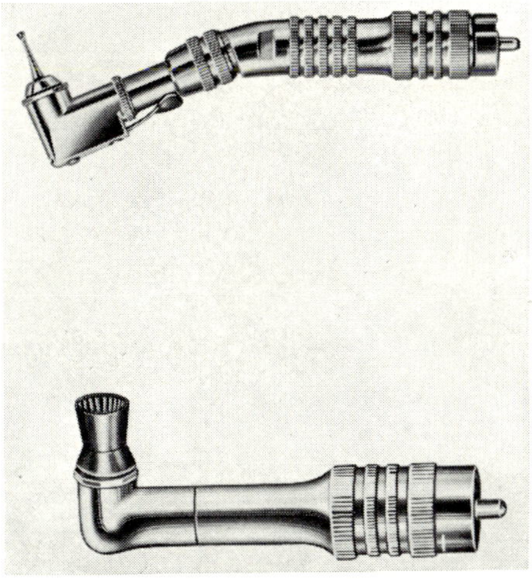

Fig. 8-9, cont'd. For legend see opposite page.

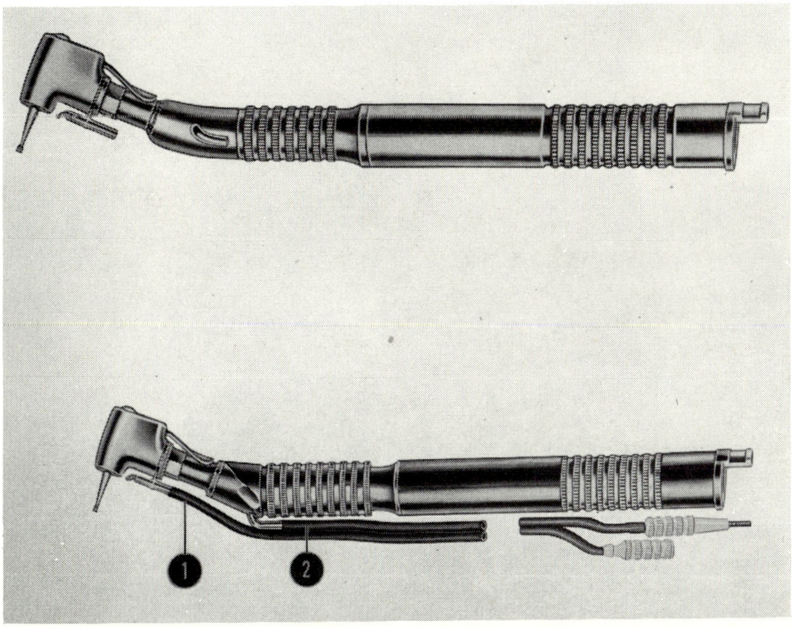

Fig. 8-10. Long sleeve contra-angles. Note 2 tubes on bottom of angle for coolant **(1)** and lubricant **(2)**. These contra-angles receive the latch type of bur shank. (Courtesy Midwest Dental Manufacturing Company.)

These handpieces and angles usually comprise one unit (Fig. 8-11). The elimination of gears makes this type of handpiece run very smoothly, but it also precludes the use of low speeds for certain operations, such as the polishing of teeth during prophylaxis. Maintenance is minimal.

Turbines

Handpieces that are not belt-driven can attain speeds of over 250,000 r.p.m. Either water or air is used as the basic propellant. The air turbine (Fig. 8-12) may receive compressed air from the central air compressor, or it may be equipped with its own special compressor. These instruments are contra-angle handpieces and high torque, low-speed straight handpieces. The assistant's responsibility in maintaining them is much less than in maintaining the conventional handpieces. The water turbine, which runs on the principle of hydraulic propulsion, is a self-contained unit.

There are numerous types of equipment available for furnishing the dental operatory. The dental team is faced with the problem of evaluating all of this equipment and choosing the kind that it will want to use in the future. The team members will not necessarily be selecting equipment that is best suited to the kind of team practice that they have been conducting in the past. They may wish to improve and change their procedures, which will mean the selection of equipment will be based upon the newly chosen methods and not upon former procedures.

BASIC FUNDAMENTALS

The influence of training and experience

The work habits of both the dentist and assistant begin to be formed early in their respective training periods. Some may even argue that the process begins even earlier than this training period, because of some previous contact with other dental personnel. Nevertheless, it is true that the dentist and assistant form lasting work habits during their educational experience, some of which are good and some poor or inefficient.

For many years, dental schools only taught students to perform dental procedures without the aid or benefit of chairside assistants. This "solo" operating method naturally required equipment that adapted itself to the single operator. It is, therefore, obvious how the bracket table, the upright dental chair, the cuspidor, and the placement of all equipment within the reach of the dentist came to be an accepted and highly desirable mode of practice. Moreover, the dental assistant, in her training, is frequently required to work with traditional equipment and finds that the equipment is not made for her, and she is not made for the equipment.

It is good to be able to report that dental schools, since the early 1960's, have been moving, although slowly, toward a clinical program that emphasizes the team approach in dental services. However, in spite of this recent movement, the influence of solo operation is still very evident in many dental schools and dental offices.

When a dentist and his assistant learn to practice in an inefficient manner, they usually find it difficult to change from these poor work habits. They feel more comfortable working with the equipment with which they learned to practice, even though it permits and encourages inefficiency. This resistance to change has a considerable influence on the selection of dental equipment. Also, there are some who resist making a change because they do not want to openly admit that they were doing something incorrectly.

Method improvement

Before proceeding to consider the selection of equipment, the dental team should conduct a thorough review of each procedure performed within the operatory. This study and the results obtained

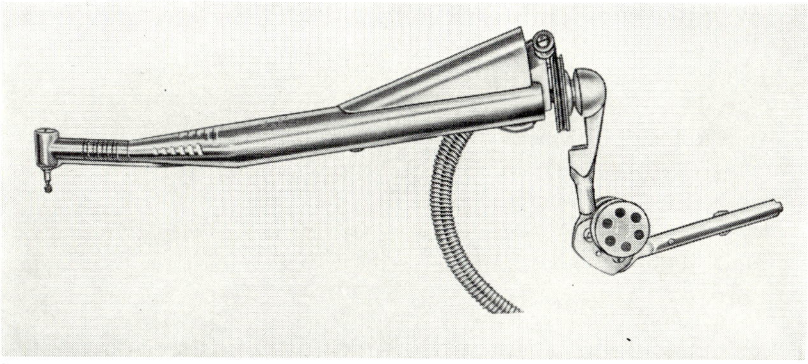

Fig. 8-11. Belt-driven high-speed angle handpiece. The friction-grip bur shanks are used with this particular handpiece. (Courtesy Chayes Dental Instrument Corporation.)

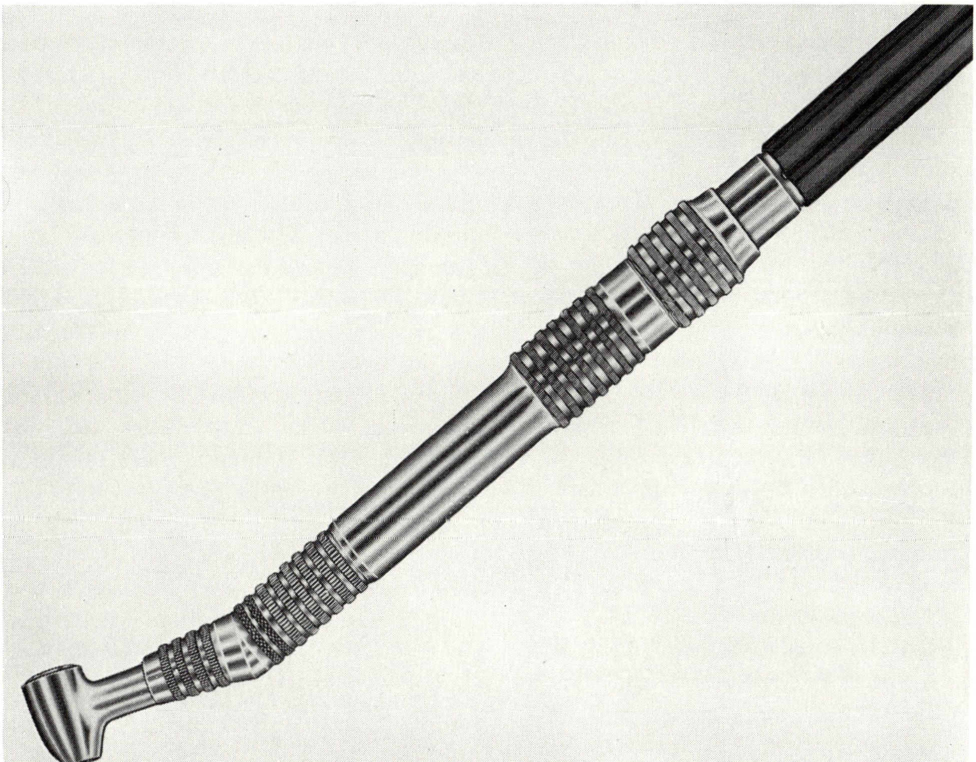

Fig. 8-12. An air-turbine contra-angle handpiece need not be taken apart for cleaning and lubrication. (Courtesy Midwest Dental Manufacturing Company.)

will be referred to as "method improvement." "Method improvement" is an organized, commonsense attack upon the way in which procedures have been done, with the intention of finding ways for doing them better. The method of attack is one of a continuing, hard-headed, questioning attitude, which takes nothing for granted. Its fundamental requirement is an open mind that approaches a problem of improvement without any preconceived ideas, bias, and prejudice. If there is any preconceived idea, it should be an assurance on the part of the team members that a new and better way can always be found. The approach should not be haphazard. To be effective, certain questions must be channeled toward 5 specific results. The basic questions are:

1. What can be combined?
2. What can be eliminated?
3. Should the sequence be changed?
4. What can be simplified?
5. What, if any thing, needs to be added?

Question five may at first appear out of place in a list of questions designed to shorten and streamline any method or procedure. However, there is always the possibility that something that has been previously eliminated needs to be reincluded. Sometimes an extra, time-consuming step may help prevent an error which could require more time to correct. Furthermore, new tests and procedures often need to be added to an old procedure.

In the method improvement approach, it is suggested that the dental team follow the outline below:

1. State objectives.
   Usually objectives can be stated in terms of saving time, increasing output, lowering cost, and improving quality.
2. Analyze present methods.
   Subdivide each method, and express the characteristics of each step necessary to the performance of the task.
3. Criticize.
   Question and criticize each step in terms of why, what, where, when, who, and how.
4. Innovate.
   Let your mind go free and dream. Then work out the details for proposed methods that appear most favorable.
5. Try it.
   If the new method appears to satisfy all of the stated objectives, it should be given a trial run.
6. Apply it.
   If the method passes all the tests established for it, do not be afraid to put the idea into practice. And do not forget to check constantly for possible refinements in any of the new methods.

After all procedures have been critically analyzed, each operator's motions and acts should be studied in detail. Time lapse photography is a method often used to study the operators' movements. In this technique the dental team is photographed while performing one or more dental procedures. The film is developed and viewed at a speed several times faster than the actual speed of the procedures, and the movements of the operators are analyzed.

If movies are not easily available, candid Polaroid pictures may be helpful in revealing awkward positions and wasted motion. Candid photographs can also be studied more easily than movies. The operator is studied to be sure that his hands are used properly, and that all hand, arm, and body actions are performed with a minimum of waste motion. The principles of motion economy should be applied to achieve this objective. These principles were originally developed by Frank Gilbreth, an American engineer, in the early part of this century. Although not developed for dental application, they are quite effective for analyzing motion economy in dental procedures. Some of the Gilbreth principles, modified somewhat for dental usage, are listed below. These principles should be used by each assistant and dentist to evaluate his or her proficiency in motion economy.

1. The two hands should not be idle at at the same instant, except during rest periods.
2. Avoid sudden and sharp motion by keeping motions continuous and curved.
3. Rhythm is essential to the smooth and automatic performance of an operation.
4. Keep motion to the least effort possible to avoid fatigue; finger motions are easier than body motions.
5. Preposition instruments and materials in definite, prescribed locations to avoid the need for searching for instruments and materials.
6. Locate all instruments and materials required for an operation within easy reach of the operator at the time they are needed.
7. Arrange instruments and materials for best possible sequence of operation.
8. Provision should be made for adequate illumination of the work area (operatory, laboratory, office).
9. Provide stools of the type and height to permit good posture for the dentist and assistant.
10. Relieve the hands of all tasks that can be performed more efficiently by the feet or other parts of the body.
11. Arrange to combine 2 or more instruments whenever practicable.
12. Design hand instruments and hand-held equipment to permit their operation with a minimum of hand and/or body exertion.

The operatory design

The selection of suitable equipment should extend to the design of the dental operatory and the entire dental office. The dentist who has the opportunity to build a new office or completely remodel his present one is indeed fortunate. The principles of time and motion economy can and should be applied in this endeavor. The arrangement of operatories within the office plan should emphasize the most important function of the dental office, the delivery of dental services. All aspects of the design should assist the dental team to achieve optimum efficiency (Fig. 8-13). The dentist is often obliged to accept available space with undesirable space limitations. The resourceful dentist may overcome constraints of limited space by utilizing an imaginative design, as illustrated in Fig. 8-14.

Developing equipment criteria

Since 1961, the United States Public Health Service, through the National Institutes of Health's Division of Dental Health, has been awarding grants to dental schools to develop techniques for teaching students to effectively utilize dental auxiliaries in a properly equipped dental operatory. This effort, known as the Dental Auxiliary Utilization (DAU) Program, has been recently joined by the TEAM Program, also sponsored by the Division of Dental Health. The TEAM Program is undertaking to teach dental students to manage and supervise a total dental health team, including various types of auxiliaries with expanded functions (see Chapter 4). One of the concepts stressed in the DAU Program is the selection of equipment that will permit the dentist to work effectively with an assistant, while applying the principles of four-handed dentistry. As an aid to individual school programs, the advisory committee to the DAU Program has developed criteria that schools could use in selecting equipment.

It is recommended that after all procedures have been analyzed and improved by the dental team, a set of specific per-

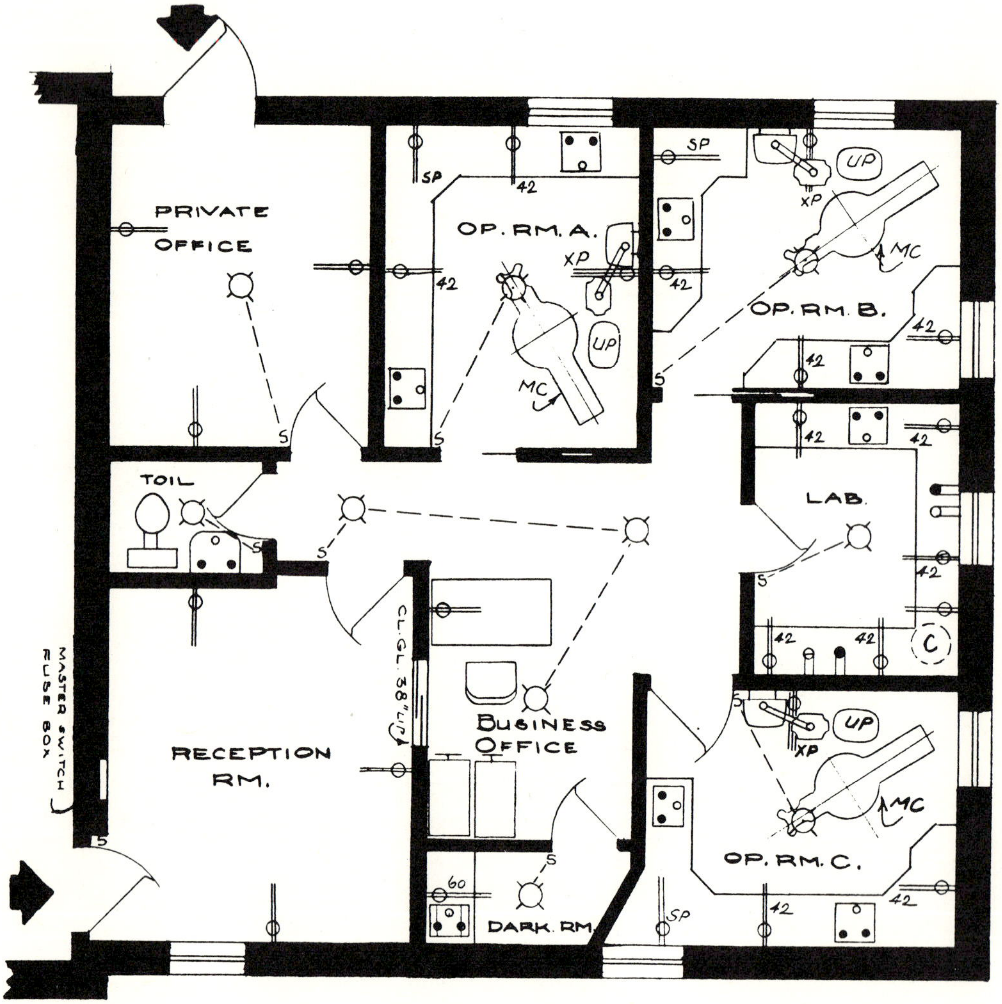

Fig. 8-13. Efficient office arrangement in 730–sq. ft. space. (Courtesy Ritter Company.)

formance criteria be developed with which to evaluate all equipment to be considered. The importance of these criteria should not be underestimated. Without them, various kinds of equipment cannot be objectively compared, and their performance cannot be objectively measured.

There are some guidelines that can be of general use in evaluating the different kinds of equipment. However, as one studies the manner in which his or her office team operates, and as one studies the new kinds of equipment that are available, he will want to include certain criteria of his own in this evaluation. In other words, if one is to have a personalized office, one must include criteria that are of particular importance to his office team.

There are many individual preferences in such decisions as whether a cuspidor or a funnel evacuator is provided for the patients. In some offices, the dental assistant may feel that a high-velocity suction is adequate. Similarly, there are dentists who want carpeted offices and operatories, and there are others who feel strongly that

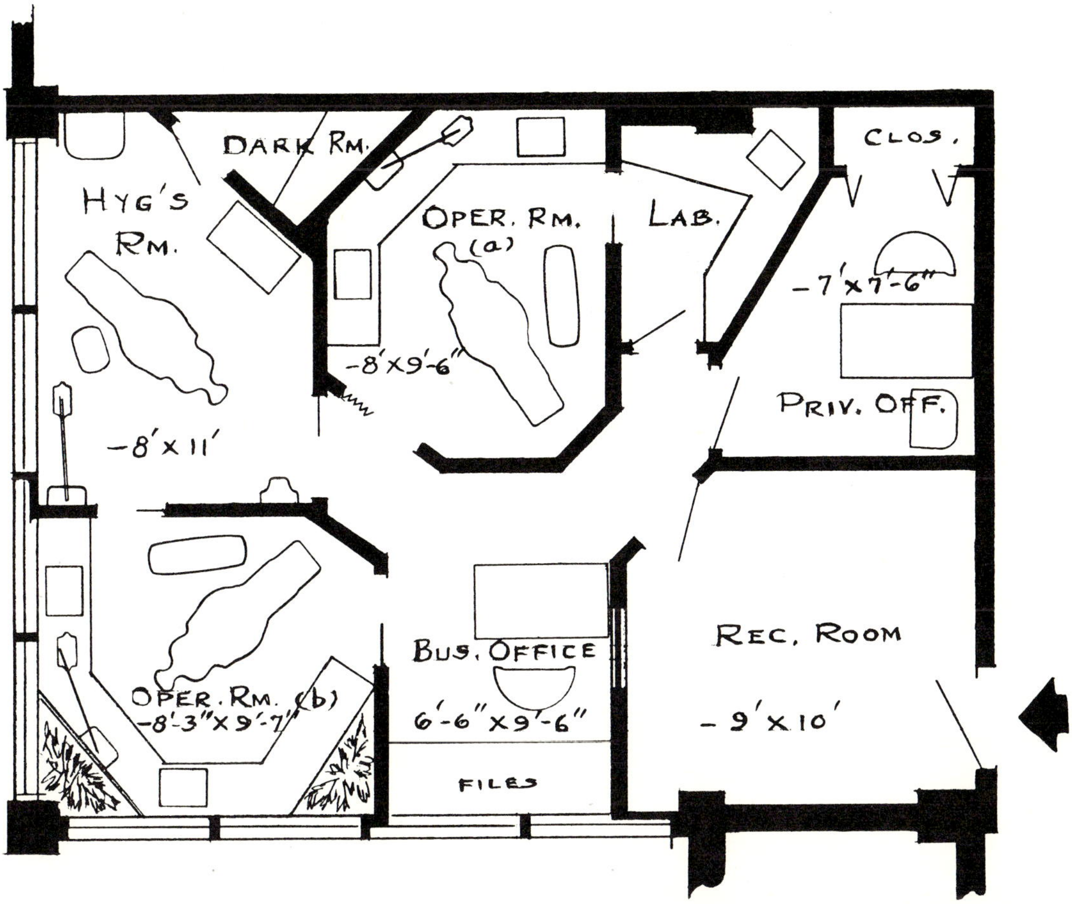

Fig. 8-14. Dental office design in 526–sq. ft. space. (Courtesy Ritter Company.)

they want a solid surface. The floor surface chosen sometimes is influenced by the kind of equipment desired. For example, the dentist may prefer the chair that glides on a platform of air; this chair only works on a flat surface and not on a carpet.

Performance criteria

The dental unit should:

1. Be located so as not to occupy space needed by the dental team.

2. Position all instruments for easy delivery to the mouth and for return with minimum motion and effort.

3. Be flexible enough for use of both right- and left-handed operation. This can be very important if one expects to invite other dentists to use the facilities from time to time or wishes to have equipment so flexible that it would be resalable to anyone, regardless of whether they are right- or left-handed.

4. Include high- and low-speed handpieces operated by a single, compact, and easily accessible foot controller capable of driving the handpieces at variable speeds.

5. Include an air-water-spray syringe that is lightweight, easily operated, and combined into one unit.

6. Contain hoses and cords with sufficient length to permit all attached instruments to easily reach the operating zone.

The dental chair should:

1. Provide power operation for frequently adjusted parts.

2. Be easily operated by both the dentist and the assistant.

3. Have a thin, narrow back.

4. Provide complete body support for the patient in a full range of positions, from upright to supine.

5. Place the operating zone (patient's mouth) at the level of the seated operator's elbow in all desired operating positions.

Dental cabinets should:

1. Be kept to the minimum number required to accommodate essential and frequently used operatory equipment and material.
2. When used as a work surface:
   a. Be movable to a position readily accessible to the dental assistant.
   b. Be of a height level with the elbow of the seated dental assistant.
3. When containing a sink:
   a. Be convenient for dentist and assistant.
   b. Be activated by controls not requiring hand operation.
   c. Be of adequate size for all operatory requirements.

As mentioned previously, it is important that the patient have the best possible image of the dental office and the care the dental team takes for the safety of the patient. Therefore, it is very important that many things be done in the presence and in view of the patient, so that nothing is left to the patient's imagination. For example, it is important to the patient that she see the dental assistant and the dentist wash their hands before touching equipment that is to go into the patient's mouth. It is important that the patient be assured that the dentist rewashes his hands after he has answered the telephone, been called away from the chair to shake hands with a visitor, or signed some papers. Sinks should be installed so that the patient can see that they are used. This effort to impress the patient with the sanitary and aseptic condition of the office also requires that the dentist and his assistant use a great deal of common sense. The team members need to refrain from touching their body, face, and clothes with hands that are going to be placed in the patient's mouth. The team should not touch equipment or adjust lights with hands that are to go into the patient's mouth, unless these adjustments are made with alcohol-drenched rags.

The dental assistant and dentist should arrange the office operatory as carefully as a stage is set for a performance, for the team is, in some ways, giving a performance. While the critic's reviews may never reach the morning paper, the evaluation and criticism of the patient in neighborhood conversation may perform a publicity function for the dental office. It can be good, or it can be bad, but the dental team should plan an office where the patient will bring home a good report on the sanitary and aseptic efforts of the whole office team.

The oral evacuation unit should:

1. Not occupy space needed by the operating team.
2. Have high velocity and low pressure.
3. Have easily operated and conveniently located controls.
4. Provide flexible, noncollapsible hoses of adequate length.

The operating stool should:

1. Be completely mobile.
2. Have adequate body support and maximum stability.
3. Be easily and conveniently adjusted in height.

The above criteria deal with only a few basic pieces of operatory equipment and are not intended to be comprehensive. They are presented to give the assistant a sample of criteria that can be expanded by the dental team.

Standby equipment

Every dentist realizes that if a handpiece becomes inoperative, his whole schedule is ruined. Therefore, he must either have a substitute or spare handpiece, or he must know that the local dealer has one that he can borrow on a moment's notice. There are many other kinds of office or operatory failures that can close down the dental office unless there is a replacement. It is important that the dentist and his assistant try to anticipate these possibilities and prepare for their eventuality. Just as hospitals have a separate gasoline engine for generating the needed electrical power in case of a local or regional electric failure, many buildings or offices try to anticipate this problem and have a standby power plant that can be switched on in case of a power failure. Even private homes may have auxiliary power plants, and it is important for an office that is concerned with the delivery of a health service to be prepared for such an eventuality.

Equipment checklist

Another technique for the selection of dental equipment is the use of an equipment checklist. This procedure may be used along with performance criteria, for they will complement each other.

As previously explained, every dentist and chairside assistant have developed operating patterns and procedures. This means that there are certain kinds of office equipment that will suit their purposes better than others. It is likely that there are certain kinds of deficiencies they have noted in their present equipment that they would like to see improved when they select equipment for their new office. Therefore, while some of the criteria most persons will want to use in critically examining a new piece of equipment can be suggested, there are many items that only the dentist and his assistant can insist must be included in the checklist of criteria.

Checklists of what the dental team wants to have and avoid are very important to develop, even before it goes to examine new equipment. After seeing 1 or 2 items, it is also a good idea for the dentist and his assistant to reexamine the list of items they will want to ask questions about when viewing new equipment.

Some persons will think that it is a waste of time to prepare a checklist, but when one is examining many different pieces of equipment, it is easy to forget to ask all questions of each salesperson. Also, it is very easy to get items confused after one has been exposed to several dozen different kinds of equipment. One type of report card or evaluation sheet for equipment might look like that on p. 186.

Equipment repair

Dentists are often reluctant to purchase equipment from a new manufacturer for several reasons. The dentist may be unsure of the reliability of the manufacturer, or there may not be enough information available to establish a life expectancy or frequency of repair record on the new equipment. Another concern that the dentist may have is the availability of service and replacement parts. The responsibility of the manufacturer goes beyond the manufacturing and marketing of dental equipment. The manufacturer must be concerned with the availability of service and access to replacement parts when needed.

There are many manufacturers of dental equipment. Some have widespread service facilities, and others do not. Fortunately, most dental equipment dealers sell and service a wide range of equipment from many different manufacturers. Moreover, new equipment that receives a favorable reaction from the dental profession usually finds its way into a wide network of dealer outlets.

Breakdown of equipment in the dental office is such a serious matter that many dentists purchase duplicates of certain kinds of equipment, as a standby in case of equipment failure. However, it can be clearly seen that this precaution can be taken only so far because of the tremendous cost involved. In any case, the dentist must be concerned about service and repair when considering the purchase of equipment.

Type of equipment ____________________

Manufacturer ____________________

Model name or number ____________________

Date examined ____________ Place ____________

Reputation of manufacturer ____________________

Ease of servicing (apparent) ____________________

Comfort to dentist or dental assistant ____________________

Comfort to patient (if applicable) ____________________

Mobility ____________________

Ease of cleaning ____________________

Location of switches or controls ____________________

Durability ____________________

Aesthetics ____________________

Where has equipment been used ____________________

Who can evaluate usefulness of equipment ____________________

Resale potential ____________________

Can equipment fit into office space ____________________

Is equipment compatible with present equipment or other new equipment to be bought ____________________

Presence of rough edges, poor finishing to ruin clothes of operators ____________

(The dental assistant and the dentist will have other items that they will wish to add to this listing.)

(Others) ____________________

SELECTION STRATEGY—PUTTING IT ALL TOGETHER

It is now time to decide precisely what equipment is most suited to a particular office, a certain dental team, and a specific group of patients. The moment of decision is near. An assumption will be made at this point. It will be assumed that the dental team is now convinced that a strategy or plan of attack is better than no plan at all. Therefore, a strategy that may be used by the dental team to select suitable operatory equipment is presented.

1. Attend postgraduate courses.
   Many courses are scheduled throughout the United States each year for

the dentist and his assistant. Some of these courses teach the dental team to work efficiently using the principles of four-handed dentistry (see Chapter 7). The dental assistant should review the Journal of the American Dental Association, the journal of the American Dental Assistants Association (*The Dental Assistant*), and the announcements of continuing education courses from nearby dental schools. Some of these include a combination demonstration and audience participation program that is very helpful.

2. Improve dental procedures.
   Use the principles of method improvement previously discussed and the knowledge acquired in the postgraduate courses as a basis for improving all dental procedures. This must be a team effort, so that both the dentist and the dental assistant understand the problems and the changes.
3. Prepare equipment criteria and checklists.
   With the knowledge acquired in the first 2 steps, develop a set of performance criteria and appropriate checklists to evaluate dental equipment.
4. Seek out and attend equipment exhibits.
   New equipment is introduced in a variety of ways, but one of the most widely used is the demonstration of equipment at state and national dental conventions. During these meetings, ample time is provided for the dental team to personally inspect the equipment and often to simulate its use. The dental team should go to the convention armed with its equipment criteria and checklists.
5. Consult local equipment dealers.
   Dental equipment dealers will have illustrations and brochures on all the equipment they sell or can procure. The dealer is experienced in the installation of equipment and may be able to give specific information on the durability and frequency of repair of several types of equipment. Frequently, the dealer will have a showroom in which equipment is displayed for customer inspection. It should be recognized that this is only a sample of all of the equipment available to him. The dealer may be able to obtain a demonstration model of a specific kind of equipment to permit evaluation by the dental team. Equipment cannot be fully evaluated from a picture and a brochure; it must be used. The dealer may also be able to take the dental team to a dental office in which there are new installations of equipment that the dealer does not have on display.
6. Observe other dental offices.
   Equipment under consideration may be in use in a nearby dental office. If this is the case, a visit to the office should be arranged in order for the team to see the equipment under conditions of actual use. The dentist and the assistant will usually be pleased to tell about their equipment and demonstrate its utility. The dental team that has done its homework (all of the above steps) before going visiting will recognize whether the equipment is being used correctly, and the visitors will be able to identify the merits and/or deficiencies of the equipment under consideration.
7. Be an independent thinker.
   In listening to the salesman praise a particular piece of equipment or another dentist praise the equipment he has chosen, be a careful listener and a good questioner. Every dealer will have his favorite products, and every dentist has a tendency to

praise highly the equipment he has purchased. It is easier to make a purchase than it is to get rid of a piece of equipment that was purchased in haste and proves to be a bad choice. There are many excellent products, and what is suitable for one office is not necessarily the best choice for every other office. Many different factors must be carefully considered before the final selection is made and the equipment is purchased.

8. Choose well.
   The wisdom of choosing well is obvious. Dental equipment is expensive and, once purchased, will undoubtedly remain in the dental office for several years. A poor choice may result in a long period of inefficiency within the dental office. Inefficiency will likely result in delivering fewer patient services, combined with harder work, while producing a lower income for the entire dental team.

Some practical considerations

Inevitably some criteria is established that no present equipment will satisfy. Therefore, the question of what to do in that event must be faced. Two suggestions are offered to the dental team when that situation arises.

First, the team should determine whether or not there is a dental manufacturer willing to build the equipment to the new specifications. The cost of this option may be prohibitive, unless the manufacturer likes the new specifications well enough to establish a new product line. One should not be discouraged too quickly, because manufacturers are constantly looking for new ideas and innovations.

When it is not practical to have new equipment constructed, a second alternative is suggested. Weights or values should be assigned to each criterion on the list developed by the dental team. These values should be determined by the relative worth of each criterion and may add up to one hundred, since that is a common scoring system. When these values are assigned, dental equipment should be evaluated and scored. The equipment with the highest score is selected.

Assigning numerical values or weightings to the different criteria is a very important exercise for the dental team to go through. It forces the team to make some value judgments concerning the comparative values or worth of the different characteristics of different pieces of equipment. It also forces the team members to realize that the various factors in the listing are not really similar, and they do not really lend themselves to being added into the total score. Some of the criteria are in terms of ease of handling and comfort for the operators. Other factors are in terms of original cost; other factors include those of appearance, comfort of the patient, resale value, compatability with other equipment, and so on. Choose equipment carefully and wisely, for it is going to be a constant companion in the office for many years. The income and salaries of the team depend upon this decision.

The interested and knowledgeable dental assistant can exert considerable influence in the selection of operatory equipment. The assistant should be on the watch for new equipment that will improve the work performed in the dental operatory and increase the productively of the team. In the dental office undergoing a transition from old to new equipment, the assistant can help analyze each piece of equipment being considered for purchase. As part of the dental team, she will play a role in applying the procedures presented in this chapter to its specific needs.

PART III SCIENTIFIC BACKGROUND

CHAPTER 9 STERILIZATION

MILTON SISKIN, B.A., D.D.S.

First impressions are easy to create and very difficult to dispel. Consequently, every effort should be made by the dentist and his ancillary personnel to provide as favorable an initial impression for the patient as possible. One thing that is essential for the accomplishment of this objective is cleanliness. In the dental office, cleanliness implies not only the absence of filth, but also freedom from disease-producing germs. Methods that may be utilized in the dental office to control and destroy microorganisms will be discussed in detail in subsequent portions of this chapter. At this point, the discussion is concerned with and directed toward physical surroundings and personnel. Most patients do not have basic or detailed information relative to the pathogenicity of microorganisms or a comprehension of methods by which disease-producing organisms are transmitted. However, almost everyone is familiar with the germ theory of disease and knows that pathogenic microorganisms may be harbored on contaminated fomites or objects containing excreta and waste. When a patient walks into a dental office and is greeted by personnel who are neat, tidy, and clean in appearance, when the sterilizing equipment is prominently displayed, and when the surroundings have an aseptic look and odor, he is given the impression that this is an office that is concerned with his welfare. A feeling of confidence that can be engendered in no other way is imparted to the patient. This confidence and the tranquility of mind that goes with it will be conveyed to all other experiences related to the dental practices. At this first exposure, the patient becomes aware that his dental problems are to be treated in a precise and professional manner, while every precaution will be taken to protect the patient's health.

RESPONSIBILITIES OF THE DENTAL ASSISTANT

It is the practice in most dental offices to delegate the responsibility of sterilization to the dental assistant. This is a confidence that must be recognized, accepted, appreciated, and never violated. The dental assistant should be thoroughly familiar with methods of sterilization used in the practice of dentistry. She needs to be aware of the operation and operating procedures for all sterilizing equipment. A knowledge of the particular method by which each item requiring sterilization can best be rendered sterile is essential. Since disease can be transmitted from patient to patient by instruments or other fomites that are not sterile, sterilizing procedures are among the assistant's most important duties.

It is the responsibility of the dental assistant, along with other members of the office team, to assure the patient that his health and welfare are of prime consideration and to reinforce this concept and impression. In the light of present knowledge, cleanliness is good, common sense and a sound practice. Negatively, it should be emphasized that carelessness and laxity can be responsible for the transmission of a communicable disease, and this in turn could have serious professional and legal consequences.

Personal hygiene

It is axiomatic that members of the dental health team must be neat in appearance and follow all of the rules conducive to good personal hygiene. In addition, there are a few specific rules relative to personal cleanliness and grooming that must be observed with special care. Obviously, the uniform and shoes must be clean. Since the assistant will be handling instruments and supplies that will be used in the patient's mouth, care of the hands is of paramount importance. The following rules concerning care of the hands must be followed:

1. The sink to be used for washing the hands should be in a prominent place, and clean towels always available.

2. The hands must be thoroughly scrubbed before each patient is treated. It is desirable to perform this act in the view of the patient. After the hands are washed, the assistant must not touch equipment or instruments that have not been sterilized.

3. Detergents that have a good hexachlorophene content will greatly minimize the number of organisms to be found on the skin. When such detergents are used repeatedly, it has been demonstrated that the hexachlorophene will produce a water-insoluble film that will remain adherent to the hands; thus, a continued and long acting bacteriostatic effect is achieved.

4. In the event that it becomes necessary for the assistant to leave the operatory to attend other office duties, the hands must be washed again before contacting the patient or before handling instruments to be used in the patient's mouth.

5. Fingernails must be kept short and clean.

6. When nail polish is worn, it should be clear or of a conservative shade.

7. If the assistant has a sore or a wound on one of her fingers, she must not handle instruments or assist at the chairside, unless a finger cot is used.

Terminology

In all areas of human endeavor, precise methods of communication are extremely important. This is particularly true in fields of the healing arts. One's comprehension of terms related to his field of interest is essential, and knowledge of the meaning of these words is mandatory, if communication is to take place. The assistant should be able to say what she means and mean what she says. There are a group of terms that are an integral part of the vocabulary related to cleanliness and sterilization; those in most frequent usage are listed here.

antisepsis The destruction of germs that cause disease, fermentation, or putrefaction.

antiseptic A substance or agent that has the capacity to inhibit bacterial growth and reproduction.

asepsis A condition or state in which living pathogenic organisms are absent.

aseptic Characterized by a state of asepsis.

aseptic technique The utilization of those procedures and precautions that will prevent the access of viable microorganisms.

asepticize To render aseptic or sterile.

bactericide An agent that will cause the death of bacteria.

bacteriostatic An agent or drug that will arrest the growth of bacteria. This term has essentially the same meaning as antiseptic and is used in its stead.

disinfectant An element or chemical compound capable of destroying organisms that cause disease, fermentation, and putrefaction.

fumigation Exposure to the fumes of sulfur or to the action of a disinfectant gas. (This method of sanitation of premises is presently believed to be ineffective.)

fungicide An element or compound capable of inducing the destruction of fungi.

germicide Any agent capable of destroying germs or microbes. This term is essentially a synonym for disinfectant.

in vivo In vivo refers to vital processes occurring in the living being.

pasteurization A process for destroying living bacteria in liquids without appreciably affecting the flavor or the bouquet of the liquid. The process consists of heating the liquid in question at 140 to 155 degrees F. for 30 minutes, and then immediately cooling it to 50 degrees F. or lower. Spores are usually unaffected by the temperature but are kept from developing by the sudden cooling. This process is used to destroy pathogenic bacteria in milk, wines, beer, fruit juices, and other liquids.

sterile The state of being free of living organisms.

sterility The condition of being sterile.

sterilization The process by which all forms of life are completely destroyed in a given circumscribed area.

sterilization temperature Temperature at which microorganisms will be destroyed.

sterilizer Any apparatus used to produce a sterile state.

STERILIZING ROOM OR ALCOVE

Every dental office should have a site designated for the purpose of carrying out sterilizing procedures. This room or alcove needs to be centrally located in the floor plan and easily accessible from all parts of the office. The area should be well lighted, easy to keep clean, and conveniently arranged. It should contain a spacious sink, equipped with hot and cold water. There must be ample facilities for the storage of supplies, instruments, and equipment after sterilization. The sterilizing area should be equipped with a sonic or ultrasonic cleaner, a pair of transfer forceps, a container for chemical or cold sterilization, a hot water sterilizer, and an autoclave. A hot-air or dry-heat sterilizer is optional.

Every instrument and dressing or any other item to be placed in the mouth must be sterilized. Considerable time may be conserved, and the sterilizing procedure disposed of with dispatch, if a definite routine is empirically established and followed. Each item used in caring for the patient should be assigned a specific method of sterilization. Storage methods must be devised and utilized to maintain sterility of supplies, instruments, and equipment until they are needed.

ULTRASONIC CLEANER

All instruments must be carefully and thoroughly cleansed before any method of sterilization is employed. It is possible to accomplish this by manual scrubbing with a stiff brush. However, compared to other techniques, this method is relatively time-consuming and somewhat ineffective. The old method of scrubbing cannot compare with the efficiency and thoroughness of the ultrasonic cleaner (Fig. 9-1, *A* and *B*). The ultrasonic cleaner is a relative newcomer to the dental armamentarium, but it is a piece of equipment that should be commonplace to every dental office. If instruments are to be rendered completely sterile, they must be free of extraneous material prior to sterilization. The ultrasonic cleaner accomplishes this thoroughly, effectively, and consistently. Also, the process requires a minimum of effort on the part of the assistant.

The ultrasonic cleaner is composed of an electronic generator and a bath solution. When the generator is in operation, it places the liquid of the bath in a state of high-frequency vibration. While in this state, the solution undergoes cavitation of an order that produces myriads of submicroscopic bubbles, which are formed and collapse almost instantaneously. The formation and collapse of the bubbles produce intense pressure changes, which result in a mechanical scrubbing action. Instruments are placed in a basket and then immersed in the cleaning solution. Vibrations set up in the solution will initiate the cleaning action, thus freeing the solid objects of extraneous material and leaving them clean and free of surface contaminants. The cleaning cycle is automatically controlled, and the process requires a time interval of

A

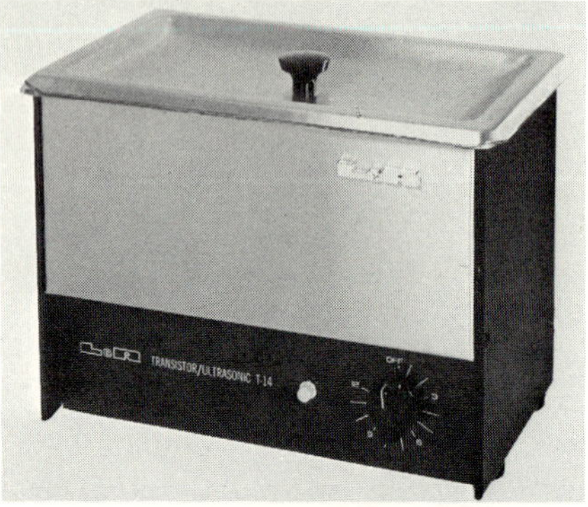

B

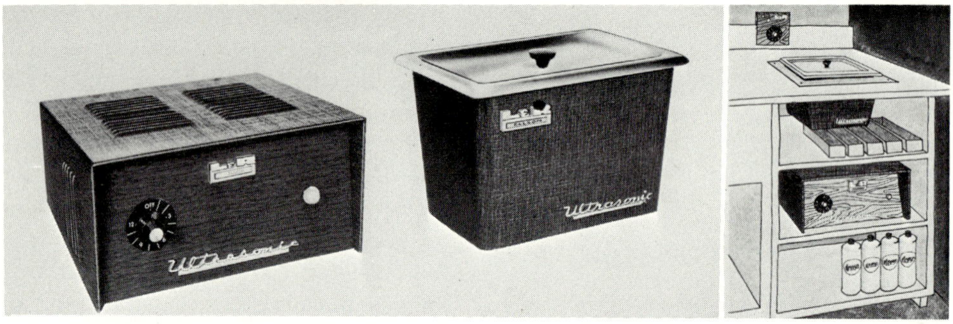

Fig. 9-1. A, Transistorized ultrasonic cleaning machine with solid state circuitry; **B,** table top model. (Courtesy L & R Manufacturing Co.)

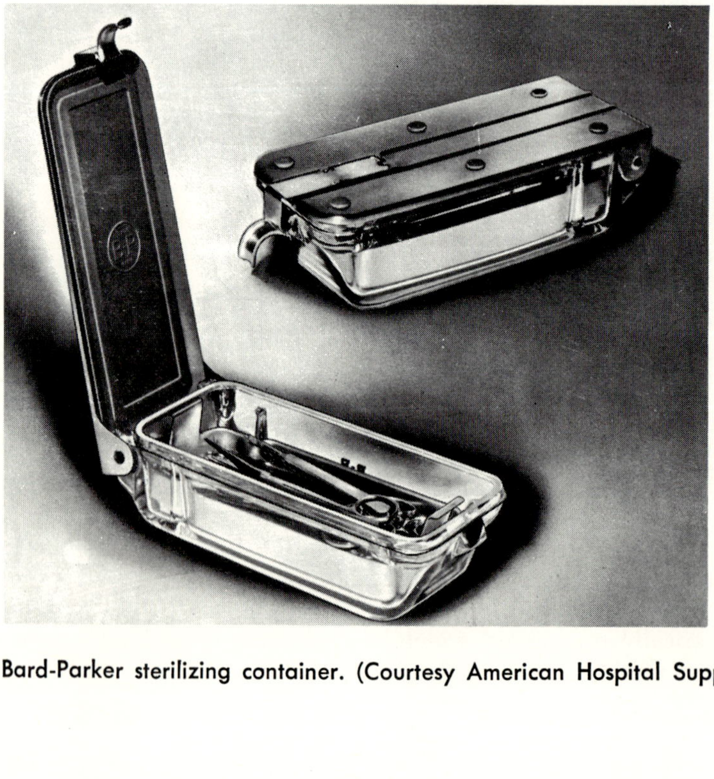

Fig. 9-2. Bard-Parker sterilizing container. (Courtesy American Hospital Supply Corp.)

2 to 10 minutes. The value of this instrument has been conclusively demonstrated.

METHODS OF STERILIZATION

Methods of sterilization can be categorized as physical, chemical, or mechanical, or any combination of the aforementioned. The most significant and important procedure for sterilization is the application of heat, a physical process. Chemicals must be regarded as disinfectants. Only in special instances is complete sterilization accomplished by chemical means. An example of a mechanical method of sterilization is filtration. This process is used primarily for the purpose of removing microorganisms from liquids or solutions.

Chemical method or cold sterilization

In comparison with the several methods of sterilization available in the dental office, the chemical method is the least effective. It is a very unreliable precedure for destroying organisms with spores, and it has several other disadvantages that surely limit the effectiveness of this type of sterilization. In most instances, the use of cold sterilization should be limited to instruments that do not lend themselves to other methods of sterilization and to instruments that have sharp cutting surfaces that must be maintained. Disinfectant solutions should never be used in an attempt to sterilize needles.

When a chemical disinfectant is to be used for sterilization, it is necessary to follow a rigid regimen. The solution should be placed in a dry, clean container that has a well-fitted top (Fig. 9-2). The lid should be kept closed at all times, except during the placement and removal of instruments. Forceps should be used for the transfer of instruments to and from the solution (Figs. 9-3 and 9-4). Since the effectiveness of the solution may be altered by air-borne organisms or by those contained upon the hands, the precautions just described should be followed without exception.

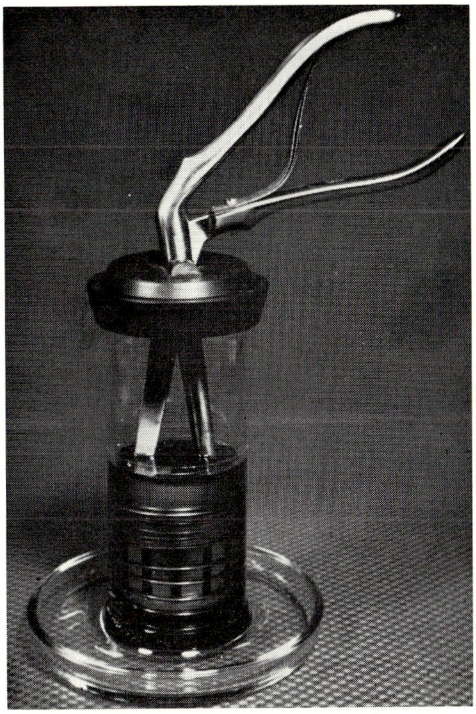

Fig. 9-3. Bard-Parker transfer forceps.

Keeping the container sealed has the added advantage of minimizing evaporation from the solution. The solution should be changed at frequent and regular intervals, since the concentration may be altered and the effectiveness diminished by evaporation or dilution. Before instruments are placed into a chemical solution, they should be carefully cleansed or scrubbed, rinsed, and dried. Should foreign material be left upon the instruments, it might act as a protective shield and prevent the disinfectant from coming in contact with the organisms that lie between the instrument and the encrusted matter. To be sterilized, the instruments must be dry, in order to obviate an alteration in the concentration of the solution. Once the sterilizing cycle has begun, the instruments should be left in the solution for 20 to 30 minutes. If additional instruments are placed in the sterilizer after a cycle has begun, the timing must be restarted.

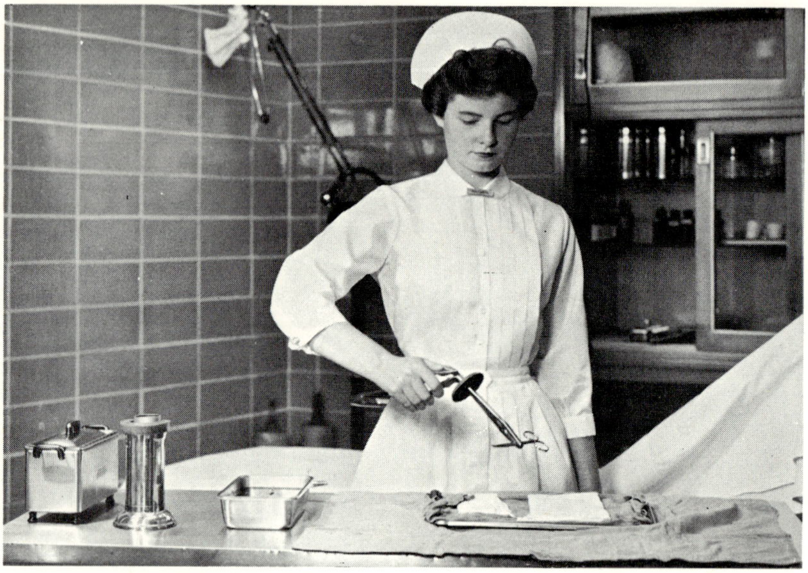

Fig. 9-4. The use of sterilized transfer forceps for moving sterile instruments. (From Swanson, M. E.: Health **4**:32, 1958.)

Many compounds are marketed as chemical disinfectants. To list them all, or even those in common usage, is impractical. However, most of those in frequent use are quaternary ammonium compounds, aldehydes, chlorine compounds, phenols, mercurials, and alcohols. Since all chemical disinfectants do not have the same capacity for destroying organisms, their germ killing potential is usually compared to a known quantity. The standard was developed by Rideal and Walker and is known as the "phenol coefficient." The phenol coefficient is an index or a measurement of the ability of a solution to destroy living organisms. Thus, by being aware of the coefficient, one is able to determine the effectiveness of various solutions and the dilutions that are used as chemical disinfectants. It should be remembered that most chemical disinfectants are effective against the vast majority of vegetative forms of bacteria if allowed to remain in contact with the organism for 30 minutes; 14 to 15 hours are required for spores, and most are unreliable against the various species of Mycobacterium.

Instruments ordinarily cared for by the chemical disinfecting procedures are as follows:

1. Mirrors
2. Explorers
3. Cotton pliers
4. Orthodontic pliers
5. Impression trays
6. Instruments for cavity preparation
7. Amalgam instruments
8. Plastic instruments
9. Suction tips (except surgical tips)
10. Water syringe tips
11. Air syringe tips
12. Burs (except surgical burs)

Some items of equipment do not lend themselves to the various methods of sterilization in common usage, but these items are likely to come in contact with the patient, with instruments to be used in the mouth of the patient, or with the hands of the operator. These include such pieces of equipment as the water and air syringes, bracket table, and light handles. These objects should be carefully wiped or swabbed down with an alcohol sponge prior to seating the patient.

Heat

Microorganisms are generally extremely responsive to temperature. It is a well-established point that metabolic activity in bacteria is at a minimum at 0 degrees C. Reproduction of organisms at this temperature ceases completely. The optimum temperature for microbial metabolism and reproduction is near body temperature. The range of temperatures for reproduction may be from 15 to 38 degrees C. As a general rule, the more pathogenic the organism, the more specific the optimum temperature requirements and the closer that temperature approaches 37.5 degrees C. Temperatures of 60 degrees C. or greater are totally destructive to bacteria. The most efficient method of utilizing heat for the destruction of microbial organisms is in the form of moist heat.

All organisms do not manifest the same degree of susceptibility to destruction by heat. Bacteria that are nonsporeformers and the vegetative forms of the sporulating organisms are least resistant to elevations in temperature. These organisms may be destroyed by moist heat at temperatures ranging from 55 degrees to 65 degrees C. applied for periods of 10 to 60 minutes. All organisms except spores can be killed by moist heat in 60 minutes at 80 degrees C. Spores are extremely resistant to heat. When attempting to eliminate bacterial spores, it should be noted that dry heat is less effective than moist heat. Some spores are able to resist boiling for three hours. Because of this, one should not rely on boiling alone to accomplish the purpose. The most effective method for killing spores is by using steam under pressure. This can be effected in 30 minutes at a temperature of 121.5 degrees C. It is interesting to note that only the bacilli produce spores, and that there are approximately 150 species with this potential.

The manner by which death of microorganisms is accomplished when using heat for sterilization is dependent upon the application. When moist heat is used, the proteins of the protoplasm of the bacteria will undergo denaturation and coagulation. Death of bacteria produced by dry heat is attributable to dehydration and the resulting oxidation.

It is essential to note that when heat is utilized to produce a sterile state, there are two factors that are of paramount importance, time and temperature. For sterilization, the requirement of each is inversely proportionate to the other: the greater amount of time used in the sterilizing process, the lower the temperature requirement; the higher the temperature used in sterilization, the shorter the amount of time needed to complete the process.

Boiling water

Of all the methods available for sterilization, boiling water is probably the most commonly used agent for sterilizing instruments in the dental office (Fig. 9-5). Boiling water is also one of the most efficient, effective, and satisfactory methods of disinfecting instruments. This process requires no elaborate equipment, is not expensive, and is most effective, except in instances where spores are involved. As previously mentioned, some spores may be resistant to boiling for periods up to 3 hours. The bactericidal action of boiling water can be enhanced by the addition of an alkali, 3 percent of saponated cresol solution or 5 percent phenol, to the water. Alkalies and boiling water are effective not only against all vegetative organisms, but against viruses as well. This is of particular importance in guarding against the spread of infectious hepatitis.

Sterilization by boiling does have limitations, since it tends to dull sharp instruments and to rust some metals. Boiling should not be used for those instruments that are expensive or adversely affected. In most instances, the deleterious effects of boiling can be minimized by the addition of antirust preparations, the use of

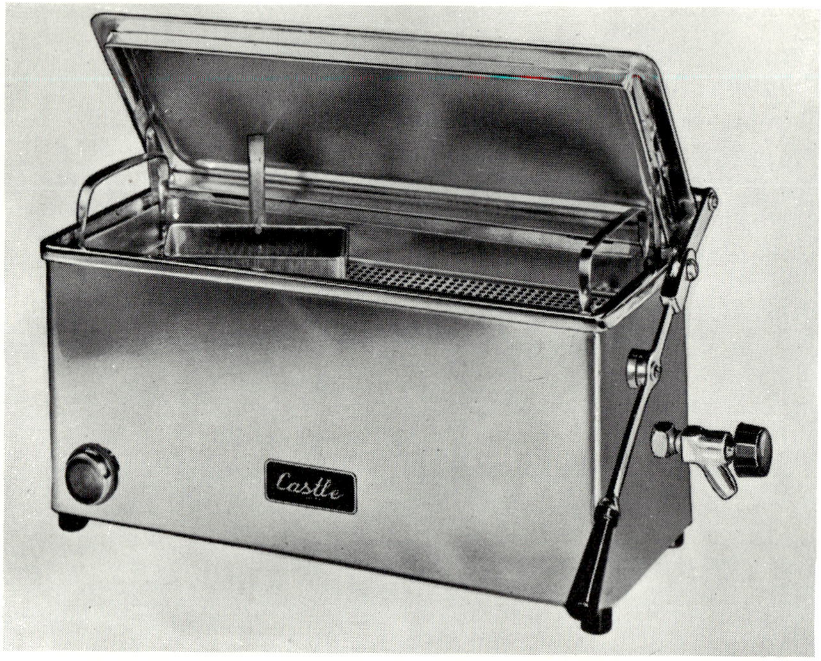

Fig. 9-5. Castle's instrument boiler. (Courtesy Ritter Company.)

distilled or mineral-free water, the addition of alkalies, the elimination of scale from the boiler, and the removal and drying of instruments at the completion of the boiling cycle.

Instruments to be sterilized by boiling must be freed of debris prior to placing them in the water bath. Should needles be included, a stylet must be passed through the lumen to dislodge any trapped material. The water must be boiling before the instruments are inserted into the tank. In the event that the placement of the instruments lowers the temperature of the water below the boiling point, the timing of the sterilizing cycle cannot begin until the water returns to a vigorous boil. The instruments must be completely submerged in the boiling water. The cycle should not be broken by the addition of more instruments. The most commonly accepted duration for the sterilizing cycle by boiling is 20 minutes. Since this interval is not long enough to be effective against spores, as was previously thought, 10 minutes may be long enough to accomplish disinfection exclusive of spores.

After sterilization, instruments are to be removed from the water immediately. The transfer is accomplished by the use of sterile forceps, and the instruments are placed between a sterile towel and then thoroughly dried. At this point, instruments with moving parts may be lubricated with sterile oil. The lubricant can be applied with a sterile cotton applicator or toothpick. Storage of the instruments in such a manner as to prevent recontamination should be effected. It is essential that sterilized instruments not be touched with the hands.

The instruments that lend themselves to sterilization by boiling are:

1. Syringes
2. Hand instruments without sharp cutting surfaces
3. Surgical instruments
4. Needles
5. Impression trays
6. Glass slabs

A

B

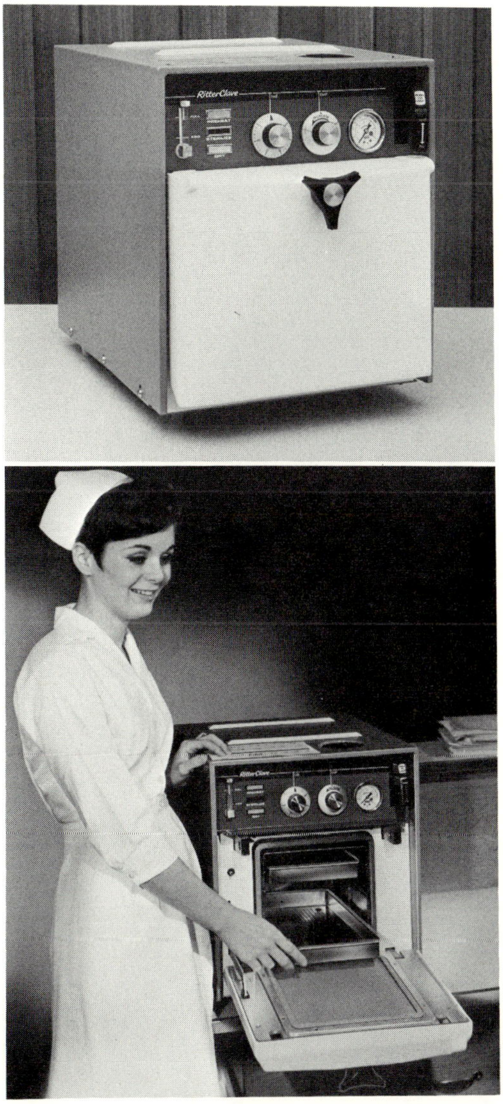

Fig. 9-6. A, Ritter autoclave, Ritter-Clave. This is a general purpose autoclave, designed for use in a dental office; **B,** interior design and construction of the chamber of this general purpose autoclave. (Courtesy Ritter Company.)

7. Scalers and other periodontal instruments
8. Suction tips

Steam under pressure (autoclave)

There are several methods of sterilization available to the dentist. However, the most effective and efficient is steam under pressure. The apparatus that provides this method of sterilization is known as the autoclave. The autoclave, in principle, is the same as a pressure cooker. Steam under pressure can be raised to temperatures that are higher than free-flowing steam or boiling water. It is the heat that sterilizes (Figs. 9-6 to 9-10). This method of providing heat has several advantages:

1. The desired temperature can be attained with ease and in a short period of time.
2. Anything that is not adversely affected by heat can be sterilized in an autoclave.
3. The damage to instruments is minimal.
4. Sterilization is effective and complete.
5. Spores are destroyed in a relatively short period of time.
6. Dissipation of heat into the room is minimal.

Sterilization in an autoclave is routinely accomplished at 250 degrees F. (121 degrees C.). This temperature is attained when the steam pressure is under 15 lbs. per square inch. The duration of the sterilizing cycle is 15 to 20 minutes at this temperature. However, the cycle can be shortened by elevating the temperature, and this may have some practical value when emergencies arise (Table 1).

When using an autoclave, the following essential steps must be observed:

1. Heat apparatus until steam is generated.
2. Insert material to be sterilized.
3. Seal the door tightly.
4. Evacuate air.
5. Elevate the temperature within the chamber to the desired level.
6. Provide adequate exposure time to the sterilizing temperature.
7. Release steam.
8. Allow for drying time.

Several aspects of sterilization by the use of the autoclave deserve special at-

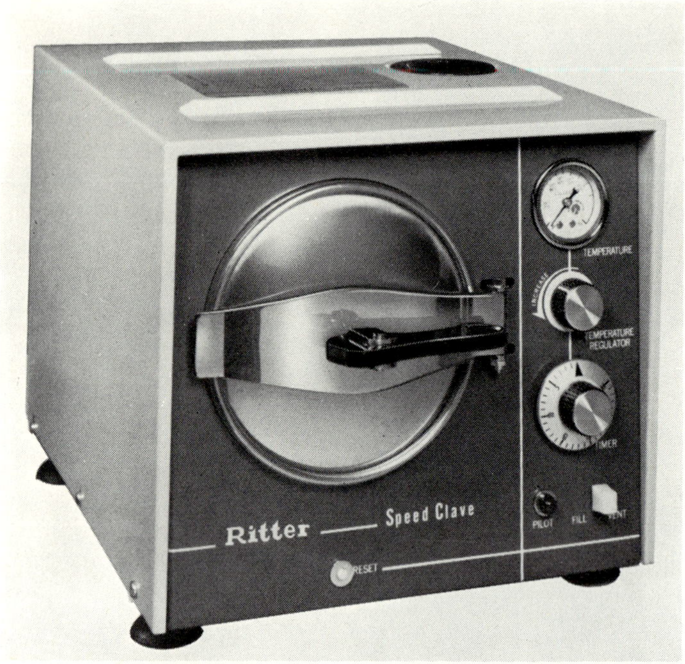

Fig. 9-7. Ritter Speed clave. This autoclave is designed to sterilize instruments and small packages. (Courtesy Ritter Company.)

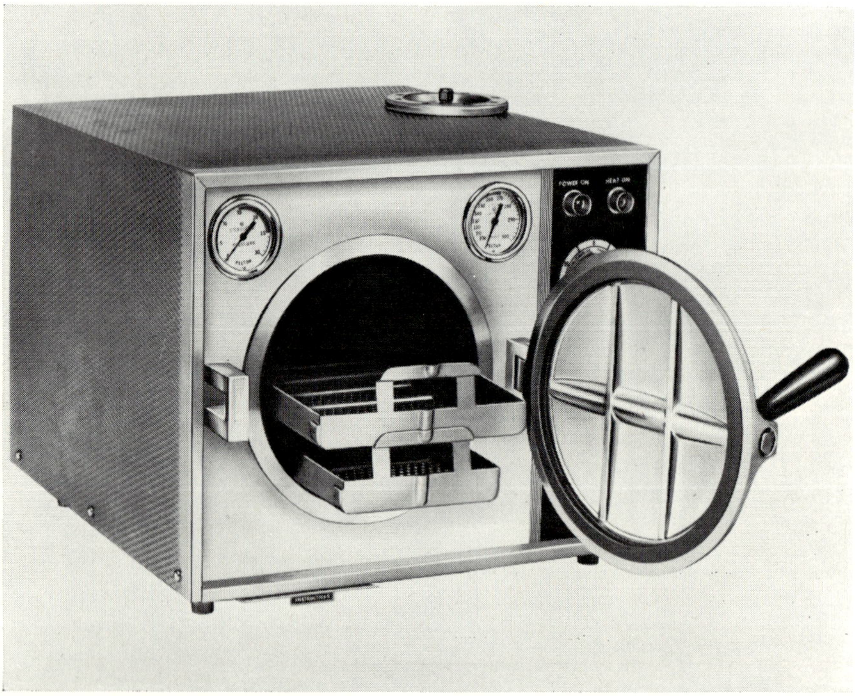

Fig. 9-8. Omniclave. The apparatus may be used for both autoclaving and dry heat sterilization. (Courtesy Pelton & Crane.)

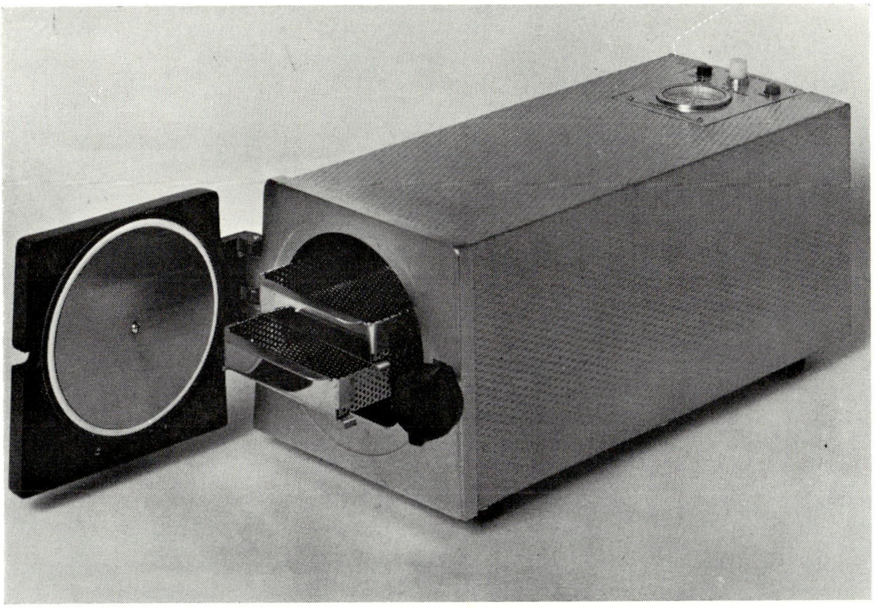

Fig. 9-9. Instru-Clave. A compact autoclave used to sterilize dental instruments. (Courtesy Pelton & Crane.)

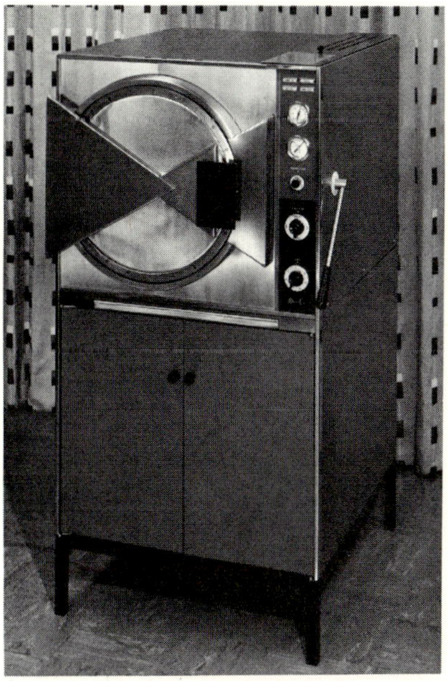

Fig. 9-10. Magna-Clave, a large general purpose autoclave. (Courtesy Pelton & Crane.)

tention and mention. Before instruments are placed into the autoclave, they must be cleansed meticulously. Since the temperature of the autoclave is evenly distributed by the penetration of the steam, the apparatus should never be packed too tightly. If the materials are packaged prior to sterilizing, they should be wrapped in a paper or cloth towel. In the event that tubes or metal containers are used for packaging, they must never be sealed tightly and must be placed on their side to prevent the accumulation of moisture. Metal objects do have a tendency to undergo corrosion when exposed to the action of steam. This needs to be taken into account, with necessary precautions taken. One method available for the protection of metal instruments is the use of Proclave. This regimen utilizes 2 solutions, one a detergent and the other an emulsion. The instruments are first placed into the deter-

Table 1. Temperature, exposure time, and load arrangement for steam pressure sterilization*

Article	Arrangement of load	Temperature in Fahrenheit degrees	Exposure time in minutes
Instruments	Layer of muslin placed in bottom of tray; instruments arranged so as to not contact one another; covered with second layer of muslin	250	15
Instruments (alternate method)	Layer of muslin placed in bottom of tray; instruments arranged so as to not contact one another; covered with second layer of muslin	270	3
Surgical dressings, small packs, other textiles	Flat compact packages wrapped with double-thickness muslin; packages placed in tray on end, never tightly packed together	250	20
Rubber gloves, rubber dam material	Flat compact packages wrapped with double-thickness muslin; packages placed in tray on end, never tightly packed together; dusting powder sprinkled between two layers of rubber	250	15
Empty glassware and utensils	Wrapped in muslin and inverted or placed on side	250	15
Solutions	Sealed in 50 ml. Pyrex flasks or test tubes up to 100 mm. long	250	15
	Sealed in 125 to 200 ml. Pyrex flasks	250	20

*From Kanterman, Cyril B.: W. Virginia D. J. 29:154, 1948.

gent; this step helps to cleanse and lower the surface tension. They are then submerged into the emulsion, which coats them with a layer that acts as a lubricant and thin protective film. When needles or objects with long thin lumens are to be sterilized in an autoclave, they should not be covered by a cotton roll, since the cotton will prevent the steam from gaining access to the lumen and thus prevent adequate sterilization. It is permissible to sterilize the needle and the cotton roll independently and then cover the needle by inserting it into the cotton roll before completely removing it from the autoclave.

Instruments and objects to be autoclaved may be placed loose into the apparatus. Upon completion of the sterilization cycles, they can be removed with sterile forceps and placed into a sterile container. However, the most advantageous method is to prepackage instruments in groupings as they are routinely used. Care must be taken to use a wrap that can be effectively penetrated by steam. Once packaged, sterilization is effected. When instruments are packaged, they may be stored for relatively long periods of time without fear of breaking the chain of sterility. A label with a thermochromatic indicator may be affixed to each package. This serves two purposes, to identify the content and to indicate that the package has been sterilized.

Hot oil sterilization

Hot oil sterilization (Fig. 9-11) is used primarily for the sterilization of conventional handpieces, contra-angles, burs, and instruments that are hinged or jointed. The apparatus closely resembles a miniature hot water sterilizer. Instead of using water as the bath, oil is used. Mineral oil, silicones, and other synthetic oils are used in the disinfection process. All objects must be thoroughly cleansed before being completely submerged in the oil. The cycles most frequently used are 150 degrees C. (300 degrees F.) for 10 minutes, or 121 degrees C. (250 degrees F.) for 15 minutes. This time-temperature ratio will kill all organisms except sporeformers. However, oil can be an effective sterilizing

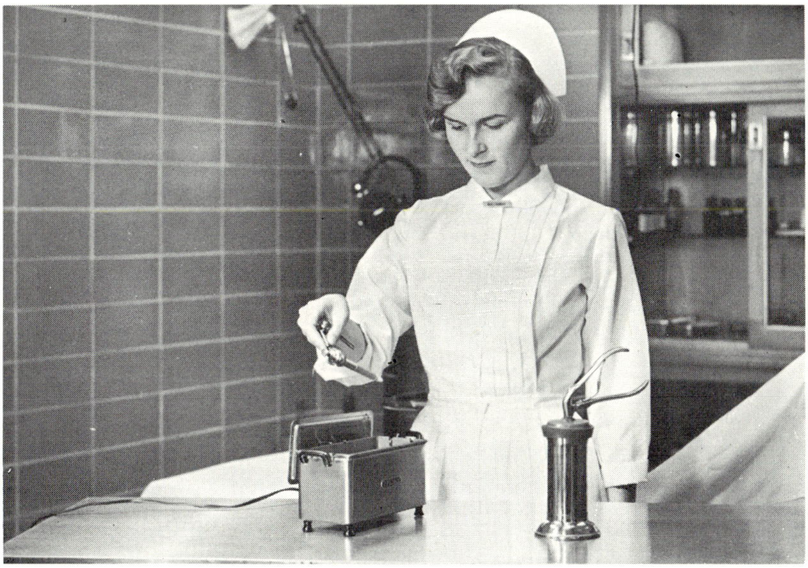

Fig. 9-11. Hot oil sterilization of a dental handpiece. The transfer forceps are used to remove the handpiece upon completion of sterilization. (From Peterson, S., editor: Clinical dental hygiene, ed. 3, St. Louis, 1968, The C. V. Mosby Co.)

agent at a temperature of 150 degrees C. (300 degrees F.) and with an exposure time of 1½ hours.

There is no one oil with all the properties that are desirable for use in hot oil sterilization. Ideally, the oil used should be nonirritating, chemically inert, and clear, have a high flash point, and be a good lubricant. The hydrocarbon oils are good lubricants, but when heated to the desired temperature, they break down and give off an offensive odor. They cannot be heated above 250 degrees C. because of their flash point. Silicones are more stable but are relatively poor lubricating agents. In spite of the inherent disadvantages and limitations, this method is recommended for disinfecting handpieces.

Dry heat sterilization

Dry heat sterilization (Figs. 9-8 and 9-12) is an effective method of sterilization, and the end results compare favorably with those achieved by the use of the autoclave. However, there are two distinct disadvantages that are ever present when using this method of sterilization. A longer sterilizing time is needed to achieve sterilization, and materials that are adversely affected by dry heat cannot be sterilized by this procedure. Dry heat sterilization is usually reserved for objects that do not lend themselves to moist heat and for those that rust readily. Root canal instruments, injection and surgical needles, and instruments with sharp-cutting surfaces are frequently sterilized with dry heat. When a minimum load is placed in the oven of the dry heat sterilizer, the sterilizing cycle is 1 hour at 160 degrees C. (320 degrees F.). However, should the oven be loaded to near capacity, the time interval must be increased to 2 hours. Timing of the cycle can begin only when the sterilizing temperature is achieved. In most instances, the high temperature that is required for this method of sterilization is injurious to fabrics. Towels and sponges can be sterilized by this technique, but the temperature is critical; 160 degrees C. must be maintained for sterilization, while anything over this amount of heat will usually produce charring.

A 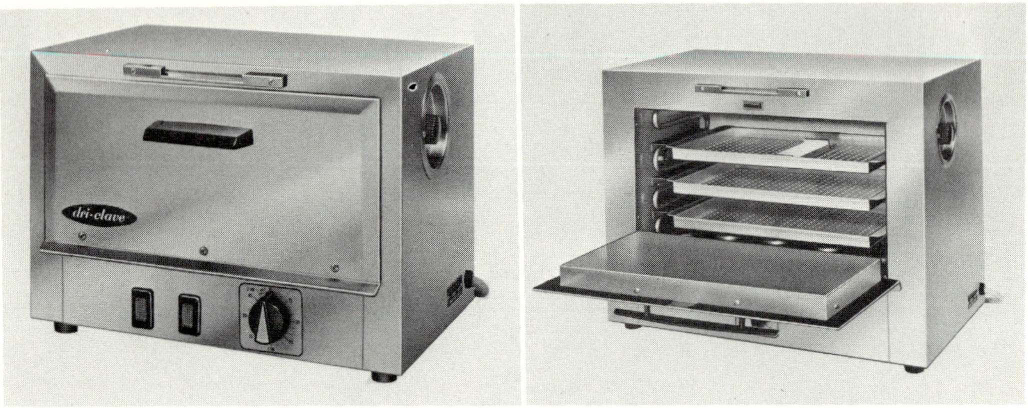 B

Fig. 9-12. A, Dri-Clave, a dry heat sterilizer, Model 75—2 tray; **B,** the interior design and construction of a dry heat sterilizer, Model 150—3 tray. (Courtesy Dri-Clave Corporation.)

The dry heat method of sterilization is usually not practical for the dental office because of the time factor and the need for sterilizing some instruments several times during the course of a single day. In addition to being used for metal objects with sharp edges, dry heat is frequently utilized in scientific laboratories and for sterilizing objects where maintaining complete dryness is mandatory.

Flaming or direct flame sterilization

Flaming, or direct flame sterilization, is accomplished by dipping an object in 95 percent alcohol and then exposing the object to the direct heat of a flame. In some instances, the alcohol dip is omitted. This method is effective in destroying vegetative forms of organisms, but it is not completely efficient for destroying all spores. It should be emphasized that direct flame sterilization includes more than just passing an object through a flame. The temperature of the object must be elevated to a minimum of 60 degrees C. Because of the effect that heat has on metals at this temperature, it is not a routinely useful method of sterilization. The only real advantage of flaming is that it allows sterilization of metal objects in a very short period of time.

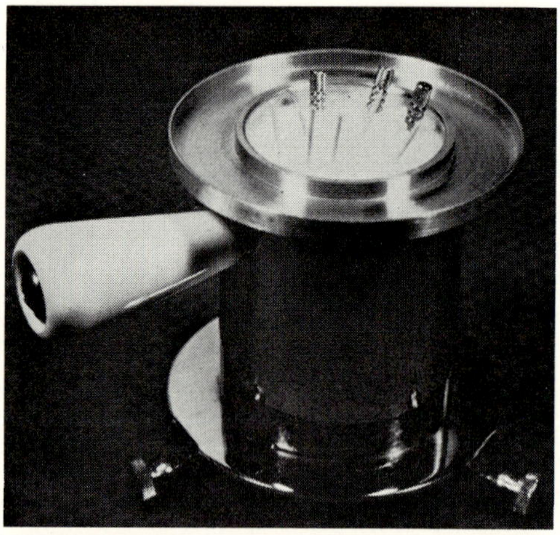

Fig. 9-13. Glass bead or salt sterilizer. This sterilizer is primarily used in endodontics. Files and paper points are inserted between the hot beads in this illustration.

Glass bead, salt, or molten metal sterilizer

This type of sterilizer (Fig. 9-13) consists of an apparatus containing a small pot in which the temperature can be maintained from 204 degrees C. (400 degrees F.) to 280 degrees C. (536 degrees F.). These sterilizers are generally of 2 types; one is electrical, and the other requires gas heat. Molten metal, glass beads, or salt is placed in the pot, and the temperature within the container is elevated to the desired level. Small objects can be inserted into the contents of the pot and left for the desired period of time. The interval is usually from 5 to 10 seconds. This method of sterilization will destroy vegetative organisms, but there is some question concerning the reliability of the device to kill spores within a reasonable time. Since the reliability of this form of sterilization is in question, and it can only be used for very small objects, it is recommended that other forms of sterilization be utilized.

This piece of equipment is used primarily in the field of endodontics to sterilize the working end of small metal instruments, paper points, and cotton pellets. Since the molten metal has the tendency to adhere, it has been discarded in favor of salt or glass beads.

Ultraviolet light sterilization

Ultraviolet light, or radiation, will destroy airborne organisms and organisms found upon exposed surfaces. It has no penetrating ability; consequently, the application of this form of sterilization is limited. Ultraviolet light is used successfully to reduce the bacterial count in a room, to sterilize drawers or cabinets, and to render sterile exposed surfaces of objects that cannot be sterilized by any other means.

Ultraviolet light is irritating to the eyes and skin. When not being used in a closed or shielded place, it should not be in use while the operator is in the room.

Gaseous sterilization

Gases have been utilized for sterilization for a number of years, and among those that have been used are sulfur dioxide and formaldehyde. However, the gas that is of primary interest in this discussion is ethylene oxide, because of its penetrating potential and ability to destroy spores. This gas is being used to sterilize many drugs, including antibiotics, biologicals, and enzyme preparations. It is also used to render sterile plastics, surgical material, processing equipment, and other pieces of apparatus. In short, ethylene oxide can usually be used to sterilize almost any object that would be adversely affected by heat or moisture. One of the several applications of ethylene oxide sterilization in dentistry is the sterilization of disposable needles.

Ethylene oxide is a colorless gas at room temperature. It is inflammable and, when mixed with air, explosive. In order that the hazard of explosion may be reduced, the gas (10 to 20 percent) is mixed with carbon dioxide and then used for sterilization. Special autoclaves are used for this type of sterilization. When the temperature and pressure conditions are ideal, the penetration of this gaseous mixture is extremely efficient. The sterilization time varies from 4 to 8 hours.

Bacterial filtration

Bacterial filtration is useful in removing organisms from thermolabile solutions. The solution is passed through special types of filters that are capable of retaining microorganisms, spores, and many types of viruses. There is some question as to the complete effectiveness of this method of cold sterilization against all viruses. However, bacterial filtration is extremely useful in sterilizing solutions when other methods are not practical or available.

HEPATITIS

There are 2 virus diseases, both of which primarily involve the liver, that are known as hepatitis. Because of the possibility of spreading these diseases from one patient to another in the dental office by the use of contaminated instruments, one should have some familiarity with them.

Infectious hepatitis is one of the most common of all infectious diseases and is transmitted by direct contact or contact with contaminated fomites or food and water. Serum hepatitis is spread by contact with blood or plasma that contains the virus. In view of the manner by which these diseases are spread, sterilization of instruments and objects that may come in contact with the patient is essential. Particular care must be taken of instruments that come in contact with blood or those that are used to penetrate the skin or mucous membranes. Autoclaving is the most reliable method available in the dental office for destroying viruses and thus preventing the transmission of these diseases via contaminated instruments.

SPECIAL CONSIDERATIONS

Storage of instruments following sterilization

After sterilization, instruments must be kept sterile until used. This may be accomplished in several ways. To maintain sterility of instruments, the following precautions must be taken:

1. Instruments that have been autoclaved or sterilized in boiling water must be removed from the sterilizer only with sterile instrument forceps; they must never be touched by the hands.

2. The instruments are then placed in designated drawers or cabinets between towels that have previously been sterilized in the autoclave. Instruments that have been wrapped for autoclaving should be left in the package until placed on the instrument tray.

3. Instruments must not be removed from the storage cabinet or container with the fingers, but they should be removed only with sterile forceps.

Instruments disinfected by chemical means are usually stored in the dental cabinet after they are rinsed and dried with a sterile towel.

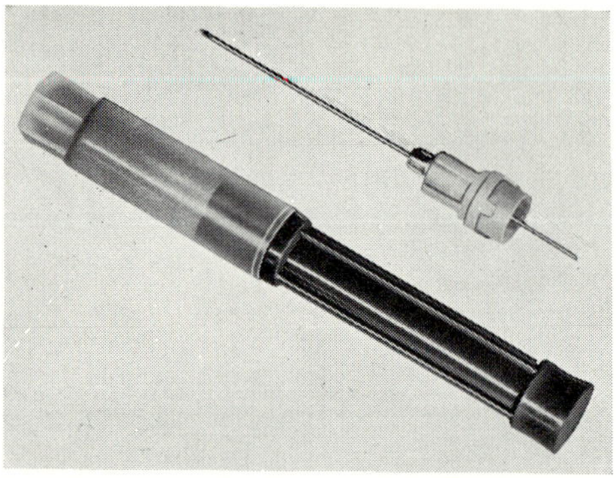

Fig. 9-14. Presterilized, disposable dental needle. (Courtesy Sherwood Medical Industries, Inc.)

Preparation of anesthetic syringe

Because it is so very important that injections be made under sterile conditions, special consideration must be given to sterilizing the syringe and preparing it for use.

After use, the anesthetic carpule is removed from the syringe and discarded. The contents of the carpule must never be saved, even though only a portion of it was used. If a disposable needle is used, it also is removed from the syringe and discarded. The syringe itself is then scrubbed with a stiff brush in warm, soapy water, rinsed thoroughly, placed in the ultrasonic vibrator, and sterilized by boiling or by autoclaving. After the syringe is sterilized, it is removed from the sterilizer with sterile instrument forceps and placed in a sterile storage area.

When needed, the syringe is removed from its sterile container, and the needle and hub are assembled, if they were sterilized separately. In this case, the hub and needle are picked up with sterile forceps, since the needle must not be touched by the hands. Many offices are now using presterilized disposable needles (Fig. 9-14). When the manufacturer's instructions concerning assembly of the syringe are followed, the disposable needle can be placed on the syringe with no danger of contami-

A

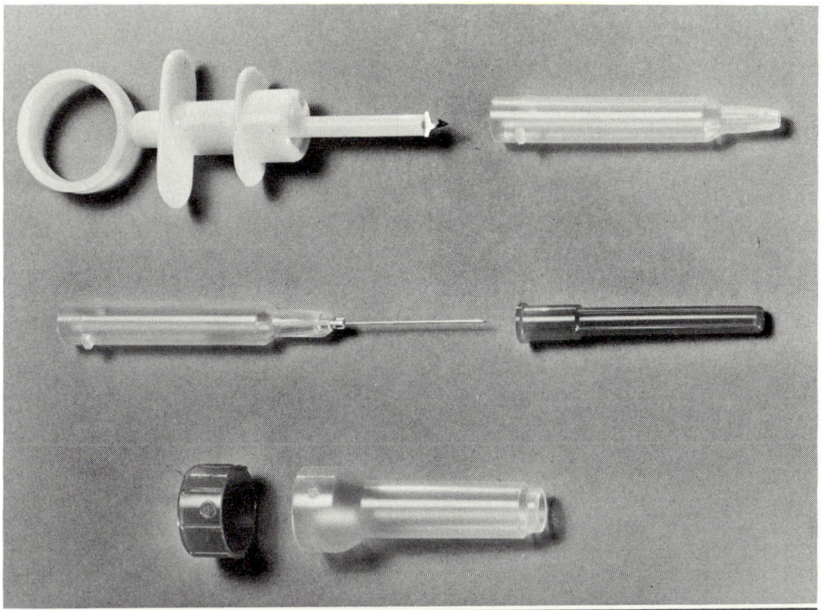

B

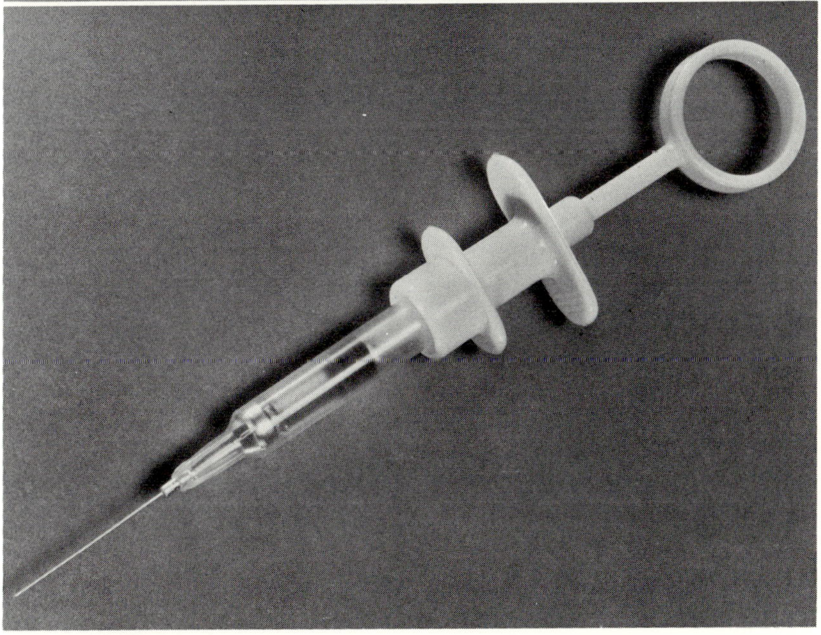

Fig. 9-15. Disposable syringe. **A,** Disassembled disposable syringe, displaying the components; **B,** assembled disposable syringe, with anesthetic carpule in place and ready for use. (Courtesy Sherwood Medical Industries, Inc.)

nation. With the needle assembly in place, the anesthetic carpule is removed from a germicidal solution and inserted in the syringe. The syringe is now ready for use, but the assistant must be extremely careful that the needle does not touch any nonsterile object before injection. Should the disposable syringe be used, the same degree of safety can be expected, and the same precautions must be exercised (Fig. 9-15, *A* and *B*). If a tray is used, it should be covered with a towel that has been autoclaved.

Tray preparation

A sterile tray setup should be used whenever practical. A container of autoclaved towels should be kept next to the sterilizer, and towels should be removed only with the instrument forceps. The tray is first covered with a sterile towel, and then sterile forceps are used to place the required instruments and supplies in proper order on the tray. If instruments have been autoclaved in individual paper containers, they should be removed and placed on the tray without being touched by the hands. A sterile towel is then placed over the instrument arrangement, and the tray is ready for use. Offices that routinely use the tray system will usually have a number of trays that have been completely outfitted and autoclaved in advance. These, of course, are available for immediate use.

SUMMARY OF STERILIZATION PROCEDURES

Upon completion of each appointment, a definite routine should be followed for the care and sterilization of instruments and equipment. In general, this routine should be as follows:

1. All instruments are removed from the bracket table or tray, scrubbed thoroughly with a stiff brush in warm, soapy water, rinsed in clear water, and then cycled in the ultrasonic vibrator.
2. Air and water syringe tips and oral evacuator tips are removed and scrubbed thoroughly, as in the case of operating instruments.
3. The instruments, syringe tips, and oral evacuator tips are then sterilized by autoclaving, boiling water, or chemical means. All surgical instruments must be autoclaved or boiled. Instruments used in examination, cavity preparation, and restorative procedures may be placed in the chemical solution.
4. Cement slabs and spatulas are scrubbed, rinsed, dried, and replaced in proper storage place.
5. Conventional handpieces, contra-angles, and prophylaxis handpieces are removed from the dental unit and placed in the hot oil sterilizer. Handpieces that cannot be sterilized by this method are wiped carefully with an alcohol sponge.
6. The bracket table or tray cover is removed and discarded (if made of paper) or placed in laundry receptacle.
7. The rim of the bracket table and the air and water syringes are carefully wiped with an alcohol sponge.

Selected readings

Addison, B. A., and others: Sterilization of surgical sutures; comparison of heat and irradiation, Amer. Surgeon **31**:242, 1965.

Antonovich, E. I.: The dry air sterilizer SS-1, Med. Promyshl. SSSR **18**:52, 1964.

Avis, K. E.: What to watch for in sterilization technic, Mod. Hosp. **100**:98, 1963.

Burrows, W.: Textbook of microbiology, ed. 16, Philadelphia, 1954, W. B. Saunders Co.

Burton, W. E.: Changing requirements for sterilization, J. Prosth. Dent. **14**:127, 1964.

Central sterile supply principles and practice, London, 1963, Oxford University Press.

Christensen, E. A.: Recent sterilization methods, Ugeskr. laeger **126**:330, 1964.

Christensen, E. A., and others: Inactivation of dried bacteria and bacterial spores by means of ionizing radiation, Acta Path. Microbiol. Scand. **58**:225, 1964.

Cleary, D. J.: Residual effects of ethylene oxide sterilization, Bull. Parenteral Drug Ass. **23**:233, 1969.

Colombo, B. M.: Sterilization on an industrial scale with ethylene oxide, Boll. Chimicofarm **103**:554, 1964.

Conte, E. A.: How to sterilize with ethylene oxide gas, Mod. Hosp. **102**:122, 1964.
Coughlin, J. W., and others: Comparison of dry heat, autoclave and vapor sterilizers, J. Ontario Dent. Ass. **45**:137, 1968.
Crawford, J. J., and others: Practical methods of office sterilization and disinfection, J. Oral Med. **22**:133, 1967.
Crowley, M. C.: Obtaining and maintaining surgical cleanliness. In Dental Clinics of North America, November, 1957, W. B. Saunders Co.
Custer, F., and others: Instrument changes during sterilization, J. Dent. Res. **49**:487, 1970.
Darmody, E. M.: The cleaning of instruments and syringes, J. Clin. Path. **18**:6, 1965.
Dittmer, H. H.: Sterilization of local anesthetics, Pharm. Prax. **2**:197, 1963.
Ehrlen, I. R.: Advances in sterilization techniques, Pharm. Weekbl. **99**:1430, 1964.
Ehrlen, I. R.: Advances in sterilization techniques, Svensk. Farm. T. **68**:818, 1964.
Eshleman, J. R.: Methods used for sterilization or disinfection of instruments, J. Dent. Educ. **32**:330, 1968.
Fallon, R. J.: Sterilization of air filters for high pre-vacuum autoclaves, J. Clin. Path. **16**:259, 1963.
Finsterbusch, W.: Experiments with cold sterilization using ethylene oxide under increased tension during one year of clinical use, Wien. Klin. Wschr. **76**:255, 1964.
Gasthalter, F. M.: Importance of sterilization in dental practice (a review of the literature), W. Virginia Dent. Ass. **36**:154, 1962.
Gillette, W. B.: Ethylene oxide sterilization in dentistry, J. Oral Ther. **2**:440, 1966.
Gimborn, H. von: Sterilization technic, Pharm. Prax. **9**:197, 1963.
Ginsberg, F.: Ethylene oxide is boon to hospital asepsis, Mod. Hosp. **102**:118, 1964.
Gould, D.: Sterilization of medical instruments with gamma rays, Elektromedizin **9**:38, 1964.
Grabar, P.: Biological actions of ultrasonic waves, Advances Biol. Med. Phys. **3**:191, 1953.
Gunther, D. A.: Balanced pressure sterilization with ethylene oxide—a new technique, Bull. Parenteral Drug Ass. **24**:193, 1970.
Haberman, S.: Some comparative studies between a chemical vapor sterilizer and a conventional steam autoclave on various bacteria and viruses, J. Southern Calif. Dent. Ass. **30**:163, 1962.
Hepatitis, Health Information Series, No. 82, Washington, D. C., 1955, U. S. Department of Health, Education, and Welfare.
Hesselgren, S. G., and others: A new method of sterilizing handpieces and contra-angles, J. Oral Ther. **3**:340, 1967.
Hok, R., and others: Ultrasonic tonometer sterilization, Amer. J. Ophthal. **58**:676, 1964.
Holmlund, L. G.: Standardization, by means of ultrasonic treatment, of test samples for laboratory steam-corrosion tests, Acta Odont. Scand. **21**:321, 1963.
Hunter, H. A., and Madlener, E. M.: Disinfection of dental instruments, Int. Dent. J. **11**:312, 1961.
Johnsen, G. N.: Our experience with a high-vacuum sterilizer, Hospitals **37**:77, 1963.
Jossel, N.: Instrument sterilization in dental practice; some limited observations, J. Soc. Dent. Res. **13**:10, 1964.
Lane, C. R., and others: High-temperature sterilization for surgical instruments, Lancet **1**:358, 1964.
Lawrence, C. A., and Block, S. S.: Disinfection, sterilization and preservation, Philadelphia, 1968, Lea & Febiger.
Lubianitskii, G. D.: Ultrasonic device type U M 2-2 for cleaning of medical instruments, Med. Promyshl. SSSR **18**:49, 1964.
McCulloch, E. C.: Disinfection and sterilization, ed. 3, Philadelphia, 1945, Lea & Febiger.
McLundle, A. C., and others: Sterilization in general dental practice, Brit. Dent. J. **124**:214, 1968.
Mercer, J. F.: The challenge of sterilization in the dental office, Dent. Asst. **38**:10, 1969.
Olander, J. W.: New facilities and equipment for radiation sterilization, Bull. Parenteral Drug Ass. **17**:14, 1963.
Opfell, J. B., and others: Penetration by gases to sterilize interior surfaces of confined spaces, Appl. Microbiol. **12**:27, 1964.
Perkins, J. J.: Principles and methods of sterilization, ed. 2, Springfield, Illinois, 1969, Charles C Thomas, Publisher.
Perkulis, B., and others: Ultrasonics and benzalkonium chloride as a method of sterilizing dental instruments, J. Dent. Child. **37**:69, 1970.
Rittenburg, M. S., and others: Preliminary evaluation of an activated glutaraldehyde solution for cold sterilization, Ann. Surg. **161**:127, 1965.
Rubbo, S. D., and Gardner, J. F.: A review of sterilization and disinfection as applied to medical, industrial, and laboratory practice, Chicago, 1965, Year Book Medical Publishers, Inc.
Shaner, E. O.: Acoustical-chemical parameters for the ultrasonic sterilization of instruments. A status report, J. Oral Ther. **3**:417, 1967.
Sterilization of surgical material; a symposium, London, 1961, The Pharmaceutical Press.
Stratford, B. C.: An ultra-violet water-sterilizing unit, Med. J. Aust. **1**(1):11, 1963.

Sykes, G.: Disinfection and sterilization, ed. 2, Philadelphia, 1965, J. B. Lippincott Co.

Taguchi, J. T., and others: Serious limitations of a portable ethylene oxide sterilizer, Amer. J. Med. Sci. **245**:299, 1963.

Trexler, P. C.: Microbic contamination control, Bull. Parenteral Drug Ass. **18**:8, 1964.

Walker, R. O., and others: The sterilization of syringes; a survey of current methods and recommendations, Brit. Dent. J. **118**:151, 1965.

Watson, D. D., and others: Sterilizing techniques with ethylene oxide, Hospitals **37**:81, 1963.

Winge-Heden, K.: Ethylene oxide sterilization without special equipment, Acta Path. Microbiol. Scand. **58**:225, 1963.

CHAPTER 10 DENTAL MATERIALS

RALPH W. PHILLIPS, M.S., D.Sc.

It is hoped that the discussion in this chapter will make the assistant increasingly conscious of the difficulties involved in making a satisfactory dental restoration or appliance. Unfortunately, too often both the dentist and the dental assistant are unaware of the rigid conditions present in the oral cavity and of the influence that the various steps taken in handling the restorative material will have on its clinical behavior.

In some mouths, restorations are subjected to biting forces of thousands of pounds per square inch. Temperature changes from hot and cold foods may cause cracking or disintegration of filling materials. The mouth is warm and humid and contains bacteria that may discolor or dissolve many types of material. The acidity or alkalinity of foods and liquids that patients eat and drink may destroy the material.

One of the greatest problems associated with the clinical use of restorative dental materials is that none of them actually bond or adhere to tooth structure. Thus, debris, acids, and microorganisms can readily penetrate around the restoration, as diagrammed in Fig. 10-1. This phenomenon is referred to as "microleakage" and may frequently be identified with postoperative sensitivity of restored teeth and with marginal caries and stain. These and other factors make it essential that all materials used in the oral cavity have highly specialized compositions and that they be handled in a standardized way to assure clinical success.

Since 1928, the American Dental Association has maintained a division at the National Bureau of Standards for establishing specifications and requirements for most of the commonly used materials. These specifications cover the essential physical and chemical properties and assure the dentist of material that is prepared to meet the rigid demands that will be made upon it in use. As present there are 22 specifications. Only products that are on the approved list of American Dental Association products should be selected. Most of the specifications of the American Dental Association have been used as guides in establishing international specifications.

In spite of this rigid control of materials by both the manufacturers and the American Dental Association, clinical failures are all too common with all types of materials. Fractures, discoloration, expansion of a material from the cavity preparation, new decay around the margins of the restoration, and severe abrasion are examples of the failures that routinely occur. These failures can no longer be blamed on the use of inferior products; rather, they must be attributed to improper manipulation of a material that was well prepared

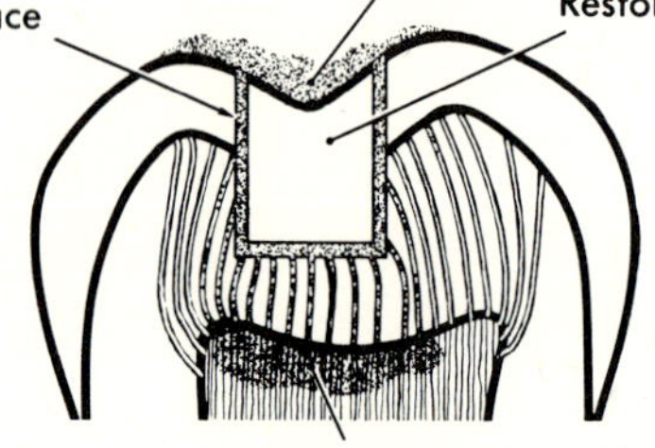

Fig. 10-1. A diagram of the "microleakage" phenomenon. In this illustration, the penetration of oral fluids and debris has penetrated the tooth restoration "interface," through the dentin itself, and into the pulp. (From Phillips, R. W., Swartz, M. S., and Norman, R. D.: Materials for the practicing dentist, St. Louis, 1969, The C. V. Mosby Co.)

by the manufacturer. Every step involved in the preparation of the restoration or appliance—such as weighing, mixing, handling in the mouth, and all laboratory steps—has a definite effect on how the material will behave in the oral cavity. In addition, patient education requires a knowledge of dental materials and their properties, in order that the assistant may aid in proper instruction to the patient. Thus, the dental assistant has a direct responsibility in controlling many of the steps that will directly influence the clinical behavior of the restoration or appliance. Such a responsibility cannot be taken lightly, and this chapter will be devoted to a discussion of the manipulative variables that the assistant controls.

Obviously, there is not sufficient space here to acquaint the student with all the background information essential to a proper appreciation of the subject, but the present discussion will make her aware of the more important factors that she must control and the reasons for the procedures outlined. It is hoped that she will be stimulated to read further in this field, since a major part of her training and her professional career will be concerned with the use of dental materials.

AMALGAM

The dental amalgam restoration is made by mixing small particles of a metallic alloy powder (composed of silver, tin, copper, and usually zinc) with mercury. In addition to the powder or filing form of the alloy, it may also be supplied as small round particles, referred to as spherical alloys. The mixing process is referred to as *trituration,* and it may be carried out either by hand or by mechanical mixers.

Approximately 80 percent of all restorations are amalgam. The widespread use of this material in the average dental office emphasizes the importance of controlling and understanding all steps involved in its use. Amalgam is obviously an excellent restorative material. Probably as much as any one single factor, the unique clinical success of this material may be associated with the decrease in the microleakage that occurs in time. Corrosion products form between the amalgam restoration and the cavity preparation; the restoration thereby tends to prevent the penetration of deleterious agents. However, daily observations in the dental office reveal large numbers of failures. These usually occur in the form of recurrent caries, fracture, or excessive dimensional change. It has been shown that faulty manipulation of the alloy or its contamination at the time of insertion accounts for approximately 40 percent of these failures. It is with this 40 percent that the assistant must be concerned.

Before the actual steps in manipulation are discussed, it is important to stress that the two physical properties that especially influence the clinical behavior of amalgam are dimensional change and strength. Proper control of these properties is essential if failure is to be avoided. Undue expansion of the material after it has been inserted in the cavity preparation should be kept to a minimum. Expansion can lead to overhanging ledges of amalgam and possible recurrence of caries from the collected debris. Likewise, contraction can lead to leakage around the restoration and to new areas of caries.

Adequate strength is also essential to the success of the restoration. Fracture, even on a small area, can lead to clinical failure, and approximately 26 percent of all failures can be attributed to fracture.

Unfortunately, both the dimensional change and the strength of the final inserted restoration are greatly influenced by the manipulative steps that are to be discussed. A standardized procedure for handling this material is essential if these important properties are to be maintained and clinical success ensured.

Proportioning

It is the unique characteristic of mercury that makes possible the amalgam restoration. The mercury, when mixed with metallic particles of a suitable alloy, forms a plastic mass that can be inserted and finished in the tooth. Subsequently, it hardens to a restorative material that serves effectively in resisting oral forces.

The exact amount of mercury used in preparing the mix is very important. There must be a sufficient amount to wet each alloy particle. Insufficient mercury will prevent a smooth mix. Excess mercury, however, is to be avoided. Proper proportioning of the mercury and alloy is one of the variables associated with the amalgam restoration that can be readily controlled. Excess mercury used in the original mix will result in a higher percentage of mercury in the final restoration. This is true regardless of the technique employed during the subsequent mixing or condensation. Since the greatest single factor that controls the strength of amalgam is the final mercury content of the restoration (the higher the percentage of mercury, the lower the strength), the use of the correct initial ratio of mercury and alloy is most important.

Since it is now recognized that the final mercury content of the restoration does dramatically influence its clinical behavior, a minimal mercury technique is popular. This procedure is often referred to as the Eames technique. With the modern fine grain alloys, it is possible to use less mercury in the original mix. Frequently, mercury-alloy ratios as low as 1 to 1 are employed. However, as previously mentioned, it is important to remember that this ratio should not be decreased too much. Insufficient mercury leads to a granular mix and causes striations and voids within the restoration.

The exact alloy-mercury ratio desired will be determined by the dentist.

A wide variety of alloy-mercury dispensers, or proportioners, are available. The type of dispenser is not so important as the proper use of the apparatus. It must be properly adjusted for the alloy being used, and the manufacturer's directions for use should be carefully read and followed. Extreme accuracy in proportioning is particularly essential when a minimal mercury technique is employed.

In addition to the particles, or grains, dental amalgam alloy may also be purchased in the form of pellets. Either type is satisfactory, but the pellet form of preweighed packets of the particles ensures consistent weights. Then all that is required is a mercury dispenser that will assure uniform "spills" of mercury. There are various brands of mercury dispensers that are accurate and dependable. A number of manufacturers have made preproportioned alloy and mercury available in disposable capsules. Although more expensive, this method of packaging is convenient and assures the proper ratio.

Trituration

The purpose of trituration is twofold: (1) to further reduce the grain size of the alloy and (2) to remove by abrasion the superficial coat of tarnish on each alloy

A

B

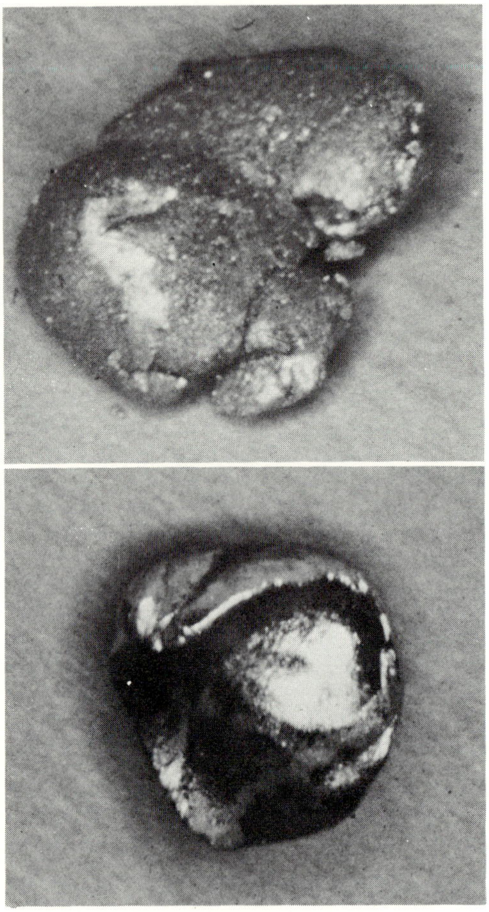

Fig. 10-2. A, An undertriturated mix of amalgam; **B,** a proper mix that will assure maximum physical properties.

particle. During and following trituration, the metal beneath this layer of tarnish is exposed and readily attacked by the mercury. Of all the variables involved in the use of amalgam, none has a greater effect upon the final restoration than the length of trituration. Research has clearly indicated that undertrituration is to be avoided. An example of an undertriturated mix may be seen in Fig. 10-2, *A*. It is impossible to remove the mercury from such a mix; hence, the restoration will have a high mercury content.

With longer trituration, the amalgam attains an appearance very much like a heavy grease, as seen in Fig. 10-2, *B*. The length of time required to attain this consistency will, of course, vary, depending on factors such as brand of alloy, type of triturating device, and size of the mix. Therefore, various mixing times should be tried under the conditions that exist in the individual office until this consistency is attained.

Regardless of the brand of alloy, undertrituration results in a drastic loss of strength and greater susceptibility to tarnish and corrosion. An undertriturated mix is also more difficult to handle, because of its rapid setting and rough carved surface that results.

A number of mechanical devices are available for trituration. Two popular brands are shown in Fig. 10-3. While they do not produce results that are superior to those achieved with *careful* hand techniques, they do standardize the mix. This is their main advantage, other than amalgamation. The capsule should be thoroughly cleared after each mix, because particles of hardened amalgam left in the capsule will contaminate subsequent mixes.

An example of the type of failure that results when the mercury content of the restoration is abnormally high can be seen in Fig. 10-4. The low strength of the amalgam has resulted in both a "ditching" effect at the margins and a fracture. Such a condition may develop if too much mercury is used in the original mix, if the amalgam is undertriturated, or if the dentist uses inadequate condensation pressure.

It is important to note that of the 3 steps that control the final mercury content of the restoration, the dental assistant is directly responsible for two.

Amalgam that is more than 3½ or 4 minutes old should not be used. When amalgam has been allowed to stand that long after mixing, it is not possible to remove the excess mercury, and a weak material results. Therefore, it should be discarded, and a new mix should be made to complete the restoration.

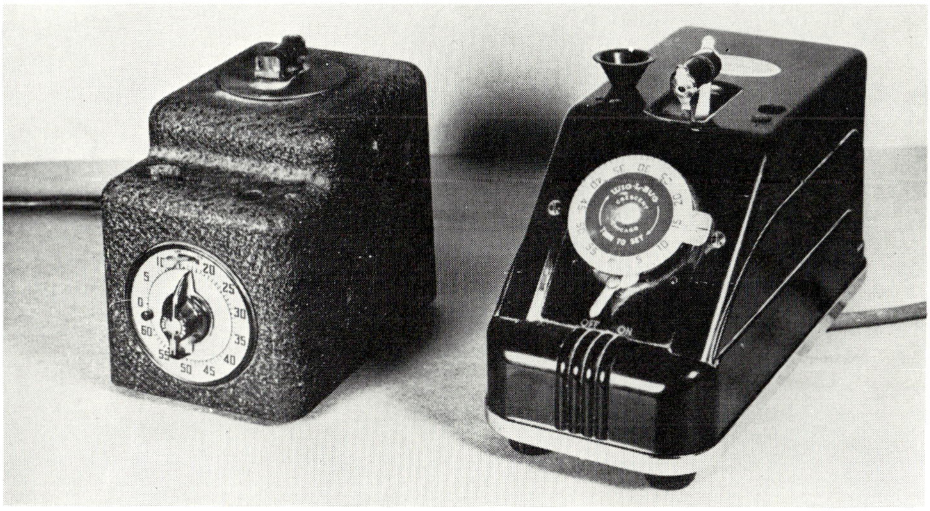

Fig. 10-3. Two mechanical amalgamators. Their main advantage over hand trituration is standardization of mixes.

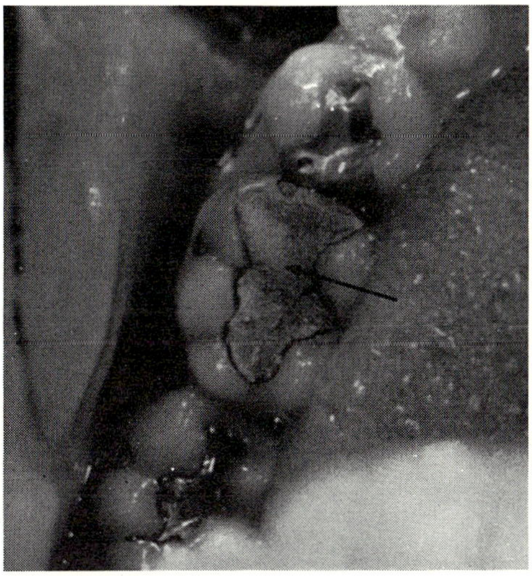

Fig. 10-4. Amalgam failure, indicated by arrow, caused by excess mercury in restoration. Correct ratio, proper trituration, and proper condensation prevent such occurrences.

Effect of moisture

Approximately 16 percent of all amalgams fail because of contamination of amalgam with moisture. Such contamination may come from perspiration on the hands or fingers of the dentist or assistant or from saliva incorporated during the time of insertion into the cavity preparation. The zinc that is present in most alloys will react with the moisture to form hydrogen gas. This trapped gas within the restoration results in severe expansion (Fig. 10-5). It may also produce postoperative pain, and the porous surface produced by the contaminant will increase the corrosion. Thus, amalgam must be handled carefully to prevent moisture contamination. Mixcd amalgam should never be touched with the fingers; if the mix is mulled, it should be done in a rubber dam.

In order to provide some safety margin in case of accidental contamination, some manufacturers have introduced alloys that contain no zinc. Most of these alloys are apparently satisfactory, but *moisture is always to be avoided,* regardless of the composition of the alloy.

Discoloration

Tarnish or corrosion on the surface of any metallic restoration is always unsightly, and amalgam is particularly susceptible to discoloration (Fig. 10-6). Certain factors, such as toothbrushing habits, diet, and flow of saliva, influence discoloration and are not directly under the control of the den-

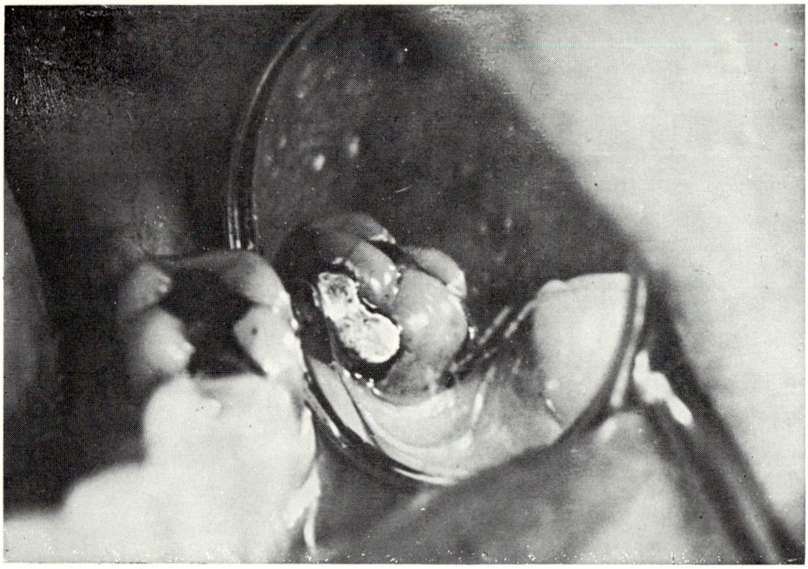

Fig. 10-5. Amalgam failure due to severe expansion caused by moisture contamination of a zinc alloy. (From Healey, H. J., and Phillips, R. W.: J. Dent. Res. **28**:439, 1949.)

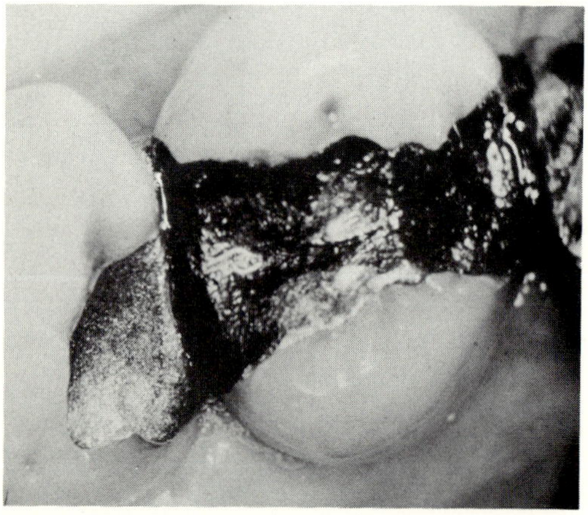

Fig. 10-6. Example of severe clinical tarnish. Oral environment and certain manipulative variables will influence its incidence.

tist or his assistant. However, manipulative variables do contribute to the maintenance of aesthetics. Generally, any step in the technique of manipulation that contributes to surface roughness will accelerate tarnish. Thus, everything possible should be done to produce a smooth final surface. This includes the use of small-grained alloys, thorough trituration, prevention of moisture contamination, and a final polishing of the surface. When these fundamental precautions are taken, the surface will usually remain lustrous in the patient's mouth (Fig. 10-7).

CEMENTS

Several types of dental cements are employed for varying purposes. A classification, based on composition and use, can be seen in Table 2. As a group, these cements are the weakest of all dental materials. They are not strong; they do not adhere to tooth structure; they will discolor; and they dissolve in oral fluids. In spite of these deficiencies, however, they possess so many desirable characteristics and are so essential to many dental operations that they are used in from 40 to 60 percent of all restorations. Recognition of their inherent weaknesses emphazies the importance of proper manipulative techniques to provide reasonable opportunity for success.

Table 2. Classes of dental cements and their respective areas of use*

Cement	Uses	
	Principal	**Secondary**
Zinc phosphate	Luting agent for indirect restorations and orthodontic bands	Temporary restorations
Zinc phosphate with copper or silver salts	Temporary restorations	
Copper phosphate	Temporary restorations	Luting agent for orthodontic appliances
Zinc oxide–eugenol	Temporary restorations Pulp capping Thermal insulating bases	Root canal restorations Luting agent for indirect restorations
Calcium hydroxide	Pulp capping Thermal insulting bases	
Silicate	Anterior restorations	
Silicophosphate	Luting agent for indirect restorations	Temporary restorations
Acrylic resin	Luting agent for indirect restorations	Temporary restorations

*From Phillips, R. W., Swartz, M. L., and Norman, R. D.: Materials for the practicing dentist, St. Louis, 1968, The C. V. Mosby Co.

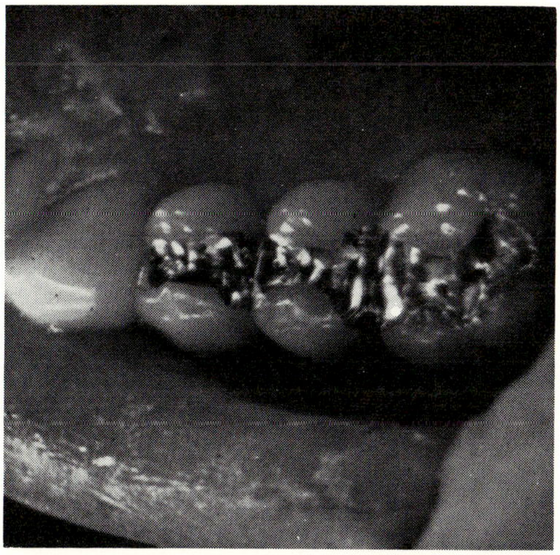

Fig. 10-7. Polished amalgam restorations. Surface remains smooth and no discoloration is apparent when proper manipulation is carried out.

Zinc phosphate cement

Zinc phosphate cement is used primarily for cementation of restorations or orthodontic bands and to provide a base under metallic restorations. The mix is made from a powder, primarily zinc oxide and magnesium oxide, and a liquid composed of phosphoric acid, water, and certain buffering agents.

The acid-water ratio in the liquid is quite critical and has been delicately balanced by the manufacturer. The setting time is seriously altered if the water content varies even slightly; every precaution should be taken to maintain this composition. If the liquid is exposed to the atmosphere, it will gain or loose water, depending upon the humidity of the room. If the liquid absorbs water, the setting is greatly accelerated. On the other hand, the loss of water slows the setting. Thus, the bottles should always be kept tightly stoppered, and tops should be replaced immediately after use.

The liquid is never placed on the slab until the assistant is ready to proceed with the mix. The liquid should never be used to the last drop. Repeated opening of the bottle over a long period of time will undoubtedly have altered the water-acid ratio of the last bit of liquid, and, therefore, the last one-fifth of the bottle should be discarded. The neck of the bottle should be kept clean and free of debris. Agitation of the liquid is not necessary. It should not be used if it becomes cloudy or gives evidence of crystallization, because this condition indicates water evaporation.

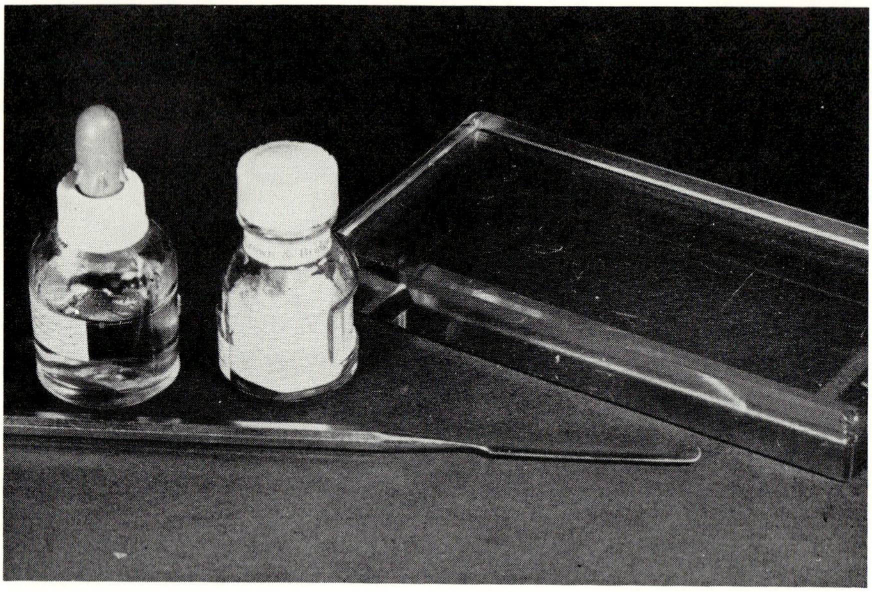

Fig. 10-8. Cement liquid, powder, slab, and spatula. The mix is made on a clean, cool slab.

The cement should be mixed on a cool, dry, heavy glass slab that is free from nicks or scratches (Fig. 10-8). The slab should be cooled to 65 to 75 degrees F., in order to slow the chemical reaction and thus prolong the setting time. This allows more powder to be incorporated in a given quantity of liquid and will, in turn, provide greater strength and lessen the chance of the cement's dissolving in oral fluids.

As mentioned earlier, the tendency of these cements to dissolve in mouth fluids is probably the primary weakness of the dental cements. It leads to recurrent caries around the cemented restoration, etching of the tooth under orthodontic bands, and staining. The portion of the cement that dissolves is the weak matrix that forms around the powder particles as the cement hardens. Thus, the more powder that can be incorporated into the mix, the less matrix will be present, and the better will be the properties of the cement.

The cool slab also assures adequate working time. In cooling the slab, care should be taken not to lower the temperature to a point where moisture will condense on the surface. If this happens, the mix will be contaminated and will harden too rapidly for proper use. Placing the slab or the powder and liquid in a refrigerator is not necessary; cool tap water is usually quite satisfactory for chilling the slab.

Although other factors, including rate and length of spatulation, affect the setting time, adequate working time can best be assured by control of the slab temperature.

Zinc phosphate cement powder should be placed on the slab and divided into 5 or 6 portions. The liquid should then be placed on the slab, and the first portion of powder added to the liquid and thoroughly mixed. Before each increment is added, the mass should be thoroughly spatulated with a rotary motion (Fig. 10-9) until it is completely homogenous. A good rule to follow is to spatulate for approximately 20 seconds after the addition of each portion; thus, the total mixing time will be 1½ to 2

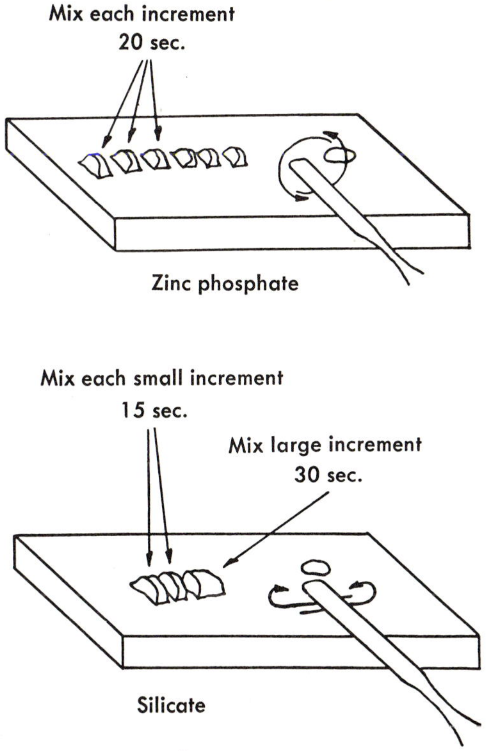

Fig. 10-9. Diagram of mixing procedures for both zinc phosphate and silicate cements. Differences in mixing technique and time of spatulation are due to the differences in chemical reactions that occur. In both cases, however, maximum powder must be incorporated. (From Peterson, S., editor: Clinical dental hygiene, ed. 3, St. Louis, 1968, The C. V. Mosby Co.)

minutes. The mix should always be smooth and free of lumps.

Silicate cement

The silicate cements, which are used primarily for restoration, also involve the mixing of a powder and a liquid. The powder consists mainly of silica, alumina, and fluoride compounds. It is the presence of fluoride that accounts for the surprisingly low incidence of recurrent caries around silicate cement restorations. It is because of this one characteristic that silicate cement is often the material of choice for patients with rampant caries. The liquid is quite comparable in composition to that of the zinc phosphate cements, and the same precautions must be taken in its care.

A silicate cement is mixed differently from a zinc phosphate cement, since the final compound formed is a gel instead of a crystalline compound. It is important to prevent any disturbance of this gel after it starts to form, or the cement will be weaker and more soluble. Therefore, the mix is completed within approximately 1 minute, and, as shown in Fig. 10-9, a large amount of powder is immediately folded into the liquid. The mix is then worked to a puttylike consistency.

As with zinc phosphate cement, the strength and resistance to disintegration of silicate cement is principally controlled by the powder-liquid ratio. Use of a warm mixing slab results in a low powder-liquid ratio that will accelerate dissolution, fracture, and stain in the oral cavity.

The two most common causes of difficulty with either zinc phosphate or silicate cement are: (1) use of liquid that has been changed by exposure to the atmosphere or by contamination, and (2) improper mixing techniques.

If the cement sets too slowly, it is probably because: (1) the mix is too thin (not enough powder incorporated in the mix), (2) the mix has been spatulated too long (increased spatulation time increases setting time), or (3) the liquid has lost water because it has not been properly cared for.

If the cement sets too fast, the cause is probably: (1) mixing on a warm slab, (2) insufficient spatulation time, or (3) too rapid addition of the powder.

Precipitation or cloudiness in the liquid denotes contamination or evaporation, and the liquid should be discarded. Addition of liquid to a mix is contraindicated. Liquid should never be added to a mix that is too stiff or has started to harden. The assistant should discard such a mix and make a new one.

Zinc oxide–eugenol and copper cements

Zinc oxide–eugenol cement is particularly advantageous as a base material under other restorations or temporary fillings, even though it is not strong enough to serve as a permanent restoration. The eugenol liquid is not acid and, therefore, is less irritating to the pulp. Because of its palliative effect, zinc oxide–eugenol is sometimes employed as a cement for fixed resorations. On the other hand, the red and black copper cements are rapidly disappearing from dentistry. They are not superior in any way, and because of their extreme acidity, they are very irritating to the pulp.

Other types of cement

As seen in Table 2, a number of other types of cements are used by the dentist. For example, cements containing calcium hydroxide are particularly effective in promoting healing of the pulp, as are the zinc oxide–eugenol cements. The silicophosphate cements are a combination of zinc phosphate and silicate cements. Their relatively high strength permits them to be used as temporary fillings and for certain types of cementation. Acrylic resin is no longer to any extent employed as a cement. Low solubility was its only asset, and the difficulty of manipulation prevented this type of cement from becoming popular.

Recently, a class of cements referred to as carboxylates has been introduced. The carboxylate cements are powder-liquid systems essentially composed of a liquid of polyacrylic acid and zinc oxide powder. Their appeal lies in the apparently good biologic characteristics and a possible adhesive bonding of the cement to tooth enamel. If the initial adhesion proves to be effective for an extended period of time, the carboxylate cements may make it possible to attach orthodontic bands directly to enamel without the use of bands.

CAVITY-LINING AGENTS

The dentist often uses lining agents to coat the cavity preparation before the permanent restoration is inserted. These agents are inert varnishlike materials that may or may not contain additives, such as zinc oxide or calcium hydroxide. Cavity varnishes serve several useful functions. They tend to inhibit the initial leakage that occurs around the amalgam restoration. Likewise, they prevent discoloration of the adjoining tooth structure produced from the penetration of ions, such as mercury, from the amalgam into the dentin. They also provide a barrier against the acid present in zinc phosphate or silicate cements.

Since a thick consistency will not properly cover the tooth surface, the liner should be kept in a tightly stoppered bottle to prevent evaporation. On occasion, the varnish may require thinning with the liquid supplied by the manufacturer.

IMPRESSION MATERIALS

Dental impression materials can be divided into 2 broad classifications—elastic and inelastic. Inelastic materials, such as plaster and compound, are not as well suited for certain uses in dentistry as the elastic materials, since they cannot be removed from around the crowns of teeth without fracture or distortion. On the other hand, the elastic materials make it possible to take impressions for bridges, inlays, and partial dentures with fewer steps and with no permanent distortion. The elastic materials are the hydrocolloids and the rubber impression materials. The following discussion concerns only some of the manipulative steps that are especially related to the impression material itself.

Hydrocolloid impression materials

As with all dental materials, the accuracy of the hydrocolloid impression materials for indirect restorations and partial or full-mouth impressions is dependent

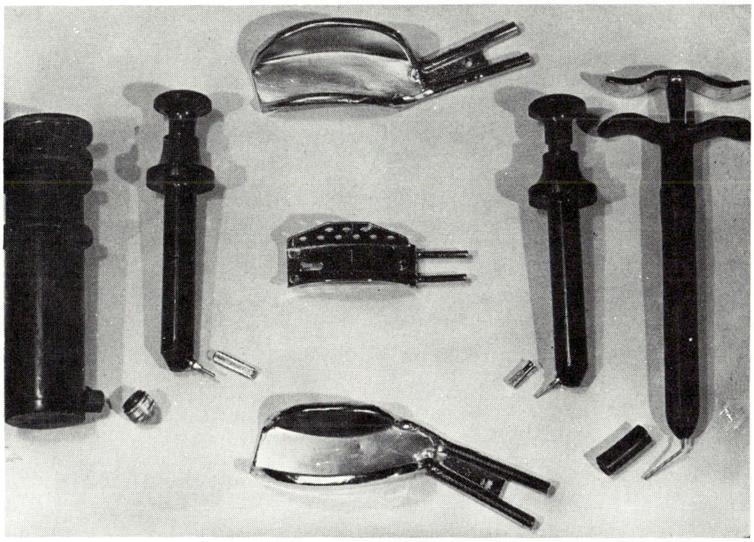

Fig. 10-10. Various trays and syringes available for hydrocolloid technique. The trays are water cooled, and the small syringes are used for injecting the material into the cavity preparation. (From Hohlt, F. A.: Dental clinics of North America, Philadelphia, March, 1957, W. B. Saunders Co.)

upon the careful control of many variables.

Hydrocolloids can be classified into 2 general types—reversible and irreversible. These materials are suspensions of aggregates of molecules in a dispersing medium of water, the water being held by capillary action. Gelation of the reversible hydrocolloids is primarily a physical change, in which a latticework of fibrils forms as the temperature is lowered. This gel can be readily dispersed by merely heating the material, hence the term *reversible.* An example of a reversible hydrocolloid is ordinary gelatin. When gelatin is dissolved in boiling water, it forms a colloidal sol that gels upon cooling. This gel can be returned to the liquid sol by heating, and reformed by cooling.

The base for dental reversible hydrocolloids is agar, a material that can be liquefied at temperatures compatible with oral tissues and then solidified to a firm but elastic gel at temperatures slightly above 100 degrees F. This gelation is accomplished in the mouth by means of water-cooled impression trays. Syringes and trays used for this technique are shown in Fig. 10-10.

The irreversible hydrocolloids, usually referred to as alginates, are not thermally reversible, and their gelation is induced by an actual chemical reaction rather than by physical means. The ingredients in the powder, when mixed with water, react to make a latticework of fibrils that form the elastic gel.

For reversible hydrocolloid, adequate boiling is essential, in order to break down the agar fibrils. A minimum boiling time of 10 minutes is required for new material, and several additional minutes should be added every time the hydrocolloid is reboiled. There is no danger in boiling too long, within reasonable limits, but insufficient boiling results in a grainy, unworkable mass. This liquefied material may then be stored at 150 to 155 degrees F. until it is needed. Proper equipment for this storage and for the subsequent tempering is essential, and inadequate armamentarium

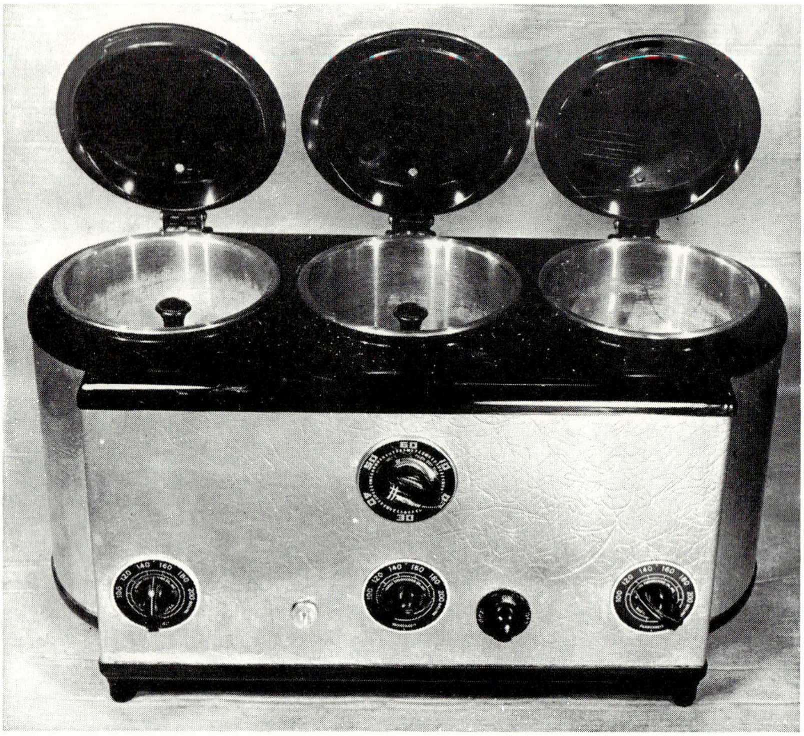

Fig. 10-11. A typical conditioner for use with reversible hydrocolloid. The 3 compartments are for boiling, storing, and tempering.

can lead only to failure. A typical conditioner is shown in Fig. 10-11. The tray material may be tempered at any temperature between 105 and 120 degrees F. for the time required to bring about adequate gelation. This tempering procedure is necessary to secure a material that is more comfortable for the patient and is easier to handle. The time and temperature combination employed depends upon the particular office routine preferred. The only precaution is not to temper for too long a period at any temperature. Obviously, the lower the water temperature, the shorter the tempering time. When tempering is unduly prolonged, gelation proceeds so far that the material becomes too stiff for use.

When a water bath is used for tempering, the top layer of water-soaked hydrocolloid should be scraped off before the tray is carried into the patient's mouth. Removal of this material assures a firm union with the hydrocolloid that has been injected into the cavity preparations.

Upon removal from the mouth, the reversible hydrocolloid impression is placed in a 2 percent solution of potassium sulfate (Fig. 10-12). This assures a harder surface on the stone model that will subsequently be poured in the impression. The immersion, which takes approximately 5 minutes, may be done while the mix of stone is being prepared. Alginate impressions should not be treated in this solution.

The alginates, of course, require less in the way of armamentarium. Usually when the alginate powder is supplied in bulk form, a volumetric cup is supplied for measuring the powder. However, the amount of packing or the fluffiness of the powder results in considerable variation from one scoop to another. Thus, it is preferable to

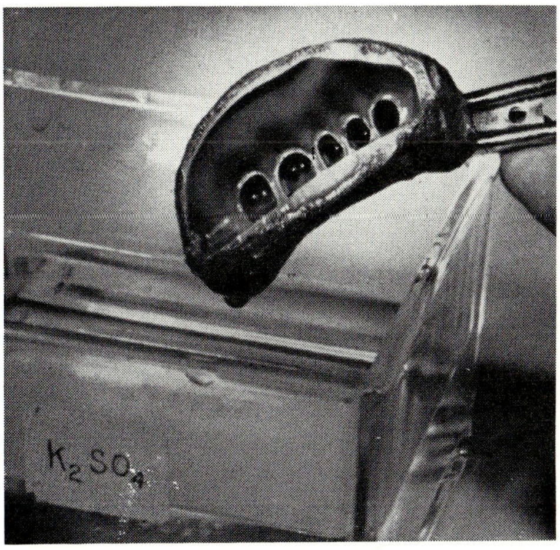

Fig. 10-12. Hydrocolloid impression being placed in 2-percent potassium sulfate solution before stone model is poured. Such treatment improves the model surface.

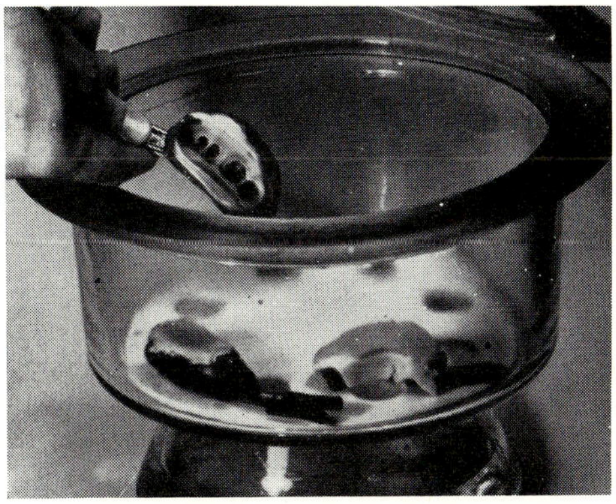

Fig. 10-13. Container that provides 100 percent humidity environment for storage of reversible hydrocolloid impression. However, impression should be poured immediately whenever possible.

weigh it. Another problem associated with the bulk packaging of alginate is the tendency of the ingredients to settle out during shipping and storage, resulting in erratic setting. Therefore, the can should be shaken periodically in order to redistribute the powder. To prevent moisture contamination, the can should be kept tightly closed when not in use.

The proper water-powder ratio must be used, since excess water will weaken the final gel. Generally, water at a temperature of 60 to 70 degrees F. should be employed in the mix. Warm water will accelerate the set and cause the mix to stiffen prematurely. The mix should be made vigorously, at approximately 200 r.p.m., and for most materials a maximum of 1 minute of mixing is sufficient. Insufficient mixing results in a grainy mass of material, whereas longer spatulation breaks up the gel and seriously weakens the material.

The impression should now be poured as soon as possible. Since both alginate and hydrocolloid impressions are approximately 80 to 85 percent water, the material will tend to lose or gain water readily, depending upon the environment in which it is stored. Loss of water is referred to as *syneresis,* and gain in water is called *imbibition.* This change in the water content is invariably accompanied by a contraction or expansion of the material and a resulting distortion. Definite distortion can be detected in only 30 minutes, if the impression is allowed to stand in air. Unquestionably, prolonged storage of the impression before pouring is the most common source of distortion with both of these materials.

Although there are no safe storage media for those cases in which the impression cannot be poured at once, the best environment for most products is an atmosphere of approximately 100 percent humidity, as in the humidifier shown in Fig. 10-13. Another simple method of storage is to wrap the impression in a wet towel and place it in a closed container. It can be seen that the humidifier (Fig. 10-13) is also useful for storage of the poured impression until the model can be removed from the impression.

Excess droplets of water or potassium sulfate solution should be gently blown from the impression before the stone or plaster model is poured, although care must be taken not to dehydrate the material. There are many commercial stones that are satisfactory for pouring the die. The newer stones (class II) have a different type of particle, are harder, and have a lower setting expansion than the older stones (class I). The manufacturer's directions with respect to the water-powder ratio for each stone should be followed. Variation in this ratio influences not only the setting expansion, but also the strength and the surface smoothness. Air voids may be minimized by the use of mechanical mixer and/or vacuum equipment, thereby increasing the strength and providing a smoother model. The stone is mechanically vibrated into the mold; mild vibration is used, and the stone is added in small increments from one area of the impression. The poured model is then allowed to harden for 1 hour before separation from the impression, since premature removal will result in a rough surface. Since the stone does not reach its maximum strength or hardness for some time, the die should not be used for 24 hours.

Rubber impression materials

More recently, 2 types of synthetic rubber-base impression materials have been introduced. The materials of one type are polysulfide polymers, while those of the other type have a silicone base. The silicone materials have a more pleasing color and odor and are somewhat cleaner to handle. Both generally come in a paste form, and the catalyst present in one of the pastes cures the material in the mouth to form an impression that is elastic and quite accurate. Different consistencies are available for the various uses to which the rubber-base materials are employed.

The surface area of the mixing slab should be large enough for extensive spreading of the pastes during mixing. If a glass slab is used, it should be thoroughly cleaned and employed only with that one type of impression material. In other words, it is not desirable to use the same slab and spatula for mixing both the polysulfide polymer and silicone impression materials. Traces of one material may remain in small scratches on the surface and thus contaminate the mix of the other material.

The setting time of these materials is important to both the dentist and the patient. There must be sufficient working time to permit mixing, injection (if the material is to be used for indirect work), and seating of the tray in the mouth. Curing should then take place rapidly enough to prevent any distortion while the tray is in position and to minimize the time that the tray must be held in the mouth.

Temperature and humidity will influence the setting time; thus, the temperature of the room and its humidity at the time of mixing may affect the setting. The higher the temperature and the humidity, the more rapid is the set. For example, one way of accelerating the set is to add a drop of water to the impression paste. Naturally, the ratio of the 2 pastes will also influence the set, and the correct ratio should be strictly maintained.

The spatula is first wetted with the accelerator paste, and the 2 pastes are then stirred for approximately 10 seconds. Then, by placing the blade flat to the surface of the slab, the mix is completed by spreading the combined material over the slab until no streaks appear. A mix such as that shown in Fig. 10-14 should take approximately 1 minute.

Bulk of material is never desirable with the rubber-base materials, as it is with the hydrocolloids. Use of the minimum amount of material necessary to take the impression will minimize the trapping of bubbles and shrinkage. Wherever possible, the amount of material between the tooth and the side of the tray should not exceed 2 mm. This need for minimal bulk emphasizes the importance of a carefully selected band or tray. The band or tray must be

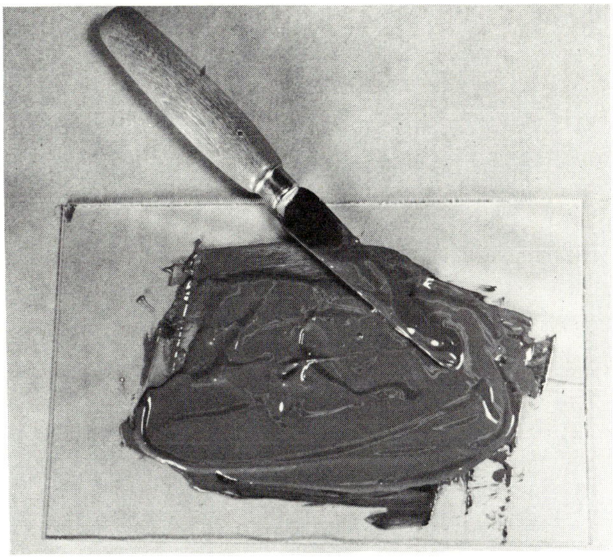

Fig. 10-14. A proper mix of a polysulfide polymer, free of any streaks. (From Phillips, R. W., Swartz, M. L., and Norman, R. D.: Materials for the practicing dentist, St. Louis, 1969, The C. V. Mosby Co.)

rigid and should be adjusted or fabricated to provide an even distribution of bulk around the cavity preparation, because nonuniform masses of material produce distortion.

It has been shown that unless the materials are held firmly by the band or tray, they will distort upon removal. Any of the commercially available rubber cements supplied with the impression materials will work nicely in holding the material to the band or tray.

One of the arguments commonly made in favor of rubber-base materials, as compared to the hydrocolloids, is that they have excellent dimensional stability and may be stored indefinitely without distorting. Recent research indicates that this view is unduly optimistic and that dimensional stability still remains a real problem with most, if not all, impression materials. There is clear evidence that storage of rubber-base materials is contraindicated. The cast should be constructed immediately.

PLASTER AND STONE

Gypsum products are among the most widely used materials in dentistry. They are employed as impression materials for the construction of casts and models and as necessary ingredients in many other products.

Although both plaster and stone are manufactured from gypsum and have the same chemical formula, they are quite different physically. The particles of the stone powder are more dense and more regular in shape than the particles of plaster. Therefore, less water is required for making the original mix. Since excess water lowers the strength and reduces the surface hardness, plaster is weaker and softer than stone.

Even at best, neither of these materials has the ideal strength that would be desired for certain dental procedures. For this reason, the ratio of powder and water is important. If too much water is employed, the set material will be weaker. On the other hand, the use of insufficient water

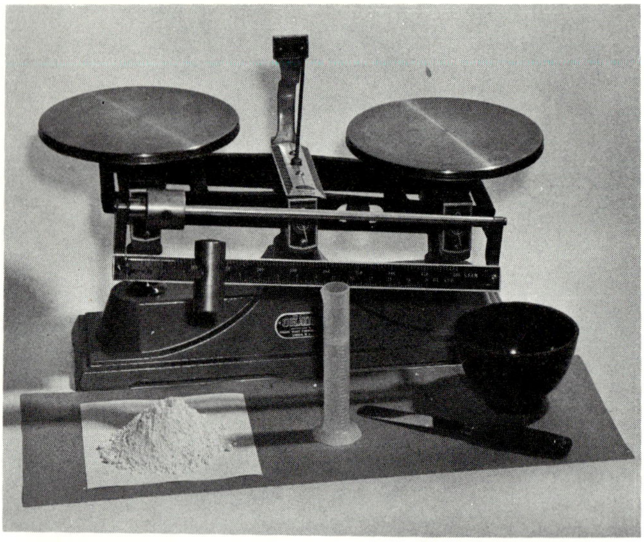

Fig. 10-15. Proper proportioning of water and stone by means of a graduated cylinder and a balance. (From Phillips, R. W., Swartz, M. L., and Norman, R. D.: Materials for the practicing dentist, St. Louis, 1969, The C. V. Mosby Co.)

will produce a granular and viscous material that will not flow into the impression or mold. Thus, the recommended ratio should be achieved by weighing the powder on a laboratory balance and proportioning the water by volume. The typical equipment needed is seen in Fig. 10-15.

The setting time must be long enough to permit the dentist to take the impression or pour the model, but it should not be so long that it will inconvenience the patient or the operator. Although the manufacturer adds accelerators and retarders to regulate the setting time, it can be altered further by changing the temperature of the gauging water. Cold water will retard the set, and warm water will accelerate it. Setting time should not be regulated by varying the water-powder ratio, for the reasons previously discussed.

Probably the most serious problem that faces the dental assistant in handling these materials is the danger of trapping air voids and bubbles. There are 3 main causes of porosity: (1) air present in the original mass of powder, (2) air incorporated during the mixing procedure, and (3) air trapped during pouring. To eliminate some of the air that is invariably present in the weighed powder itself, the powder should be gently sifted into the water. Powder should never be dumped into the water in large masses, but should be sifted in slowly in small increments. Plaster or stone powder should always be added to the water; the water is never added to the powder.

The mixing should be done with a swiping motion against the sides of the bowl. A whipping motion is to be avoided, since it entraps air. Good examples of the effects of these manipulative variables upon the density of the model are shown in Fig. 10-16.

The mixed plaster or stone is poured into the impression or mold under *mild* vibration. Excess vibration will cause internal voids or produce bubbles at the surface. The mix is also added in small increments. The technique is illustrated in Fig. 10-17.

As mentioned previously, newer stones

A

B

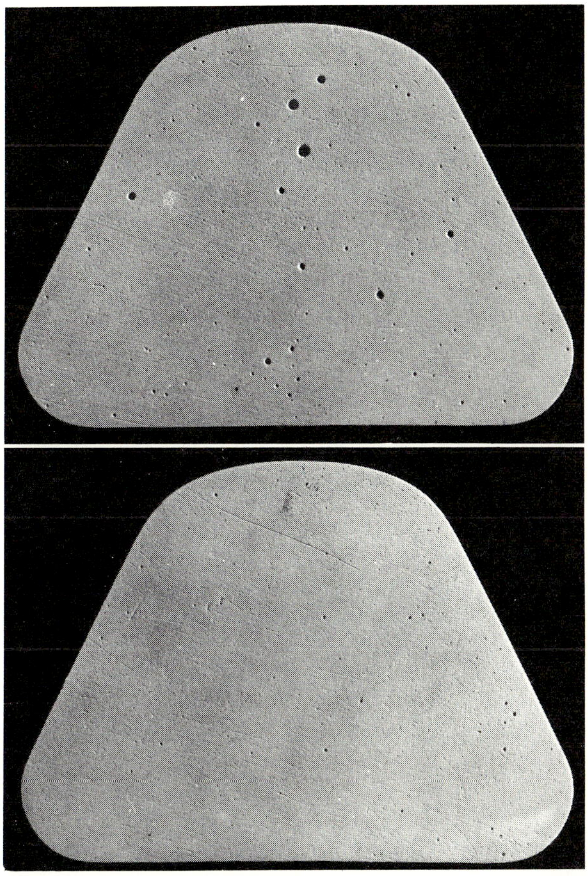

Fig. 10-16. A, Gross porosity, as seen in cross section of plaster model, that occurred when powder was merely dumped into water; **B,** porosity is minimized when plaster is carefully sifted into water and when whipping is avoided during mixing. (From Lindquist, J. I., Brennan, R. W., and Phillips, R. W.: J. Prosth. Dent. **3**:274, 1953.)

developed in recent years are harder and have less dimensional change on setting than the older materials. These class II stones are used almost exclusively for indirect inlay construction. For a still harder die upon which to fabricate a wax pattern or to finish a metal casting, the impression may be electroplated. The stone is poured into the metallic-plated impression, and upon separation, there is a hard metal surface on the die. Certain impression materials (for example, hydrocolloid) cannot be satisfactorily plated, but others, such as the polysulfide rubber materials, can be electroplated without distortion. The exact procedures for electroplating may be found in the references listed at the end of this chapter.

DENTAL CASTINGS

The object of a dental casting technique is to produce from a wax pattern a casting that will fit snugly on the preparation, but at the same time slip completely to place in response to finger pressure or very light tapping with a mallet and orangewood stick. The casting, when completed, should be minutely accurate,

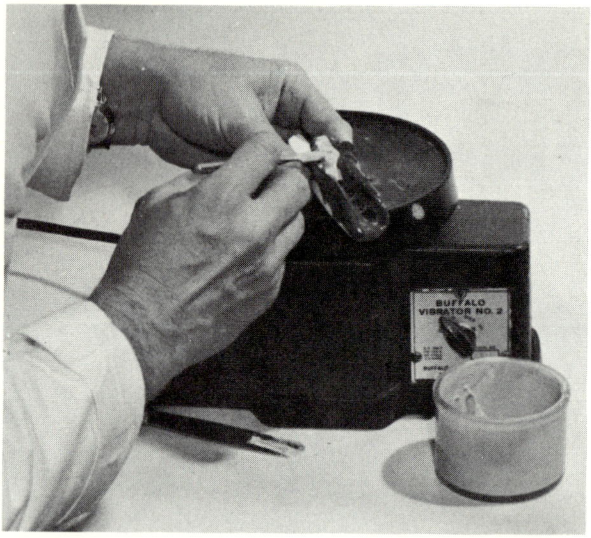

Fig. 10-17. The danger of trapping air in the poured impression is minimized by adding small increments of stone and flowing the mix into the impression under mild vibration. (From Phillips, R. W., Swartz, M. L., and Norman, R. D.: Materials for the practicing dentist, St. Louis, 1969, The C. V. Mosby Co.)

smooth, and free from bubbles and internal or surface porosity. The clinical success of the cast restoration depends primarily upon the accuracy of the final casting.

Castings that possess these qualities are not difficult to secure consistently, and casting failures are now the exception rather than the rule. The casting procedure is not a haphazard one, however, but a definite, standardized technique in which certain necessary fundamentals must be taken into consideration. These fundamentals cannot be altered, regardless of the particular technique to be employed.

In the past, the greatest impediment was change in dimension of the casting due to the contraction of a gold alloy during freezing. The exact figure for this contraction remains unknown, although values ranging from 1.1 to 1.6 percent have been published. The approximate value of 1.4 percent for dental gold alloys is most generally accepted.

Various methods have been employed in different casting techniques to compensate for this contraction, but all the currently accepted methods involve the expansion of *investment*. This material, which is used to surround the wax pattern, is composed mainly of stone to provide strength and silica to provide the necessary expansion. While it is setting, and also while it is being heated thermally, the investment expands to enlarge the mold and thus compensates for the contraction of the metal. Additional expansion may also be secured by immersing the setting investment in a water bath (referred to as hygroscopic expansion).

The essential components involved in the fabrication of the gold casting are shown in Fig. 10-18. The wax pattern, shown in the center of the casting ring, should be invested immediately after its removal from the cavity preparation or die. This wax pattern contains internal stress and will rapidly distort if not surrounded by the hardened investment.

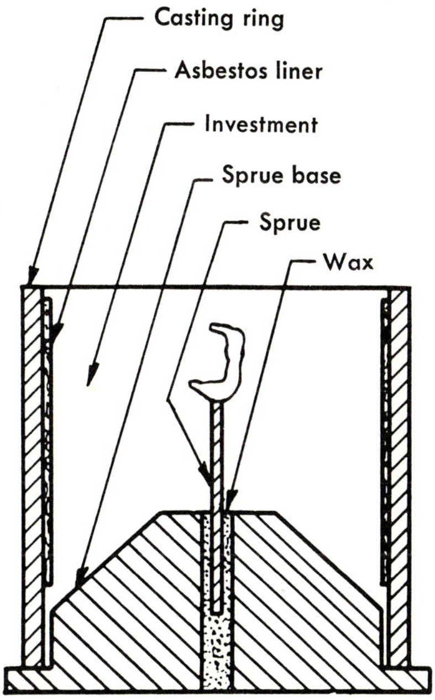

Fig. 10-18. Schematic drawing of components involved in the fabrication of gold casting. (From Peterson, S., editor: Clinical dental hygiene, ed. 3, St. Louis, 1968, The C. V. Mosby Co.)

Investing procedure

The importance of cleanliness and accuracy in any casting procedure cannot be overemphasized. The pattern should always be clean and free from oil and crumbs of wax. The investment and water should be carefully proportioned. The sprue base should be clean and covered with a thin coat of oil. The sprue should be not less than 14 gauge, unless the pattern is extremely small. Long and thin sprues are likely to cause internal porosity, commonly called shrinkage porosity. The length of the sprue should be such that the pattern is approximately ¼ inch from the open end of the ring. If a greater thickness of investment is present, "back pressure" porosity will result. This is due to the fact that the air in the mold cannot escape through the investment and thus prevents the gold from completely filling the mold. Either wax or metal sprues may be used, but metal sprues should always be made of a rust-resistant metal to prevent contamination of the mold.

The use of vacuum equipment for both mixing and investing is preferable to hand spatulation and investing. Two types of vacuum equipment are shown in Fig. 10-19.

Although it is imperative that the pattern be invested as soon as possible to prevent warpage, heating of the mold to burn out the wax may be started at any time after the sprue has been removed. This may be done immediately, or it may be postponed indefinitely. Once the heating is started, however, the casting should be completed without allowing the mold to cool. Reheating a previously heated mold causes marked loss in strength.

Slow heating is advised until the free water is forced from the mold. If heating is too rapid, steam may form and cause small pieces of the investment to explode off the inside of the mold, resulting in defective, rough, and poorly fitting castings. Thus, burnout should be slow and gradual, and it is preferable that it be done in an electric furnace. Approximately 45 minutes to 1 hour should be required for bringing the temperature up to 1300 degrees F. Care should be taken to avoid heating above 1300 degrees F., since the investment may break down at this temperature, and the sulphur that is liberated will attack the gold as it enters the mold.

Casting

When gold alloys are melted with a blowtorch, it is important to keep the tip of the reducing cone on the metal. This position of the flame will minimize oxidation, and, since this is the hottest portion of the flame, the metal will heat more quickly. When the metal is in the reducing part of the flame, it has a shiny, mirrorlike surface; when being oxidized, it is covered with a dull scum. Improper use of the flame will result in "occluded gas" porosity

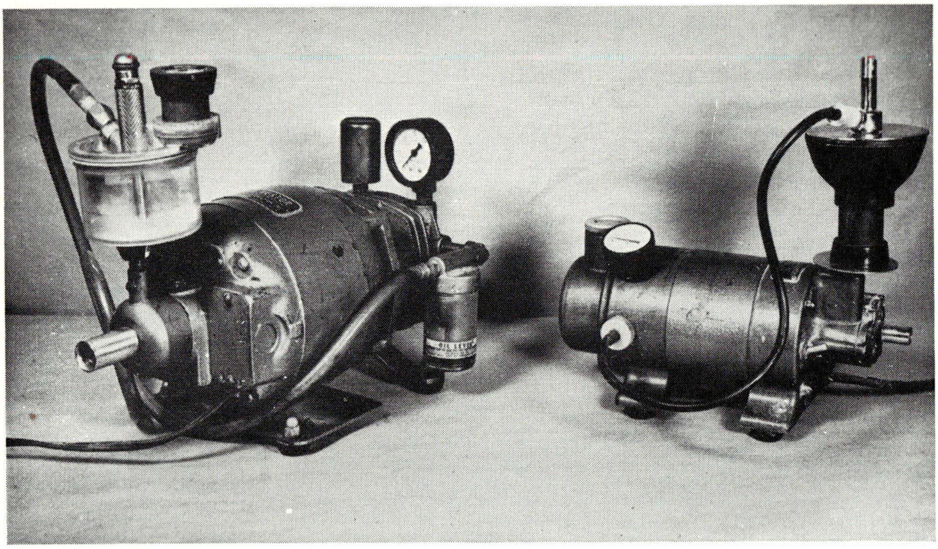

Fig. 10-19. Apparatus used for vacuum investing of wax patterns. The main advantage is standardization of procedure.

and a severe pitting of the surface of the casting.

Generous portions of flux should be used in melting the gold alloy to reduce the likelihood of oxidation and to increase the flowing qualities of the melted metal. Dental fluxes generally contain borax and finely divided particles of charcoal. Care should be taken not to overheat the alloy, but it is equally important that the metal be thoroughly melted. Experience here is probably the best teacher.

After the gold has frozen and cooled for approximately 1 minute, the ring may be plunged into cold water. This will facilitate removal of the investment, which is generally very tenacious. After the bulk of the adhering investment is removed, the casting may be "pickled" by placement in 50 percent solution of sulfuric acid to clean the metal. It will be noted that sometimes a black film remains on the casting. Often this is not a fault in the gold but just a surface oxide. It may readily be removed by pickling. All traces of acid should be thoroughly washed off before the casting is tried on the cavity preparation.

The casting should be examined with a magnifying lens, so that small bubbles or irregularities may be detected. If either are present and are not removed with a small bur before the casting is tried on the preparation, injury to the tooth or enamel margin may result, necessitating the refinishing of the margin and making of a new casting.

RESINS

Plastics, correctly referred to as resins, are continually increasing in their dental applications. They are used exclusively for dentures, and they are also used as partial dentures, filling materials and cements, and artificial teeth. With the rapidly expanding industrial use of resins, it is probable that the future of these materials in dentistry holds ever greater promise.

The fabrication of dental appliances or restorations from resin usually involves the use of a powder and a liquid. The liquid is referred to as the *monomer* and consists of unattacked, single molecules of methyl methacrylate. This liquid is combined with the powder, which is called the *polymer.*

The polymer is a long-chain molecule similar to the monomer itself, except that the single molecules have been combined. Under the action of heat or certain chemicals, these single molecules of the monomer can be joined together to form a long-chain molecule similar to that of the original powder. This process is known as *polymerization*. Thus, in the construction of a denture, the liquid and powder are mixed together to form a moldable dough, which is placed into the denture mold under compression and heated in a water bath in order to solidify the whole mass into the polymer form.

The temperature at which most of this change occurs in the resin is between approximately 150 and 175 degrees F. Since the reaction is accompanied by the liberation of heat, it is necessary that the material be carried through this temperature range slowly. If not, the liquid will vaporize, and internal porosity will develop.

Obviously, it is not possible to use heat of this magnitude in the oral cavity. Thus, chemical catalysts must be added to the liquid when the resin is to be used as a restorative or cementing material.

There are certain inherent shortcomings in the physical properties of resin that to date have limited its use for dental restorations. Certain of these, such as the tendency for the earlier materials to discolor, have been virtually eliminated. However, the low hardness and strength of this resin, as compared to amalgam or the gold inlay, have restricted its use to restorations that are not subjected to biting forces. However, the excellent aesthetic characteristics of this early type of resin and its insolubility in oral fluids make it useful in other types of cavity preparations, particularly in the anterior region of the mouth.

Another problem that is associated with resin is the relatively high coefficient of thermal expansion, or the amount of dimensional change that occurs in the material when it is subjected to temperature changes. Unfortunately, this value is considerably higher for resin than it is for tooth structure. For every degree of temperature change that occurs during the ingestion of hot or cold foods and beverages, the resin restoration may expand or contract approximately 7 times as much as the adjoining tooth. The coefficient of thermal expansion of other restorative materials is much closer to that of the tooth. Conceivably, this could lead to the continual pumping of fluids and microorganisms, for example, in and out of the marginal areas of the resin restoration. For this reason, great care must be exercised by the assistant and the dentist during the manipulation of the material, in order to provide maximum adaptation of the resin to the cavity walls and thereby minimize the tendency of it to pull away from the tooth during temperature cycling.

Recently, a new type of resin restorative material has been introduced to the profession. These products use a somewhat modified version of the older resin. However, the main difference is that a high concentration of a filler has been added. As much as 80 percent of the resin may be composed of fillers, such as glass or quartz. When present in this amount, the filler acts as a reinforcing agent. Such materials are referred to as *composites*. They have a somewhat lower coefficient of thermal expansion and are harder and stronger than the conventional acrylic resins. It has not yet been established whether the improvement in properties is sufficient to warrant the use of composite resins in stress-bearing restorations.

Suggested readings

Peterson, S.: Clinical dental hygiene, ed. 4, St. Louis, 1972, The C. V. Mosby Co.

Peyton, F. A.: Restorative dental materials, ed. 4, St. Louis, 1971, The C. V. Mosby Co.

Phillips, R. W. (consulting editor): Symposium on dental materials. In Dental Clinics of North America, Philadelphia, January, 1971, W. B. Saunders Co.

Phillips, R. W.: Elements of dental materials for dental hygienists and assistants, ed. 2, Philadelphia, 1971, W. B. Saunders Co.
Phillips, Ralph W., Swartz, M. L., and Norman, R. D.: Materials for the practicing dentist, St. Louis, 1969, The C. V. Mosby Co.
Skinner, E. W., and Phillips, R. W.: The science of dental materials, ed. 6, Philadelphia, 1967, W. B. Saunders Co.

CHAPTER 11 SHARPENING AND MAINTAINING INSTRUMENTS*

JAMES T. ANDREWS, B.A., D.D.S.

One of the many duties of the dental assistant is the maintenance and sharpening of cavity preparation and scaling instruments used by the dentist or the dental hygienist.

It is imperative that the dentist have sharp cavity preparation instruments so that he may properly prepare the cavosurface angles (margins) of the preparation, place retention and resistance forms in the cavity preparation, remove carious dentin, and finish the cavity walls of the preparation. Dull instruments will not cut the hard structures of the teeth. Unfortunately, many dentists probably have reduced their use of hand cutting instruments in cavity preparation, as a result of not having anyone in the office who is knowledgeable in instrument sharpening techniques.

One of the most important services performed in the dental office is the removal of deposits and stains from the teeth, either by the dentist or the dental hygienist. Sharp instruments must be employed in scaling procedures, as dull instruments require more time by the operator to complete a procedure and frequently result in the incomplete removal of deposits from the teeth. Dull instruments necessitate more pressure to be exerted by the operator in scaling procedures, resulting in more discomfort to the patient and more trauma to the periodontal tissues.

The objective of this chapter is to describe methods of sharpening hand cutting instruments used in cavity preparation and scaling instruments used in performing a dental prophylaxis. There are many techniques for sharpening instruments, and all will not be discussed. It is recommended that the mechanical oscillating instrument sharpener (Fig. 11-2) or a similar mechanical sharpener be used in sharpening the cavity preparation instruments, and that the prophylaxis instruments be sharpened by the use of the hand-held sharpening stones.

EQUIPMENT

Hard Arkansas oilstones are preferred for the sharpening of cutting instruments, as they produce the finest edge. These stones should be lubricated with a fine-grade light oil prior to sharpening instruments, and they should be wiped clean fol-

*Special credit for the preparation of the illustrations in this chapter is given to John Hembree, D.D.S., Associate Professor and Vice-chairman of the Department of Operative Dentistry, University of Tennessee College of Dentistry.

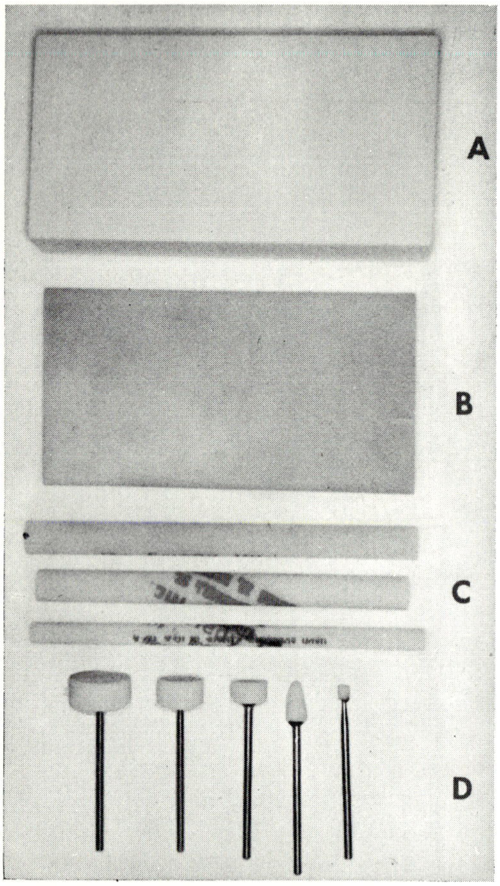

Fig. 11-1. Stones used for sharpening instruments. **A,** Flat Arkansas stone; **B,** flat, tapered Arkansas stone; **C,** cylinder Arkansas stones; **D,** composition handpiece stones. (Courtesy University of Tennessee College of Dentistry.)

lowing the sharpening procedure. Hard Arkansas oilstones may be obtained in various sizes and shapes (Fig. 11-1) for use in sharpening by hand or using the dental handpiece.

A mechanical instrument sharpener (Fig. 11-2) with oscillating sharpening stones is also available. This machine will perform most of the procedures that can be accomplished with the stones shown in Fig. 11-1. This sharpener is fairly simple to use, because it has fixed guides for holding instruments as they are sharpened. The large sharpening stone should be thoroughly coated with black emery compound while the stone is rotating to prevent burning of the instruments and destroying of the temper of the blade.

METHODS OF SHARPENING

It must be remembered that whatever method of sharpening is employed, the objectives are to produce a sharp cutting edge on the instrument, to remove as little metal as possible from the instrument, and to retain the original bevels and shape of the instrument. Therefore, it is necessary for the assistant to know the dimensions, angulations, and shapes of the instruments she is sharpening, so that they may be held in the proper relationship with the sharpening stone.

Instruments that are used routinely will not retain a sharp edge for very long; therefore, it is advisable to check all cutting instruments for sharpness after an operation and sharpen them, if necessary, prior to sterilization or disinfection. In the completion of difficult cases, it may be necessary to have duplicate scalers available, as the instruments may become dull before the operation is complete. Sharpening of instruments may be accomplished at the chair in a few seconds with the flat, tapering Arkansas oilstone (Fig. 11-1, *B*), which can be sterilized by the dry heat method of sterilization.

Flat stones

Flat Arkansas oilstones (Fig. 11-1, *A*) that are at least 2 inches by 5 inches may be used to sharpen most instruments. Instruments that have a cutting edge perpendicular to the long axis of the blade, such as enamel hatchets, chisels, and hoes, are the easiest to sharpen in this manner. The instrument is held with the thumb, index finger, and middle finger. The other 2 fingers are used for support on the side of the stone (Fig. 11-3). The bevel of the blade must approximate the stone com-

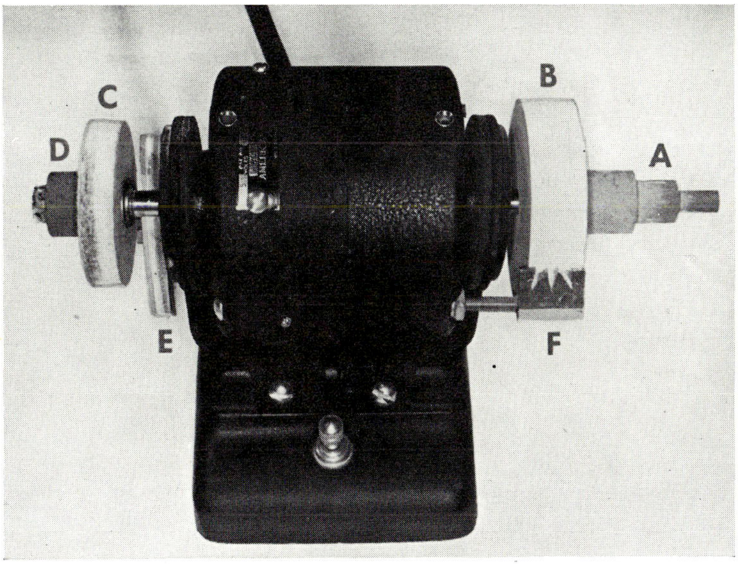

Fig. 11-2. Mechanical oscillating instrument sharpener. **A,** Stones for sharpening right-angled instruments with curved blades; **B,** large sharpening wheel; **C,** felt wheel to remove bur from instruments after sharpening; **D,** stone for sharpening left-angled instruments with curved blades; **E,** oscillating wheel; **F,** instrument guide. (Courtesy University of Tennessee College of Dentistry.)

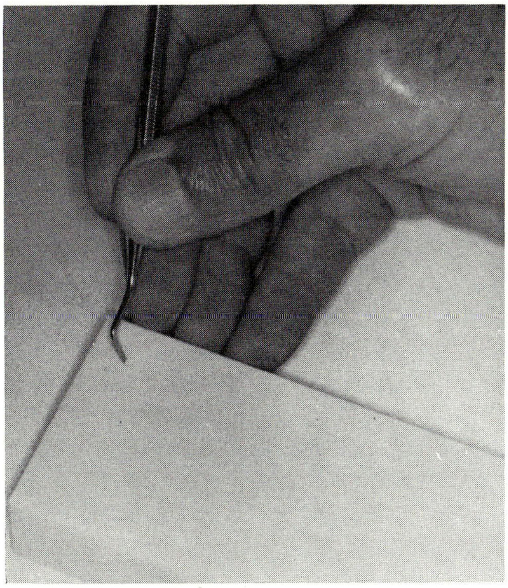

Fig. 11-3. Enamel hatchet sharpened on flat Arkansas stone. (Courtesy University of Tennessee College of Dentistry.)

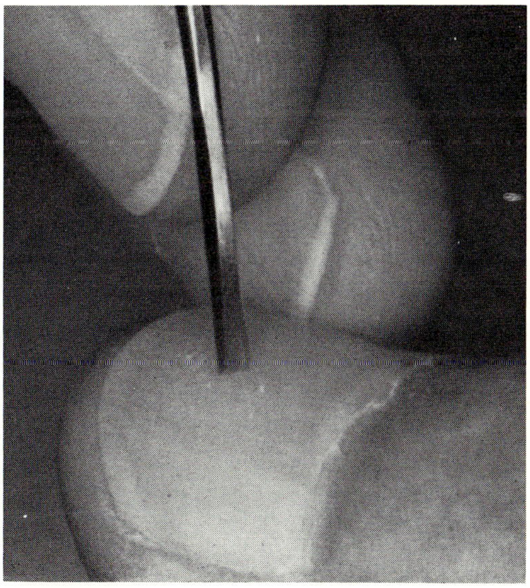

Fig. 11-4. Wedelstaedt chisel checked for sharpness by placing on thumbnail at an angle. If cutting edge does not slide, the instrument is sharp. (Courtesy University of Tennessee College of Dentistry.)

pletely, and it should retain this relationship to the stone as the assistant draws the instrument toward her. This motion may be repeated several times, if necessary. The instrument can be tested for sharpness against the thumbnail, as shown in Fig. 11-4. Gingival margin trimmers and angle formers, which are instruments that do not have their cutting edges perpendicular to the long axis of the blade, may be sharpened in the same manner.

Flat tapered stones

Flat Arkansas oilstones that are thicker on one side and taper to a lesser thickness on the other side, with both the thick and thin sides rounded (Fig. 11-1, *B*), may be used in sharpening most sizes of curets and spoon excavators. Whichever rounded edge best fits the curvature of the blade of the instrument may be used. In addition, the flat surface of the stone may be used in sharpening procedures.

Cylinder stones

Cylinder-shaped Arkansas oilstones (Fig. 11-1, *C*) of varying diameters may be used to sharpen those prophylaxis and cutting instruments that have a curved blade. A stone is selected that most nearly fits the curvature of the blade to be sharpened.

Straight handpiece stones

Straight handpiece stones are mounted composition stones. They are available in various diameters and are used in the same manner as the cylinder stones previously described (Fig. 11-1, *D*). Composition stones are not as hard as Arkansas stones; therefore, they will not produce as sharp an edge.

Mechanical sharpener

The mechanical oscillating sharpener is provided with an instrument guide, which holds the instrument stationary and allows a flat bevel to be placed on the instrument. This bevel may be increased or decreased by rotating the motor on its axis while the instrument is held parallel to the floor.

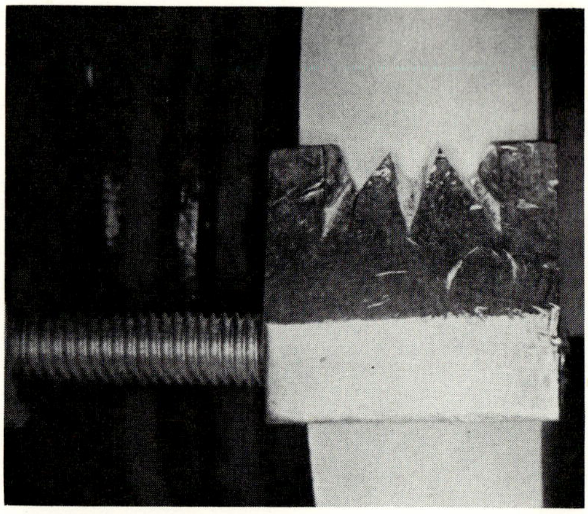

Fig. 11-5. Instrument guide on mechanical sharpener. (Courtesy University of Tennessee College of Dentistry.)

The instrument guide (Fig. 11-5) has 3 slots for the placement of instruments. The center slot is used for sharpening instruments in which the cutting edge is perpendicular to the long axis of the blade, such as enamel hatchets, chisels, and hoes; the other 2 slots are used when sharpening instruments in which the cutting edge is not perpendicular to the long axis of the blade, such as gingival margin trimmers and angle formers. Right-angle bevels are placed in the right slot, and left-angle bevels are placed in the left slot.

Sharpening wheels of 3 smaller sizes are used for sharpening curved-blade instruments with a right-angle bevel, such as spoon excavators and scalers, and for cleaning out the concave surface of gingival margin trimmers with right-angle bevels (Fig. 11-6). The sharpening wheel (Fig. 11-2, *D*) is used for sharpening spoon excavators or cleaning out gingival margin trimmers with left-angle bevels.

To stop this instrument from oscillating, a wedge is placed between the oscillating wheel and the motor. The fixation of the large sharpening wheel is necessary, so that

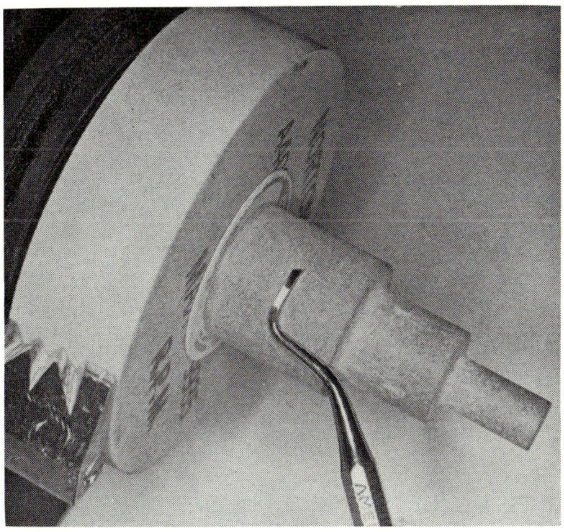

Fig. 11-6. Cleaning out concave surface of gingival margin trimmer with right-angled bevel. (Courtesy University of Tennessee College of Dentistry.)

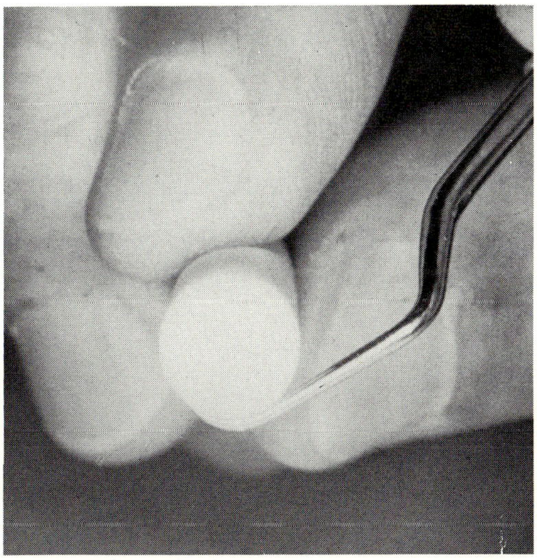

Fig. 11-7. Curet sharpened with cylinder Arkansas stone. (Courtesy University of Tennessee College of Dentistry.)

the side cutting edges of the hatchets, chisels, and hoes may be sharpened.

Prophylaxis instruments

As a rule, prophylaxis instruments, such as sickle scalers, hoes, chisels, and curets,

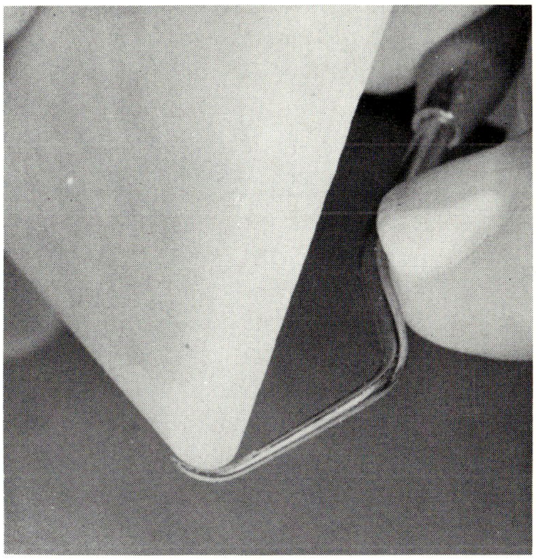

Fig. 11-8. Curet sharpened with rounded edge of flat, tapered Arkansas stone. (Courtesy University of Tennessee College of Dentistry.)

should be sharpened with hand stones because of the smallness of the blades. Mounted handpiece stones and the sharpening wheel of the mechanical sharpener will remove too much metal from the blade, unless they are in the hands of experts.

Curets may be sharpened with a cylinder Arkansas stone of appropriate size to fit the curvature of the blade by holding the instrument with the flat part of the blade parallel to the floor and moving the stone at right angles to the length of the blade, while maintaining the stone in contact with the flat surface of the blade (Fig. 11-7). A flat, tapered Arkansas stone with rounded edges may be used to sharpen curets in the same manner as with the cylinder stones (Fig. 11-8).

Curets also may be sharpened by using a flat stone and sharpening the outer surface of the blade. In this technique, the blade is again held parallel with the floor, and the stone is moved downward, following the curvature of the blade (Fig. 11-9).

Mounted handpiece Arkansas stones may be used to sharpen curets. A stone fitting the curvature of the instrument is se-

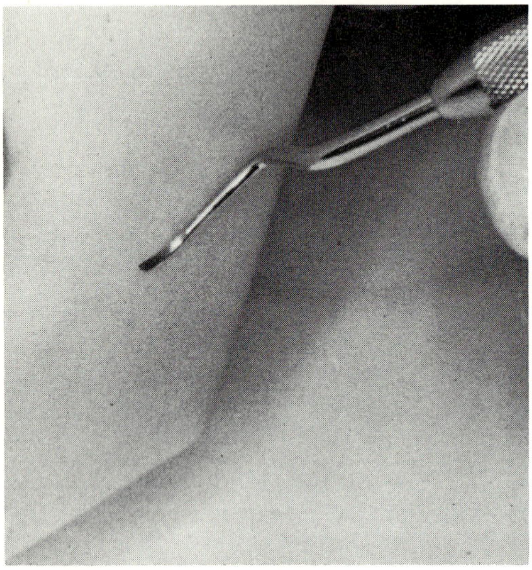

Fig. 11-9. Curet sharpened with flat, tapered Arkansas stone. (Courtesy University of Tennessee College of Dentistry.)

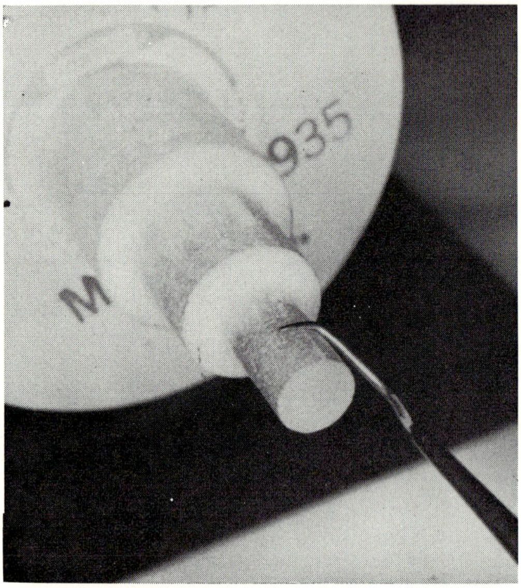

Fig. 11-11. Curet sharpened on mechanical sharpener. (Courtesy University of Tennessee College of Dentistry.)

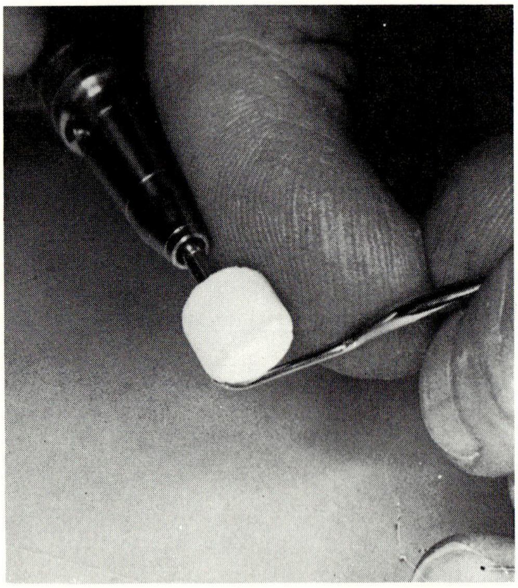

Fig. 11-10. Curet sharpened with composition handpiece stone. (Courtesy University of Tennessee College of Dentistry.)

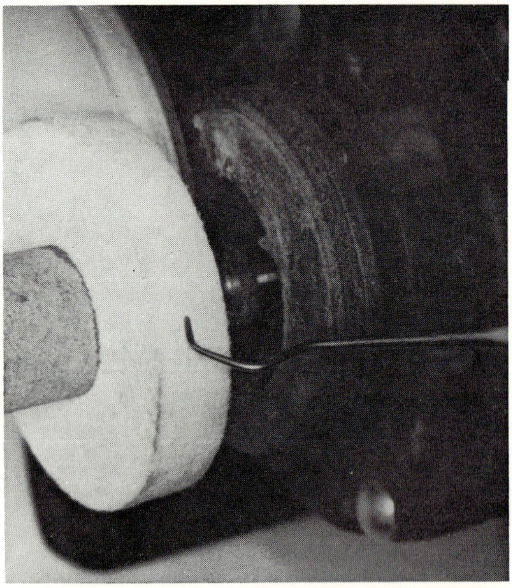

Fig. 11-12. Bur on cutting edge of curet removed by felt wheel of mechanical sharpener. (Courtesy University of Tennessee College of Dentistry.)

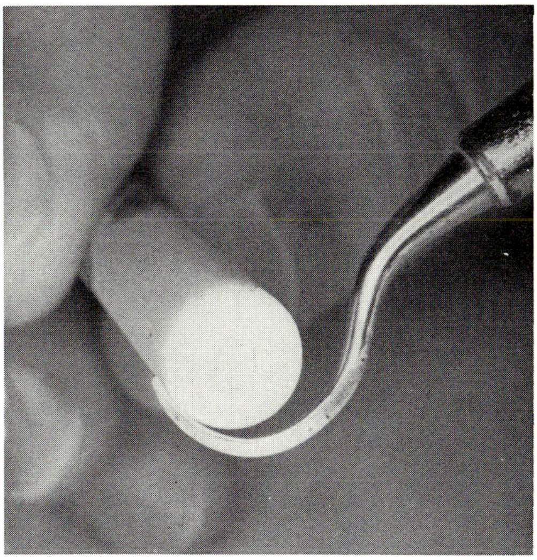

Fig. 11-13. Sickle type of scaler sharpened with cylinder Arkansas stone. (Courtesy University of Tennesse College of Dentistry.)

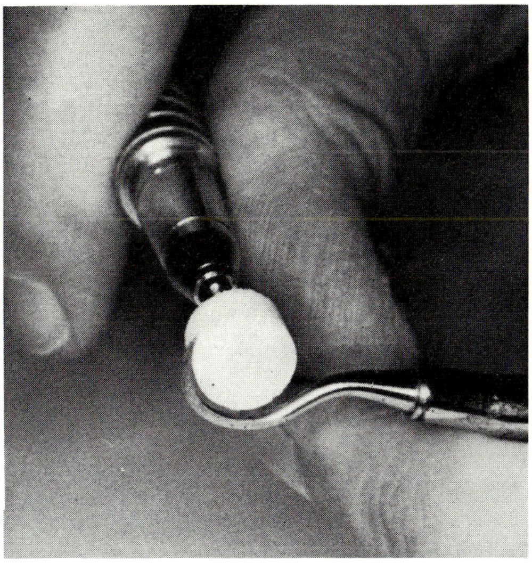

Fig. 11-14. Sickle type of scaler sharpened with composition handpiece stone. (Courtesy University of Tennessee College of Dentistry.)

lected and positioned in the straight handpiece; it is then placed in contact with the concave portion of the blade (Fig. 11-10). The stone should be moved back and forward slightly to prevent grooving the blade.

The small stone on the mechanical sharpener can be used to sharpen curets. This is accomplished by placing the concave surface in contact with the stone while using light pressure (Fig. 11-11). The bur produced in sharpening is removed by holding the convex surface of the blade against the felt wheel (Fig. 11-12).

Sickle scalers of large size can be sharpened by techniques described for curets, using cylinder Arkansas stones (Fig. 11-13) or large cylindrical stones mounted in a straight handpiece (Fig. 11-14). Scalers of the Jaquette type can be sharpened with a small stone in the straight handpiece (Fig. 11-15) or by use of the flat tapered stone (Fig. 11-16).

The hoe type of scalers is best sharpened with the large, flat Arkansas stone. The bevel of the blade is placed in apposition to the surface of the stone, and while using the remaining fingers to stabilize the instrument in this position, the instrument is drawn toward the assistant (Fig. 11-17). The sharpening movement is from the shoulder, since the fingers, hand, wrist, and elbow should remain as fixed as possible while the instrument is moved across the stone, in order to place 1 bevel on the blade instead of several bevels. This procedure may need to be repeated several times, in order to produce a sharp edge.

The chisel type of scalers is sharpened in the same manner as that described for the hoe type of scalers (Fig. 11-18), or they may be sharpened with the mechanical sharpener (Fig. 11-19).

Files used in prophylaxis usually cannot be satisfactorily sharpened in the dental office, so they should be returned to the manufacturer for this procedure.

Cavity preparation instruments

Cavity preparation instruments may be sharpened with flat Arkansas stones, cylinder stones, and the mechanical sharpener. The flat Arkansas stones may be used in sharpening hatchets and other instruments of this type. The use of the mechanical

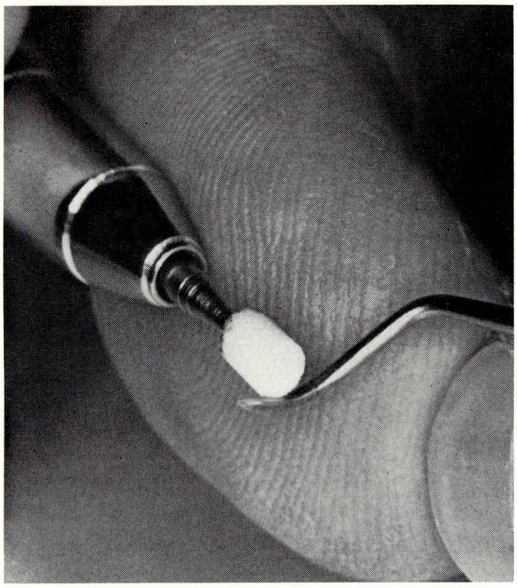

Fig. 11-15. Jaquette type of scaler sharpened with composition handpiece stone. (Courtesy University of Tennessee College of Dentistry.)

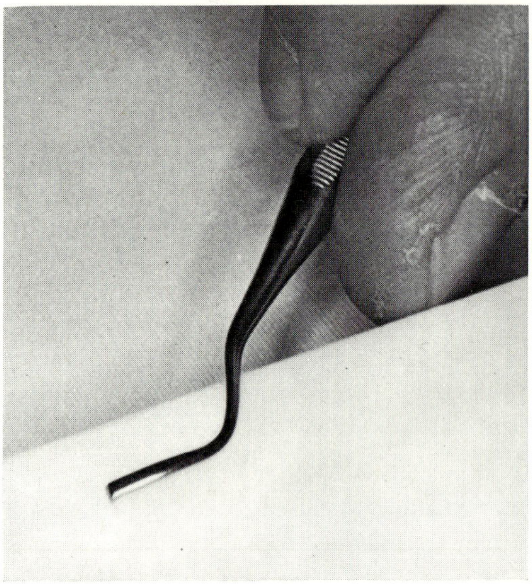

Fig. 11-17. Hoe type of scaler sharpened on flat Arkansas stone. (Courtesy University of Tennessee College of Dentistry.)

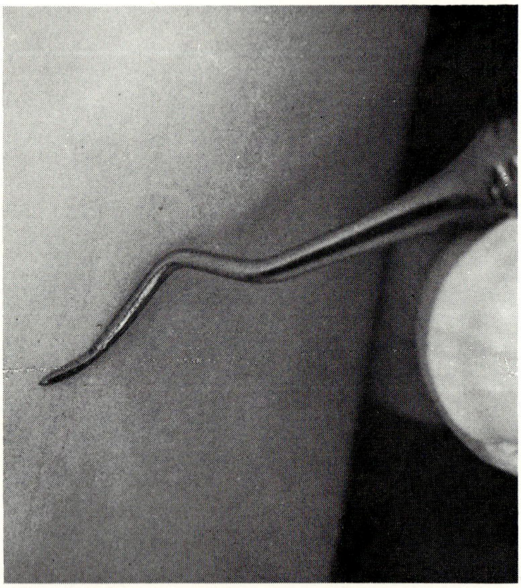

Fig. 11-16. Jaquette type of scaler sharpened with flat Arkansas stone. (Courtesy University of Tennessee College of Dentistry.)

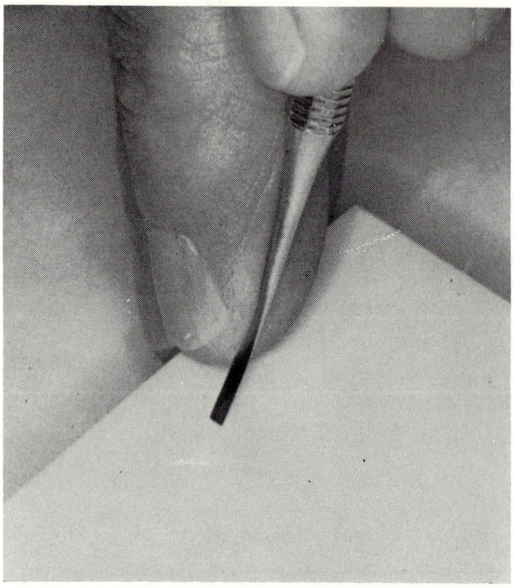

Fig. 11-18. Chisel type of scaler sharpened on flat Arkansas stone. (Courtesy University of Tennessee College of Dentistry.)

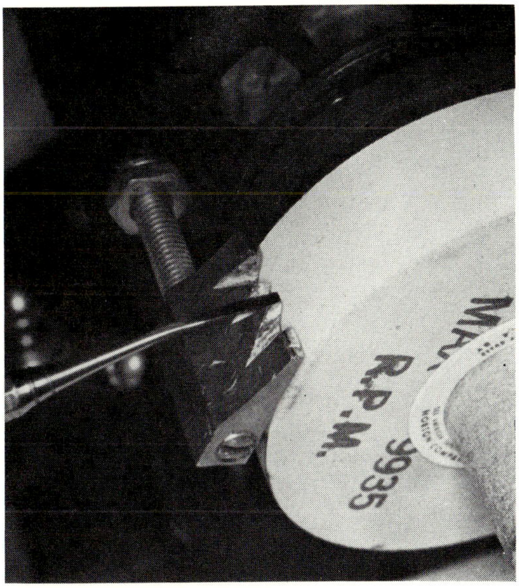

Fig. 11-19. Chisel type of scaler sharpened on mechanical sharpener. (Courtesy University of Tennessee College of Dentistry.)

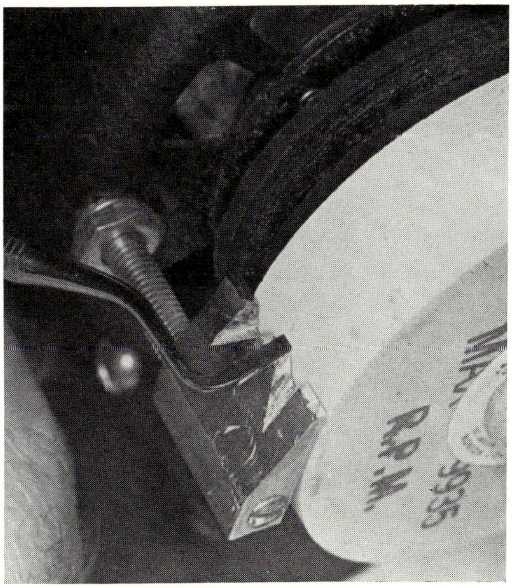

Fig. 11-20. Enamel hatchet sharpened in center slot of instrument guide of mechanical sharpener. (Courtesy University of Tennessee College of Dentistry.)

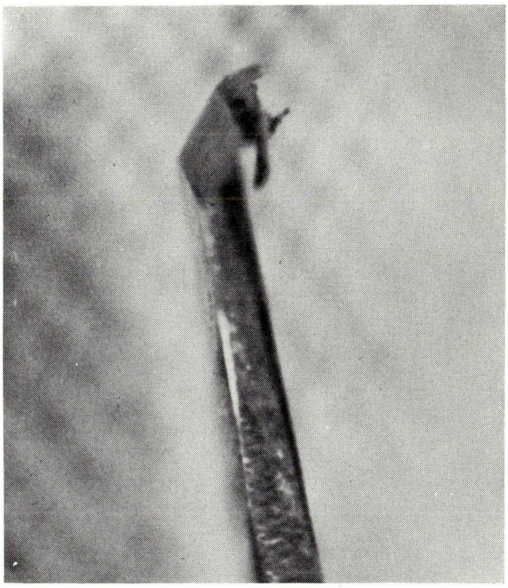

Fig. 11-21. Bur on cutting edge of instrument after sharpening on mechanical sharpener. (Courtesy University of Tennessee College of Dentistry.)

sharpener is recommended for sharpening cavity preparation instruments, because of the ease of placing a single accurate bevel on the instruments and the facility with which the sharpening operation may be accomplished.

Hatchets, chisels, and hoes are all instruments that have the cutting edges of the blades perpendicular to the long axis of the blade. These blades are sharpened in the center slot of the instrument guide of the oscillating mechanical sharpener (Fig. 11-20). While holding the blade of the instrument parallel to the floor in the center slot of the instrument guide, the assistant should rotate the motor either forward or backward, until the bevel on the cutting edge of the instrument is duplicated when the instrument approximates the sharpening stone. She should apply gentle pressure, until she can see the entire cutting edge in close approximation to the stone. A slight bur (Fig. 11-21) will be produced on the cutting edge of the instrument. This

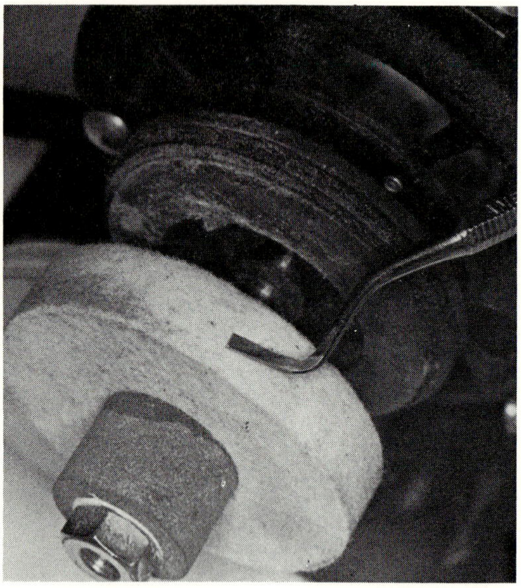

Fig. 11-22. Bur on cutting edge of enamel hatchet removed by holding the bur against the felt wheel. (Courtesy University of Tennessee College of Dentistry.)

A

B

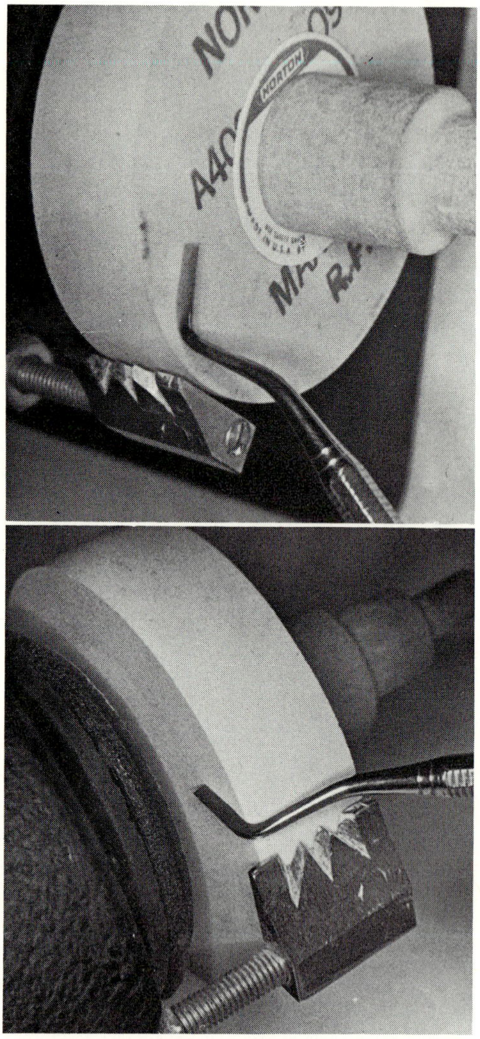

Fig. 11-23. A, Distal side bevel of enamel hatchet sharpened on mechanical sharpener; **B,** mesial side bevel of enamel hatchet sharpened on mechanical sharpener. (Courtesy University of Tennessee College of Dentistry.)

is removed by turning the blade over and holding it against the felt buffing wheel for a few seconds (Fig. 11-22). The blade is then removed and checked for sharpness, as illustrated in Fig. 11-4.

Instruments with cutting edges on the sides of the blades may be sharpened on the large sharpening wheel, after placing a wedge between the oscillating wheel and the motor to prevent the sharpening wheel from oscillating (Fig. 11-23).

Gingival margin trimmers and angle formers are instruments with cutting edges that are not perpendicular to the long axis of the blade. These instruments are sharpened in the left and right slots of the instrument guide, with the left slot being used for left-angle bevels and the right slot being used for right-angle bevels. The instruments are approximated to the stone and sharpened, and the bur is removed as described for hatchets, chisels, and hoes (Figs. 11-24 to 11-25).

Spoon excavators are sharpened on the smaller stones (Fig. 11-26). If the spoons are not very dull, they can be sharpened by holding the convex side of the blade against the felt buffing wheel (Fig. 11-27). Small discoid spoon excavators are best sharpened by this method (Fig. 11-28).

Gold knives may be sharpened on the felt wheel (Fig. 11-29) or on a flat Arkansas stone.

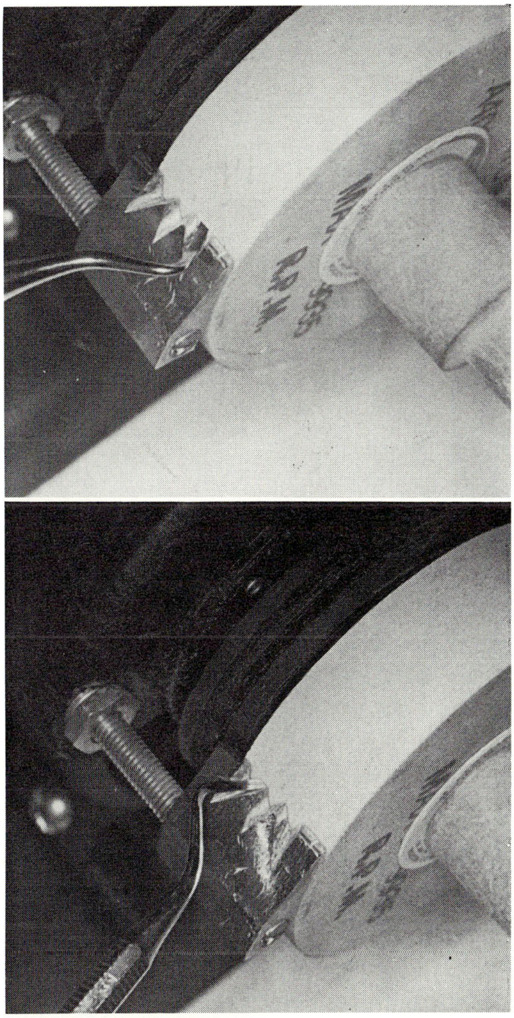

A

B

Fig. 11-24. A, Gingival margin trimmer with right-angled bevel sharpened in right slot of the instrument guide of mechanical instrument sharpener; **B,** gingival margin trimmer with left-angled bevel sharpened in left slot of instrument guide of mechanical instrument sharpener. (Courtesy University of Tennessee College of Dentistry.)

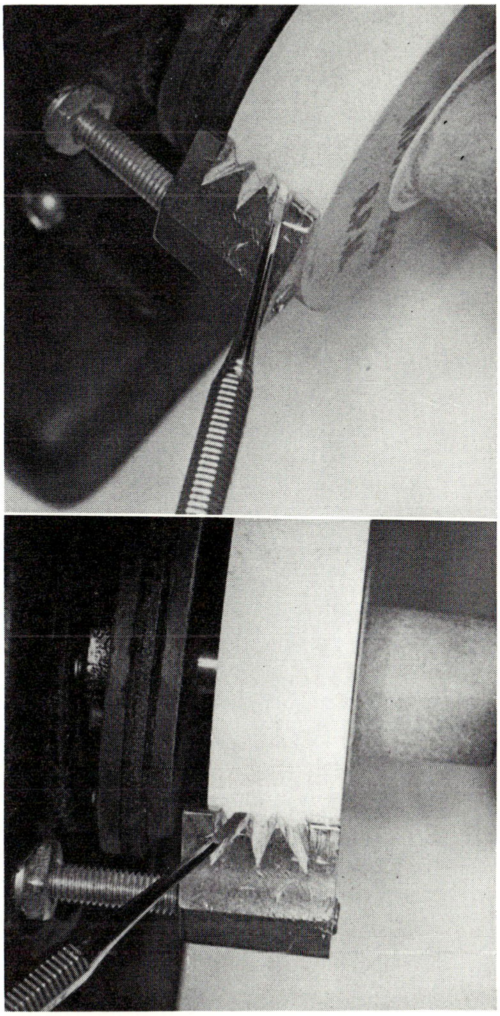

A

B

Fig. 11-25. A, Angle former with right-angled bevel sharpened in right slot of instrument guide of mechanical sharpener; **B,** angle former with left-angled bevel sharpened in left slot of instrument guide of mechanical sharpener. (Courtesy University of Tennessee College of Dentistry.)

After the use of prophylaxis instruments at the chair, the dental assistant should check all instruments for sharpness, and those that are dull should be sharpened and recleaned.

Most dental cutting instruments are made of carbon steel, and they can be sharpened to a finer cutting edge than instruments made of stainless steel. Carbon steel instruments cannot be sterilized by the autoclave or boiling methods of sterilization, as these methods will dull the cutting edges of the instruments; therefore, carbon steel instruments should be disin-

A

B

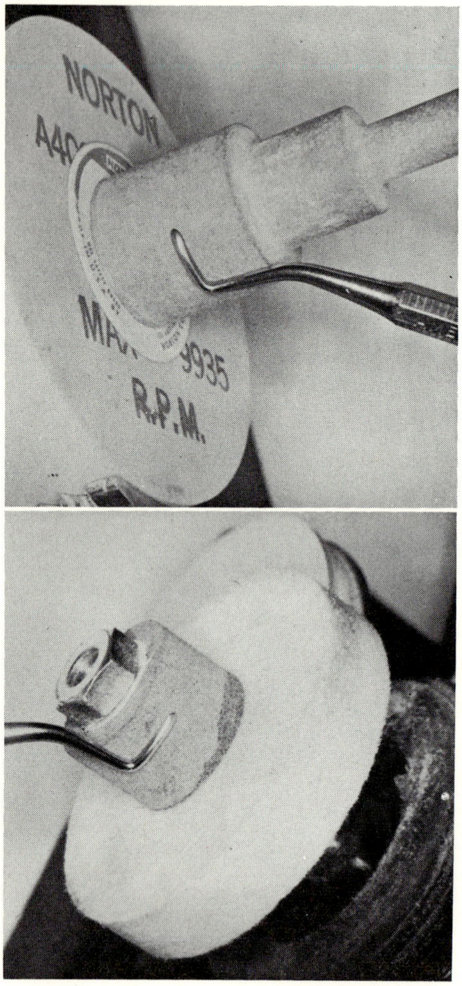

Fig. 11-26. A, Spoon excavator sharpened on small stone of mechanical sharpener—right-angled blade; **B,** spoon excavator sharpened on small stone of mechanical sharpener—left-angled blade. (Courtesy University of Tennessee College of Dentistry.)

fected in a chemical solution to prevent damage to the cutting edges (see Chapter 9). The dental assistant never should forget to place antirust tablets in the disinfecting solution, if they need to be added to the particular solution being used, or the instruments will be damaged.

Dry heat sterilization at a temperature of 160 degrees C. for 1 hour is an effective

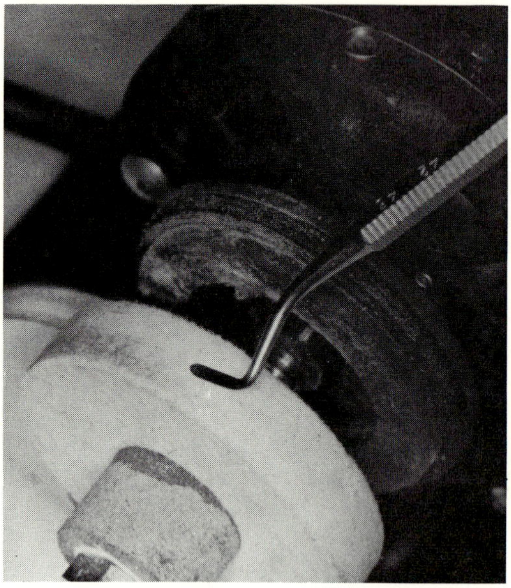

Fig. 11-27. Spoon excavator sharpened on felt wheel of mechanical sharpener. (Courtesy University of Tennessee College of Dentistry.)

method of sterilizing cutting instruments without damaging the cutting edges; however, if this method of sterilization is used, more duplicate sets of instruments will be necessary.

Stainless steel cutting instruments can be sterilized in the autoclave without damage to the cutting edges; however, one must sacrifice cutting efficiency when using instruments made of this material.

After sterilization or disinfection, instruments should be removed and dried with a sterile towel and placed in the instrument cabinet.

CARE AND MAINTENANCE OF EQUIPMENT

All equipment should receive routine preventive maintenance, and the equipment in the dental office is no exception. Considering the cost of equipment in a dental office and the fact that this expensive equipment will perform satisfactorily for many years if it is cared for, it is imperative to properly maintain it.

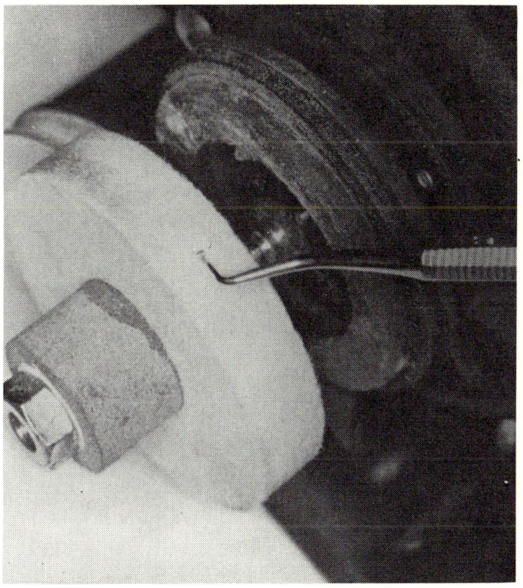

Fig. 11-28. Discoid spoon excavator sharpened on felt wheel of mechanical sharpener. (Courtesy University of Tennessee College of Dentistry.)

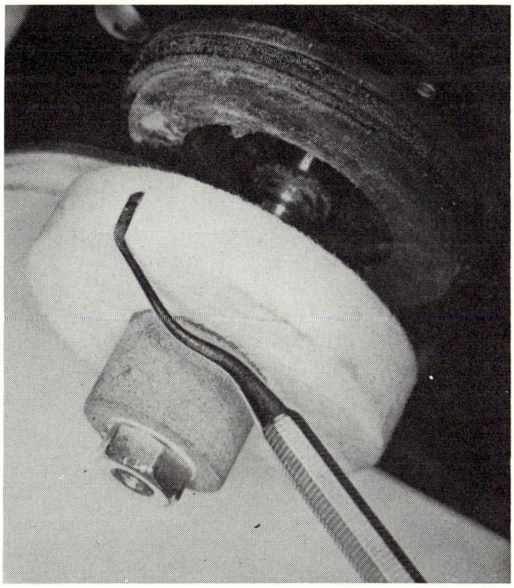

Fig. 11-29. Gold knife sharpened on felt wheel of mechanical sharpener. (Courtesy University of Tennessee College of Dentistry.)

A good, safe procedure in the care and maintenance of all equipment is to follow the manufacturer's recommendations, as the equipment has been operated and thoroughly tested before it is sold. Many hours of lost time can be saved by routine preventive maintenance as recommended by the manufacturer.

A schedule of periodic maintenance operations should be set up for all pieces of equipment in the dental office, and one or more of the auxiliary personnel should be assigned to perform these tasks. This may be accomplished by an index card file, typed schedule, calendar, or some other arrangement.

One of the more important aspects in the care and maintenance of equipment is an appreciation of what can be done in the dental office with respect to the repair of equipment, and when a dental repairman should be called in to care for the equipment. Most manufacturers provide a manual of instructions on the operation and maintenance of their equipment, together with some instructions on how to locate and correct malfunctions of equipment as they occur. Extra copies of these manuals may be obtained from local dental dealers. If the equipment malfunctions cannot be located and corrected after following these suggestions, it is best to call the dental equipment repairman. Dental equipment has become highly specialized and complicated and requires special knowledge and training in its repair; therefore, most repairs will require the services of a trained repairman.

Contra-angles

Prophylaxis angles

In the armamentarium of the dentist and the dental hygienist, the prophylaxis angle (Fig. 11-30) is one of the items of equipment requiring routine care and maintenance. Since this instrument is exposed to saliva, blood, debris, and polishing agents when used for cleaning and pol-

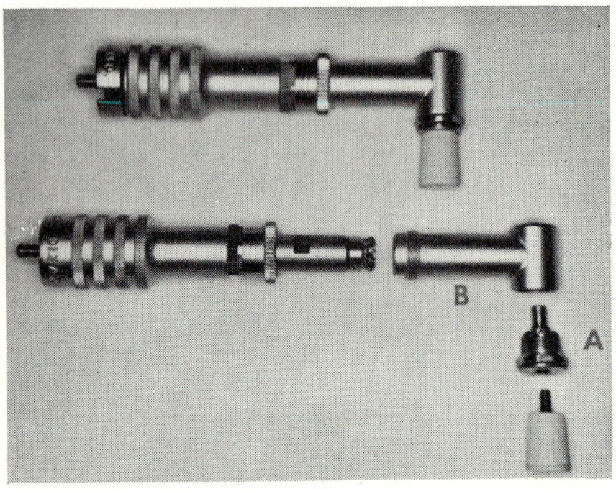

Fig. 11-30. Prophylaxis angle disassembled. **A,** Gear barrel assembly; **B,** head of angle. (Courtesy University of Tennessee College of Dentistry.)

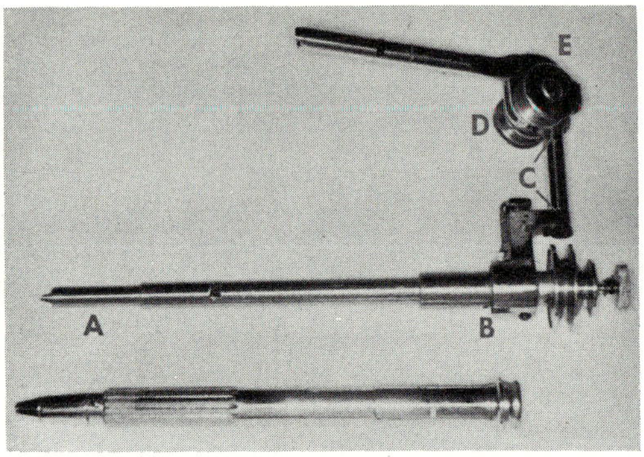

Fig. 11-31. Friction type of handpiece with sheath removed. (Courtesy University of Tennessee College of Dentistry.)

ishing procedures in the oral cavity, it must be cleaned, sterilized, and lubricated after each operation to ensure a long period of use. A number of prophylaxis angles should be available in the dental office, so that dentist or dental hygienist does not have to pause between patients, waiting for the angle to be cleaned.

The cleaning of these instruments is best accomplished by running the complete angle on the straight handpiece in a cleaning solution. The gear barrel assembly (Fig. 11-30, *A*) should be removed and the remainder of the angle run in the cleaner to dissolve old grease. Old grease should be removed from the gear barrel assembly with cleaner and a brush, and the inside of the head of the angle should be blown dry with air. The head shell (Fig. 11-30, *B*) should be removed and the remainder of the angle again run in the cleaning solution to dissolve old grease. The gear barrel assembly should be replaced in the head shell and tightened. The head shell then is filled with grease and screwed back on the body of the instrument. The instructions for cleaning and greasing a prophylaxis angle are those recommended in Fig. 11-30 for the particular instrument, but in all cases the dental auxiliary assigned this task should follow the instructions provided by the manufacturer for the instrument being cleaned, sterilized, and lubricated.

In the event that these instruments are to be sterilized in oil, the instrument should be placed in the sterilizer with the head removed and greased after sterilization.

Friction angles

Friction angles are low-speed instruments that are primarily used for cavity preparation and finishing restorations, and they will need lubrication after each use. They should be cleaned and lubricated at the end of the day, following the manufacturer's recommendations for the type of angle used in the office.

Ball-bearing angles

Ball-bearing angles are precision-built, high-speed instruments requiring strict compliance with the manufacturer's recommendations for cleaning and lubrication. All ball-bearing angles, both long and short sheath, should be lubricated after each use. Cleaning the instrument, followed by lubrication, should be done at the end of each day, or more frequently if recommended by the manufacturer. Always use the type of oil specified in the instructions with the handpiece.

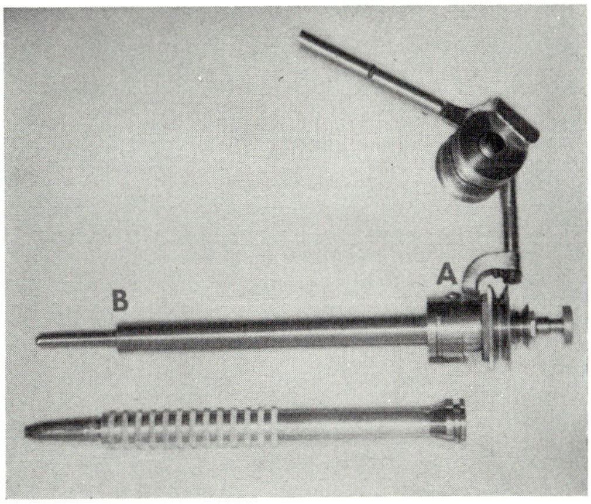

Fig. 11-32. Ball-bearing handpiece with sheath removed. **A,** Rear bearing; **B,** front bearing. (Courtesy University of Tennessee College of Dentistry.)

Handpieces

Friction handpieces

Many hygienists and dentists will be using a low-speed, friction-type straight handpiece. This instrument will be in routine use daily and will require constant cleaning, lubrication, and sterilization or disinfection.

The handpiece shown in Fig. 11-31 with the sheath removed should be oiled several times a day by placing a drop of oil at points *A* and *B*. At the end of the day, the handpiece should be thoroughly cleaned and lubricated. The inside of the sheath should be cleaned with a bristle brush, dipped in cleaning solution, and dried off with air. The spindle should be cleaned with a piece of cloth and cleaning solution. The chuck is cleaned with a pipe cleaner dipped in cleaning solution. A drop of oil is placed at points labeled *A, B, C, D,* and *E* in Fig. 11-31, and the handpiece is reassembled.

Ball-bearing handpieces

The handpiece shown in Fig. 11-32 is a high-speed, ball-bearing handpiece with sealed ball bearings that requires little lubrication. The rear bearing never requires lubrication, and the front bearing should be lubricated twice a month with 1 drop of oil. Since the spindle of the handpiece does not rotate against the sheath, no lubrication is necessary for the spindle. At the end of each day of use, the sheath should be removed and cleaned with a brush and cleaning solution, and the spindle should be wiped clean with a small piece of clean cloth that is wet with cleaning solution. The chuck should be cleaned with a pipe cleaner that is dipped in cleaning solution and 2 drops of oil and placed down inside the bur hole.

Ball-bearing handpieces are precision instruments, and the manufacturer's recommendations should be rigidly followed, including the use of the type of lubricant recommended. The sheath may be sterilized by any means except immersion in a chemical disinfectant. The driving unit of the handpiece should not be placed in any type of sterilizer, because the sealed bearings will be damaged.

Ultraspeed handpieces

Air turbine handpieces (Fig. 11-33), or airotors, require little lubrication of the handpiece, as most of them have built-in lubricating systems; however, at the end of each day, air only should be run through the handpiece for 30 seconds, in order to remove any water in the head of the handpiece. The manufacturer's instructions for the particular type of ultraspeed instrument used in the office should be followed with respect to cleaning, lubrication, and routine maintenance.

Most air turbine handpieces have a built-in lubricating system, with the oil reservoir located either in the dental unit or in an attached control box. It is imperative that the oil level be checked daily or even more frequently to ensure that a proper oil level is maintained in the oil reservoir to prevent damage to the handpiece. The type of oil recommended by the manufacturer

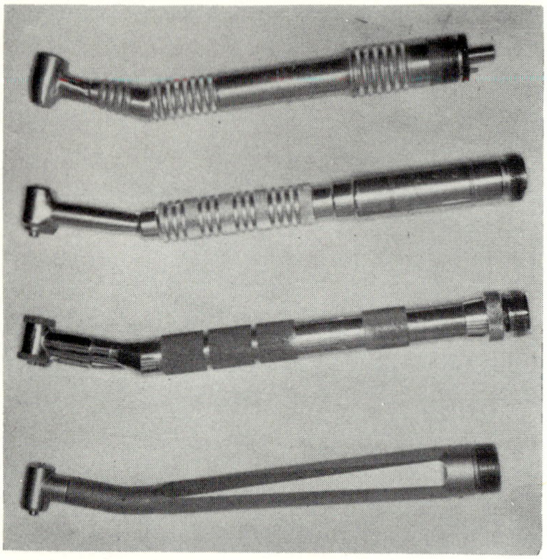

Fig. 11-33. Several types of airotor handpieces. (Courtesy University of Tennessee College of Dentistry.)

should always be used, because an oil of a different viscosity will result in a different lubrication rate for the instrument and may damage the handpiece. The oil reservoir should be periodically removed and cleaned according to the manufacturer's recommendations.

The air supply to turbine handpieces contains an air filter to remove both moisture and minute particles of dust from the air before it reaches the bearings in the handpiece, because either moisture or dust will damage the bearings. The air filter should be purged daily by pressing a small, spring-loaded purging valve at the base of the air filter.

The new dental units being manufactured may be purchased with a built-in lubrication system for the air-driven handpieces, as previously described, or they may be obtained without a lubricating system. When the unit in the dental office does not contain a lubricating system for the air-driven handpieces, it is necessary for one of the auxiliaries in the dental office to perform this required, routine maintenance by hand. Strict compliance with the manufacturer's recommendations for cleaning and lubrication of air-driven handpieces is necessary. This applies to frequency of lubrication as well as type of lubricant.

Cavitron unit

The Cavitron unit (Fig. 11-34) is an ultrasonic instrument designed for use in oral prophylaxis. It requires no preventive maintenance other than the removal of the insert from the handpiece after its use. Inserts may be dismantled (Fig. 11-35) for cleaning and sterilization and may be autoclaved, providing the temperature is not allowed to rise above 121 degrees C. (250 degrees F.).

GENERAL MAINTENANCE

Most pieces of equipment in the dental operatory will need regular maintenance, either at short intervals or over longer periods of time. It will be the purpose of this section to state in general terms the maintenance procedures as they apply to equipment in the dental operatory, since there are so many different types of equipment on the market today.

Dental unit

The unit, including engine arm and pulleys, should be wiped clean with a dry cloth to remove dust and debris and should be cleaned and waxed periodically according to the manufacturer's recommendations.

The cuspidor bowl should be cleaned daily to prevent staining and formation of odors. The cuspidor trap should be removed and cleaned at least twice a week.

Several cups of warm water should be flushed through the saliva ejector once a day, or more frequently if a large number of metal restorations have been removed in daily operations. The metal strainer in the head of the saliva ejector should be removed and also cleaned daily.

Air, water, and multiplex syringes should be checked daily for proper function or leaks. If any irregularities are noted,

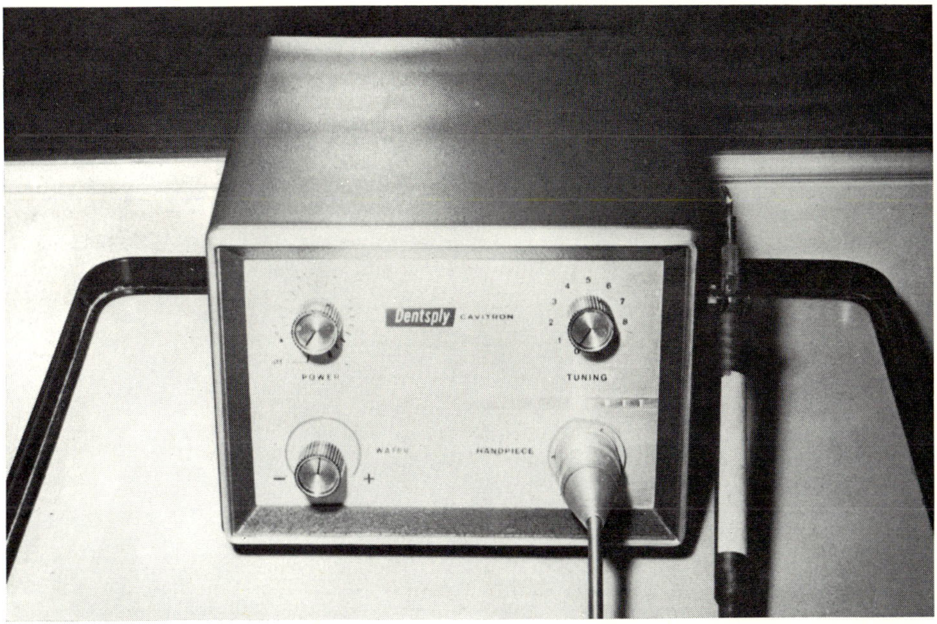

Fig. 11-34. Cavitron unit. (Courtesy University of Tennessee College of Dentistry.)

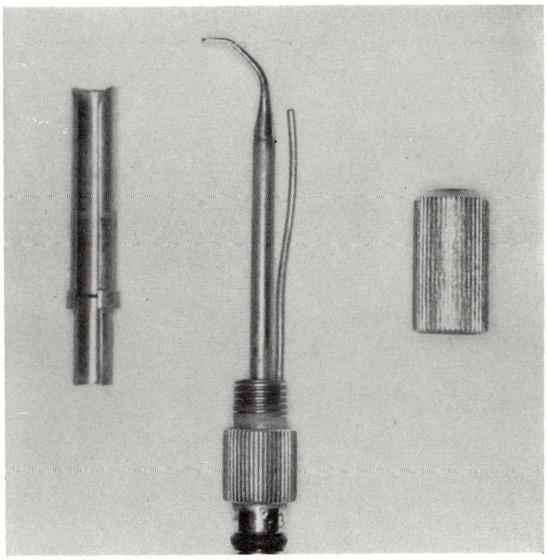

Fig. 11-35. Insert for Cavitron handpiece disassembled. (Courtesy University of Tennessee College of Dentistry.)

they should be brought to the attention of the dentist.

The engine, engine arm, and engine arm pulleys require periodic oiling. The manufacturer's recommendations concerning the time interval for lubrication and the type of oil used should be followed. When the engine cover is removed for oiling the engine is a good time to check the condition of the brushes in the engine and replace them if necessary.

The movable joints in the tray arm or bracket table arm and the operating light should be lubricated, if necessary, according to the manufacturer's recommendations.

The water supply strainer located in the unit should be removed and cleaned periodically, depending upon local conditions.

Foot rheostats should be checked and lubricated periodically. The manufacturer's instructions should be followed.

Oral evacuators

Oral evacuating units must be kept clean to prevent the formation of unpleasant odors in the operatory. Suction hoses should be rinsed with 1 or 2 cups of water following each use and when used in surgery; the hose should be rinsed before and after removing blood from the mouth. A germicidal spray may be sprayed into the suction hoses once a day while the machine is operating, and, at the end of the day, the hoses should be rinsed with several cups of water.

If the evacuator has a collection tank that is not self-emptying, it should be drained twice a day, and the collection tank should be removed and cleaned twice a week, following the manufacturer's instructions.

Suggested readings

1. Blackwell, R. E.: G. V. Black's operative dentistry, ed. 9, South Milwaukee, 1955, Medico-Dental Publishing Co., vol. II.
2. McGehee, W. H. O., True, H. A., and Inskipp, E. F.: A textbook of operative dentistry, New York, 1956, McGraw-Hill Book Co.
3. Peterson, S.: Clinical dental hygiene, ed. 3, St. Louis, 1968, The C. V. Mosby Co.
4. Schultz, L. C., and others: Operative dentistry, Philadelphia, 1966, Lea & Febiger.

CHAPTER 12 ROENTGENOLOGY

HARRISON M. BERRY, Jr., M.Sc., D.D.S.
JAMES E. PHILLIPS, A.B., M.Sc., D.D.S.

When Professor Roentgen, in 1895, discovered invisible rays that could penetrate the body, he called them "x rays," using the symbol for an unknown quantity. They are now known more formally as *roentgen rays,* and x-ray films are known as *roentgenograms.* They are used extensively in the the health professions to detect disease processes and fractures and to kill cancers; in industry they are used to discover flaws in metal castings.

Today every dental patient knows about roentgen rays. They are used to determine the growth and development of the teeth and jaws in children and to reveal impacted teeth, early dental decay, diseases within the jaws, fractures, and rate of healing of the bone. These films are taken (exposed) and developed (processed) by either the dentist, his dental assistant, or his dental hygienist. A few states require that the dentist expose the films, but others permit the properly educated dental assistant and/or dental hygienist to do this, under the dentist's supervision.

When it is permissible for the dental assistant to operate the x-ray machine, it is necessary for her to know the basic facts about this machine and its adjustment. She must know how to position the patient and the film and how to direct the x-ray beam. She must understand both the benefits and the dangers of roentgen rays to herself and to others.

NATURE OF ROENTGEN RAYS

Roentgen rays are highly penetrating, invisible "electromagnetic" rays. They are similar to light rays or radio waves, but they have shorter wave lengths and, therefore, are able to pass through objects with density up to that of lead. Fig. 12-1 shows the several kinds of electromagnetic radiations; as their wave lengths become shorter or longer, their physical behavior changes.

PRODUCTION OF ROENTGEN RAYS

Roentgen rays are produced when a stream of high-speed electrons (negative particles of electricity) bombards a target (focal area) that is made of the element tungsten. This takes place in a glass x-ray tube, as shown in Fig. 12-2. The tube is enclosed within a metal shell, called the tube housing, which has 1 small opening. The rays that pass through this opening to the patient are called *primary* rays. As the primary rays pass through the patient's cheek, jawbone, and teeth, some strike the film, and some are bent and scatter in all directions from the patient's face. These latter are called *secondary* rays; if they

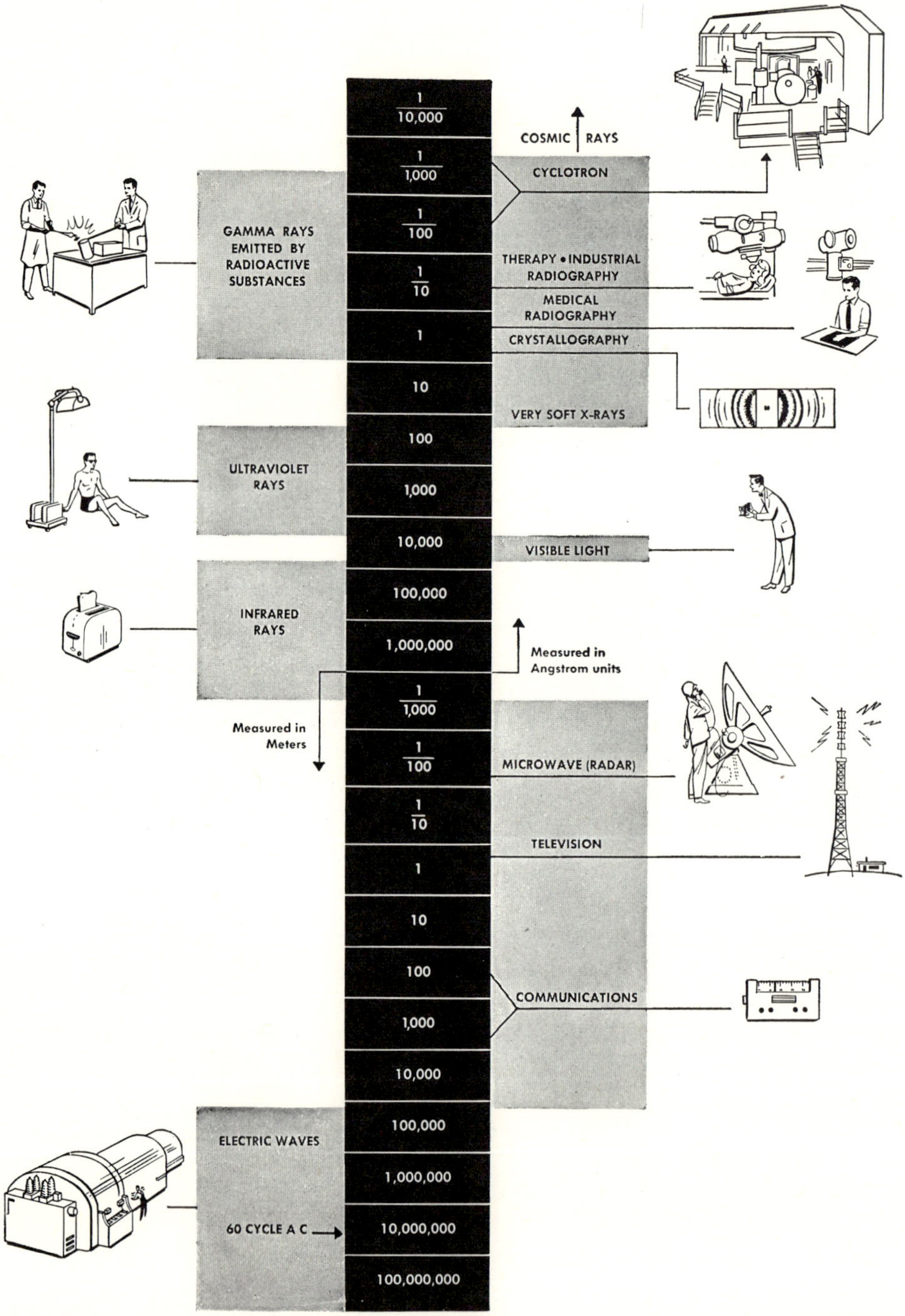

Fig. 12-1. Radiations as depicted by the electromagnetic spectrum. (From The fundamentals of radiography, ed. 9, Rochester, New York, X-ray Sales Division, Eastman Kodak Co.)

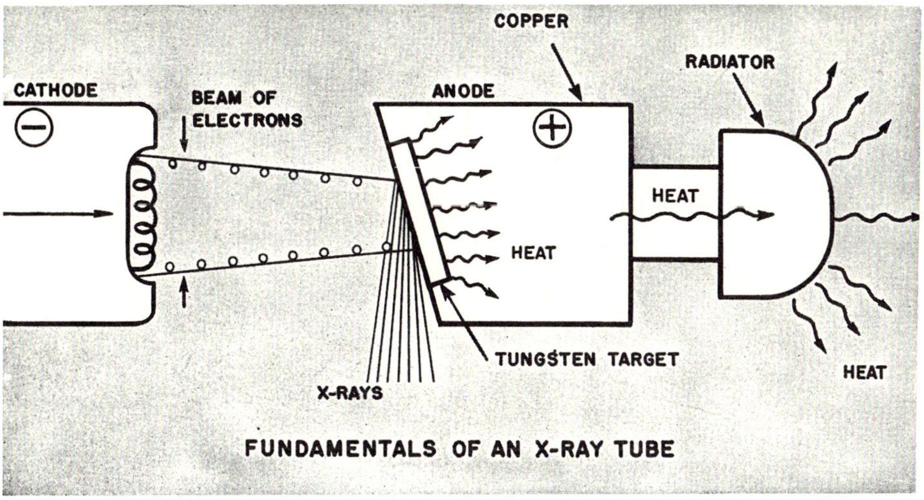

Fig. 12-2. Fundamentals of an x-ray tube. (From Principles of dental x-ray generation, Milwaukee, Wisconsin, General Electric Co.)

were visible, the patient's head would appear to glow like an electric light bulb!

DANGERS OF ROENTGEN RAYS

These highly energized, penetrating rays can damage tissue and change the characteristics of living cells. The damage is cumulative, or additive. This does not mean that the body stores roentgen rays, but rather that the damage done to the body cells remains, so that damage is added to damage. The amount of radiation required for taking roentgenograms of the teeth is not sufficient to cause harm to the patient's face; primary concern in this atomic age is the radiation received by the reproductive cells. Too much radiation to these cells could produce sterility, and lesser amounts, which do not produce any demonstrable changes in the person receiving the radiation, could be passed on to produce changes in future generations. These are known as *genetic changes*. In view of the many sources of radiation to which the earth's population is now subjected (atomic bomb fallout, cosmic rays, radium, and uranium), the National Academy of Sciences has recommended a limit to the amount of radiation to which the reproductive cells of every person in the world should be exposed—10 roentgen units from conception to the age of 30 years.

Radiation is measured in roentgen units (R). A dental x-ray unit operated at 65 kv., 10 ma., and with filtration equivalent to 2 mm. of aluminum, gives about 1 roentgen unit (R) of radiation to the patient's jaw during a 1-second exposure. The total exposure time for a full-mouth examination (16 films), when a fast film is used, is about 5 seconds. Therefore, the patient's jaws receive about 5 R of radiation. Secondary radiation scattering from the jaws during the full-mouth examination delivers about .0005 R to the reproductive cells of an adult male patient.

Protection from radiation

The operator of the x-ray machine (the person who uses it every day) must *never hold a film in the patient's mouth.* Such continual exposure could cause ulceration and cancer of the operator's finger. Mechanical film holders are available, when needed. If the patient is too young, too old, or too infirm to hold the film himself,

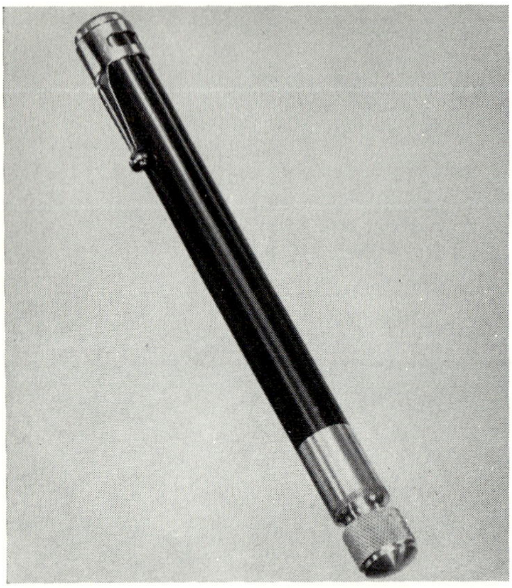

Fig. 12-3. "Pen" type of ionization chamber for monitoring of stray radiation. (Courtesy Victoreen Instrument Co.)

the person who accompanied him to the office should be asked to hold it; this person is not being continually exposed.

Furthermore, by standing close enough to the patient to hold a film in his mouth, the operator is exposing herself to the secondary rays scattering from the patient's face. The maximum permissible dose (MPD) to the operator's body from secondary radiation is 0.3 R per week; 3 R per 13 weeks; and 5 R per year. If the 5 R yearly dose limit is divided by 50 working weeks in a year, the *average* weekly limit becomes 0.1 R.

How may the operator determine her exposure from secondary radiation? Secondary radiation exposure may be monitored by means of either a "pen type" of ionization chamber or a radiation film badge. The ionization chamber, which is

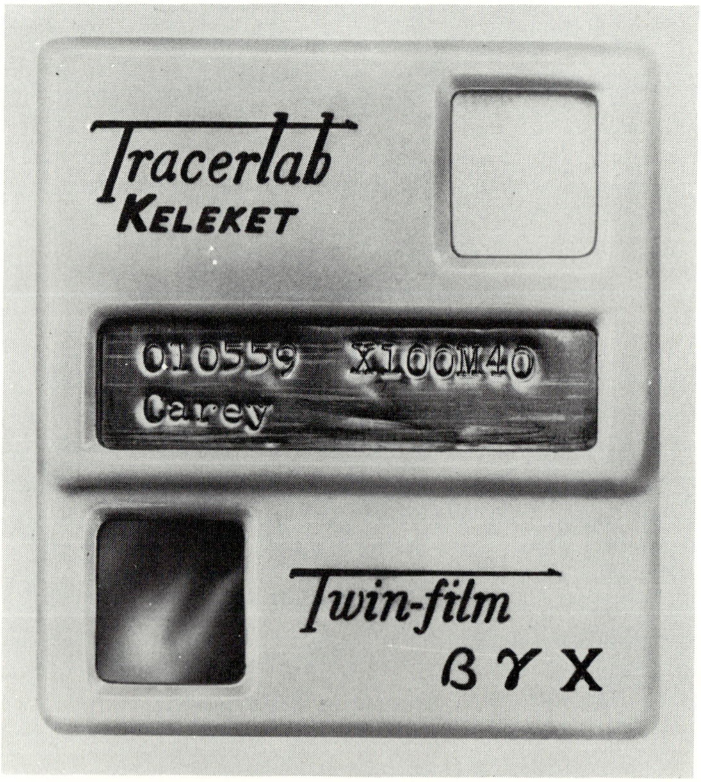

Fig. 12-4. Radiation film badge. One film is replaced each week, giving a weekly reading of secondary radiation to the operator; the other is worn for 12 weeks, giving the accumulated dosage. (Courtesy Tracerlab-Keleket, Inc.)

shaped like a fountain pen, is worn in the pocket for a period of time and then placed in a charger-reader, where the roentgen dosage is read (Fig. 12-3). The radiation film badge (Fig. 12-4) consists of a case containing 2 dental films. It is clipped to the uniform, and at weekly intervals, it is mailed to the company supplying the service. There the films are developed and compared with films exposed to known amounts of radiation, and a report of the exposure received is mailed to the subscriber.

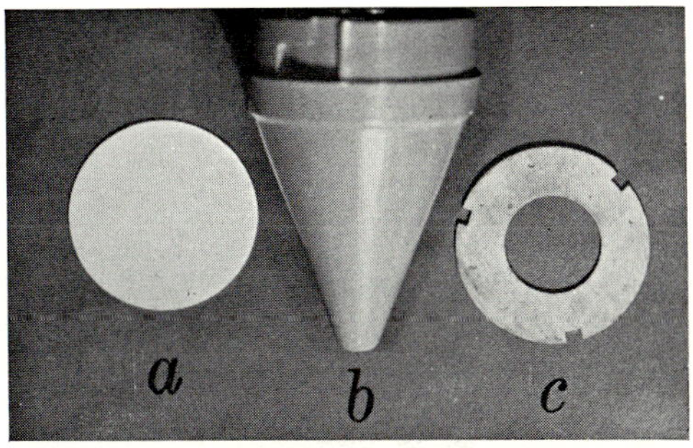

Fig. 12-5. A, Aluminum filter; **B,** plastic pointer cone; **C,** lead diaphragm. (From Peterson, S., editor: Clinical dental hygiene, ed. 3, St. Louis, 1968, The C. V. Mosby Co.)

Control of radiation

Since the chief danger to the operator is radiation scattering from the patient (secondary radiation), it stands to reason that the less radiation the patient receives, the less the radiation to which the operator will be exposed. The x-ray beam, starting from a spot on the target in the x-ray tube, comes out in the shape of an ever-enlarging cone. The diameter of this beam must be controlled, so that when it reaches the film, it is no larger than necessary; a larger beam merely gives the patient unnecessary radiation. Limiting of the beam diameter is called *collimation* and is accomplished by placing a *lead diaphragm* over the opening through which the rays leave the tube housing. This lead disk (Fig. 12-5) has a hole in the center, and the size of the hole determines the size of the x-ray beam. The diaphragm should limit the diameter of the beam at the tip of the pointer cone to a maximum of 2.75 inches. Actual measurement has shown that when the diameter of the beam at cone tip is reduced from 3.5 inches to 2.75 inches, the patient receives 38 percent less primary radiation to the face and 30 percent less secondary radiation to the reproductive cells. There is a corresponding decrease in scattered secondary radiation to the operator.

The waves in the x-ray beam are not all the same length. The short wavelengths have greater penetrating power than the longer wavelengths; in fact, some of the long waves cannot even get through the patient's cheek to reach the film. Thus, since they do not contribute to the image on the film, they only give the patient unneeded radiation. Aluminum has the same ability as the cheek to absorb these longer waves. When a solid disk of aluminum (Fig. 12-5) is placed over the hole in the lead diaphragm, these longer rays never reach the patient's face. Such a disk is called an *aluminum filter,* for it filters out (absorbs) the long waves, but has no effect on the short waves, which pass through to register on the film. The effect of the filter is to reduce the primary radiation to the patient's face, which, in turn, results in less secondary radiation scattering to the patient's own reproductive cells and to the operator. The recommended thickness of the aluminum filter ranges from 1.5 mm. to 2.5 mm. The thicker aluminum filters may cause the films to be somewhat light, so that a slightly longer exposure time is necessary; even so, the patient will still receive considerably less radiation. (At the present time, each state has a radiation code; the dental assistant should ascertain the thickness of aluminum filter required in her state.)

Although reduction of the radiation reaching the patient also reduces the amount of secondary radiation scattering to the operator, the operator can protect herself even more by either (1) standing behind a lead protective screen or (2) standing so far from the patient's head that the rays are unable to harm her. Table 3 shows the number of seconds the operator may expose films each day while standing at various distances, without receiving more than the maximum permissible dose. She should make it a rule never to stand closer than 5 feet from the patient's head.

Finally, a most effective means of reducing x-ray exposure to the patient, and thereby less scatter to the operator, is the use of *fast* film. Such a film is more sensitive to roentgen rays, and it requires only one-fourth to one-fifth as much exposure time as a medium-speed film.

OPERATION OF THE X-RAY MACHINE

Dental x-ray machines consist of 3 basic elements: (1) the control circuit, (2) the generating circuit, and (3) the x-ray tube.

The control circuit controls the generating circuit, which provides the power for the x-ray tube, which in turn produces the roentgen rays. The dental assistant must understand the dials of the control circuit. For details concerning the generating circuit, the reader is referred to the suggested readings at the end of this chapter, particularly the books by Ennis and Berry and by Peterson. Specific details concerning the operation of a particular machine will be found in the operating manual supplied by the manufacturer.

Control circuit

Dental x-ray machines are of 2 general types, fixed and variable. In the fixed type, the tube current is fixed and cannot be changed. In the variable type, the tube current is selective; hence, this type has more control dials than the fixed machine.

Tube current

Tube current is the current of electricity (stream of electrons) that flows through the x-ray tube to strike the target (Fig. 12-2). The amount of current (number of electrons) is measured in milliamperes (1 milliampere = 0.001 ampere). The force driving the electrons is measured in kilovolts (1 kilovolt = 1,000 volts). The more electrons flow per second (milliamperage), the more roentgen rays will be produced per second. The greater the speed of the electrons (kilovoltage), the more penetrating will be the rays produced. When either higher milliamperage or higher kilovoltage is used, the time of the exposure must be shortened.

Controls

The controls in the fixed machine are as follows:

1. On-off switch. This switch simply

Table 3. Permissible workload for operator's safety*

Distance between patient and operator in feet	Permissible daily workload with 65 KVP in seconds	Permissible daily workload with 90 KVP in seconds
2	60	25
3	140	60
4	240	105
5	380	165
6	540	240
8	960	425
10	1,500	665

*From Richards, A. G., and others: Report of committee on radiation protection of the American Academy of Oral Roentgenology, J. Amer. Dent. Ass. 56:514, 1958.

turns the machine on so that it is ready for use; it does not generate roentgen rays. The switch may be of the ordinary toggle type, such as a light switch in the home, or it may be a lever on which the timer switch hangs.

2. Circuit-breaker switch. This type of switch is a spring switch that automatically shuts off if the circuit becomes overloaded. It protects the tube against a sudden surge of current.

3. Timer. The timer consists of a dial on which the operator sets the number of seconds for the exposure and a button that, when pressed, energizes the generating circuit and produces roentgen rays.

4. Voltmeter. This control indicates the amount of house current coming into the machine. It should read 110 during the exposure.

5. Voltage regulator, or voltage compensator. This dial can be turned to regulate the incoming voltage and make the voltmeter read 110. In an office building, or even in a home, other electrical appliances (air conditioners, elevators, for example) will drain off electricity and cause a drop in the line current. With a 110-volt line current, the transformer in the generating circuit of the x-ray machine will produce the kilovolts needed to produce a proper roentgenogram. A lesser current will produce a light film; a greater current will produce a dark film.

6. Milliammeter. A meter that indicates the amount of current flowing through the tube is known as a milliammeter. A current of 10 milliamperes is required; less will produce a light film, and more a dark film.

The controls in a variable type of machine are as follows:

1. The same 6 controls listed for the fixed machine.

2. Kilovoltage selector. This selector is a dial, or a series of push buttons, whereby any kilovoltage from 60 to 90 may be selected. Exposure time must be correlated with changes in kilovoltage.

3. Milliampere selector. This control is a dial whereby any desired milliamperage from 2 to 20 may be selected. Exposure time must also be correlated with milliampere changes.

Operational hints

The operator should position herself during the exposure so that she can see the meters and be sure that they are registering properly. The timer button must be firmly pressed. The operator must never hold the tube housing or the cone of the machine with her hands during an exposure; not only can radiation leak through the metal tube housing or around the cone, but, by being in position to hold the housing or cone, the operator is too close to the patient's head and will subject herself to his field of secondary radiation.

DENTAL X-RAY FILM

A dental x-ray film consists of a clear or blue-tinted cellulose acetate base, coated with a light-sensitive photographic emulsion. The emulsion consists of sensitive silver bromide salts suspended in gelatin. Intraoral films (periapical, bitewing, and occlusal) are purchased in film packets in which the film is surrounded by light-proof paper with a thin piece of lead foil behind the film. The back of each packet has a colored tab (black or green); the front (or the side facing the tube of the x-ray machine) is white.

A periapical film is used to show the teeth in a certain area of the mouth and the area surrounding their apices.

The bite-wing film (Fig. 12-19) packet has a tab, or "wing," upon which the patient bites; this film shows only the crowns of the teeth and the edge of the supporting bone.

The occlusal film (Figs. 12-6 and 12-7) measures about 2 by 3 inches and is used to show the entire maxillary or mandibular arch, any large segment of the arch, or the floor of the mouth.

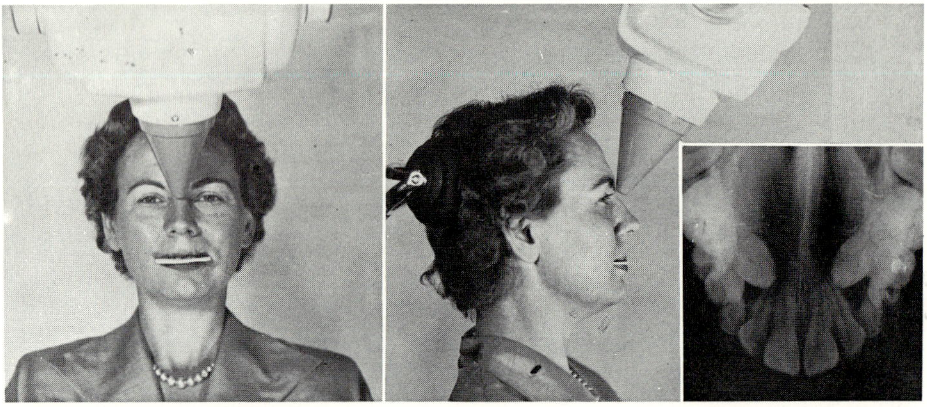

Fig. 12-6. Frontal and lateral views of the maxillary midline occlusal technique and maxillary midline occlusal film. (From Peterson, S., editor: Clinical dental hygiene, ed. 3, St. Louis, 1968, The C. V. Mosby Co.)

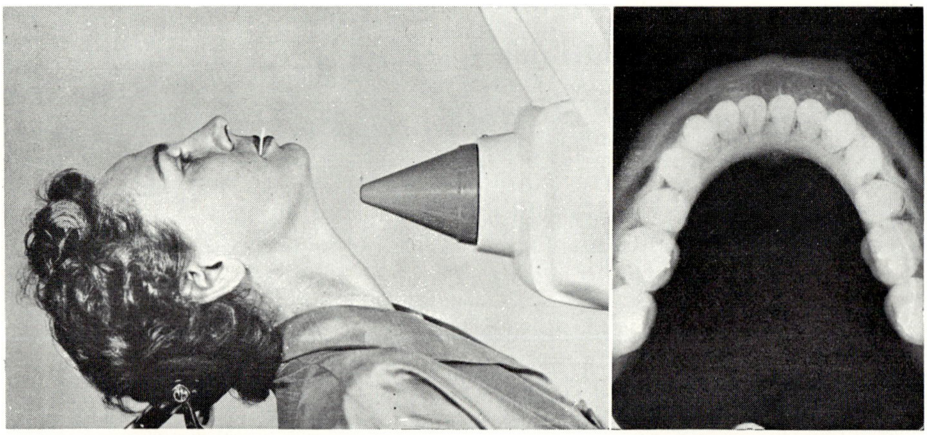

Fig. 12-7. Mandibular floor-of-the-mouth occlusal technique and film. (From Peterson, S., editor: Clinical dental hygiene, ed. 3, St. Louis, 1968, The C. V. Mosby Co.)

Extraoral films are large films (5 by 7 inches or 8 by 10 inches), which are held beside the face. Some are available in packets; others are sold as individual sheets, which must be placed in an exposure holder (in the darkroom) to protect them from visible light. "No-screen" film is used in a cardboard exposure holder; this produces a sharp, fine-grain image, but requires a longer exposure. "Screen" film is used in a "cassette" and requires only a short exposure, but it yields a grainier image. A cassette has hinged front and back covers made of either aluminum or plastic. Inside each cover is a piece of cardboard coated with phosphorescent crystals that give off a bluish visible light when roentgen rays strike them. The x-ray film, being sandwiched between the cardboard screens, receives not only roentgen rays, but also visible light for its exposure. Hence, the x-ray exposure delivered to the film is intensified

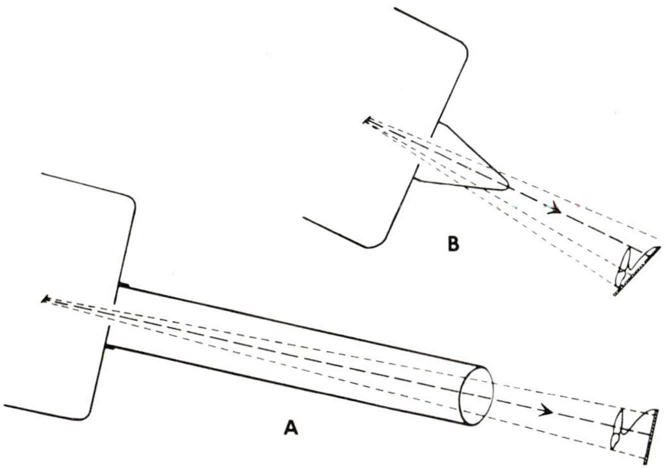

Fig. 12-8. A, Paralleling technique; **B,** bisecting technique. (From Peterson, S., editor: Clinical dental hygiene, ed. 3, St. Louis, 1968, The C. V. Mosby Co.)

by the visible light from the screens. From this action comes the name "intensifying screens."

Intensifying screens are available in the following speeds: slow or high definition, par or intermediate speed, and fast. The detail of the resulting image decreases as the speed of the screen increases.

It should be noted that the manufacturers of dental films are producing new emulsions at such a rate that the user must pay special attention to the recommended exposure on each box of film and the expiration date of the given box.

Periapical film technique

In every phase of dental practice, a given objective may be accomplished in a variety of ways. If he were to select 5 oral surgeons at random, one would probably see 5 different techniques for the extraction of teeth; the important thing is that in each case the teeth would be successfully removed. In other words, attainment of the basic objective is the important consideration. The basic objective of using periapical film is to produce a good image of a tooth, or group of teeth, and the supporting structures. A good image may be described as one that records the size and shape of a tooth as accurately as possible.

Two basic periapical techniques have been devised and are widely used, the bisecting technique and the paralleling technique. Each technique has advantages and disadvantages; neither is perfect. Only the bisecting technique will be described here. (For discussion of paralleling technique, see suggested readings.)

In preparing for an examination, the patient is greeted, informed that he will hold the films in his mouth, and given an opportunity to wash his hands. Such items as eyeglasses and dentures are removed.

The following steps should be performed in the order listed for each film.

1. Position patient's head.
2. Place film in patient's mouth.
3. Have patient retain film in mouth.
4. Check patient's head position; readjust, if necessary.
5. Adjust tubehead for correct vertical angulation.
6. Adjust tubehead for correct horizontal angulation.
7. Adjust tubehead for correct point of entry.
8. Set timer, and make exposure.

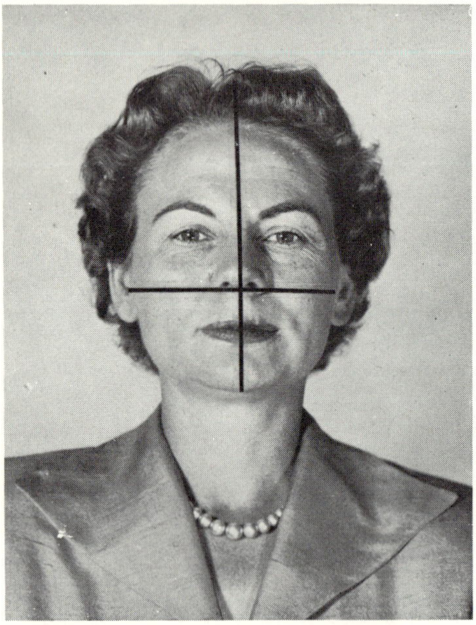

Fig. 12-9. Head position for maxillary films showing midsagittal plane perpendicular to the floor and "line of orientation" parallel with the floor. (From Peterson, S., editor: Clinical dental hygiene, ed. 3, St. Louis, 1968, The C. V. Mosby Co.)

Head position

The occlusal plane of the teeth under examination must be parallel with the floor. For the maxillary periapical and posterior bite-wing examinations, the occlusal plane of the maxillary arch is placed parallel with the floor. A line from the ala of the nose to the tragus of the ear, the *ala-tragus line,* is anatomically parallel with the maxillary occlusal plane. Therefore, if the head is positioned so that the ala-tragus line is parallel with the floor, the maxillary occlusal plane will be in the proper position. For the mandibular teeth, the lower occlusal plane is sighted and made parallel with the floor when the mouth is opened comfortably (not wide). In both instances, the midsagittal plane of the head must be perpendicular to the floor (Fig. 12-9).

Film placement

A full-mouth examination (Fig. 12-10) consists of a minimum of 14 periapical films: upper and lower incisor regions, upper and lower right and left canine regions, upper and lower right and left pre-

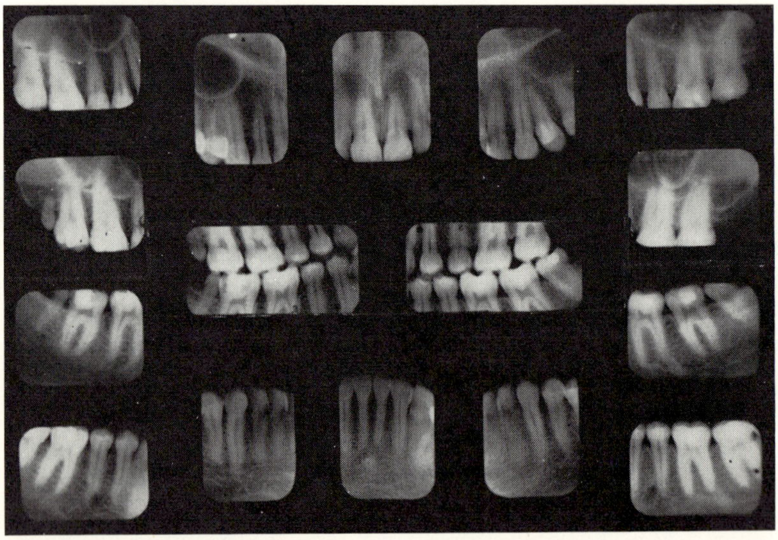

Fig. 12-10. Basic full-mouth films. (From Ennis, L. M., and Berry, H. M., Jr.: Dental roentgenology, ed. 6, Philadelphia, 1967, Lea & Febiger.)

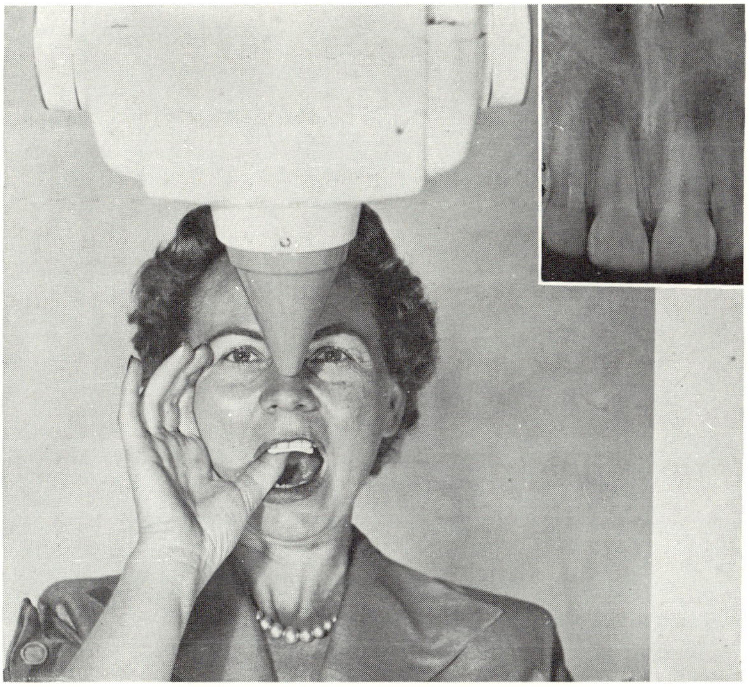

Fig. 12-11. Maxillary incisor periapical technique and film. (From Peterson, S., editor: Clinical dental hygiene, ed. 3, St. Louis, 1968, The C. V. Mosby Co.)

molar regions, and upper and lower right and left molar regions. Posterior bite-wing films are usually included in a full-mouth examination.

Maxillary incisor film

Place the film packet against the incisal edges of the incisors; then slide it posteriorly until about ¼ inch of the film is visible. The packet is centered in the midline. Rotate the posterior end of the packet upward until it touches the palate.

Maxillary canine film

Place the center of the film packet against the incisal edge of the canine and slide it diagonally across the arch until just ¼ inch of the film is visible. The packet is centered on the canine. Rotate the portion of the packet that extends across the arch up to the palate. The upper front corner of the packet will usually bend, because of the slope of the palate. This is acceptable, provided that the remainder of the packet remains flat.

NOTE: In children and in adults with narrow arches, it may be necessary to place the incisor and canine films without rotation to the palate, in order to avoid excessive bending of the film packet. In such cases, the vertical angulation must be increased to 60 to 65 degrees.

Maxillary premolar film

Place the packet flat against the occlusal surfaces of the premolars and canine. The lateral edge of the packet should be just beneath the median grooves of the premolars; the anterior edge should be just beneath the mesial surface of the canine. Rotate the packet upward, until the upper edge rests against the palate; the lower portion will rest against the lingual cusps of the premolars and first molar. Not more

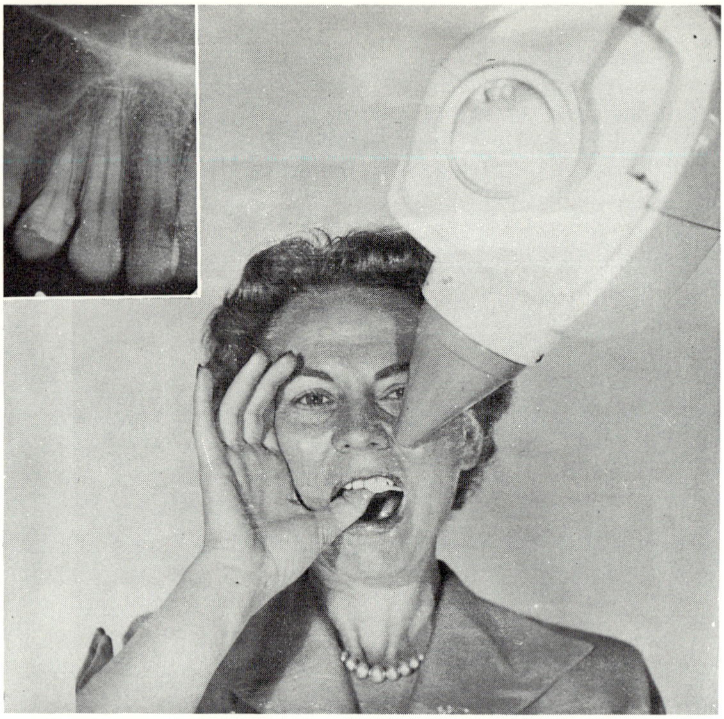

Fig. 12-12. Maxillary canine periapical technique and film. (From Peterson, S., editor: Clinical dental hygiene, ed. 3, St. Louis, 1968, The C. V. Mosby Co.)

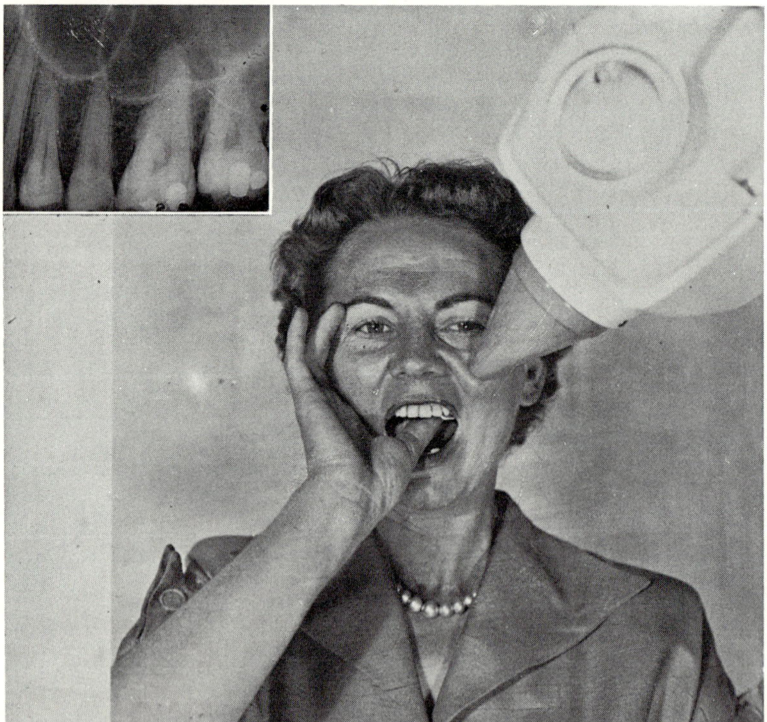

Fig. 12-13. Maxillary premolar periapical technique and film. (From Peterson, S., editor: Clinical dental hygiene, ed. 3, St. Louis, 1968, The C. V. Mosby Co.)

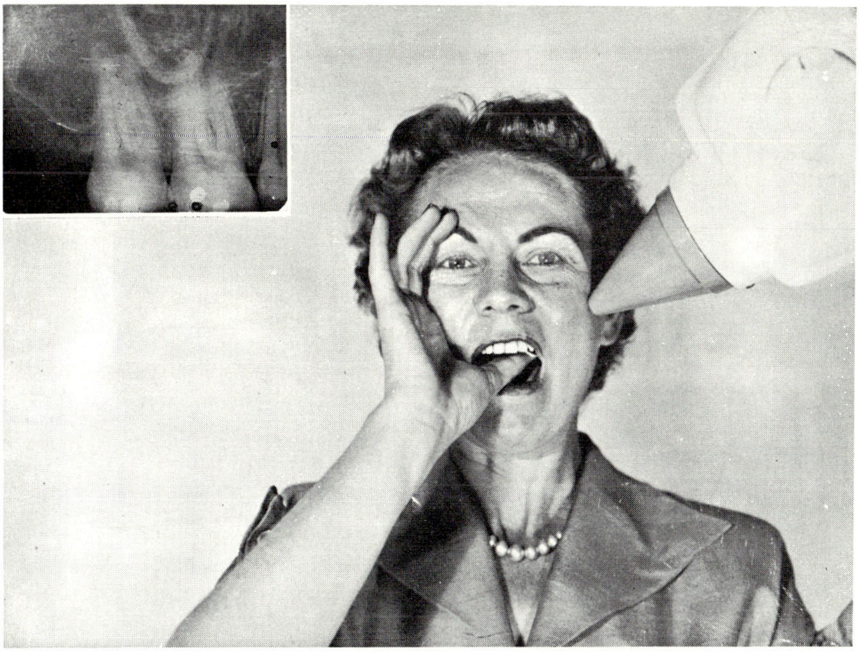

Fig. 12-14. Maxillary molar periapical technique and film. (From Peterson, S., editor: Clinical dental hygiene, ed. 3, St. Louis, 1968, The C. V. Mosby Co.)

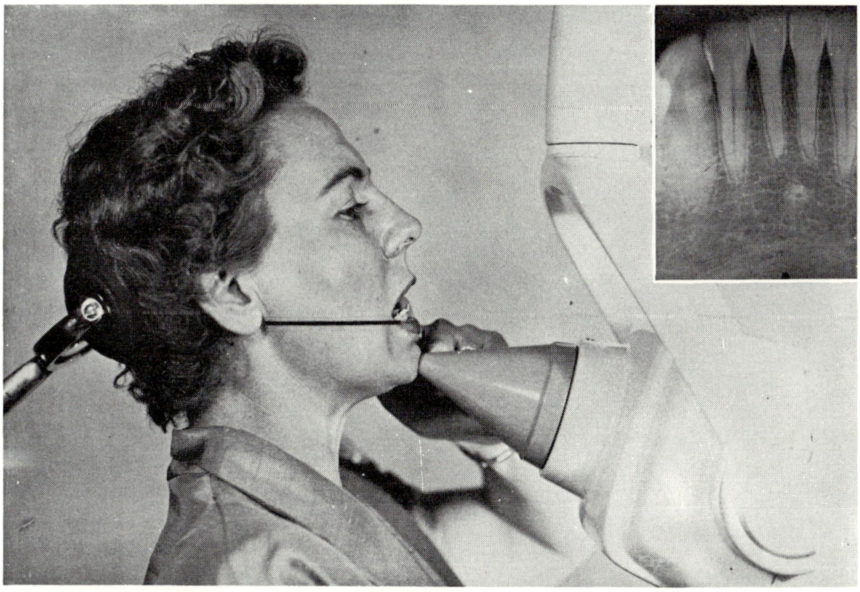

Fig. 12-15. Mandibular incisor periapical technique and film. Note that the occlusal plane of the lower teeth is parallel with the floor. (From Peterson, S., editor: Clinical dental hygiene, ed. 3, St. Louis, 1968, The C. V. Mosby Co.)

than ⅛ inch of the packet should extend below the cusps of the teeth.

Maxillary molar film

Place the packet flat against the occlusal surfaces of the premolars and canine, with the lateral edge of the packet just beneath the median grooves of the premolars. (This step is the same as for placing the premolar film.) Slide the packet posteriorly, until the front edge is just beneath the mesial surface of the first molar. Rotate the packet upward, until the upper edge rests against the palate; the lower portion will rest against the lingual cusps of the molars. Not more than ⅛ inch of the packet should extend below the occlusal surfaces of the molars.

Mandibular incisor film

Adapt the packet over the index finger so that it has a U shape when viewed from the end of the packet. Grasp the packet so that the U shape is maintained. Place the lower edge of the packet in the floor of the mouth against the frenum of the tongue; allow the upper edge to rest against the lingual surfaces of the incisors. The upper ¼ inch of the packet should extend above the incisal edges of the teeth. The packet should be centered in the midline.

Mandibular canine film

Prepare and grasp the packet as directed for the preceding mandibular incisor film. Place the lower edge of the packet in the floor of the mouth, against the frenum of the tongue. The packet should be centered on the canine and rest against the lingual surfaces of the teeth. Adjust the height so that ¼ inch extends above the incisal edges of the incisors and canine. (The portion adjacent to the premolars will extend more than ¼ inch above these teeth, but this is acceptable.)

Mandibular premolar film

Roll the lower anterior corner of the packet around the index finger so that when it is placed in the mouth, it will curve gently toward the midline. Place the lower edge of the packet into the floor of the mouth, between the side of the tongue and the lingual surfaces of the teeth. The anterior edge of the packet should be adjacent to the mesial surface of the canine. Tilt the lower edge of the packet toward the center of the mouth, and slide it gently downward, until only ⅛ inch extends above the teeth.

Mandibular molar film

Place the lower edge of the packet into the floor of the mouth in the premolar–first molar region. Gently slide the packet posteriorly and downward, until the front edge is even with the mesial surface of the first molar and only ⅛ inch of the pack extends above the teeth.

Posterior bite-wing film

The lower anterior corner of the packet should be rolled around the index finger so that when it is placed in the mouth, it will curve gently toward the midline. Grasp the tab with the thumb and index finger. Place the lower half of the packet down between the tongue and the lingual surfaces of the posterior teeth. The front edge of the packet should be adjacent to the middle of the canine crown. Hold the tab firmly against the occlusal surfaces of the teeth, using one index finger; use the other index finger to tilt the upper portion of the packet toward the midline. Instruct the patient to close slowly on his back teeth. When the upper teeth touch the finger holding the tab, rotate the finger outward and downward so that the tab is now held against the buccal surfaces of the teeth. As the patient continues to close the mouth, keep the upper portion of the packet tilted toward the midline, until the teeth touch the finger. Then remove the finger, and have the patient continue to close until he is biting firmly on the tab. The index finger holding the tab may then be removed.

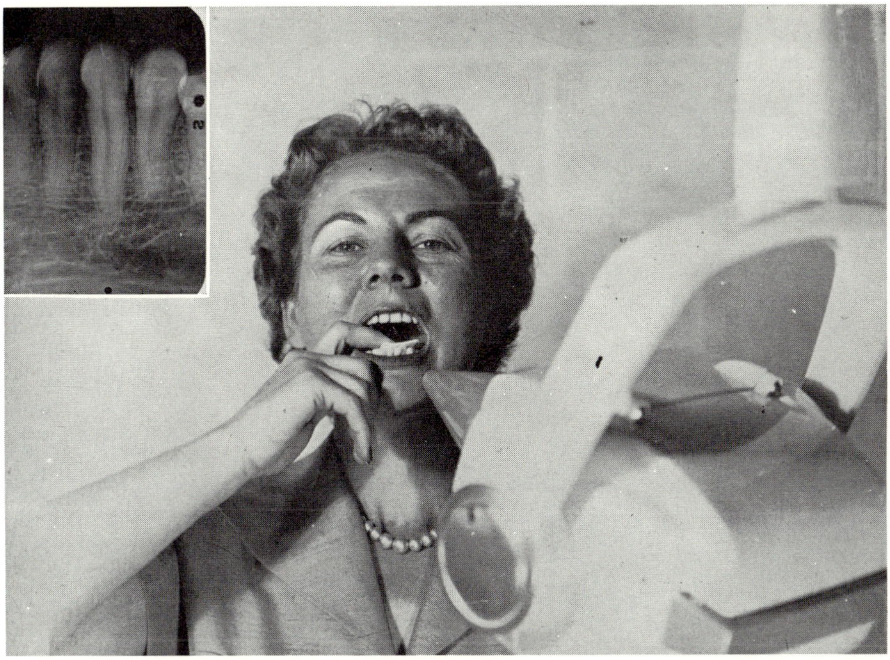

Fig. 12-16. Mandibular canine periapical technique and film. (From Peterson, S., editor: Clinical dental hygiene, ed. 3, St. Louis, 1968, The C. V. Mosby Co.)

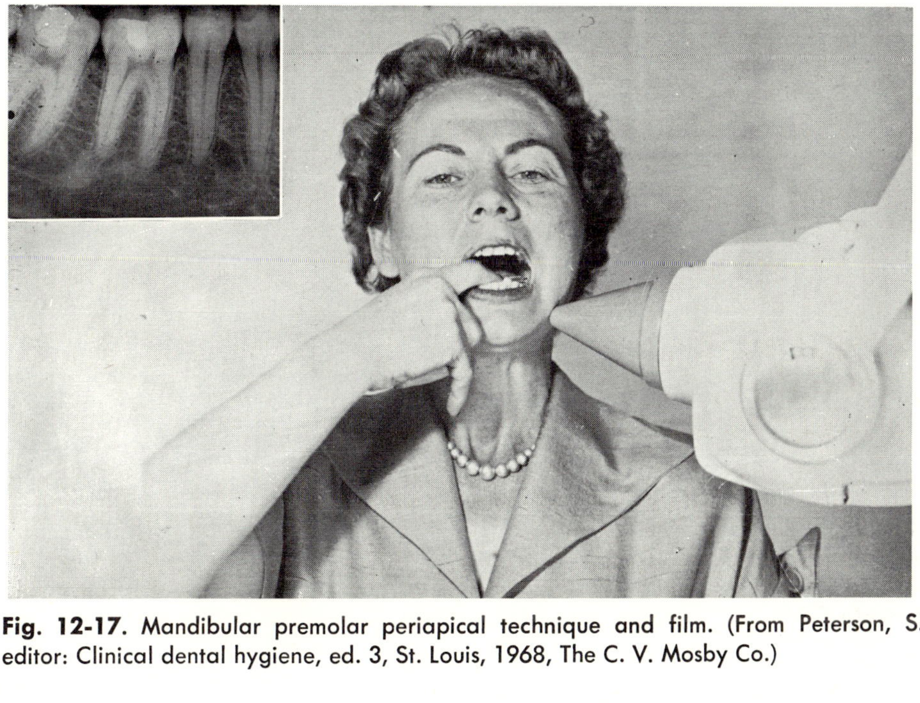

Fig. 12-17. Mandibular premolar periapical technique and film. (From Peterson, S., editor: Clinical dental hygiene, ed. 3, St. Louis, 1968, The C. V. Mosby Co.)

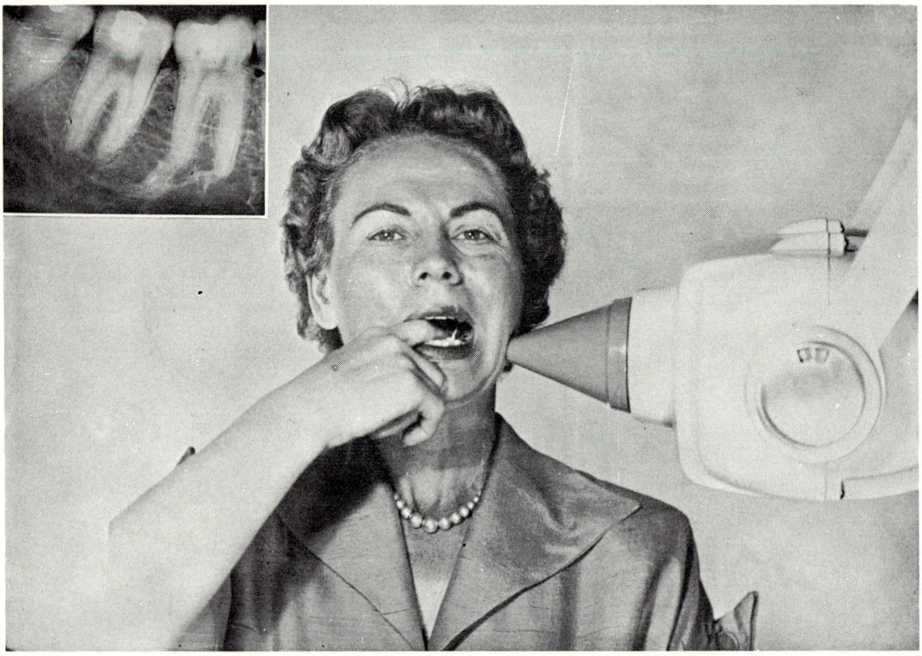

Fig. 12-18. Mandibular molar periapical technique and film. (From Peterson, S., editor: Clinical dental hygiene, ed. 3, St. Louis, 1968, The C. V. Mosby Co.)

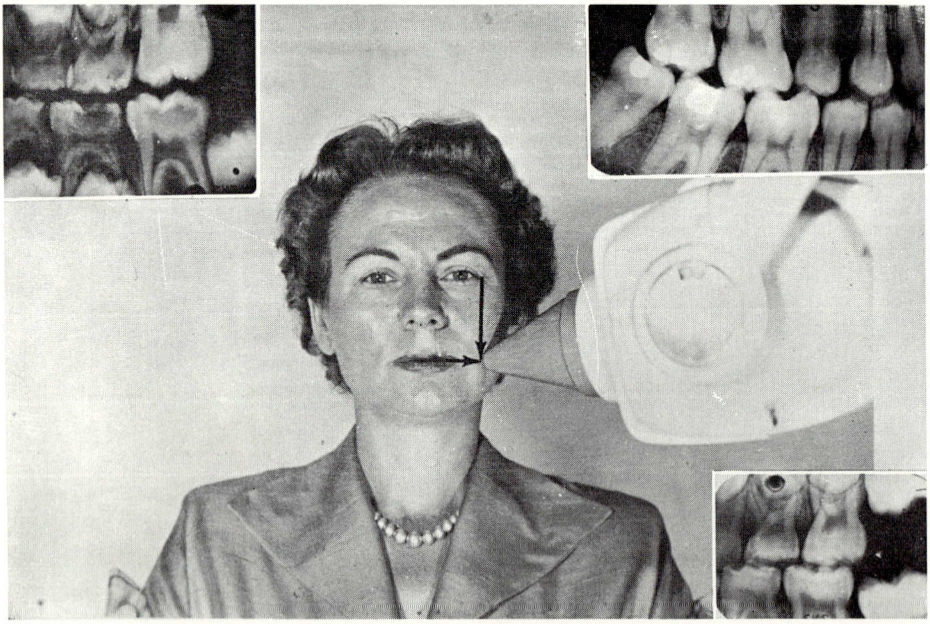

Fig. 12-19. Bite-wing technique. **Inset upper right,** adult (Type 3) bite-wing film; **inset upper left,** child (Type 2) bite-wing film; **inset lower right,** child (Type 0) bite-wing film. (From Peterson, S., editor: Clinical dental hygiene, ed. 3, St. Louis, 1968, The C. V. Mosby Co.)

Retention of films

Maxillary periapical films are retained by placing the patient's thumb to hold the packet against the crowns of the teeth. For the incisor film, either thumb may be used. For other films, the thumb from the opposite side is used. If the film is in the right premolar region, for example, the left thumb is used to retain it. The side of the retaining hand should be placed against the side of the patient's face for added stability. Mandibular periapical films are retained by placing the patient's index finger to hold the packet against the crowns of the teeth. Either index finger may be used for the incisor film. For other films, the finger from the opposite side is used. The remaining 3 fingers should be folded against the palm of the hand. The thumb of the retaining hand should be placed beneath the lower border of the mandible for added stability. For the incisor film, the elbow of the retaining hand should be raised so that it is level with the shoulder.

In all cases, the operator should guide the patient's retaining finger or thumb to the proper position. Verbal directions should be avoided, because the patient cannot see into his own mouth and, therefore, has difficulty in carrying out verbal instructions.

Checking patient's head position

Frequently, when the film packet is being placed or retained, the patient's head will move and, therefore, will not be in the correct position. When this occurs, it is necessary to readjust the head to the correct position, as previously described, before proceeding to the next step.

Vertical angulation

Vertical angulation refers to the up-and-down tilting of the cone of the x-ray tubehead. When the cone is parallel with the floor, the vertical angulation is said to be 0 degrees. When the cone is directed downward, there is "positive angulation"; conversely, the angulation is "negative" when the cone is directed upward. A scale on the side of the tubehead, calibrated in degrees as a circle, may be used to adjust the vertical angulation accurately to the desired figure.

From the preceding description of film placement, it can be seen that in all areas of the mouth (except the mandibular molar area), the film packet and the crowns of the teeth meet to form an angle. It is necessary that the vertical angulation of the x-ray tubehead be adjusted so that the image of the tooth on the radiograph is the same length as the tooth itself. If the vertical angulation is insufficient, the tooth image on the radiograph will show elongation; if the vertical angulation is excessive, the tooth image will be foreshortened. Correct vertical angulation is achieved by using the so-called bisecting principle, or Cieszynski's rule, of isometry.

The bisecting principle is based on the geometric theorum that states that 2 triangles having 2 equal angles and a common side are equal triangles. This principle is utilized in vertical angulation as follows. The angle formed by the tooth and film is bisected. The bisection creates 2 equal angles. The central ray of the x-ray beam is directed through the ape of the tooth, perpendicular to the bisecting plane. This creates 2 right angles, which are equal. The bisecting plane is a common side for both triangles. Thus, we have fulfilled the requirements of the theorum and have 2 equal triangles. Therefore, the length of the tooth and the length of the image on the film are also equal.

The bisecting principle must be thoroughly understood and applied for best results in taking intraoral radiographs. Obviously, the angle formed by the teeth and film will vary from one film area to another and from one patient to another, and the vertical angulation will vary from one patient to another. From the beginning, the operator should try to visualize the correct

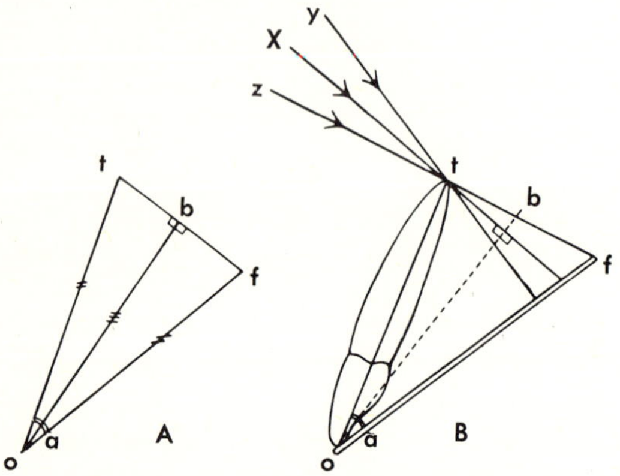

Fig. 12-20. A, Bisecting principle. Angle **a** is bisected by line **ob;** line **tf** is perpendicular to **ob;** therefore, triangle **tob** equals triangle **fob,** since each has right angles at **b,** equal angles at **a,** and a common side, **ob.** Thus, **to** equals **fo. B,** Cieszynski's law of isometry. Angle between tooth, **to,** and film, **fo,** or angle **a** is visually bisected by line **ob.** Central ray, **X,** is directed perpendicular to the bisection, **ob.** Thus, 2 equal triangles are formed, as in **A,** and side **to** (length of tooth) of **tob** equals side **fo** (length of image) of **fob.** (From Peterson, S., editor: Clinical dental hygiene, ed. 3, St. Louis, 1968, The C. V. Mosby Co.)

vertical angulation for each film of an examination.

Frequently, the inexperienced operator may have some difficulty in establishing the correct vertical angulation because of difficulty in visualizing the proper application of the bisecting principle. Therefore, a knowledge of "average" vertical angulations, which will produce acceptable results in most patients, is helpful for the beginning operator. Average vertical angulation values, suitable for this purpose, are given in Table 4.

Table 4. Average vertical angulation

Film	Average vertical angulation in degrees
Maxillary incisor periapical	+50
Maxillary canine periapical	+50
Maxillary premolar periapical	+40
Maxillary molar periapical	+30
Mandibular incisor periapical	−25
Mandibular canine periapical	−25
Mandibular premolar periapical	−10
Mandibular molar periapical	0
Posterior bite-wing	+10

Horizontal angulation

Horizontal angulation refers to the lateral positioning of the x-ray tubehead. Correct horizontal angulation is necessary to avoid overlapping images of tooth crowns and to produce distinct root images. As a general rule, the x-ray beam should be directed perpendicular to the labial or buccal surfaces of the teeth being examined. In the central incisor region, for example, the x-ray tubehead is placed directly in front of the patient, so that the x-ray beam is perpendicular to the labial surfaces of the incisors.

The correct horizontal angulation is easily visualized when the mandibular regions are examined. It is somewhat more difficult, however, to visualize the correct horizontal angulation for the maxillary regions. Therefore, it is helpful for the inexperienced operator to learn the average horizontal angulations that are given for these regions (Fig. 12-21).

Point of entry

"Point of entry" is the term used to indicate the spot where the center of the x-ray beam should strike the patient's face. The term "central ray" refers to the center of the x-ray beam. If the point of entry is not correct, a portion of the film may not be exposed by the x-rays. When such a film is processed, it will show a clear area where it was not exposed. "Cone-cutting" is the term used to describe a radiograph that shows such an unexposed portion.

As a general rule for periapical films, the central ray should be directed through the root apex of the tooth nearest the center of the film, in accordance with the bisecting principle. The following specific points of

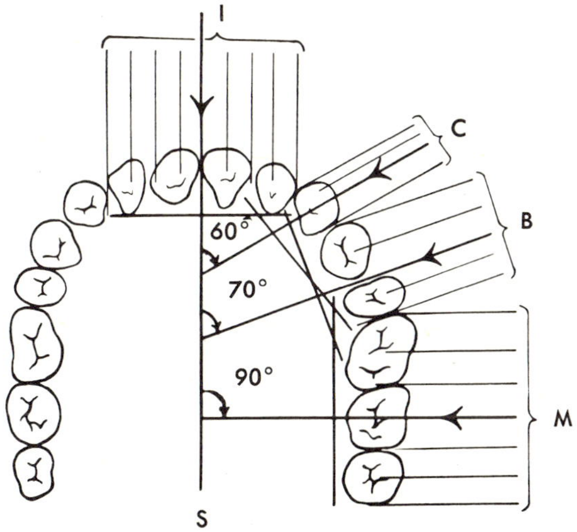

Fig. 12-21. Horizontal tube movement around the head. For each film the central ray must be perpendicular to the mean tangent of the teeth under examination. **S,** Midsagittal plane; **M,** horizontal rays for molar film; **B,** horizontal rays for premolar film; **C,** horizontal rays for cuspid film; **I,** horizontal rays for incisor film. (From Peterson, S., editor: Clinical dental hygiene, ed. 3, St. Louis, 1968, The C. V. Mosby Co.)

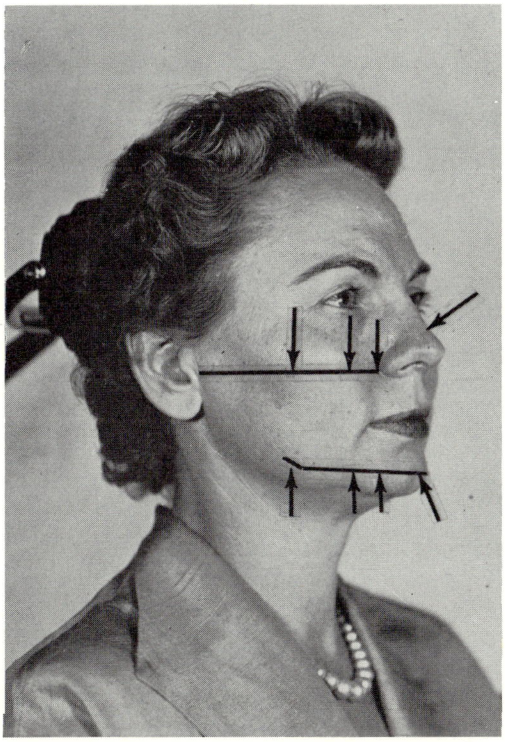

Fig. 12-22. Points of entry for periapical films. (From Peterson, S., editor: Clinical dental hygiene, ed. 3, St. Louis, 1968, The C. V. Mosby Co.)

entry are used for periapical films (Fig. 12-22).

Maxillary incisor. The central ray is directed through the lower one-third of the nose; it passes through the midline at the level of the root apices of the central incisors.

Maxillary canine. The central ray is directed to a point ¼ inch from the ala of the nose, on the ala-tragus line; it passes through the root apex of the canine.

Maxillary premolar. The central ray is directed to a point ¾ inch from the ala of the nose, on the ala-tragus line; it passes through the root apex of the second premolar.

Maxillary molar. The central ray is directed to a point on the ala-tragus line directly beneath the outer rim of the orbit of the eye; it passes through the root apex of the second molar.

Mandibular incisor. The central ray is directed through the midline of the chin and about ½ inch above the lower border of the mandible; it passes through the midline at the level of the root apices of the central incisors.

Mandibular canine. The central ray is directed through the canine region and about ½ inch above the lower border of the mandible; it passes through the root apex of the canine.

Mandibular premolar. The central ray is directed through the second premolar region and about ½ inch above the lower border of the mandible; it passes through the root apex of the second premolar.

Mandibular molar. The central ray is directed through the second molar region and about ½ inch above the lower border of the mandible; it passes through the root apex of the second molar.

Bite-wing film. The central ray is directed through the cheek at a point about 1 inch posterior to the corner of the mouth (Fig. 12-19); it passes through the occlusal plane of the first molar region.

Setting timer and making exposure

The timer must be set to deliver the correct exposure for a given film. Also, be sure that the kilovoltage and milliamperage settings are correct. The exposure switch must be firmly pressed and held until the exposure is terminated by the timer.

FILM PROCESSING

When roentgen rays strike the light-sensitive emulsion of the film, a latent image is formed. Only when the film is immersed in certain chemicals does the image appear. The procedure by which a permanent image of the teeth is produced on film is known as film processing. It is accomplished in a darkroom (Fig. 12-23) and consists of developing, rinsing, fixing, washing, and drying.

The requirements of a dental darkroom are as follows:

1. It must be dark. The reader may consider this a facetious statement, but in many so-called darkrooms, light is allowed to lead around the doors and windows, and films are consistently fogged.

2. The safelight must be a *safe light.* A 10-watt bulb in a safelight with a 6B Wratten filter is suitable for all x-ray films. However, other filters that provide increased illumination can now be used with most intraoral films. The package of film usually contains instructions concerning the permissible safelight for the film. The safelight is normally placed 4 feet above the loading bench.

3. The darkroom must be clean. Whenever a drop of solution is spilled, it must be wiped up with a clean cloth soaked in clear water.

4. There must be sufficient enamelware or plastic utensils for measuring ingredi-

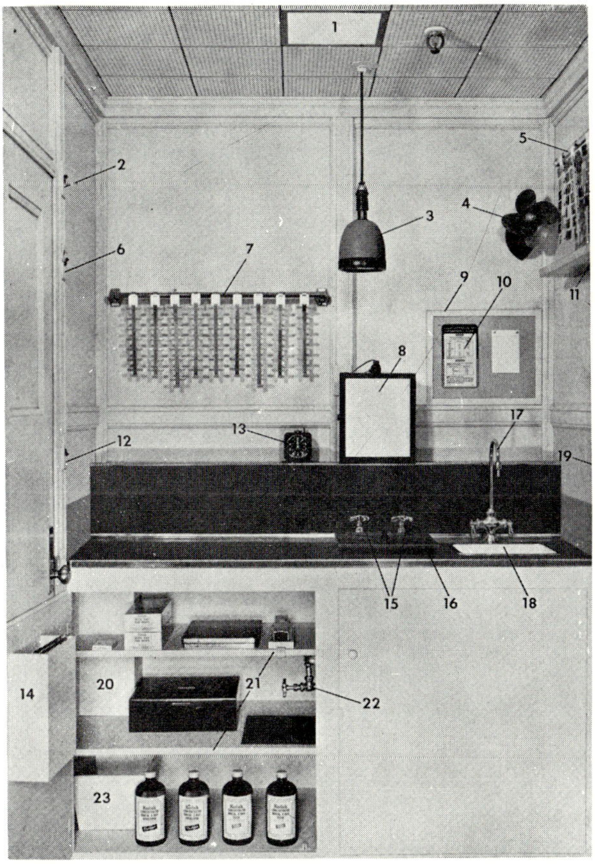

Fig. 12-23. Model x-ray darkroom. (From X-rays in dentistry, Rochester, New York, Eastman Kodak Co.)

ents. A thermometer and a timing clock are other essential items of equipment for the darkroom.

The processing of films involves the following steps:

1. The film packets must be unwrapped carefully, so that fingernail marks are not imprinted.

2. The films must be carefully clipped to the film hanger. The tanks must not be so crowded that films touch each other.

3. The hanger is placed in the developer for 5 minutes at 68 degrees F. At higher temperatures, the films will be dark; below 68 degrees F., they will be light.

4. The films are rinsed in running water.

5. The films are immersed in the hypo (fixer) for 5 minutes.

6. The films are washed in running water for 20 minutes or in still water for 40 minutes.

7. The films are dried in a lint-free, warm, dry space.

The dental assistant is obligated to assume the double responsibility of professional competence and spotless housekeeping; this applies to her darkroom procedures as well as to her work at the chair. Have you ever "snapped" a roll of film and anxiously awaited the moment when you could see the pictures? And have you ever been disappointed because that one big snapshot did not turn out as you had hoped? To the dentist, every x-ray film that he takes is a big one. For him, it may mean the way he diagnoses and treats a case, and for his patient, it means time and money. Therefore, the assistant must be just as careful in every step of her procedures as the dentist is in every step of his examination, diagnosis, and treatment procedures.

Darkroom procedure, care, and operation

The foregoing procedures are a rough outline of film-processing steps. Since the quality of each film delivered to the dentist will largely rest in the assistant's hands, the information that follows can be of the utmost importance.

Processing solutions

Solutions for processing dental x-ray films may be procured in 2 forms: (1) liquid concentrate and (2) mix-it-yourself powder. The liquid concentrate is quicker to prepare, lasts a shorter time, and is more expensive. The powdered chemicals require a few more minutes for preparation, but they last longer and cost less.

Tanks

The tanks into which the processing chemicals are placed must be spotlessly clean. As a rule, 3 complete rinsings with water plus vigorous brushing with a mild soap, followed by ample rinsing, will clean a developer tank. If deposits accumulate on the tank walls, the following cleaning solution should be used:

Commercial hydrochloric acid—1.5 oz.
Cold water—16.0 oz.
Lukewarm water to make 1.0 gallon

This formula is for a 1-gallon tank. First, the old developer is drained, and the walls of the tank are wiped with clear water. The cleaning solution is mixed in the tank and allowed to soak for 30 minutes. Then the tank is drained and rinsed thoroughly with fresh water. Addition of tablets to control algae is also recommended.

The proper level of solutions should be constantly maintained by replenishing each morning, but the tanks should be drained, cleaned, and refilled every 3 weeks.

Time and temperature

The processing of an x-ray film is a chemical reaction, and all chemical reactions require the proper and precise ingredients reacting at a critical temperature and for a critical length of time. Since the manufacturers of chemicals dispense the ingredients in correct proportions, the dental assistant's chief concern is time and temperature. The latter can generally be controlled easily in the winter, but it may be a problem in the summer. One should never add ice directly to a solution, for ice will obviously dilute and weaken the solution. One way to rapidly lower the temperature of a solution is to put ice in a rubber glove, tie the glove at the wrist, and float the glove on the surface of the solution. The recommended temperature is 68 degrees F. (20 degrees C.), and the optimum time (usually 5 minutes) is printed on each given container.

Washing

The washing of a film is also a chemical process. The gelatin of the emulsion has soaked up a great quantity of processing chemicals. Unless washed in running water for 20 minutes, sufficient chemicals will remain to form a brown stain at a later time and ruin the film.

Wetting agents

Wetting agents reduce the surface tension on the film. That is, if oils from the fingers should contact the surface of the film, the wetting agent will remove them, so that the processing chemicals will contact the film evenly. A capful of wetting agent added to the developer will assure even development of the film. When added to the rinse water, the wetting agent will produce swift and clear washing. By adding the wetting agent to a bucket of still rinse water after the 20 minute running water wash, it is possible to save half of the usual drying time.

Cutting reducers

Occasionally, a film will come out slightly dark, as a result of overexposure to roentgen rays or overdevelopment. In these cases, Farmer's Reducer may be employed to advantage. This compound is a silver solvent that removes silver deposits from the film, layer by layer. Dark areas of the film will become lighter, but so will light areas; great care must be exercised so that light areas will not be completely removed from the film. The two solutions used in Farmer's Reducer rapidly deteriorate when combined; thus, only the needed quantity should be mixed at a time. Farmer's Reducer is prepared as follows. One oz. potassium ferricyanide is dissolved in 16 oz. water (solution A); one oz. hypo crystals is dissolved in 16 oz. water (solution B); and equal parts of solutions A and B are mixed. The water-soaked film is dipped in the combination for a few seconds, rinsed in running water, examined, and rinsed again if necessary, until the desired density is achieved. The film is then washed in running water for 20 minutes and dried. The room need not be dark for this procedure.

Faulty roentgenograms

Shadows on x-ray films that were not cast by the body tissues are called "artifacts." They may best be described as mistakes in the technical chain of events. Some of the more common artifacts are as follows:

1. Reticulation ("fish-net" or "orange-peel" crinkled lines)
   Cause: Wash water too warm, causing shrinking and cracking of gelatin emulsion
   Remedy: Have wash water the same temperature as processing solutions
2. "Blotchy," fogged, dull film
   Cause: Outdated film
   Remedy: Carefully check expiration date of each batch of film
3. Dark splash marks
   Cause: Film splashed with developing solution before being immersed in developer, causing overdevelopment in splashed areas
   Remedy: Care and good housekeeping in darkroom
4. Light splash marks
   Cause: Film splashed with hypo before being immersed in developer, silver bromide salts dissolved in these areas so that no silver deposits remain
   Remedy: Care and good housekeeping in darkroom
5. Splash marks, same density as rest of film, circular hairline outline
   Cause: Processed, dried film splashed by water
   Remedy: Rewash in running water for 20 minutes
6. White spots on film
   Cause: Granules of chemical powder on film when it is placed in developer or dust particles on film
   Remedy: Absolute cleanliness in darkroom; use of wetting agent in developer
7. Black lines, straight
   Cause: Bending of film packet
   Remedy: Never bend the packet during film placement
8. Black marks, elliptical
   Cause: Pressing fingernail against packet when opening
   Remedy: Strip off back of packet without pressure from fingernails
9. Outline of another film, light
   Cause: Contact with another film in developing tank; pressure of contacting films prevents development in that area
   Remedy: Do not overcrowd films in tank
10. Light, bizarre-shaped spots
    Cause: Dust, lead slivers in plastic pointer cone
    Remedy: Periodically unscrew cone and clean it out
11. Partial image, arc-like cut across film
    Cause: "Cone-cutting," failure of x-ray beam to cover entire film
    Remedy: Refine technique in film placement and check point of entry
12. Stretched, blurred image
    Cause: Bending of film packet

Remedy: In film placement, never bend packet

13. Thin (light) image
    Cause: Too little exposure to roentgen rays, cold developing solution, too little time in the developer, film packet placed into mouth backward (with lead foil side toward tube), failure to stir developer before placing film in solution
14. Dense (dark) image
    Cause: Overexposure to roentgen rays, prolonged development, or developer too warm
15. Fogging
    Cause: Unsafe storage of film before and/or after exposure at chair; outdated film, lack of filtration (with aluminum filter) of useful beam, diaphragm opening for useful beam too large, light leak in darkroom, or unsafe safelight in darkroom

Suggested readings

Ennis, L. M., and Berry, H. M., Jr.: Dental roentgenology, ed. 6, Philadelphia, 1967, Lea & Febiger.

Fitzgerald, G. M.: Dental roentgenology. I. An investigation in adumbration, or the factors that control unsharpness, J.A.D.A. **34**:1-20, 1947.

Fitzgerald, G. M.: Dental roentgenology. II. Vertical angulation, film placement, and increased object-film distance, J.A.D.A. **34**:161-170, 1947.

Fitzgerald, G. M.: Dental roentgenology. III. The roentgenographic periapical survey of the upper molar region, J.A.D.A. **38**:293-303, 1949.

McCormack, F. W.: A plea for a standardized technique for oral roentgenography, with an illustrated classification of findings and their verified interpretations, J. Dent. Res. **2**:467, 1920.

McCormack, D. W.: Dental roentgenology; a technical procedure for furthering the advancement toward anatomical accuracy, J. California Dent. Ass. **13**:89, 1937.

McCormack, D. W.: Mechanical aids for obtaining accuracy in dental roentgenology, J.A.D.A. **40**:144-153, 1950.

National Council on Radiation Protection Report No. 35, Dental x-ray protection, Washington, D. C., 1970, National Council on Radiation Protection and Measurements.

National Research Council: The biologic effects of atomic radiation; a report to the public, Washington, D. C., 1960, National Academy of Sciences.

Peterson, S., editor: Clinical dental hygiene, ed. 3, St. Louis, 1968, The C. V. Mosby Co.

Radiation protection, regulation 433, Harrisburg, Pa., 1956, Commonwealth of Pennsylvania.

Richards, A. G.: Roentgen-ray doses in dental roentgenography, J.A.D.A. **56**:351-368, 1958.

Richards, A. G., and others: Report of committee on radiation protection of the American Academy of Oral Roentgenology, J.A.D.A. **56**:514-521, 1958.

Silha, R. E.: Paralleling long cone technic, Dent. Radiogr. Photogr. **41**:3-19, 1968.

Spear, L. B., and Hannah, R.: Practical and improved periapical technic, Dent. Radiogr. Photogr. **26**:21-25, 1953.

Waggener, D. T.: The principles of the long tube technique, J. Nebraska Dent. Ass. **24**:3, 1947.

Wuehrmann, A. H., and Manson-Hing, L. R.: Dental radiology, ed. 2, St. Louis, 1969, The C. V. Mosby Co.

CHAPTER 13 PREVENTIVE DENTISTRY

RICHARD E. JENNINGS, D.D.S., M.S.D.

The obligation of the dental profession to the citizens of the United States is to maintain, in as realistic a manner as possible, an adequate state of dental health. Since the dental assistant is a recognized member of the dental profession, the objective of this chapter on preventive dentistry is to aid in an understanding of prevention, how it can be applied in a modern dental practice, and, in particular, how the dental assistant can most efficiently fulfill her role in a preventive dental practice.

Fundamentally, there are 2 ways to cope with any medical or dental disease or health problem, treat it or prevent it. The bulk of dental education, and consequently of dental practice, has been traditionally oriented toward treating the damage resulting from disease, with too little emphasis upon efforts to prevent dental diseases from occurring. In a 1960 survey by the National Opinion Research Center of the University of Chicago, the majority of 757 dentists interviewed did not apply topical fluoride solutions to their patient's teeth, did not use a patient recall system, and used no salivary tests to determine susceptibility to dental caries. The Survey of Dentistry,* impressed by the potentially overwhelming magnitude of dental disease in the United States, estimated in 1960 that the people in the United States had accumulated at least 700,000,000 unfilled cavities. One out of every 10 5-year-old children had 8 or more cavities. Advanced periodontal disease affected half of the population by the age of 50, and almost everyone by age sixty-five. It would be totally impossible today to correct all damage that has been produced by dental disease in the United States. It is doubtful that dental manpower can ever cope with the disease, if the sole emphasis is placed upon a reparative or restorative program. The continued increasing emphasis on the prevention of these dental diseases offers hope for a future time, when the amount of damage to the mouths of our patients will be reduced to a practical level. The dental assistant can and must play a major role in a dental practice oriented toward preventive dentistry.

In essence, all procedures performed in a dental office are oriented toward prevention. The placement of a restoration in a tooth is preventive as well as reparative, in that it is performed *to prevent* further damage to that tooth. A pulpally involved tooth is treated endodontically *to prevent* the subsequent development of periapical infection and loss of the tooth. The prosthetic replacement of a missing tooth is *to prevent*

*American Council on Education Commission on the Survey of Dentistry in The United States, The Survey of Dentistry: The Final Report, Washington, 1961, American Council on Education.

harmful and disease-producing drifting of teeth adjacent to the edentulous area. The removal of all the teeth in a patient with severe, untreatable periodontal disease is *to prevent* potential harm to his health by orally initiated systemic infection; the placement of complete dentures is *to prevent* any serious effects occurring functionally, nutritionally, or emotionally, due to the lack of teeth.

The utilization of preventive principles in a dental practice can be arbitrarily divided into 3 distinct phases—primary, secondary, and tertiary. Primary prevention refers to those procedures that are applied prior to the inception of a disease. It could perhaps be more aptly called "prepathogenic prevention." The goal of secondary prevention is to diagnose and stop a disease process in its early stages, so that damage and subsequent repair are minimized. Secondary prevention can be considered "pathogenic prevention." Tertiary prevention is the application of reparative (restorative) procedures in a sound way *to prevent* any damage from the restoration itself. Perhaps a label of "postpathogenic prevention" is suitable for this tertiary stage.

Fig. 13-1 illustrates this concept of prepathogenic, pathogenic, and postpathogenic stages of preventive dental treatment. It is interesting to note that following the arrestment of a disease process and the repair of its damage, the patient has completed this circle and returned to the "no disease" category. Prepathogenic (primary) prevention is now the major goal of treatment for this patient.

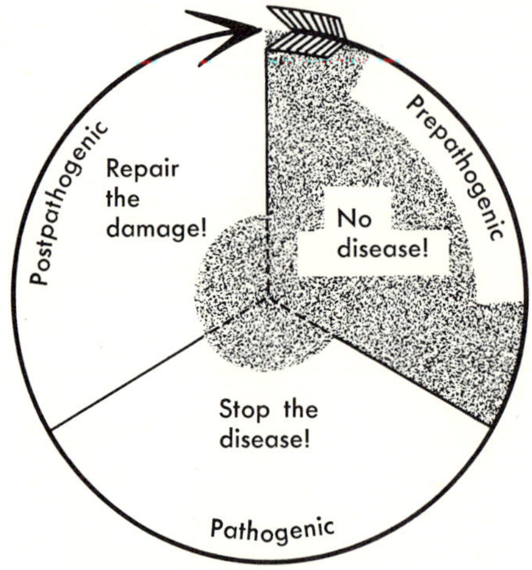

Fig. 13-1. Patient treatment.

PREPATHOGENIC PREVENTION

Promotion of dental health

Promotion of dental health should be an integral function of every dental office. It is the responsibility of the dental team to educate every patient in the importance of good oral health and the methods available to obtain and maintain it. The dental assistant has a unique opportunity in the dental office for patient education, since practicing dentists must utilize most of their office hours in delivering dental treatments. The dental assistant should be totally informed, so that she can give patients dental health information and answer specific questions relating to treatment procedures. Numerous articles supplying general information are available from such organizations as the American Dental Association and the American Society of Dentistry for Children. Dental health information must also be disseminated outside the dental office. National Children's Dental Health Week is a good example of a public information program that has been initiated by dentists (American Dental Association) and is promoted each year by all local dental organizations. During this period of time, many dental assistants and dentists are called upon to talk at schools or in other special programs. Sponsoring newspaper articles, supplying speakers to service clubs and PTA programs, and supporting science fair projects are also examples of dental health promotion at a community level.

Specific treatment procedures

Many specific treatment procedures for prepathogenic (primary) prevention are available today to aid in the prevention of dental disease. Some of those more commonly used will be discussed in the following sections.

Oral hygiene

It has been stated many times that tooth decay affects over 95 percent of the population of the United States, and that most people age 65 years and older suffer from advanced periodontal disease. These are recognized as rather startling statements, when one considers that both diseases are produced by microorganisms that live on the teeth, and that with thorough and complete oral hygiene procedures, it is possible to remove them. The problem, of course, rests not only with the ability or inability of the dental team to teach correct oral hygiene procedures to patients, but also with the necessity of motivating them to practice these procedures faithfully. Without motivation, teaching is of questionable value.

The microorganisms live on the surfaces of the teeth in almost invisible colonies known as dental plaque. Arnim describes dental plaque as an adherent colonized microbial mass consisting of motile and nonmotile bacteria, protozoa, leucocytes, desquamated epithelial cells all enveloped and permeated by a thick, viscous, serous exudate that helps hold these elements and their noxious end products in contact with the tooth and the gum.* These bacteria are capable of producing acids that will cause dental caries to occur on the tooth surface under the plaque and toxic poisons that damage the gingival tissue and tooth-supporting membranes, causing peridontal disease. Daily removal of this dental plaque by every patient will greatly reduce, if not eliminate, both of these diseases.

*Arnim, S. S.: Thoughts concerning cause, pathogenesis, treatment and prevention of periodontal disease, J. Periodont. **29**:217, July 1958, p. 217.

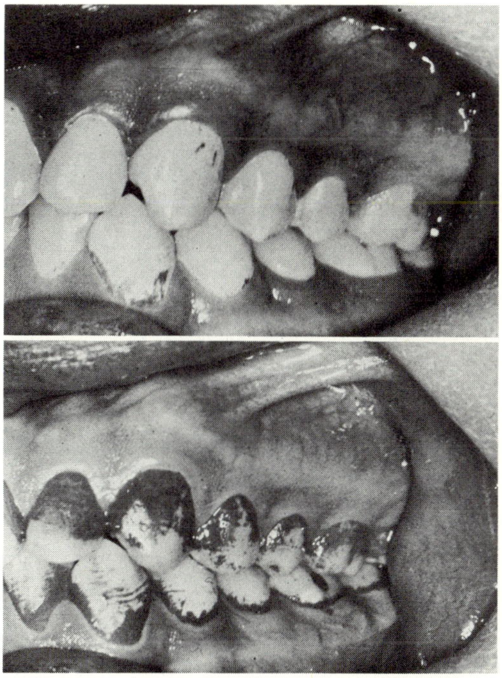

A

B

Fig. 13-2. A, Appearance of unstained teeth; **B,** dental plaque seen after being stained with disclosing wafer.

Disclosing wafers

One of the major difficulties in motivating a patient to follow correct oral hygiene procedures rests in his inability to see the dental plaque on his own teeth. Dentists and dental hygienists have for years applied chemical solutions (disclosing solutions) to a patient's teeth in the dental office to color the dental plaque and make it easy to see for removal during a dental prophylaxis. Only in recent years, however, have disclosing wafers been available for patients to use at home. One of the more popular is made with a red food dye (erythrosin, F.D.C. Red No. 3) and can be used by a patient to see the bacterial plaque prior to cleansing of the mouth. After cleaning the teeth, a new tablet should be used to check the thoroughness with which cleaning has been performed. Fig 13-2, *A* and *B* illustrates how dental plaque is more easily seen after it is stained.

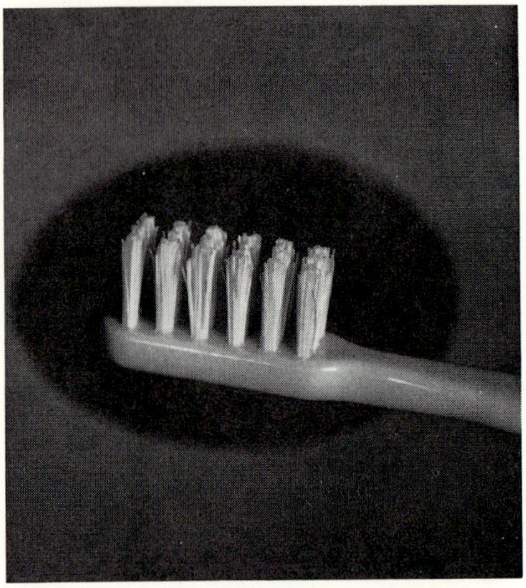

Fig. 13-3. Toothbrush with small head; bristles are trimmed in a straight line.

A 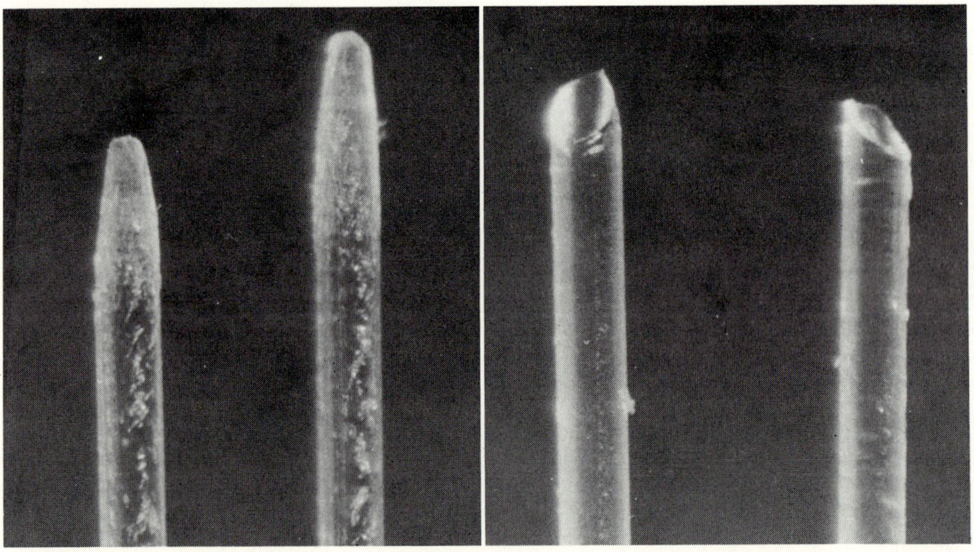 B

Fig. 13-4. Microscopic view of bristles of toothbrush. **A,** Good toothbrush has bristles that are round and smooth; **B,** poor toothbrush has jagged bristles that can injure gingival tissue.

Toothbrushing

Although minor details of a toothbrush may vary, it is generally agreed that it should have a straight handle approximately 6 inches long, with a small in-line head not over 1 inch long. The bristles should be trimmed in a straight line (Fig. 13-3), vary in stiffness from medium to soft, and have *round* and *smooth* ends (Fig. 13-4, *A*). Uneven and jagged bristles (Fig. 13-4, *B*) may scratch and injure the gingival tissue around the teeth, as dental plaque growing on the tooth next to the gingival tissue is removed.

A

B

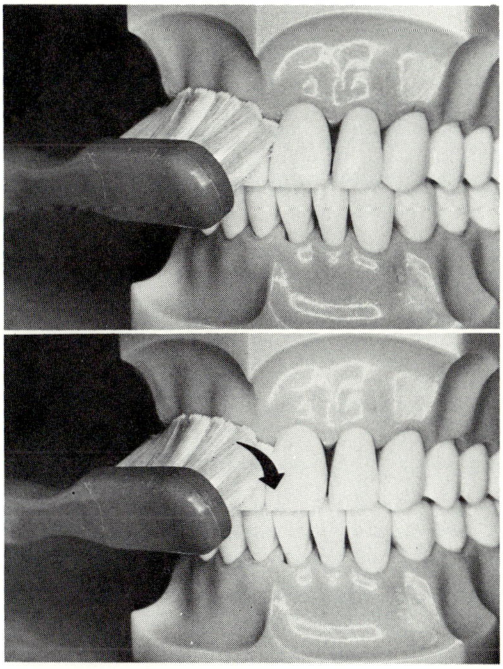

Fig. 13-5. Modified Bass technique for brushing teeth. **A,** For brushing facial and lingual surfaces, brush is placed at base of teeth at a 45-degree angle away from chewing surface of teeth; **B,** using firm pressure, brush is rotated with vibratory motion, so that bristles move toward occlusal surface of teeth.

Many techniques of adequate toothbrushing are described in the dental literature. Charles C. Bass, a physician-teacher at the Tulane University School of Medicine, New Orleans, designed and described a method of personal oral hygiene after years of research upon the causative factors of dental caries and periodontal disease. Bass's method of tooth cleansing utilizes a brush with polished and round-ended bristles, so that the ends of the bristles can be forced into the gingival crevice without damaging the soft tissue. He has also recommended the use of unwaxed dental floss, consisting of many fine nylon threads twisted together.

The following, modified Bass, technique, using a soft brush with round-ended bristles, is recommended. When brushing the facial and lingual surfaces, the brush is placed against the junction of the tooth and the gingival tissue at a 45-degree angle, away from the chewing surface of the tooth (Fig. 13-5, *A*). Using firm pressure, a vibratory motion is started, and the brush rotated, so that the vibrating bristles move toward the occlusal surface of the teeth (Fig. 13-5, *B*). This stroke should be repeated, until the tooth surface is clean. By using a disclosing wafer after brushing, one can determine how many strokes are necessary. The ends of the bristles will reach into the gingival sulcus and interproximal areas with this technique. All the facial and lingual surfaces of all the teeth are cleaned in this manner. The occlusal, or chewing, surfaces can be cleaned with a forward and backward stroke, permitting the ends of the bristles to more or less scrub these surfaces. Regardless of the particular technique taught in any office, as long as the prime objective of removing dental plaque without damaging the teeth or soft tissues is achieved, the method used should be satisfactory.

Electric toothbrushes

Electric toothbrushes are becoming more popular each day. It should be emphasized that they can clean the teeth as well as a manual brush, but offer no particular advantage to patients who develop a satisfactory hand brushing technique. However, for those individuals who do not have the capability for manual dexterity, such as a child with cerebral palsy, the electric brush has definite advantages. It may also appeal to people who are fascinated by gadgets and, in this way, serve as another motivational device.

Flossing

Even the most efficient toothbrushing technique fails to remove all dental plaque from adjacent surfaces of teeth, as it is physically impossible for the bristles to reach deep into these areas. For this reason,

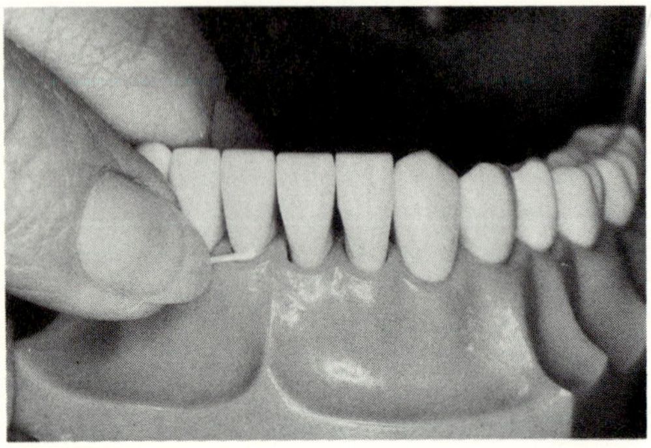

Fig. 13-6. Dental floss is passed gently between teeth and underneath edge of gingival tissue to ensure complete removal of plaque in inaccessible areas.

the use of dental floss is recommended to remove all dental plaque from the approximating sides of the teeth beneath the contacting area. The floss is passed gently between the teeth and underneath the edge of the gingival tissue (Fig. 13-6). While being held tightly against the proximal surface, it is pulled slowly toward the occlusal surface of the tooth. Both sides of every tooth should be cleaned with dental floss in this manner. Cleanliness and removal of plaque are readily evidenced by a squeaking sound, as the floss slides along the tooth surface.

It should be mentioned that the incorrect or careless use of dental floss may be harmful to the patient. It must be emphasized to patients that the floss should be placed carefully and not moved in labiolingual directions in a sawing fashion. The correct use is exacting and must be thoroughly taught to patients.

Mouthwashes and irrigators

Following the use of the toothbrush and dental floss, the mouth should be thoroughly rinsed to remove any loose dental plaque or food particles. A mouthful of tap water should be satisfactory for this purpose. In special cases, the dentist may wish to recommend one of the irrigators available today. In recent years, these devices have become increasingly popular, although the use of forced water irrigation to clean debris from subgingival spaces has been recommended for over 50 years. Irrigators may vary from simple hose and nozzle devices that fasten to a water faucet to relatively expensive electric pumps that pulsate water from a storage reservoir. All, however, have a small nozzle to permit the patient to direct the spray alongside and between the teeth to remove *loose* debris. Forced water irrigation is not usually suggested as a routine procedure for all patients, but it is valuable where mouthrinsing is not effective. Irrigation may help to rinse debris from under bridges, around fixed orthodontic appliances, or between the teeth of patients who have undergone periodontal surgery. Mouthwashes may be used for their pleasant taste, although they should be considered as mechanical cleansers only.

Dentrifices

Regardless of the many claims made in dentifrice advertising, these products must still be considered primarily an aid in the toothbrushing procedure. The toothbrush bristles actually do the cleaning. Patients generally find the pleasant taste to their liking, and dentifrices are presumed to be effective in helping the brush to remove stains and to keep the mouth clean and pleasant tasting.

The use of a toothbrush and water alone will remove stains from some individual's teeth. The addition of a mild abrasive, such as sodium bicarbonate, is more effective. Most of the dentifrices on the market today contain some sort of abrasive, and the product's ability to remove stain is thought to be related to the harshness of the abrasive used. The type of flavoring agent and detergent used will also affect the cleaning capability. For certain patients whose teeth are sensitive to hot and cold foods, a dentist may wish to recommend one of the desensitizing dentifrices that are available. For children and for adults whose teeth are susceptible to dental caries, most dentists will recommend one of the fluoride-containing dentifrices that have been approved by the American Dental Association.

Fluoride

Many years ago, dentists learned that people who drank water containing fluoride compounds had much less tooth decay than those drinking water that contained no fluoride. The United States Public Health Service studied many communities where the water did and did not contain this element and concluded that the presence of the fluoride ion reduced tooth decay by about 65 percent. Over 25 years ago, studies were undertaken in several large cities where fluoride was added to the drinking water. Control cities of approximately the same size and in the same area, where the water did not contain fluoride, were also studied, and the results were conclusive that tooth decay could be reduced 60 to 65 percent by adding 1 ppm. (part per million) fluoride to a community's water supply. Since that time, 4,834 communities, with over 80,000,000 residents, have taken advantage of this prevention method. Adding the 8,378,824 people who use drinking water with fluoride naturally present, a total of more than 88,000,000 people are now receiving this benefit. Twenty-three percent of the people in the United States live in areas without a central water supply.

Controlled fluoridation can be described as a conscious maintenance of the optimal concentration of fluoride in a water supply. This can be achieved by adding the chemicals to a water supply that is deficient in fluoride or by removing fluoride where the concentration is in excess of the optimal level. It is also possible to blend 2 different water supplies that contain natural fluoride to achieve the optimal concentration. The optimal concentration will vary from 0.7 ppm. to 1.2 ppm., depending upon the annual average of daily maximum air temperatures in the community.

The fluoride ion combines chemically with the forming tooth structures to produce a tooth that is more decay-resistant. Maximum benefits are received by the child who drinks this water throughout his tooth-forming years, but some benefits may occur even in adults (who did not drink fluoridated water as a child), from a topical effect of the water passing over the teeth. Community fluoridation programs have been described as "a classic example of a public health procedure since it serves the entire population, requires no conscious and sustained effort on the part of the individuals with the community and automatically restricts individual consumption of the fluoride supplement to levels which have been shown to be safe."*

Topical fluoride

Since not all people drink water from a central source, other ways have been sought to bring the benefits of fluoride to those people who have no central supply. In the late 1940's, the use of topically applied fluoride-containing solutions was investigated. Since that time, it has been generally believed that the topical application of a fluoride solution at regular 6- or 12-month intervals can reduce tooth decay by approximately 50 percent. The fluoride ion will form a loose chemical bond with the outer enamel layer, but over a period of time, the fluoride leaves the tooth. For this reason, it is recommended that the fluoride be reapplied at frequent intervals. Two fluoride solutions are commonly used today, and both require that the teeth be thoroughly cleaned just prior to application. The teeth are then isolated, dried, and kept free of saliva while the solution is painted on them.

---

*Muhler, J. C.: Current evaluation of fluoride therapy, J. Amer. Pharm. Ass. NS3:133, 1963, p. 133.

The 8-percent solution of stannous fluoride (SnF_2), applied for ½ minute, or a 2-percent solution of sodium fluoride buffered with phosphoric acid (A.P.F.), applied for a 4-minute period, seem to be equally effective. Shannon has recently reported a method using 2-percent stannous fluoride in a water-free prophylaxis paste for polishing the teeth, followed by use of a mouthrinse containing 0.5-percent stannous fluoride.* In laboratory tests, the solutions in this procedure seem to be as effective in combining fluoride with tooth enamel as the 2 previously mentioned, topically applied solutions. The addition of fluoride compounds to polishing pastes and the development of self-applied fluoride pastes or solutions for daily use at home offer much promise for the future. Even though a patient is drinking fluoridated water, it has been demonstrated that the use of regular topically applied fluoride is still beneficial.

Fluoride dentifrices

In the early 1960's, the Council on Dental Therapeutics of the American Dental Association granted approval to a toothpaste manufacturer to use the following statement in advertising: "Crest has been shown to be an effective decay-preventive dentifrice that can be of significant value when used in a conscientiously applied program of oral hygiene and regular professional care." The endorsement was granted after review of research data from clinical trials of the dentifrice. The results indicated that this dentifrice imparted anticariogenic benefits to the patients in these study groups. Since that time, the same approval has been granted to 4 other dentifrices.†

*Shannon, K. L., and others: Clinical application of stannous fluoride solutions in caries prevention and control of root sensitivity, J. S. Calif. State Dent. Ass. 33:520, 1965.

†Cue, Fact, Super Stripe, and Colgate with MFP.

Fluoride tablets

The prescribing of fluoride supplements has been suggested for children who live in an area where little or no fluoride is present in the drinking water. The suggested daily allowance for fluoride administration is 1 mg. For children under the age of three, half this dosage is suggested. However, the procedure for fluoride supplement administration is not quite as simple as prescribing 1 mg. each day.

The dentist must be positive that the drinking water contains little or no fluoride. If this information is not available from the local health department or the state board of health, a sample of drinking water must be collected for fluoride analysis. Most city and state health departments are prepared to assist the dentist in this procedure. If it is found that the water contains at least 0.7 ppm. of fluoride, supplemental fluoride is not recommended. If the drinking water contains from 0.2 to 0.6 ppm. fluoride, the amount administered must be adjusted accordingly to arrive at a maximum daily intake of 1 ppm. (Table 5).

Once a recommended daily level has been determined, the dentist must write a prescription. If the amount desired is exactly 1 mg. per day, any of the tablets that have been approved by the Council on Dental Therapeutics may be prescribed. However, if less than 1 mg. is desired, it is necessary to prescribe a liquid supplement. The parent is then instructed to administer

Table 5. Adjustment of fluoride administered based on fluoride content of drinking water (reduced to half for children ages 2 to 3)

Fluoride in drinking water	Adjusted allowance (fluoride mg. per day)
0.0	1.0
0.2	0.8
0.4	0.6
0.6	0.4
0.7	Not needed

a specified number of drops of the solution to reach the desired dosage level. It is usually recommended that the tablet be dissolved in a glass of water or fruit juice for administration to the child. If drops are used, they are added to water or juice also.

For children under 2 years of age, no recommended daily dose is suggested. A dentist may help the parent prepare water that contains fluoride at a concentration of 1 ppm. to use in making the formula or to use as the child's drinking water. Administration of dietary fluoride supplement must be consistent and continuous from birth until 12 to 14 years of age, if presumed benefits are to be realized. Very few clinical studies reporting the effectiveness of this method of fluoride administration are available.

Preparations containing sodium fluoride and vitamins in fixed combinations are *not* recommended by the Council on Dental Therapeutics. The effect of a fluoride-vitamin combination on dental caries has not been adequately studied. Also, any alteration in the amount of fluoride ingested to adjust the level to the intake of fluoride from natural sources would also produce an alteration in the vitamin intake. This is not believed to be a logical method of fluoride administration.

Caries susceptibility tests

Tests to determine the current state of caries susceptibility for a particular patient in an attempt to predict future incidence of dental caries have been used in dentistry for many years. Snyder's test is a colorimetric method for determining acids formed in a carbohydrate medium by oral microorganisms. It measures the quantity of oral microorganisms present in the patient's mouth that are capable of converting these foods to acids. Since the number of these microorganisms increases proportionate to the frequency of eating freely fermentable carbohydrates, the test becomes a valuable tool for monitoring a patient's diet.

Snyder's test as modified by Albans* is more practical for routine office use. The patient drools unstimulated saliva into a test tube containing Snyder's media. This test tube is then incubated at 37 degrees C. for 4 days, and daily observations are made. The depth of color change from blue-green to yellow, and the speed with which this change occurs reflect the ability of this saliva to produce acids. Other caries activity tests that have been suggested are the lactobacillus colony count, enamel solubility test, Wach test, and amylase test. Even though the degree of correlation of the results of these tests with the caries activity found in the patients' mouth is not always reliable, many dentists are finding the tests useful as a motivational tool in an office patient education program.

Dietary counseling

Dental health is greatly influenced by food habits, and it is a dental responsibility to counsel patients in this area. It is always good to encourage proper eating, even though there is no apparent deficiency that is causing either general or dental disease. Since new knowledge is not easily acquired with only one exposure, the dental team is in a unique position for dietary counseling, in that patients are usually seen in a series of appointments over a period of time, and information can be given at all these appointments. A repetition of educational exposures over a period of time allows for greater assimilation of new knowledge.

Two facets of the diet are important from a dental standpoint, nutritional adequacy and frequency of sugar ingestion. During the period of childhood, when the teeth are forming (birth to 12 or 14 years of age), an adequate diet is necessary. This is true not only for the teeth, but also for all other growth that is taking place. A very good method for counseling is to utilize the

*Albans, A.: An improved Snyder's test, J. Dent. Res. 49:64, 1970.

National Dairy Council's Guide to Good Eating,* in which all foods are divided into 4 basic groups. It is relatively simple to compare a patient's food record with the recommended servings for these groups. A 5-day food record can be kept by the patient and then evaluated for nutritional adequacy. Several studies using this approach have been reported, and it was found that less than 50 percent of all the children studied were receiving a nutritionally adequate diet. In one of these studies (in a high socioeconomic group), only 13 percent of the children were found to be eating a diet that could be considered good.

Of particular interest to the members of the dental profession is the relationship of the refined carbohydrates (sugars) eaten and the amount of tooth decay present in the mouth. A direct relationship definitely exists between the number of in-between-meal snacks containing sugars and the incidence of tooth decay. A person normally eats 3 meals each day. This results in 3 exposures to refined carbohydrates and represents a certain amount of acid production in the dental plaque. If this same individual snacks another 3 times each day on a refined carbohydrate food, the exposures have been doubled. The repeated eating of foods containing a high degree of refined carbohydrates furnishes more material for dental plaque to use and changes the microflora balance of the mouth. As more of this food is eaten, more of the microorganisms that are thought to be involved in dental caries can be found. The frequency of exposure is more important than the total amount consumed in 1 day. The nature of the sugar-containing food is also of importance. A liquid form of sugar does not seem to produce an increase of dental caries activity as readily as sugars that are combined with sticky or other highly retentive food forms.

*National Dairy Council, Chicago, Illinois.

If we can aid our patients to eat all the foods necessary for a nutritionally adequate diet, there should be less tendency for between-meal snacking. For those patients who do snack between meals, foods with low refined carbohydrate content should be recommended.

Mouth protectors

Another facet of a dental practice that is frequently overlooked as a preventive element is the recommendation to wear a mouth protector for contact sports. A very serious and frequent problem in children is the fracture of a tooth during rough activity. Since 1962, the National Alliance Football Rules have required that a player wear a tooth and mouth protector. It is interesting to note that during the first year this rule was in effect, Texas high school football players displayed a 48-percent reduction in dental injuries. Three types of mouthguards are available for use—stock, mouth-formed, and custom-made. The stock guard fits all mouths and is held in place by keeping the jaws closed. The mouth-formed guard is fitted over the upper teeth directly in the mouth, whereas the custom-made protector is fabricated over a cast of the teeth made from a dentist's impression. Needless to say, the latter mouthguard (Fig. 13-7) is by far the most satisfactory. Many college and professional football players use mouth protectors routinely.

PATHOGENIC PREVENTION

Pathogenic prevention (secondary prevention) consists of those phases of prevention (Fig. 13-1) that are applied during the early diagnosis and prompt arrestment of a disease process. The concept during this stage is that a disease is already existent, and the earlier the diagnosis is made, the quicker treatment can be instituted. Early treatment in most situations will be simpler, more expeditious, and more satisfactory than if treatment were delayed.

No one will disagree that the earlier a

A

B

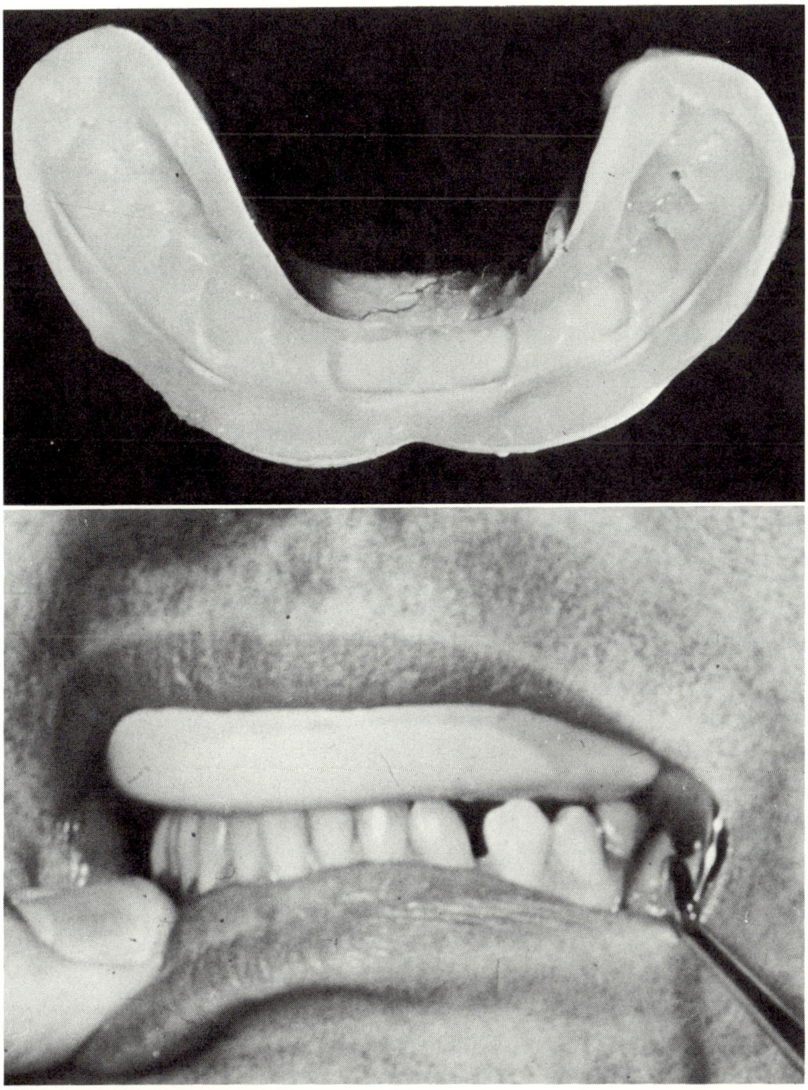

Fig. 13-7. Custom-made mouthguard, made from dentist's impression.

carious lesion is discovered, the smaller and simpler will be the restorative procedure necessary to replace the damaged tooth structure. Compare, if you will, the placement of a simple occlusal amalgam restoration in the first permanent molar with the placement of a full cast-gold crown on that same tooth. The amount of the tooth that has been destroyed by the caries process is the principal determinant of the type and size of the restoration placed. The development of the x-ray machine, its subsequent refinements, and the newer techniques for its use have been major aids in the early diagnosis of carious lesions. Routine and regular use of cavity-detecting (bite-wing) x-rays is among the major tools in the dental office for prevention in the pathogenic phase.

Regardless of the capability for early diagnosis of dental caries and the ability to place durable restorations, the treatment of dental caries goes much farther than just its discovery, the removal of the damaged portion of the tooth, and its replacement by a restoration. Massler has stated, "If the mouth harbors cariogenic flora, the most beautiful restorations will break down."* This introduces the idea that dental caries must be treated as both an infection and a restorative problem. The correct application of prepathogenic (primary) prevention is as important for the tooth with a restoration as for a tooth that has never suffered a caries attack. In cases of rampant dental caries, temporary anticariogenic restorations (rather than permanent restorations) are placed, until oral hygiene procedures and dietary changes have affected the oral environment to preclude the continuation of this rapid and severe caries attack upon the teeth. Another consideration of dental caries that should be stressed is the recommendation that all children receive their first dental examination *prior to* their third birthday. Most authorities will agree that the usual starting time for dental caries is during the second year of life. Again, early diagnosis and prompt treatment leads to the simplest and most satisfactory result.

Recall appointment system

Early diagnosis of dental caries, periodontal disease, and developing malocclusions can most easily be made if a patient visits a dental office regularly and routinely. Following the completion of any necessary treatment, it is good preventive policy to advise that patient when to return for another examination. The time interval should be determined individually and will vary according to the patients needs. A recall system can vary from advising the patient when to return to actually scheduling the appointment months in advance. Some dental offices prefer to mail a reminding card or letter, and others telephone the patient at the suggested time.

The procedures performed at the recall appointment will vary according to the patient's needs. A typical recall appointment may include a prophylaxis, topical fluoride treatment, and bite-wing x-rays for a patient susceptible to dental caries and periodontal disease. Personal oral hygiene practices can be evaluated, and the previous teaching reinforced. Nutritional advice and other patient information procedures can also be reemphasized. The objectives of the recall appointment are to prevent diseases and, if they already exist, to diagnose early and make treatment simpler.

Periodontal disease

Practically all cases of severe periodontal disease existed at some earlier time as a simple gingivitis. This could have been treated by a routine dental prophylaxis (scaling and polishing) and the use of good personal oral hygiene procedures at home. Both office treatment and home care are the important procedures that will prevent the continuation of damage to the periodontal tissues. Poor dental restorations and a poor functioning occlusion of the teeth will add to the severity of disease. Again, early diagnosis and prompt treatment, followed by the development of good home oral hygiene practices, can prevent the continuing development of periodontal disease to a state of damage so severe it results in loss of the teeth.

Prevention of malocclusion

The prevention of malocclusion in child patients is a new and rapidly growing area of dentistry. As more is learned of the normal growth process, dentists are better able to intercept a developing malocclusion, institute some form of relatively simple correction, and then maintain this altered pattern until dental maturity. The most important area to consider is the maintenance of space for permanent teeth.

---

*Massler, M. M.: Changing concepts in pedodontic education, J. Dent. Child. 33:157, 1966, p. 158.

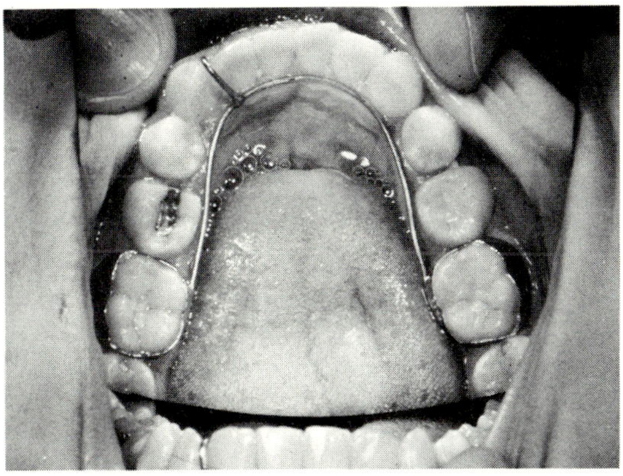

Fig. 13-8. Lingual arch, in position.

A

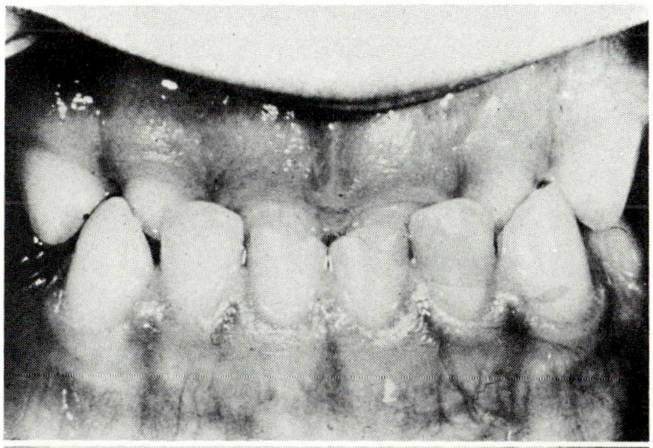

B

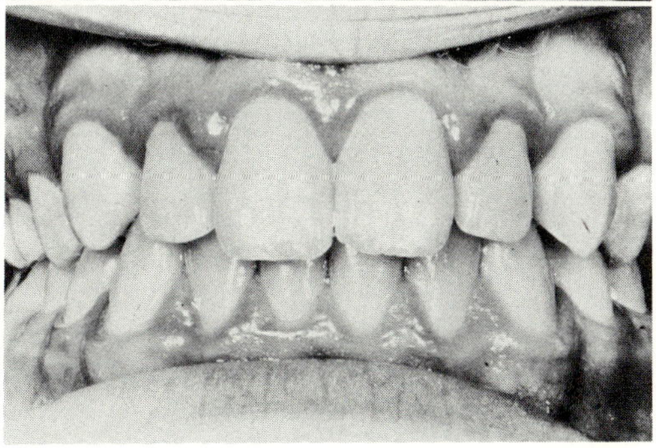

Fig. 13-9. A, Anterior cross-bite in 5-year-old child. This condition was corrected in 1 month with simple appliance; **B,** same patient at age 17.

Primary teeth have many functions in children's mouths. One function is to preserve space in the dental arch for the permanent teeth that will replace these deciduous teeth. Premature loss of primary teeth plays a major role in the subsequent development of malocclusion due to lack of sufficient space for the permanent teeth. Fig. 13-8 illustrates a lingual arch, one type of a space maintainer designed to prevent unwanted migration and tipping of the adjacent teeth following premature loss of the primary molars. With few exceptions, the early removal of a primary tooth requires that space maintenance procedures be instituted.

The second most important area for preventive orthodontic treatment is the diagnosis and early treatment of a functional disorder in a child's mouth. Most commonly, this is manifested as an anterior crossbite, a posterior crossbite, or sometimes a combination of both crossbites. The etiologic factors that may produce this malposition of the mandible during occlusion are many and varied. Among the known factors are discrepancies in proper exfoliation of the primary teeth and abnormal eruption patterns of the permanent teeth, both of which may result in occlusal interference. The child will then shift his mandible forward or sideways to achieve a comfortable occlusion. Differential diagnosis must confirm that it is truly a functional malocclusion and not a skeletal growth problem. Once the functional diagnosis is confirmed, treatment should be promptly instituted, as these malocclusions are seldom self-correcting. Fig. 13-9, *A* illustrates an anterior crossbite of a 5-year-old child that was corrected in 1 month with a simple appliance. Fig. 13-9, *B* is the same patient at age 17. Fig. 13-10, *A* illustrates a lateral crossbite in a 4-year-old child. The correction seen in Fig. 13-10, *B* resulted solely from occlusal equilibration to remove some premature contacts that existed as the child closed his teeth together in centric position.

Many malocclusions cannot be prevented. Most notable are the abnormal skeletal growth patterns (Class II and III malocclusions) and those cases where a discrepancy exists in the size of the permanent teeth (arch size–tooth mass discrepancy).

A

B

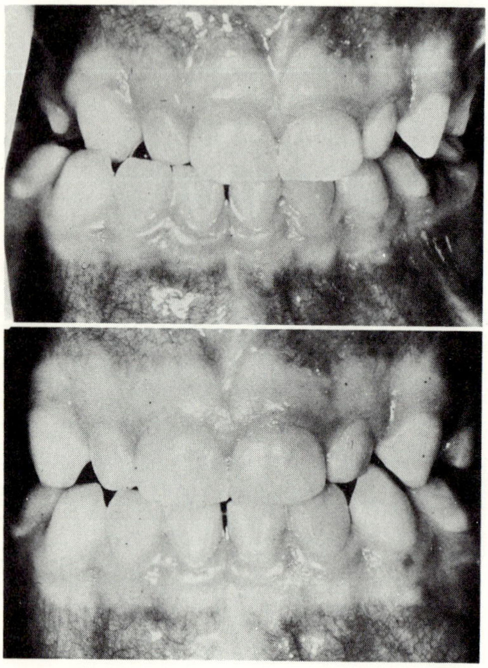

Fig. 13-10. A, Lateral cross-bite in 4-year-old child; **B,** correction resulted from occlusal equilibration to remove premature contacts that existed with teeth closed in centric position.

Careful use of those diagnostic aids that are today available to dentistry must be made by the dentist in general practice in determining which cases he can treat and which should be referred to the orthodontist. A set of well-trimmed study casts are an important diagnostic aid in the analysis of a patient's occlusion.

Examination and history

It has been said many times that the mouth is the mirror of systemic health and disease. A major part of dental prevention is early tentative diagnosis of local and systemic diseases, discovered by a careful and thorough examination of the soft tissues of the mouth and surrounding areas. Adding a well-taken history to this clinical examination, a dentist may discover the beginning symptoms of many different systemic illnesses. Prompt referral to a physician may contribute to early and perhaps life-saving treatment.

Early detection and prevention are the most effective weapons for combatting oral malignancies. It is the dentist who bears the principal responsibility for this early detection, since his work centers in the oral cavity, and he is familiar with normality and abnormalities of the soft tissue in the mouth. In its early stages, oral cancer does not exhibit pain, swelling, or bleeding. The American Cancer Society feels that the dentist's role is crucial in discovering the cancer lesions early, so that prompt treatment can be effected. In some countries of the world, oral cancers represent as much as 47 percent of all cancers; however, in the United States, oral lesions comprise approximately 6 percent of all cancers. At the present time, 14,500 cases of oral cancer are annually diagnosed. Thirty-eight percent of these patients will show a 5-year survival rate. The earlier the diagnosis and treatment, the higher the rate of survival will be. The exfoliative cytologic smear (Papanicolaou test) may be used as a screening test for oral lesions. If the dentist suspects that oral cancer is present, microscopic examination of a biopsy section of tissue is mandatory.

Many other general diseases display symptoms in the mouth that can be detected during an oral examination. The oral manifestations of congenital syphilis may be the only clinical signs of the disease in a child. The permanent incisors may look like screwdrivers and be notched on the biting edge. These are known as Hutchison's incisors and result from a hypoplastic defect during the acute infection period shortly after birth. The first permanent molars may also be affected and are described as "mulberry molars." Acquired syphilis displays a variety of signs in the mouth. The lower lip and tongue are frequent sites of syphilitic chancres. In the secondary stage of syphilis, mucous patches are seen in the mouth. If untreated tertiary syphilis is present, gummas are commonly seen in the oral cavity. Perforation of the hard palate, resulting in a communication between the oral and nasal cavities, may result from a gumma.

All the common forms of the blood dyscrasia diseases have definite oral signs and symptoms, and, in most cases, a careful oral examination and adequate history will result in early detection. Signs of icterus (jaundice) in the oral mucosa are common early diagnostic findings in sickle-cell anemia. Osteoporosis, osteosclerosis, and a ladder arrangement of interseptal bone can also be seen on intraoral radiographs. Enlargement of gingival tissue with edema and hemorrhage is an early sign of leukemia. A smooth, red, and painful tongue may be indicative of pernicious anemia. Spontaneous bleeding from the gingiva is common in thrombocytopenic purpura.

Diabetes mellitus is another disease that has definite oral signs. Dryness of the mouth, coupled with intense thirst and a sweet smell to the breath, are typical signs. The lack of protective secretions that result in the dry mouth lend a greater susceptibility of the soft tissue to local irritants. Periodontal abscesses and putrescent exudates occur more frequently in diabetics with periodontal disease. Marked destruction of the tooth-supporting alveolar bone may result in extreme loosening of the teeth.

The destruction of bone in the maxilla or mandible in a typical "punched out" pattern, discovered in a routine dental x-ray examination, may be the first clinical sign of one of the reticuloendothelial diseases. Gaucher's disease also displays large destructive bony lesions on dental x-rays.

Even though the dental office is planned to facilitate the diagnosis and treatment of diseases of the oral cavity, the dentist and dental assistant are members of the health team. History and examination of all patients must include a consideration of diseases other than those occurring just in the mouth. As Hine has so aptly stated, "Failure to locate a small area of dental caries may result in the loss of a tooth, but failure to locate a small cancer may result in the death of a patient."

POSTPATHOGENIC PREVENTION

This stage of prevention (tertiary) consists of the restoration of the damaged portion of the teeth, dental arches, or mouth in such a way that function of these structures is maintained in a healthy manner. This process can be as simple as occlusal amalgam restoration of one tooth or as complicated as placing immediate complete dentures.

The term "iatrogenesis" should be introduced here. Iatrogenesis is literally defined as "generated by a physician." It can be related to dentistry as the use of poorly executed reparative procedures, so that the reparations themselves are capable of producing disease. All restorative dental procedures in this postpathogenic stage of patient treatment must be performed with the prevention of future disease in mind. A proximal amalgam restoration that is not properly extended to self-cleansing areas will be more susceptible to recurrent caries. An over-extended denture flange will produce a sore spot and ulcer of the soft tissue. A concept of prevention of future dental disease must be foremost in mind when restorative procedures are being performed. As previously mentioned, following the postpathogenic stage of patient treatment (Fig. 13-1), the patient has returned to the prepathogenic stage. All tissues are now healthy, and primary prevention is of first importance for the future.

The utilization of prevention in a dental practice is principally a philosophy of the method of approach to dental disease. In the dental office of many years ago, the practitioner waited until a disease was clinically visible and then concentrated his efforts on correcting the damage that had occurred. However, since it is possible today to prevent most of the common dental diseases, emphasis in a modern dental practice must be placed upon prevention.

Patient education programs explaining the causes of dental caries, periodontal diseases, and malocclusion can be entirely conducted by the dental auxiliary. These may be formal programs in the dental office utilizing audiovisual aids, or casual conversations while placing patients in the dental chair. Dietary counseling and teaching of oral hygiene can be performed by the dental assistant. Most dental offices perform prepathogenic procedures, and the dental auxiliary has many opportunities to reinforce this through efficient patient education procedures.

Pathogenic prevention depends upon early diagnosis of an existent disease. An efficient recall system, with the routine use of bite-wing x-rays, is a major factor in early interception of carious lesions and periodontal disease. Importance of proper home oral hygiene procedures and dietary counseling can be reemphasized at these recall visits. In this way, damage correction is accomplished rapidly and with the greatest ease to both the dental team and the patient. Treatment procedures are now so easily and satisfactorily accomplished for the patient that an ever increasing amount of time can be spent in patient education procedures urging both the use of all known prevention practices and frequent and early dental visits to minimized development of disease.

Suggested readings

American Council on Education Commission on the Survey of Dentistry In The United States: The survey of dentistry; the final report, Washington, 1961, American Council on Education.

American Dental Association: Teeth, health and appearance, Chicago, 1957, American Dental Association.

Arnim, S. S., Diercks, C. C., and Pearson, E. A.: What you need to know and do to prevent dental caries (tooth decay) and periodontal disease (pyorrhea), J. North Carolina Dent. Soc. **46**:296, 1963.

Arnim, S. S., and Sandell, P. J.: How to educate high school students in oral hygiene, J. Health Phys. Educ. Rec. **31**:33, 1960.

Bass, C. C.: An effective method of personal oral hygiene, J. Louisiana State Med. Soc. **106**:100, 1954.

Blayney, J. R., and Hill, I. N.: Fluorine and dental caries, J. Amer. Dent. Ass. **74**:234, 1967.

Bohannon, H. M.: Oral physiotherapy. In Goldman, A. M., and Cohen, D. W., editors: Periodontal therapy, St. Louis, 1968, The C. V. Mosby Co.

Cartwright, H. V., Lindahl, R. L., and Bawden, J. W.: Clinical findings on the effectiveness of stannous fluoride and acid phosphate fluoride as caries reducing agents in children, J. Dent. Child. **35**:36, 1968.

Culpepper, R. T., and Jennings, R. E.: Extradietary fluoride, Texas State J. Med. **60**:482, 1964.

Leavell, H. R., and Clark, E. G.: Preventive medicine for the doctor in his community, ed. 2, New York, 1958, McGraw-Hill Book Co.

McClure, F. J.: Fluoride drinking waters; a selection of public health service papers on dental florosis and dental caries; physiological effects, education, and welfare, Bethesda, Maryland, 1962, Public Health Service, National Institute of Dental Research.

Muhler, J. C.: Current evaluation of fluoride therapy, J. Amer. Pharm. Ass. **NS3**:133, 1963.

CHAPTER 14 POURING MODELS

ROGER E. BARTON, D.D.S.
BILLY E. RIGSBY, D.D.S.

The well-trained dental assistant plays an important and time-saving role in the taking of impressions and the pouring of models. The assistant must become familiar with the various materials employed in impression taking, and she must learn how to prepare the materials for use by the dentist. The assistant does not actually take the impression, but her duties begin again after the impression is made.

The preparation of impression materials is discussed in another part of this book; therefore, the present chapter will be concerned only with construction of the cast or model from the impression.

It may be advantageous at this point to define the terms *mold, impression, cast,* and *model.* A *mold* is a matrix, form, or cavity in which an object is shaped. An *impression* is a mold of a dental arch (a negative reproduction). *Cast* and *model* are interchangeable terms that refer to the object formed or shaped from the mold or impression.

POURING THE MODEL

It is advantageous for the assistant to form the habit of pouring the model as soon as possible after the impression is made. Some impression materials have better dimensional stability than others. For most accurate results with any material, however, it is best for the assistant to pour the model immediately or as soon as possible, being careful not to exceed the time limit recommended by the manufacturer.

Impression materials

One of the materials most commonly used in taking impressions for study models is the alginate, or irreversible hydrocolloid material. After the impression has been removed from the mouth, it is washed with running water to remove all mucus, saliva, and debris (Fig. 14-1). The assistant should note whether the particular alginate material being used requires a fixing or hardening solution. If it does, the impression must be allowed to soak in the fixing solution for the recommended time before pouring (Fig. 14-2). If the alginate requires no fixing, the model can be poured immediately.

If the model cannot be poured immediately, it is possible to store the alginate material satisfactorily by carefully wrapping the impression in a damp paper towel and placing it in a humidor (Fig. 14-3). The impression should not be allowed to remain in this atmosphere for more than 20 minutes, however, if accuracy is an important factor.

When reversible hydrocolloid impression material is used, the fixing procedure recommended by the maufacturer should

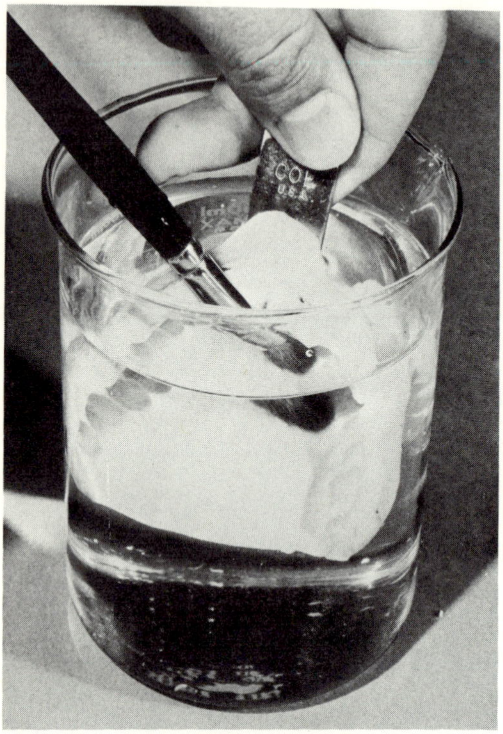

Fig. 14-1. Alginate impression washed under running water. (Courtesy The University of Texas Dental School at San Antonio.)

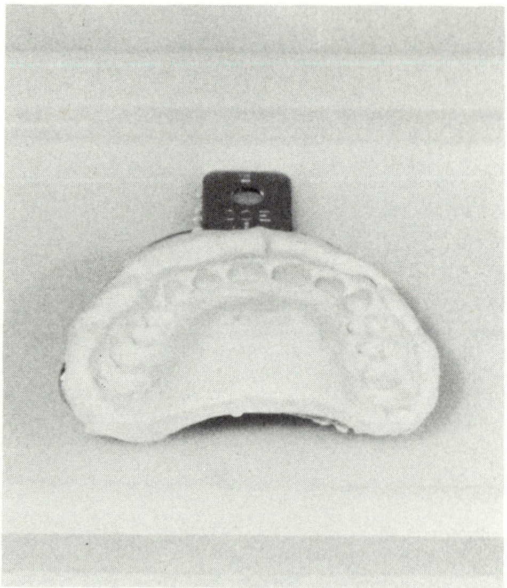

Fig. 14-2. Impression washed in fixing solution of 2-percent potassium sulfate for 10 minutes. (Courtesy The University of Texas Dental School at San Antonio.)

be followed. This material has many of the same physical properties as the irreversible material and must be treated with the same precautions when storing and pouring the impression.

Other impression materials, such as impression compound or the rubber-base materials, should be poured as soon as possible, although the time limit for accuracy can be extended beyond the 20 minutes recommended for reversible and irreversible hydrocolloid impressions. These materials, however, are very seldom used to take impressions for study models.

Methods

Depending upon the type of work to be done on the model, either plaster of paris or dental stone can be used in pouring. Study models, however, are usually made of plaster, since no actual fabrication is done on this type of model. The same principles apply in the manipulation of the gypsum product and in the pouring procedure for either material.

There are 3 basic methods for pouring models: (1) boxing method, (2) inverted method, and (3) double-pour method. Each of these methods may be altered to suit the individual operator.

Boxing method

The term "boxing" applies to a method of preparing the impression to receive plaster or stone. This technique is used more for preparing models on which prosthetic appliances are constructed than for making study models. It is difficult, and sometimes impractical, to employ boxing methods on impressions taken with reversible or irreversible hydrocolloids, because of the nature of these materials. Where applicable, the boxing method does have the following advantages: (1) it helps produce a more dense model; (2) it develops a uniform

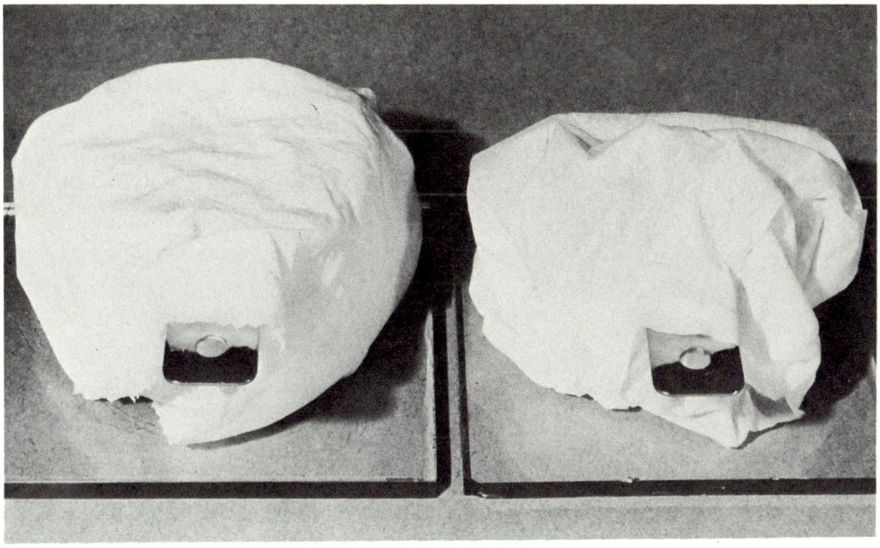

Fig. 14-3. Impressions wrapped in damp paper towels ready to be poured. (Courtesy The University of Texas Dental School at San Antonio.)

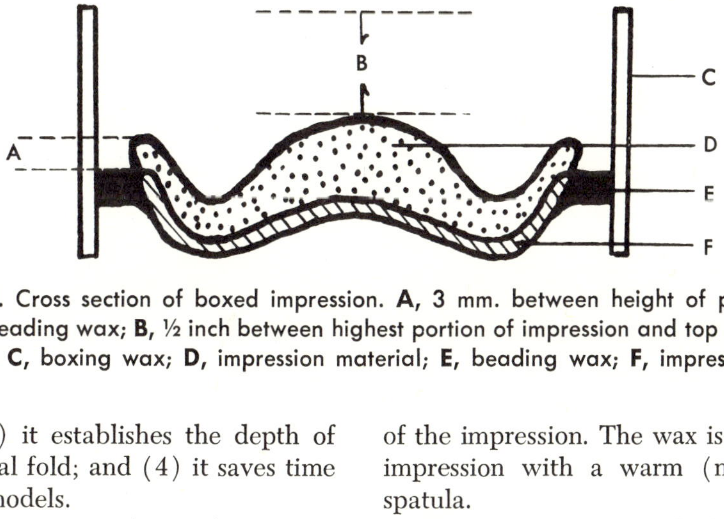

Fig. 14-4. Cross section of boxed impression. **A,** 3 mm. between height of peripheral roll and beading wax; **B,** ½ inch between highest portion of impression and top of boxing wax wall; **C,** boxing wax; **D,** impression material; **E,** beading wax; **F,** impression tray.

land area; (3) it establishes the depth of the mucobuccal fold; and (4) it saves time in trimming models.

The boxing process consists of "beading" the impression and applying a side wall around it (Fig. 14-4).

A strip of square rope utility wax is placed around the outside of the impression, parallel to the height of the peripheral roll and 3 mm. below it. This beading should continue across the posterior border of the impression. The wax is sealed to the impression with a warm (not hot) wax spatula.

The side wall is made by adapting a strip of thin boxing wax to the beading and sealing the two firmly.

The model should be no more than ½ inch thick in its thinnest portion. To obtain this thickness, the assistant should measure ½ inch from the highest part of the impression and mark the boxing wax. The wax

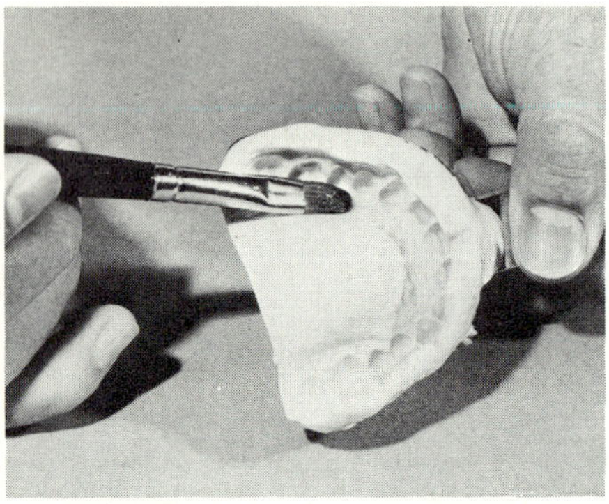

Fig. 14-5. Impression dryed with sable brush. (Courtesy The University of Texas Dental School at San Antonio.)

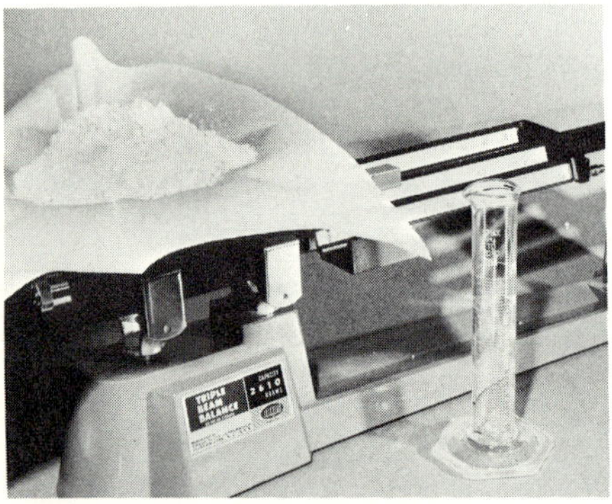

Fig. 14-6. Graduated cylinder, weighed plaster, and scale. (Courtesy The University of Texas Dental School at San Antonio.)

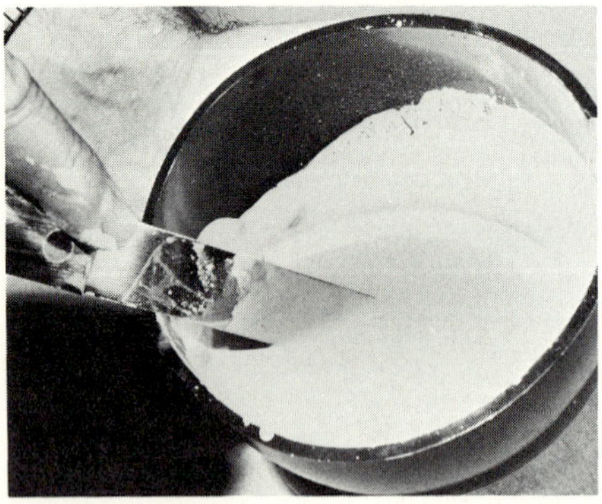

Fig. 14-7. Creamy mix of plaster. (Courtesy The University of Texas Dental School at San Antonio.)

may be cut down to this mark, or several markings may be made to indicate the amount of plaster or stone to be used.

Throughout the boxing procedure, caution must be exercised not to apply pressure to the sides of the impression, not to apply excessive heat during the luting, and not to touch the surface of the impression with an instrument or with the fingers.

When a lower impression is boxed, the beading is continued around the entire periphery, including the lingual area. A piece of baseplate wax is cut and adapted to the lingual beading to act as a tongue-space filler. This prevents excess material from flowing into the lingual area and creating a removal problem.

The model is then poured according to the prescribed methods of manipulating gypsum products.

Inverted method

The impression is washed clean of any saliva and debris, and all excess water is removed from the impression by drying with a sable brush (Fig. 14-5). Care must be exercised not to go to extremes in removing this water, especially in the reversible and irreversible hydrocolloid impressions.

The correct water-powder ratio (60 ml. water per 100 grams plaster, or 30 ml. water per 100 grams stone) is used to assure proper physical and working properties of the plaster or stone (Fig. 14-6). The mix is made in a clean plaster bowl according to instructions (Fig. 14-7). Mechanical spatulation and vibration of the mix reduce the amount of trapped air.

The impression (contained in the tray) is held on the vibrator, and a small amount of plaster is placed on the palatal portion adjacent to the last molar on the upper arch or the lingual flange on the lower arch. To vibrate this small amount into the indentations made by the teeth, the impression is tilted on the vibrator (Fig. 14-8), allowing the plaster to run from one tooth indentation to the next, until all are filled. This

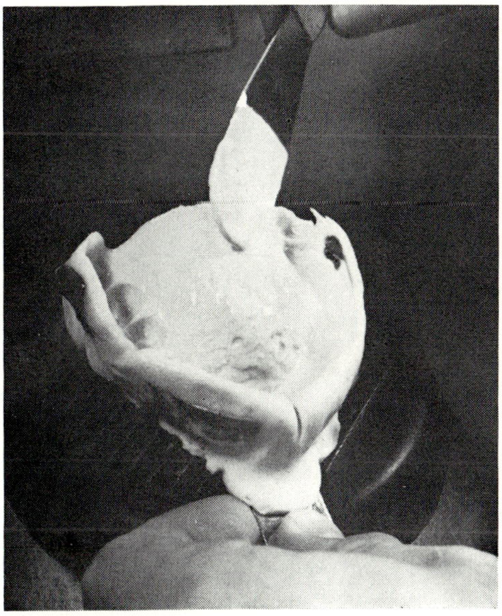

Fig. 14-8. Addition of small amounts of plaster until all the tooth imprints are filled aids in elimination of voids on the tooth surfaces of the models.

method will require the addition of several small amounts of plaster and will help eliminate trapped air. One large addition of plaster will trap air in the tooth indentations, even if vibration is used, and thus produce voids in the cast. The tooth indentations are completely filled before any large amounts of plaster are applied.

After the tooth imprints are filled, larger amounts of plaster are added, until the impression is filled up to and covering the peripheral roll or mucobuccal fold (buccal and labial extensions or borders). After this is accomplished, additional plaster is heaped on the surface to provide material for a base. The remaining plaster is placed on a glass slab, and the impression is inverted on this mass. The sides of the base portion are smoothed with a spatula, and the case is allowed to assume a final set.

Double-pour method

The double-pour method is exactly the same as the inverted method up to and including the filling of the impression and covering of the mucobuccal fold. At this point, the top surface of the plaster is left in a rough, undercut condition (Fig. 14-9). The base portion of the model is then made as the second pour, after either the initial set or the final set has occurred.

If the original pour has assumed the final set, it must be soaked in water for 5 minutes before the second pour is made. The material need not be soaked if only the initial set has occurred.

The second mix is made under proper conditions and placed on a glass slab. A thicker mix than that made for the first pour is desirable, so that it will hold the weight of the first pour while the side of the base are being formed with the spatula. The mass should be about ¾ inch thick and should spread over a large enough area to receive the original pour. The tray is then inverted and held in contact with this second pour, while the sides of the second pour are shaped with a spatula (Fig. 14-10). The poured impressions are then covered with a wet towel until the final set has occurred (Fig. 14-11). If the tray is pressed into the second pour with too much force, the initial pour will sink into the fresh mix, and not enough material will be left for a sufficiently thick base portion.

After the plaster has thoroughly set, the assistant removes it from the glass slab by allowing water to run over the slab and then sliding the model off.

In the double-pour method of making study models, the least distortion results if slight discrepancies occur during the pouring process.

When lower models are poured, the area between the inside of the lingual flanges of the tray may be filled with wax or packed with moist paper to prevent the building up of plaster in this area. In the double-pour process, this area may be shaped at the time the sides are shaped, before the second pour becomes set.

Two other methods of forming the base

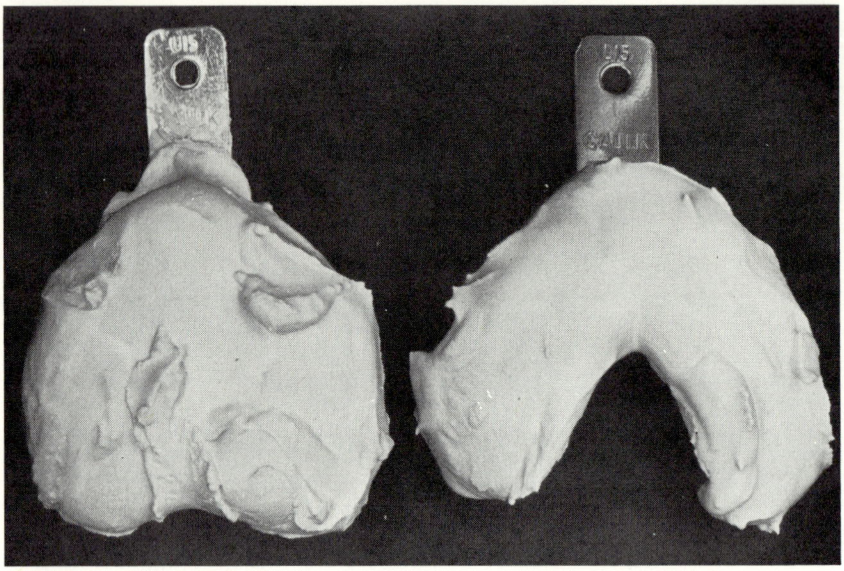

Fig. 14-9. Maxillary and mandibular impressions filled with plaster in first pour that covers the entire impression, including the impression borders. Surface is left rough to assist in mechanical bond with second pour.

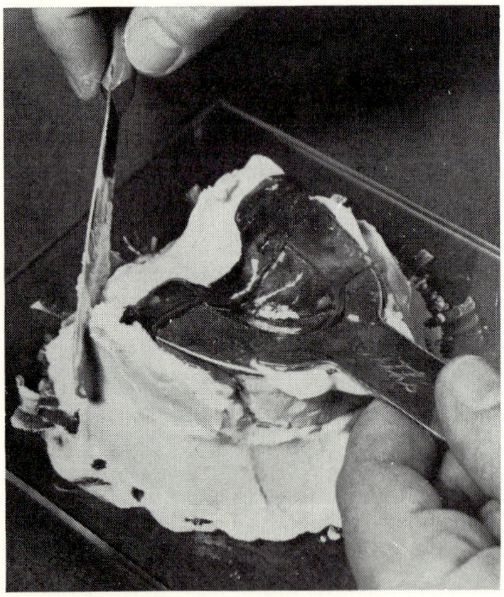

Fig. 14-10. When inverting the impression and first pouring into the plaster for the base, one must continue to hold the tray while forming the sides with the plaster spatula. This will assure sufficient thickness of base material for the art portion of the model.

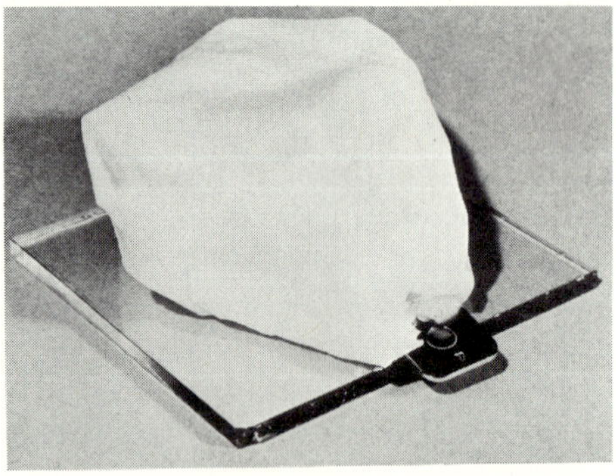

Fig. 14-11. Poured impressions covered with wet towel until final set. (Courtesy The University of Texas Dental School at San Antonio.)

portion are as follows. A matrix of boxing wax is sealed to a glass slab; then it is filled with gypsum. The poured impression is inverted into the matrix and allowed to set (Fig. 14-12). The other method is to use a flexible base-former, instead of the wax matrix (Fig. 14-13).

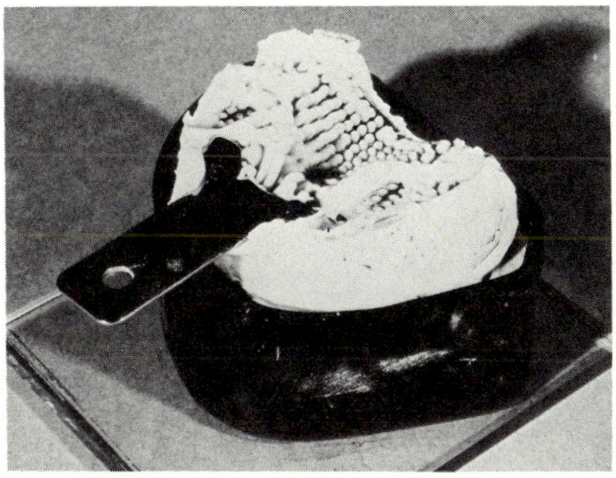

Fig. 14-12. Poured impression inverted into wax matrix. (Courtesy The University of Texas Dental School at San Antonio.)

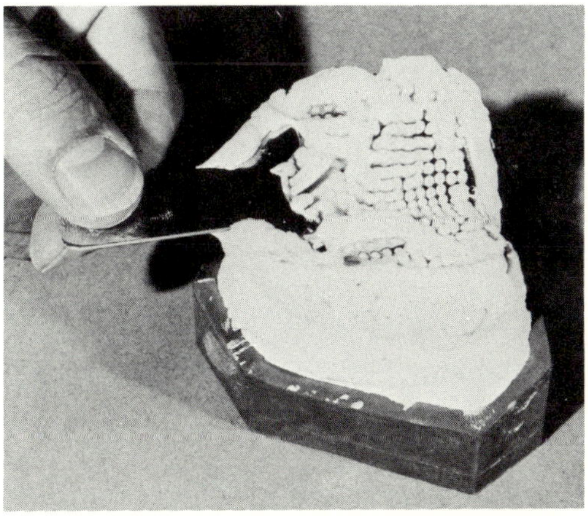

Fig. 14-13. Poured impression inverted into flexible base former. (Courtesy The University of Texas Dental School at San Antonio.)

SEPARATION OF THE CAST AND IMPRESSION

Separation of the model from elastic impression materials is different from separation from plastic impression materials. In all cases, care must be exercised during separation to prevent breaking of the teeth.

Separation of the model from elastic materials is begun by the removal of any plaster from the tray, so that the tray edges are free and visible. The anterior portion of the tray is first loosened and slightly raised. The entire impression should be freed by pressure applied in the anterior region. When the entire model is loose, the impression is lifted off with a straight pull. A rocking motion will tend to fracture the teeth on the model.

In the separation of plastic impression materials, such as impression compound, the material must be heated to 95 degrees F. This will soften the impression material enough to allow the cast to be easily removed. Heating to a higher temperature will cause the compound to stick to the cast as it is removed. Again, a straight pull, with no rocking motion, is used.

When the impression is boxed, the boxing material is removed before any attempt is made at separation.

TRIMMING THE MODELS

Study models prepared with a sense of aesthetics present a pleasing appearance and often reflect the quality of work that the patient can expect. The patient will certainly think more of a dental practice after seeing well-finished models than after seeing crude models that have been constructed in a haphazard manner.

The cast or model is composed of 2 parts—the anatomic portion and the art portion. The anatomic portion is a reproduction of the anatomic landmarks represented in the impression. The art portion, which is an additional part constructed as a base, adds an artistic and balancing effect. The art portion should be no less than one third the height of the entire model.

There are a multitude of shapes and relationships in dental arches, and not all the rules for producing the art portion can be followed in every case. However, there are a few fundamental procedures that when coupled with aesthetic considerations, will result in a well-balanced and nice-looking model.

Fig. 14-14 illustrates the symmetric trimming of the art portion of the maxillary

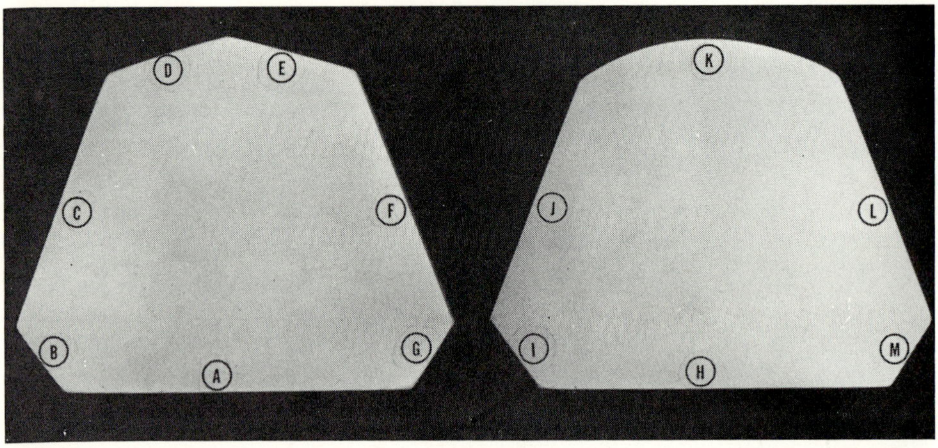

Fig. 14-14. Symmetric base forms for the maxillary (**left**) and mandibular (**right**) art portions of study models. **A** and **H** represent back cuts; **B, G, I,** and **M** are heel cuts; **C, F, J,** and **L,** are side cuts; and **D, E,** and **F** represent the anterior cuts.

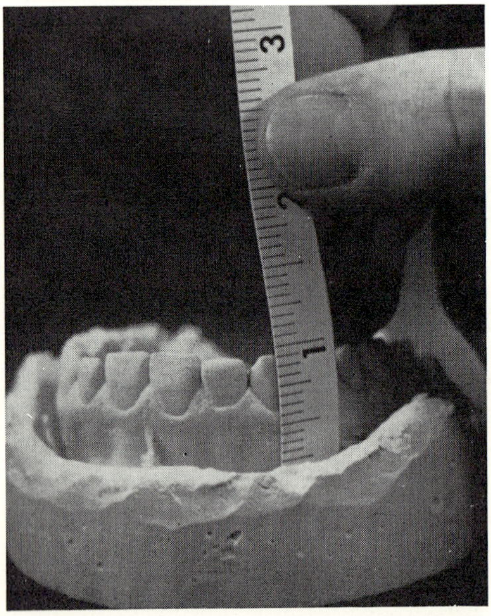

Fig. 14-15. The height of the anatomic portion is measured from the mucobuccal fold or border to the incisal surface of the canine. The flexible ruler is useful for this procedure. Voids on the base portion are the result of improper mixing of the gypsum product.

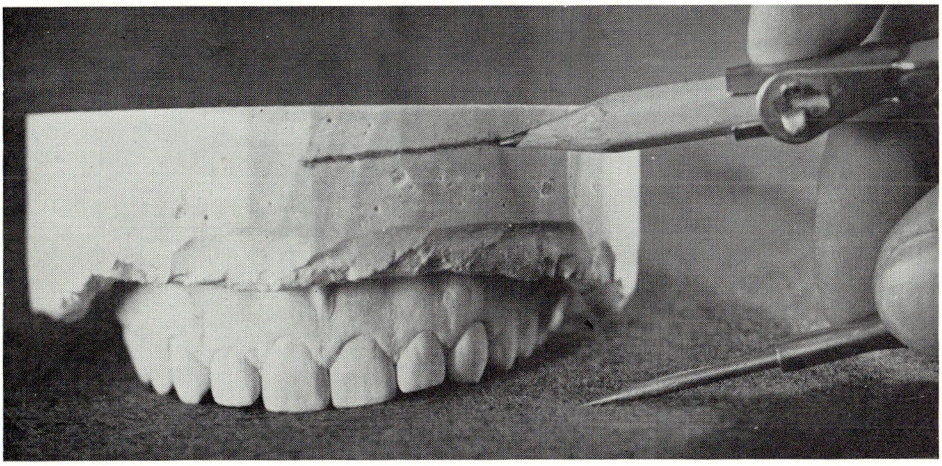

Fig. 14-16. The total height of the model is 1⅓ times the anatomic height and is marked with a set of dividers. The model is placed, tooth surface down, on a flat surface.

(*left*) and mandibular (*right*) models. For clarification in describing the procedure, the letters represent the adjacent sides; therefore, *A* and *H* are back cuts; *B*, *G*, *I*, and *M* are heel cuts; *C*, *F*, *J*, and *L* are side cuts; *D*, *E*, and *K* are anterior cuts.

The procedure for trimming the models is as follows:

1. The models are soaked in water for 5 minutes.

2. The sides of the maxillary and mandibular models are roughly trimmed on the model trimmer to produce a flat surface for the markings to follow. One should not remove too much material from the sides at this time.

3. Dividers are used to determine whether the maxillary or the mandibular model has the greater anatomic width and length, and trimming of the larger of the 2 models is begun.

4. Any excess in the posterior region that might prevent the teeth from resting on a flat surface when the model is inverted is trimmed.

5. The greatest height of the anatomic portion (from the height of the vestibule or mucobuccal fold to the occlusal or incisor portion of the teeth) is measured with a flexible ruler. This is usually in the area of the canines (Fig. 14-15).

6. One third of this measurement is calculated and added to the original measurement. The dividers are set to this figure, which represents the total height of the model.

7. The model is placed, tooth surface down, on a flat surface, with the plane of occlusion parallel with the flat surface, and a line is inscribed around the base of the model (Fig. 14-16). This line will be parallel to the flat surface and, therefore, parallel to the plane of occlusion (Fig. 14-17).

8. The base is trimmed to this line on the model trimmer.

9. On the trimmed model, which is the larger of the 2 models, the point of the dividers is placed at the lingual interproximal of the central incisors, and a mark is inscribed on each heel ¼ inch distal to the last molars or ¼ inch distal to the last anatomic registration, whichever is greater. The same divider opening is used for both back markings.

10. These markings are bisected with lines sighted through the mesiodistal centers of the molars or the centers of the ridges. Allowance must be made for badly

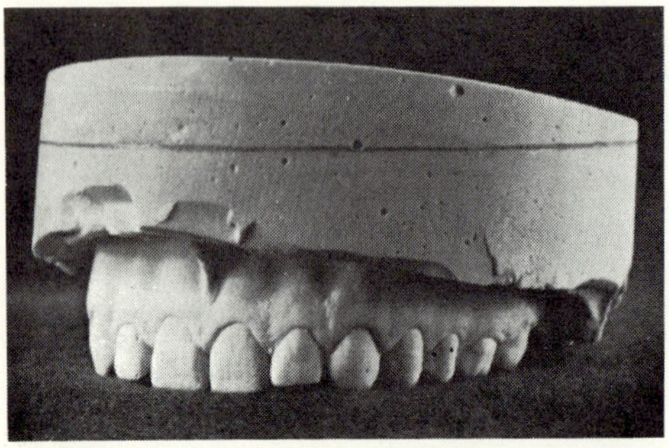

Fig. 14-17. The height marking is carried around the entire rough-cut surface of the model.

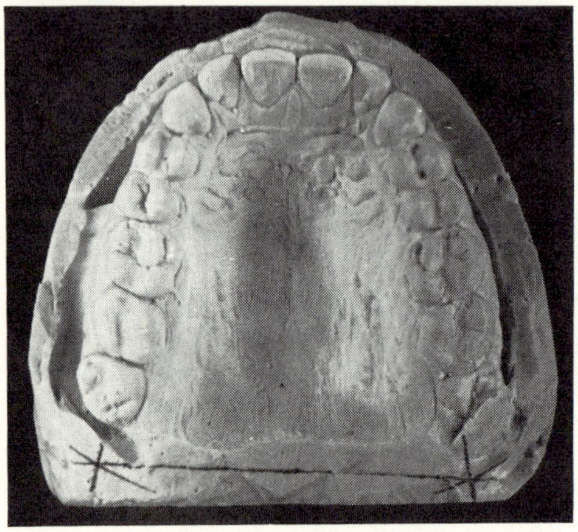

Fig. 14-18. Connection of the back markings produces the line to which the back of the model is trimmed.

rotated teeth. These points of bisection are connected (Fig. 14-18), and the model is trimmed to the connecting line.

Check point: The base should be parallel to the occlusal plane, and the back (*A* or *H*) should be at a right angle to the base and perpendicular to the median line.

11. On the other model, any excess that may interfere with proper occluding of the models is trimmed. This trimming includes removal of blebs on the occlusal surfaces of all teeth.

12. The greatest height of the anatomic portion is measured. One third of this measurement is calculated and added to the original measurement to give the height of the model. The second model is placed, teeth down, on a flat surface, and a mark corresponding to this measurement is made on the anterior portion of the model.

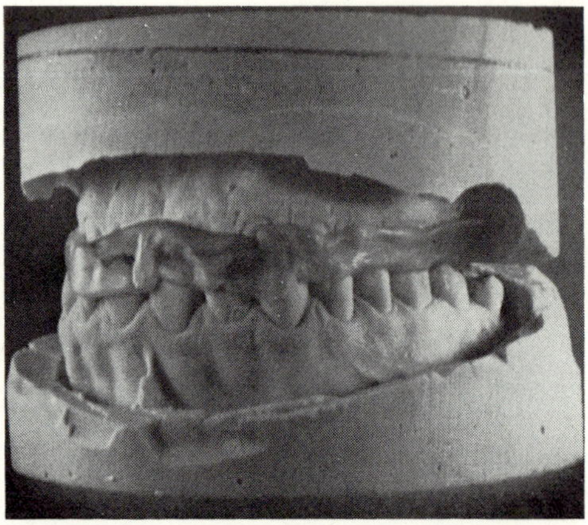

Fig. 14-19. Base line of the occluding model is marked parallel to the occlusal plane and the opposing model base.

13. The wax bite (obtained by the dentist at the time of the impressions) is placed in position, and the models are occluded. The occluded models are placed on a flat surface, with the previously trimmed base on the flat surface.

14. The dividers are set from the flat surface to the marking on the anterior surface of the top model, and a line is inscribed around the model (Fig. 14-19).

15. Two cuts are then made on the model trimmer. The models are separated, and the second one is trimmed back to the base line. Then the models are occluded, and the back is cut to the same plane as the previously trimmed occluded model (Fig. 14-20). The wax bite should always be in position when the occluded models are placed on the trimmer.

Check point: Bases of both models should be parallel to each other and to the plane of occlusion. Backs (*A* and *H*) of both models should be perpendicular to and on the same plane as the median line, and at right angles to the bases.

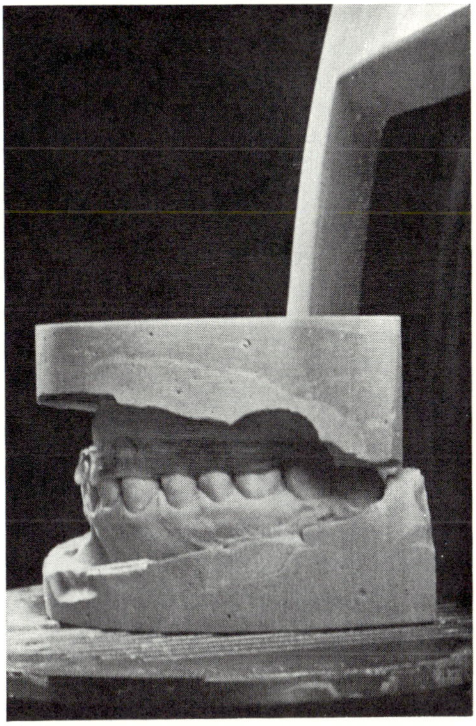

Fig. 14-20. The back of the model on the model trimmer platform is trimmed to the plane of the back of the occluding model. Note wax bite in position to protect the teeth and ensure proper occlusion.

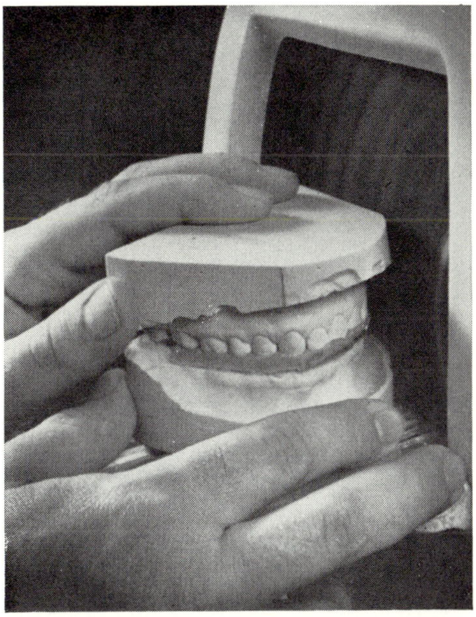

Fig. 14-22. When occluded models are being trimmed to the same plane, the wax bite is in position, and the uncut model is placed on the platform.

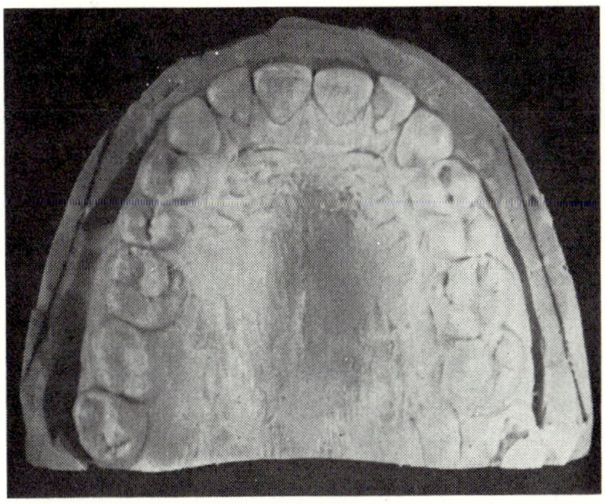

Fig. 14-21. The markings for the side cuts are parallel to the mesiodistal planes of the premolars and ¼ inch away from the bony ridge of the premolars.

16. On the model with the wider anatomic portion (the model that was trimmed first), a flexible ruler is used to inscribe a line parallel to the mesiodistal plane of the premolars ¼ inch buccal to the bony ridge, just below the gingival margins of the premolars. This marking is made on both sides of the model (Fig. 14-21). Malpositioned or missing teeth must be considered, and allowances must be made in marking this line.

17. The model is trimmer back to these lines on the model trimmer (*C* and *F* or *J* and *L*).

18. The heels are trimmed, with a cut ½ inch wide made parallel to the mesiodistal plane of the canine, on the opposite side of the arch (*B* and *G* or *I* and *M*).

19. Again the models are occluded (with the wax bite), and the sides and heels of both models are trimmed to the same planes (Fig. 14-22). To facilitate manipulation and provide a better view, the

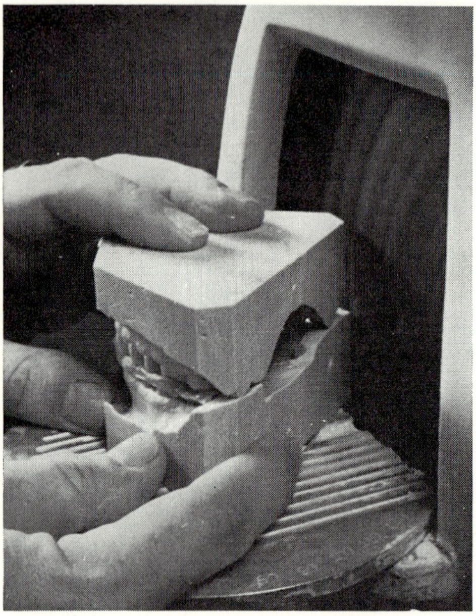

Fig. 14-23. When heel cuts are being trimmed on the same plane on the model trimmer, both models are held firmly, but they are not pressed against the revolving wheel with too much force.

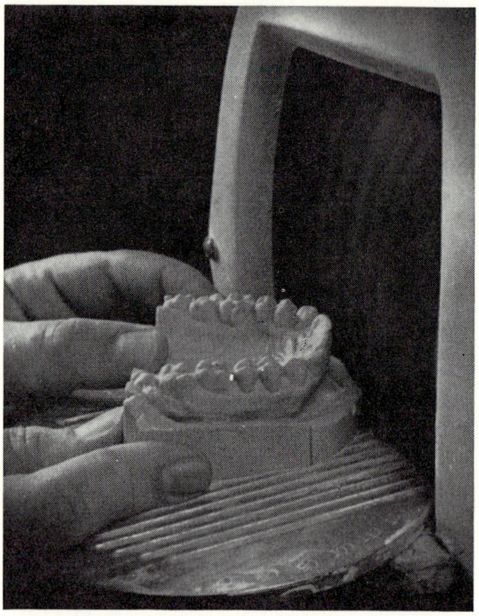

Fig. 14-24. In making the anterior cuts, care must be exercised not to trim the labial surfaces of the anterior teeth. Note the marking on the base that represents the distal extent of the anterior cut.

uncut model is placed on the model trimmer platform, with the trimmed model occluded on top (Fig. 14-23).

Check point: At this stage, all maxillary and mandibular side cuts and heel cuts should be on the same planes and at right angles to the bases (*C* on same plane as *J*, *B* on the same plane as *I*, and so on).

20. On the maxillary model, a mark is inscribed on each side of the model, corresponding to the mesiodistal center of the canines. Also, a mark corresponding to the median line is inscribed on the anterior portion of the model. The canine markings are joined with the median line marking. This line should be ¼ inch from the labial bony ridge, just below the gingival margins of the central and lateral incisors.

21. The canine markings are repeated on the mandibular model.

22. The anterior portion of the maxillary model is trimmed, with cuts brought back to ¼ inch from the labial bony ridge of the central and lateral incisors (Fig. 14-24). This part of the trimming procedure following the canine and median line markings, produces 2 flat surfaces (*D* and *E*). If anterior teeth are malpositioned or missing, the 2 anterior cuts should be made equal in length, rather than following exactly the markings dictated by the previously mentioned landmarks. When trimming the anterior portion of the maxillary cast, one must be careful not to mar the labial surfaces of protruding anterior teeth.

23. The anterior portion of the mandibular model is trimmed back to ¼ inch from the labial bony ridge of the central and lateral incisors. This cut is made in form of an arc (*K*) from the mesiodistal centers of the mandibular cuspids.

24. The land area is trimmed with a

knife back to a point where the depth of the fold is easily observed (Fig. 14-25). The lingual area of the mandibular model is trimmed to produce a smooth, aesthetic appearance (Fig. 14-26, left).

25. All defects and discrepancies in the models are filled in with a small amount of plaster that is conveyed with the finger or a camel's-hair brush. The models must be throughly soaked, or these additions will not stay in place. A piece of fine-grit sandpaper is placed on a flat surface, and the trimmed surfaces of the models are rubbed over the sandpaper to produce a smooth surface (Fig. 14-27). Each side is tilted to form a 45-degree angle with the flat surface, and the model is drawn across the sandpaper for about 4 inches. This will produce a very small, but definite bevel on the edges of all sides of the base of the model.

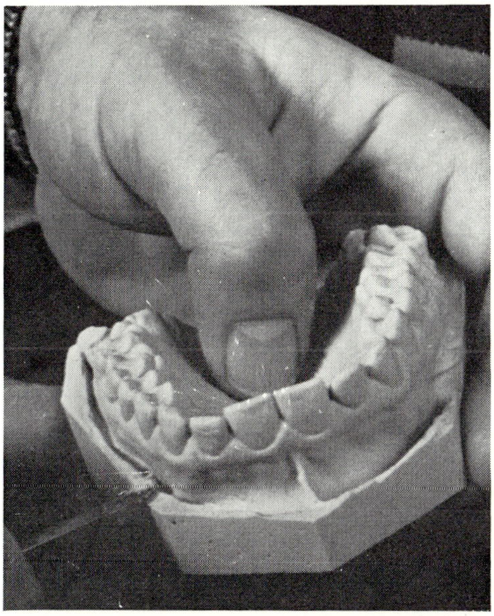

Fig. 14-25. The model should be reduced to where the mucobuccal roll is clearly evident, and a land area should be established, wherever possible.

26. After the models have thoroughly dried (usually 48 hours), they are soaked in a warm (165 degrees F.) concentrated soap solution for 20 to 30 minutes. Then they are removed and rubbed with a soft cloth to produce a smooth glossy surface. A plastic spray coat may be used instead of the soap bath to produce the finish on the models and to protect the surface. The spray is applied as several thin coats. If too much is applied at one time or in one place, it will run and produce an uneven surface.

27. A uniform method of identifying models is to place the patient's age on the left maxillary and mandibular heels, the patient's name on the backs of the maxillary and mandibular models, and the date the impressions were made on the right maxillary and mandibular heels (Fig. 14-

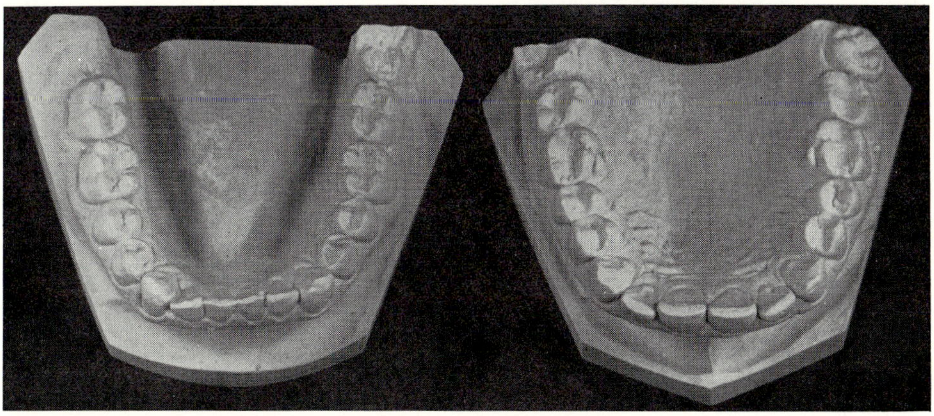

Fig. 14-26. Maxillary and mandibular models completely trimmed, including lingual area of mandibular model.

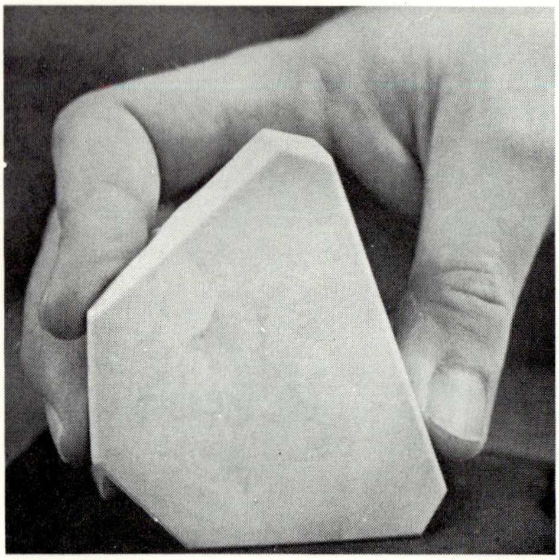

Fig. 14-27. The cut surfaces are smoothed on fine-grit sandpaper, and a small bevel is produced on the base.

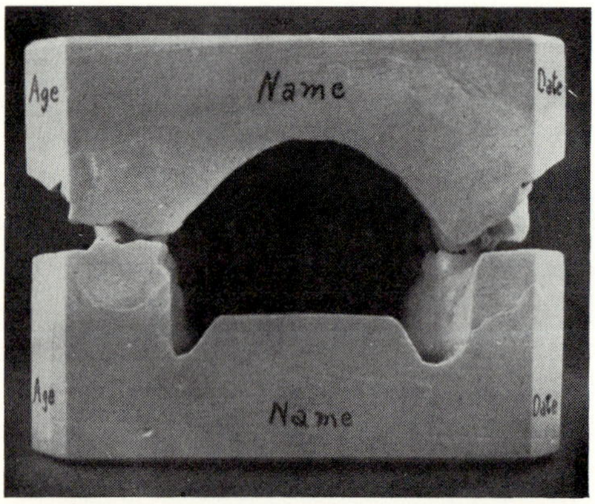

Fig. 14-28. Markings for identification of models. Rubber type may be used for these markings.

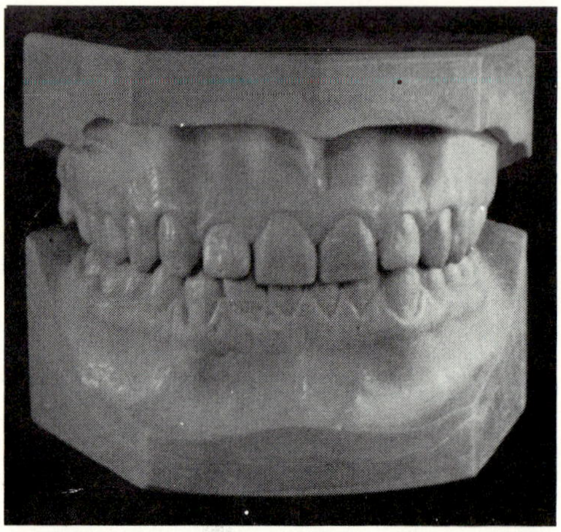

Fig. 14-29. Completed maxillary and mandibular models.

28). This information may be printed with a pen or pencil, or it may be stamped with rubber type.

Models prepared according to the foregoing procedure present complete and aesthetic reproductions of the dental arches and are valuable adjuncts in the progressive dental practice (Fig. 14-29).

Suggested readings

Phillips, R. W., and Skinner, E. W.: Elements of dental materials for dental hygienists and assistants, Philadelphia, 1965, W. B. Saunders Co.

Strang, R. H. W.: A textbook of orthodontia, ed. 3, Philadelphia, 1950, Lea & Febiger.

Swenson, M. G.: Complete dentures, ed. 4, St. Louis, 1958, The C. V. Mosby Co.

Swenson, M. G., and Terkla, L. G.: Partial dentures, ed. 2, St. Louis, 1959, The C. V. Mosby Co.

PART IV SUPPORTING THE OFFICE PRACTICE

CHAPTER 15 THE OFFICE RECEPTIONIST AND SECRETARY

SHAILER PETERSON, B.A., M.A., Ph.D.

It is impossible to overemphasize the importance of a good secretary-receptionist. It is also impossible to overemphasize the harm that can be done in any office by a poor secretary-receptionist.

The receptionist is vital to the success of the office for a number of reasons. The first contact that the new patient has with the office is with the receptionist, either by telephone or when the patient enters the front door. This first contact is very important, for some patients are frightened away by this first visit and never see the dentist. The image of the office is on display in the reception room, because it is here that many patients spend a great deal of time. It is also in the reception area where all visitors to the dentist spend enough time to learn how the receptionist treats other people, how she spends her time, how she speaks to other employees and her employer, and how she approaches her duties and responsibilities.

HELP OR HINDRANCE

While the secretary-receptionist is important to any office, there is probably no place where this importance can be more easily demonstrated than in a dental office. Some have said that the receptionist either makes or destroys the professional image of the dental office. A poor—or even an average—receptionist can drive patients away from an office even before they have seen the dentist. Some receptionists create situations that result in a patient not returning, even though the patient was very pleased with the dentist and the dental service he received.

Usually, the dentist never knows how many patients have never gotten as far as his operatory, even though they waited in his reception room. Also, he often never knows that many patients who do not return for their appointments were discouraged from returning because of a poor receptionist.

The dentist does not usually know how much money and how many patients he has lost because of inefficiency in his reception room. Months or even years may go by before a dentist realizes that his declining practice is because of his secretary. Of course, some dentists do not realize that their rapidly growing practices may be attributed, in a large part, to an efficient and conscientious receptionist or secretary.

The employers, whether they be dentists, physicians, or business executives, are usually too busy in their own operatories or offices to observe and supervise what is going on in a reception room. When they do hear about a discourteous employee, it is usually only after considerable damage in public relations has already been done and after a major problem has arisen.

Most employers are sufficiently busy that they do not have the time to educate and train their new employees, and they hope that the new employee will have a great deal of interest in the new position and a real dedicated desire to become expert in it. Too few employees look at a new position as even a temporary "career" and as a new challenge. Too few employees have ever thought of studying their new position to determine how they fit into the operation of the entire office. Too few try to define and understand what they are expected to do and what they could do to make themselves more valuable to the office. Too few employees have ever thought that they might develop a position that is not only extremely important, but also one of which they can be extremely proud.

There are really no unimportant jobs or positions, but there are many positions in which the employee has never discovered either her importance or her responsibilities. Her position may seem routine, until she realizes how costly even the simplest of mistakes can be to other people and to her employer.

FORMS OF ADDRESS

All secretaries and receptionists in a dental office recognize that they should and must address their employer in a formal and professional manner. Even the wife or sister of the dentist who may be helping in a dental office must remember that she must always use formality and address the dentist as "Dr. Jones" and not by his initials or first name.

Employers will vary in the manner they address their employees. Some think that informality encourages a close working relationship; therefore, they call their assistants and receptionists by their first names or even by their nicknames. Some employers will even make age distinctions and will address their middle-aged employees as "Miss Smith" or "Mrs. Olsen" and refer to their new and younger employees as "Jane" or "Suzie." Normally, this is not recommended, for it seems to categorize the personnel, and some might think that the formal address is restricted for those with the major responsibilities in the office—and responsibility is not always related to the age of the individual.

Most professional offices use the formal approach entirely, with the dentist always addressing his secretary or his receptionist as "Miss Jones" and refraining from calling her by her first name—either in private or in front of patients. A girl who has worked in a store where she has been called "Jill" may, at first, feel strange to have her new boss in the dental office always refer to her as "Miss Jones." It is comparable to graduating from a high school where she was called "Jill" by her instructors and then entering a university where her instructors call her "Miss Jones."

Most dentists have found that the patients prefer to call the receptionist by her last name and also to have their children use the formal manner of address. However, this is purely a matter of choice that the dentist-employer must determine for himself. What is spontaneous and better for one office is not always the same for another office.

There are times when the dentist and his assistant have relatively little to say about the forms of address they should use in their office. Sometimes all of the professional men in a certain building are very informal, and when the new dentist with his new assistant move into the building, they feel that they should conform to the policies and practices that have already been established. However, even here they may wish to decide for themselves what they wish to do, even if it means showing some originality and independence.

STUDY, LEARN, AND MASTER

A desire to learn and improve does not automatically make one a top dental assistant. Reading this book will undoubtedly make the reader much more knowledgeable about many things that will improve her efficiency in the dental office. However, to improve and to grow as much as a student is capable of growing, she must study and be anxious to learn.

No matter how much schooling one has had, and no matter how much experience one has had working in the offices of various dentists, this previous education and past experience do not mean that one will automatically be an expert dental assistant in the new office. Every new position that an employee holds requires that she adjust to the wishes of the new employer and the needs of the new office. The girl who accepts a new position must also accept the responsibility of studying the new position and asking her new employer for help and guidance in acquiring the new skills and knowledge that she will need if she is to be successful.

Many girls who have been efficient in one office have failed completely in a new position, because they had false feelings of self-assurance and an almost conceited attitude that they had nothing more to learn. Adjusting successfully to a new position is as important and often almost as difficult —as learning the basic skills in the first place.

Many girls who take on a new position obtain false notions of their own success and of their own security, because most employers are inclined to be understanding and patient with the new employee, realizing that she has many new things to learn in a new and complex office situation. The employer cannot afford to be lenient and easygoing forever, and he soon wonders why his new employee is not making progress in learning the operation of the office. He will soon wonder why she does not decide for herself that she must come early and stay late at her own expense to learn rapidly. Many secretaries have won positions by giving the impression that they were able to type, only for the employer later to find that it took them a whole day to type 4 or 5 double-spaced pages. A girl who finds that her work is this poor or rusty owes it to herself and her employer to spend hours of time at night and on weekends practicing her typing, if she wants to hold her job.

If a position is worth holding, it is also worth working to hold, and this means (1) evaluating one's own deficiencies, and (2) studying and practicing to remove these deficiencies.

Unfortunately, it is the rare dental assistant, receptionist, or secretary who takes enough interest in her own position that she will really work to (1) discover if she is as efficient and successful as her employer expected her to be, (2) improve herself and her efficiency, (3) admit her own deficiencies even to herself, and (4) ask for advice and help from her employer. In regard to this last item, there are many new and old employees who have a fear of asking questions of their employers. They sometimes rationalize their silent attitude with the excuse that their employers do not want to be bothered. It is true that employers do not want to be bothered by useless and needless chattering. However, every employer would much rather have the opportunity to answer a question and explain to his employee how he prefers to have something done than to have her do things incorrectly and unwisely.

Some employees have the notion that they do not need to bother their employers, for they think that they can learn all of the facts by making inquiries of other employees, the girls in neighboring offices, or friends. Nothing could be so incorrect or so unwise. *Only* the employer knows exactly the way that he wants things done in his office, and the information given by another employee may be completely incorrect, for the following reasons:

1. She does not know what is expected of a new employee.

2. She may not want the new employee to succeed.

3. She may want to appear more efficient and thus withhold information.

Do not depend too much on your colleagues in the office to give you tips on how to do a better job, when you can go directly to your boss for the answers. He not only can give you the best answers, but he also needs to know that you have an interest in improving.

Common sense and good judgment

In any office, whether it be a dental office, or a physician's office, or the office of a dental school administrator, there is no substitute for plain common sense and good judgment. One can be the best stenographer, the best clerk, or the best bookkeeper, and yet fail miserably as a receptionist, secretary, or dental assistant, if one fails to use common sense and good judgment. There are so many illustrations that show the lack of good judgment and the lack of thinking before acting or speaking. The following are a few examples of acts of thoughtless secretaries and receptionists:

1. Miss X tells 3 other dental assistants at their meeting that Internal Revenue representatives have been in to question her employer all week.

2. Miss X tells a patient that her employer makes 3 times as much money as the dentist next door.

3. Miss X tells a patient that he must have cash for his treatment, because the dental laboratory will not deliver the prosthodontic appliance unless it is paid for immediately.

4. Miss X tells several patients that their appointments will need to be postponed, as her employer has a dental meeting to attend in New York that she knows will be a "blast."

5. Miss X fails to tell her employer about his phone calls she received before he arrived in the office.

6. Miss X explains to the patients that the dentist has not arrived yet, but that "he is always late on Monday mornings."

7. Miss X explains to a waiting patient that the patient who has just left had much work to be done because she had neglected her teeth for so long.

8. Miss X explains to the patients and the representatives of dental dealers that she is underpaid and that her talents are not appreciated.

9. Miss X fails to mail her doctor's personal mail for a week, because she cannot find any stamps.

10. Miss X leaves the office at 3:00 PM, without telling anyone that she had a call to pick her child up early from the nursery.

11. Miss X fails to make a list of the people whom her doctor asked her to call and invite for a committee meeting at his office.

12. Miss X tells her friends that her doctor has loaned her the money to pay for her new automobile.

13. Miss X rushes into the office or operatory and disturbs everyone with an announcement that her work will be held up if the doctor does not take the time, immediately, to sign the statements and letters that need to go out.

14. Miss X opens and reads all mail, including the letters marked "personal" and "confidential" addressed to her doctor.

15. Miss X interrupts a private conference with a patient to loudly announce that a bothersome collector or salesman is back again to see the doctor.

16. Miss X is given a note by her employer with instructions to place the dates on his calendar and to keep him reminded of the deadlines involved. She misplaces the note and forgets the whole incident, and

her employer misses his meetings and fails to prepare his reports.

17. Miss X follows her doctor's request to send a clipping of a journal article to Dr. Y, but fails to insert any note to indicate to Dr. Y who has sent him the material.

18. Miss X encloses in Dr. W's letter, by error, some handwritten notes that her doctor made from confidential information received over the telephone.

19. Miss X sends to Dr. Y a carbon copy of a letter that was intended for Dr. W.

20. Miss X loans a file to Dr. Y's secretary, without checking the file to see if it contained confidential information that should not go out of the office.

21. Miss X fails to doublecheck the plane tickets that she has picked up for her doctor, only for him to discover when he gets to the airport that they are made out for the following day.

22. Miss X tells all the people who call on the telephone that the doctor is not in, but quickly volunteers that he can be reached at his club—without remembering that he does not wish to be disturbed and without discovering if the call is important enough to warrant locating the doctor.

23. Miss X tracks her doctor down through emergency calls and paging while he is at a meeting, only to let him know that there are no problems at the office and everything is going along fine.

Many of the preceding mistakes in judgment are serious enough to warrant instant dismissal. Not all of these mistakes would be made by a malicious person, but a serious mistake that is made by an innocent, careless, and thoughtless person is just as damaging as if it had been made maliciously. *There are no excuses for thoughtlessness or carelessness.*

Too few secretaries and receptionists make a thorough study of their own positions. Those who take their positions seriously and who want to make themselves worthy of their present salaries and worthy of raises in the future do make an effort to study their jobs and become efficient at them.

The following suggestions, ideas, and comments should be of help to every secretary and receptionist. The list is not complete, for every girl will find that her office involves additional problems and solutions. Also, some of the suggestions given here may be more applicable in certain types of offices and for some particular responsibilities than for others. Also, it must always be remembered that when one adopts a new idea or adapts an old one to fit a new office, it is wise to discuss this with the employer. Not only will he be pleased to know that his employee has the interest and enthusiasm to want to improve her work and to systematize it, but he will also want to pass judgment on it and help her to determine whether it should be adopted in exactly that fashion. Many of the following suggestions and recommendations are applicable in a medium-sized business office or in a office of a dean of a dental school, and they have equal usefulness in a dental office that has a volume of correspondence and an employer who has many meetings to attend and many records to maintain.

General office suggestions

A receptionist should develop her own card file or rotary file system to help her remember the names of the following:

1. Doctor's friends who often call on the telephone and who come for visits
2. Patients and their sons and daughters (if patients or visitors)
3. Doctor's business acquaintances who frequently call or correspond
4. Professional persons and their secretaries who are located in the same building
5. Business firms (local and distant) with whom business is routinely conducted
6. Clubs, associations, and societies of which the doctor is a member
7. Relatives who should be contacted in the event of illness of the doctor or members of his family
8. Doctor's personal physician, attorney, in-

surance broker, and banking consultants
9. Persons to be contacted in case of emergencies
10. Former and current employees of the office
11. Officers of local, state, and national dental associations
12. Officers of local, state, and national American Dental Assistants Association and American Dental Hygienists Association

To associate names with faces, the receptionist and her doctor may wish to plan a method for taking pictures of all new patients or visitors. These pictures can also be helpful when attached to the personal data sheet or treatment-planing sheet. This practice is useful for study, and it helps the doctor who goes out into a reception room to be greeted by a sea of faces, some of whom he may not have seen for a couple of years. Patients expect the receptionist and the doctor to remember them.

A new employee is unwise to ask endless questions the first few days she is employed, for any employer is sensitive about being placed in a position of answering a formal list of questions by a new employee —or anyone else for that matter. However, there are some things that the new secretary or receptionist must know quickly, such as the following:

1. Regulations and rules of the office—office hours, who opens and closes the office, customs on coffee breaks, and lunch hours.

2. Persons to call in case of emergency —for example, interruption in electrical power, or leakage or flooding caused by gas or water lines, as these things could occur when the dentist is not in the office.

3. Whether the dentist wants to call the dental dealer in the event that some piece of equipment does not function, or whether this is something expected of the secretary.

4. Responsibilities in relation to other employees in the office, so that she does not shirk what she is supposed to do and yet does not appear to be taking over someone else's position.

5. Whether employer wants to be interrupted when representatives from dental dealers visit the office, and if he wants the receptionist to handle other sales persons and delivery personnel.

6. Customs that the dentist wants observed with telephone calls from other dentists and physicians, his family, friends coming through town, and so on.

7. Operation of the fancy array of telephone buttons—several extensions with buttons, flashing lights, hold buttons, and buzzer buttons.

Every employee (both *old* and *new*) should make a list of her duties. This will seem meaningless to many, who think their duties are so simple and natural that there is no need for such a list. Those who do make such lists will find them invaluable if reviewed periodically, and they will also find these lists important in observing how the responsibilities and duties of an efficient employee increase and expand the longer she holds her position.

A new employee should learn the vocabulary of the office. She should make a planned study of the terminology used by the dentist with his patients. She should use the glossary and index of this textbook and check the terms her dentist uses. These terms should be reviewed every week or so, until she has mastered them.

The receptionist may learn from her dentist what her responsibilities to the sales personnel who visit the office are to be—for example, whether she is expected to learn about their products, handle inventory, do the purchasing, or make recommendations for purchasing.

The new secretary-receptionist who takes pride in learning about the accomplishments and achievements of her employer will not only please her employer, but will also give herself additional reasons for being proud of the position that she holds in this important office.

New secretaries and receptionists must learn how to make long-distance calls efficiently. Dentists who have accidentally overheard their secretaries place a long-distance call may have been very irritated to listen to the lengthy, verbose discussion that she carries on with the telephone operator. The dentist who makes frequent long-distance calls from his home or when he is out of town becomes accustomed to giving just the pertinent information, and he cannot understand why anyone else should use superfluous words.

In this day and age of direct dialing and area codes, long-distance calling has become very simple. A dentist can be away from home at a hotel and complete a call to his home by only (1) telling the hotel operator, "I want to make a long-distance call and will place it on my credit card," and (2) telling the long-distance operator, "I want to make a 'credit-card' call. My number is 628-2925-KO87. (pause) I want to call Memphis, Tennessee, area code 901, and the number is 682-2900. I am Dr. Jones in Room 606." Then when he is in his outer office and hears his secretary giving a lot of extraneous information, he is driven to distraction.

If he is calling Dr. Smith of the American Dental Association in Chicago, he may hear his secretary say, "Operator, this is Dr. Samuel Jones' office in the Medical Arts Building, Room 783, on the corner of Broad and Central, and we want to make a person-to-person call to Chicago, Illinois. Oh yes, our number here is 242-0779, and our area code is 414. We want to talk with Dr. William Smith, who is Secretary of the Council on Dental Materials of the American Dental Association at 211 East Chicago Avenue, Chicago, Illinois, zip code 60611. The number there is Whitehall 4-6730, and we want to talk with Dr. Smith. Oh yes, and the area code for Chicago is 312."

All she would have to have said was, "We want to call Chicago, where the area code is 312. The number is 944-6730, and we want to speak with Dr. William Smith. Our number is 242-0779."

This is cutting the wordage down from 105 words to 28 words, or down to one-fourth its original length; more important, the shorter version is businesslike and saves the operator and everyone else a great deal of writing time. The lengthy directive not only contains extraneous and confusing information, but also some of the important information is hidden at the end of the conversation. When one confuses the operator with a lot of extraneous and useless information, she may presume that this is important and take the time to write it down, only to find out later that the secretary has had all of the pertinent information all of the time.

It is the new secretary's responsibility to develop a resource book that contains the information needed for various emergencies and for different types of situations.

She should develop a notebook—aside from her appointment book— in which she could list the date and the time of every person who visits the office and every telephone call received or placed. There are many occasions in which her employer will want to know when it was that Dr. X called him, to enable her employer to know what time he suggested sending Miss B for a consulation. Her employer may want to know when Mr. Y, a salesman, was in the office, for he recalls that he ordered a certain item at that time, and it still has not come.

A receptionist is expected to develop a listing of names and phone numbers to keep at home, for there are times when her dentist will need to call her at home and ask her to make a series of calls for him before the start of the new day.

She should be sure that she has at her home the names, phone numbers, and addresses of her employer and the other employees in the office, for in the event of illness, she will need to keep her office informed about her inability to come to work.

Fig. 15-1 shows a secretary using 2 different type of card index or filing system

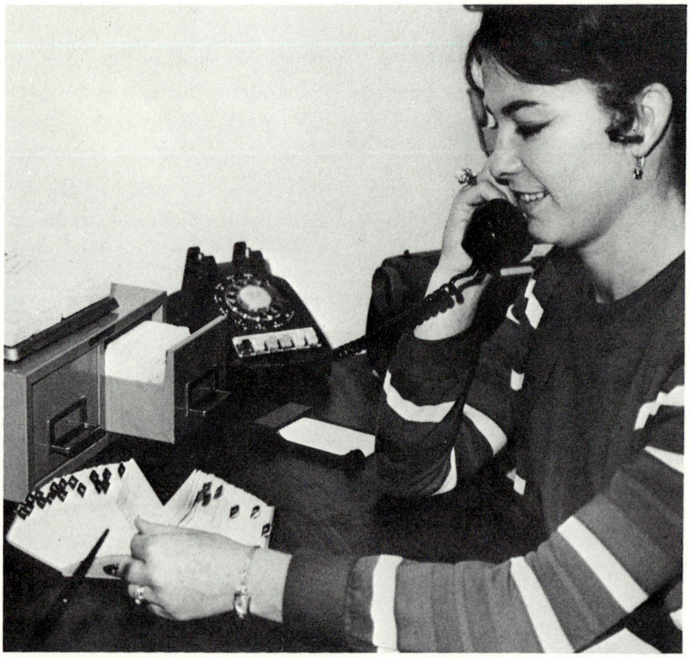

Fig. 15-1. Secretary uses a quick reference file for those telephone numbers and addresses that are frequently needed and for the names of the officers of the local dental society. (Courtesy The University of Texas Dental School at San Antonio.)

on her desk. One of these has been set up for patients, with their names, addresses, phone numbers, names of their children, and so on. The other, flip-type of card index is for names and phone numbers of the persons who frequently call or names of persons whom the boss may ask her to call. This latter file takes a bit of ingenuity to develop, for it cannot be the usual type of alphabetical file based only on last names. While Joe, the janitor, will have a card file under his last name, which the secretary finds difficult to pronounce and to remember, she has a card for "janitor," which lists both his name and his phone number in the building and at home (in case of emergency).

Her filing system will largely depend upon her own association of words, names, and functions. She might have a card for "repair" or "service," to let her know the name and number of a company to be called to repair the dental unit or the dental chair. She might list the legal firm that handles her doctor's affairs under "lawyer," "attorney," or "legal." In short, every secretary should have her own little set of "Yellow Pages" to assist her in remembering names and in using the telephone.

The employer's travel plans should be known by the secretary, so that she would be able to reach him in an emergency, and she must know what constitutes an emergency.

Every dentist wants to know if his dental assistant, receptionist, or secretary is learning and progressing. She also should be interested to know if she is growing in her position. If she is not growing at a reasonable rate, the dentist will need to let her know, so that he can seek a new person, and so that she, in turn, can begin looking for a new position. If she is growing and developing, then both the dentist and the dental assistant will feel rewarded in knowing that she is able to meet the challenges and the demands of the new position.

It would be convenient if one could develop a simple paper-pencil examination that could be used for this evaluative purpose, but every office and every responsibility are so different that it is not practical to prepare a single examination to serve everyone's purpose. Some suggested items for a self-made test are given later in this chapter.

Considerable space could be devoted to the discussion of the dress and the grooming of both the dentist and his assistant. Nearly every dental assistant, receptionist, secretary, and dental hygienist automatically recognizes that she is working in a professional office, where attractiveness, neatness, and good taste are tremendously important.

Few girls can afford expensive clothes and daily trips to the hairdresser, but there are attractive white or colored uniforms that are decorative, and it takes only a little time and care to be an attractive addition to the office. The receptionist and secretary in a dental office will dress differently and apply makeup differently than the girls on a movie set or the girls getting ready to go to a dance or a ball. Heavy makeup, eye shadow, false eyelashes, and conspicuous shades of lipstick are usually frowned upon by the dentist-employer.

The new employee will usually be observant and follow the patterns already set by the other people in the office. While this is normally a good guide, it would still be advisable to discuss the matter of dress and makeup with the dentist to see what it is that he feels would be appropriate for his own taste and that of his patients. It is always possible that the dentist will welcome some brightening of his office and encourage his employees to use more makeup than they have been using or more than is being used in some of the neighbor offices.

OBSERVATION

A great many other evaluations of the office operation can be made only by direct observation. Just as the girls in the outer office may not realize how they get in the habit of chattering and wasting time, they often also may not realize that their own office gets to look like a stock room or a rummage sale, instead of like an orderly, professional office.

Some girls come from homes with no flowers or plants to water, and others come from homes where maids or servants take care of these duties. Consequently, some dental assistants have never had the responsibility of arranging an office with good taste and keeping it looking attractive and neat. While the dentist will surely not want to be bothered with the housekeeping chores, he certainly will need a receptionist or a secretary who has sufficient pride in her office surroundings to render this service for him.

How many dentists or dental assistants have ever taken the time to sit in the operating chair or survey the whole office from a patient's point of view? Smudges or cobwebs on the ceiling or at the top of the draperies might escape the view of the cleaning personnel for months, if the dentist or his assistant did not sit in the dental chair once in a while. Only the patient can see the wad of gum that some child has quickly stuck under the bracket table, and it might remain there for a long time, if the dentist and his assistant only looked at things from above.

TEAM APPROACH

Most dentists have weekly conferences with their employees, and even if the dentist has only 1 employee, he ought to set aside some time to discuss with her the operations of the office and the progress or lack of progress that she is making. Some employers like to have their suggestions made in writing, so that the girls can develop a loose-leaf booklet of ideas, and it is expected that the girl will then discuss with her employer the reasons for these suggestions. Unfortunately, some girls are unwilling to accept suggestions and merely assume a defensive attitude when their employer is trying to help them and improve the overall office procedure.

Helpful suggestions cannot always be given in a calendared meeting, because there are times when something critical occupies all of the allotted time. Also, there are instances in which the dentist discovers, when he is working at the office late at night, that the girls have made some mistakes, so he makes a written note of it and draws it to their attention when they come in the next morning. The writing of notes can help the office develop a set of rules and regulations and helpful suggestions that could never be anticipated by trying to write them all at one time.

The dentist who has meetings with his employees will probably want to develop a series of questions that he can ask new employees as he watches them grow. Unless the dentist has employed a series of individuals, he will not understand that one can never take things for granted and assume that every new employee will have the ingenuity to get the answers to many important questions.

Unfortunately, there will always be petty jealousies and feelings of insecurity, but the well-operated offices are those in which everyone realizes that everyone looks good when there is a fine appreciation for the team approach. Imagine what would happen to patients on an operating table if the anesthesiologist thought he was not getting enough attention for his responsibility, and he resented the surgeon getting so much of the praise for the successful operations. If surgeons, anesthesiologists, nurses, and other aides can work successfully as a team when lives are at stake, certainly the members of a dental office should be able to work as a team, for here again patients and even their lives may be at stake.

Consider the matter of emergencies in a dental office. How many receptionists and secretaries would know what number to dial in the case of a fire or a broken water pipe? How many secretaries would know what physician to call if her own boss suffered a coronary failure—or if one of the patients presented special problems that the boss could not handle, and the patient needed help immediately? How many secretaries would have to go to the telephone book to find her employer's home telephone number, so that she could relay a message to his wife?

It is not the difficult duties that cause the problems in the office, for if the secretary has not anticipated something of a difficult nature, this can usually be forgiven. More often, the problems arise when the secretary has made a mistake on something that her employer considered so simple he did not bother to mention it. Therefore, it is the simple things with which the dentist should concern himself and, if possible, even make a list of them for use by his new staff members. Even in the interview prior to employing a new secretary, it might be interesting and helpful to know how she would answer certain basic questions about the operation of an office. This will not only give the dentist some insight of the office training she has previously had, but also will give him some notion as to whether she is frank about admitting that the answer to some questions would have to depend upon the individual office and its special rules and customs.

A few questions that might prod the imagination of a prospective receptionist are as follows:

1. Do you open the boss's personal or confidential mail when he is out of the city?
2. If the boss is attending a dental meeting out of the city, how do you explain this to a patient who has an emergency problem, and how do you see that the patient is cared for?
3. If you were to learn on a Sunday at home that your boss's child had met with a

serious accident, and he is out of the city attending a meeting, what procedures would you follow in an effort to get in touch with him?

4. If you became too sick to come to work one morning, and yet you knew that you were being depended upon to be at the office early to open it up and that the boss would be late getting to the office, what steps would you take?

5. If a dentist in a neighboring office came in to borrow an instrument during the noon hour, and your own boss was not yet back from lunch, how would you handle the situation?

6. If a patient whom you have known as a close friend for many years before coming to work wants to discuss her dental treatment and the estimated fees that she thinks are too high, how would you handle the situation?

7. If a wife of another professional man calls and asks you if your employer will be in the city on a certain date because she is giving a party to which she would like to invite your dentist and his wife, what kind of an answer would you give?

8. If you came to open the office and found that you had forgotten your keys, what would you do?

9. If some national incident occurred that caused the radio announcers and the newspapers to proclaim a holiday for the next day, would you plan to go to work as usual, and what would you do about the scheduled patients?

10. If another dentist in the city were to offer you a position with a $25 per month increase in salary, how would you handle the situation?

Communication

If the dentist-employer expects his secretary-receptionist to type letters of any kind, he ought to take the precautions to have the prospective employee type some letters as a demonstration. This should enable him to know whether she knows how to write a letter, and whether it will be neat and orderly. He may have the habit of drafting some of the significant data and expecting her to locate the details and to set it up for his signature. If his drafts are done hastily, as is often the case, he will also expect her to fill in the missing words, correct the punctuation and grammar, and complete the letter. A rough draft such as shown in Fig. 15-2 might be given to the applicant. She is instructed that this is a very rough draft, and that she is to use her knowledge and skills to correct the spelling and grammar, eliminate duplicated words, insert words that have been omitted, and set the letter up in a neat fashion, ready for the doctor's signature. She may use a dictionary and telephone directory.

Much needs to be done to help receptionists and secretaries to perform a better job in the use of the telephone. The local telephone company usually provides a service that will help receptionists and secretaries, and they also have booklets that give some suggestions and help.

However, it is not only a case of using the right words and the proper sentences; the manner in which the conversation takes place is important. A girl may use the proper words, but her tone of voice may indicate a lack of interest or even be an insulting tone that can and will drive patients away. Curtness and lack of patience, along with slovenly or garbled speech, will also destroy the professional image of the office.

Some receptionists routinely make recordings of the 2-way conversation, or at least of her own part in the conversation. This often proves useful. Also, the employer can learn a little about his own office by calling and learning how the first part of the conversation is conducted prior to identifying himself or being recognized. Patients will often give reports on the way that their telephone problems are handled; these reports can be helpful to both the receptionist and the dentist-employer.

Everyone has mannerisms that they may not recognize without actually hearing, and,

(use current date)

Dr. Joseph Smith
(use residence address)
Savannah

Dear Dr. Smith:

Dr. Wayen johnson; president of the Savannah dental SOCiety, has
asked me to be ehare charemen of a new standing Committee of Post-
graduate Dental Educatin. As yo u know, you and Dr. Johnson,
Dr. Hudson, and Dr. Jones are to be on my committee.
Out first meeding will be on sunday afternoon, December 12, 1965,
at 3 'clock. We shall meet at my home which is at 1283 Akerswood
Road. This will be an introductory meeting and shall try meke it
brief, ending by by 4:30.
With kind personal regards, I remain
Cordially yours,

Walter Weber,ph. D
Dean

Fig. 15-2. Sample rough draft of letter that doctor or his secretary hands to new secretarial applicant for correcting and typing.

therefore, the dentist, as well as his receptionist, may want to make use of recorders to determine how they can improve their own methods of communication. The receptionist might ask a friend to call when she least expects it and ask for an appointment or ask for strange information and then see how she handles the situation.

Tests

While there are many types of examinations and tests that can be used by both the dentist and his assistant to determine the growth of a new employee, most of the growth that takes place will be her knowledge of facts that are related to the office in which she practices and her acquaintance with the people with whom she is working. Therefore, the most effective and most valid tests will probably be those that the dentist or the dentist with his assistant can construct themselves. These tests should include some basic facts that she would be expected to know even before she begins her work, but most of the items will be those that she will be expected to learn as she works in the office and comes in contact with her associates, with other dentists, with the patients, and with sales personnel.

The sample examination on pages 320 to 322 is one that a dentist might use to pattern a test of his own construction.

Responsibility

Fortunately, most employers, whether they be dentists, deans of dental schools, or business executives, are optimistic and hope that the office details that they do not see everyday are going along smoothly. The dentist may happen to come into his office over the weekend and find that his secretary has left a stack of stamped and addressed letters on her desk. Looking at them, he discovers that some are airmail letters about a speech that he was to give. It was important that these go out airmail, so that the letters would be received on Monday. All of the extra work and effort to get the letter dictated, typed, addressed, and stamped has been lost, for it will not arrive in time. Inquiry later shows that his secretary remembered that the mail slot in the building would not take the large-sized envelopes, so she did not mail them. She did not bother to consider the possible importance of the letters, and it did not occur to her to be imaginative and remember that there was a mailbox a block down the street, where she could drop them and where they would be picked up shortly thereafter.

Mistakes such as the foregoing are often irreparable and costly. They are foolish and thoughtless, and yet these things are done more often than one might imagine. Also, they are often made by extremely dedicated persons who would never knowingly do anything to harm their employers or disrupt the office harmony. Mistakes can be and are made by loyal employees and also by the very capable employees. The stupid and malicious people have no patent on making mistakes, but unfortunately a mistake made by a loyal and dedicated person can hurt her employer just as much as a mistake that is done intentionally by another person.

Sometimes, it seems as though an office worker or secretary must be accident prone or mistake prone, judging by the repeated mistakes that she makes. This will often happen with an employee who has been showing good progress and who has been almost a model employee. Rather than being mistake prone, the receptionist in such a case usually, for one reason or another, has become so overly conscious of details that she has lost sight of the overall job she should be trying to do. Some people become so worried and tense about their jobs that they seem to lose all of their efficiency and just sit and shuffle papers. It is often much easier to diagnose such a situation than it is to cure it. Even the girl involved may recognize that she is literally "spinning her wheels" and worrying needlessly about everything in general and nothing specifically, but still she may not be able to pull herself out of the worrying state. Frequently, an excellent secretary will become overly sensitive about every suggestion and every correction that her employer makes, even though she has previously accepted criticism, knowing that it was meant to be constructive and helpful. The secretary may become overly sensitive about the careless remarks of other employees and let these worry her to the extent that she can not do her job as efficiently as she formerly did. Again, many employees even realize what their problem is and yet seem to be unable to correct the situation by simply ignoring the problem.

It is very easy for one to say that when one has excellent teamwork in an office, the office will be very efficient and pleasant to work in. This is not only a good theory, but it is also very true. The difficulty is that every worker is human, and an office is the combined effect of all of the employees. If one knows the problems that one of the employees may be having at home, it may be understandable why she cannot help but have her work at the office influenced by these outside worries. However, one usually does not know this at the time that she makes some unkind or thoughtless comment, and this may set off a series of misunderstandings and hard feelings. The employer has not the time to become a constant counselor and advisor to each of his employees, or he would not get any of his own work done, and he hopes that his employees will be mature and understanding enough to leave their personal problems at home and to try to work harmoniously together at the office.

If everyone in the office could only remember that the things that seem to be problems today will seem insignificant and unimportant 6 months from now, there would be fewer upheavals and crises.

If everyone could also realize that in

Name ______________________ Date ____________

Months of experience in dental office ______________________

Months of experience in this office ______________________

Nomenclature

1. What is meant by each of the following abbreviations?
   a. D.D.S. ______________________
   b. D.M.D. ______________________
   c. M.D. ______________________
   d. D.V.M. ______________________
   e. B.A. ______________________
   f. C.D.A. ______________________
   g. R.D.H. ______________________
   h. C.D.T. ______________________
   i. F.A.C.D. ______________________
   j. F.I.C.D. ______________________
   k. A.D.A. ______________________
   l. A.M.A. ______________________
   m. A.D.A.A. ______________________
   n. A.D.H.A. ______________________
   o. R.N. ______________________
   p. R.Ph. ______________________

2. What is meant by the following?
   a. Orthodontics ______________________
   ____
   b. Pedodontics ______________________
   ____
   c. Prosthodontics ______________________
   ____
   d. Periodontics ______________________
   ____
   e. Oral surgery ______________________
   ____
   f. Endodontics ______________________
   ____

3. Define:
   a. Amalgam ______
   b. Calculus ______
   c. Caries ______
   d. Articulator ______
   e. Benign ______
   f. Biopsy ______
   g. Buccal ______
   h. Cavity ______
   i. Denture ______
   j. Edentulous ______
   k. Exodontics ______
   l. Distal ______
   m. Enamel ______
   n. Fissure ______
   o. Gingiva ______
   p. Anesthetic ______
   q. Fracture ______
   r. Fluoridation ______
   s. Incisor ______
   t. Inlay ______
   u. Interproximal space ______
   v. Mandible ______
   w. Malocclusion ______

4. Give the name of the following:
   a. President of local dental society ______
   b. President of state dental society ______
   c. Secretary of local dental society ______
   d. Secretary of state licensing board ______

e. President of local dental assistants' society ______________________

____

f. President of local dental hygienists' society ______________________

____

g. Dental school from which your employer is a graduate ______________________

____

h. City in which the next state dental association meeting will be held ______________________

____

i. City in which the next national meeting of the American Dental Assistants' Association will be held ______________________

____

j. Mayor of the city ______________________

____

k. Employer's personal physician ______________________

____

l. The civic clubs of which employer is a member ______________________

____

m. The national organizations of which employer is a member ______________________

____

almost every instant, the person who has made the mistake or who has made the cutting remark either has some significant problems, or that some unimportant misunderstanding or lack of communications has caused the problem, there would be less retaliating. If even the first person involved did not try to retaliate and teach someone a lesson, there would not be any serious misunderstandings at the office.

There is not space or time in this chapter to fully explain how to squelch the office rumors or how to successfully ignore the statements that seem critical, even though they were not intended in that way.

Office personnel who have a dedication to the office and what it stands for and who are proud of their responsibilities will find that they will always be able to work harmoniously as a team.

When the people in an office know the meaning of the word "teamwork," there will be no caste system in the office. Just as the quarterback may be selected to call the plays in a football game, this does not mean that he or anyone else thinks that he is so important that he could win the game without the other 10 men on his team there to do their respective assignments. The same applies in a dental office. Even the most menial task of answering a telephone is an important part in keeping that office in business and letting it make the money that will pay everyone's salary. Remember that even the boss has to do some menial tasks. While his "image" is that of a dental practitioner or surgeon in a spotless operatory, he often takes time away from this role to visit with a worried patient or an upset child. He often works on the adjustment of equipment in his office, even though he could easily have had the service man repair it; he may "peck out" a note to an old friend on the office typewriter, rather than dictating it to the secretary. The doctor may help seal the envelopes before the mail is picked up, when he finds that all of the girls are busy. In a successful dental office, no one stands on ceremony, and no one feels that they are too important to perform some simple, routine task that is usually done by a beginning clerk.

Each secretary, each receptionist, and each person who has some of these responsibilities in the office from time to time should be proud of the fact that she is a key person in that office. This is the one position in any office that never really becomes routine or uninteresting. Every day brings new people, new problems, new challenges, and new chances to make her an even more important cog in the wheel of that whole office operation.

If is true that an employer cannot always be noticing all of the fine things and important bits of public relations that a secretary does for the office, and he cannot be complimenting her continuously. However, he knows the worth of a good secretary-receptionist. She should be proud of the office, of her employer, and of the job that she can do for both of them.

Remember, as mentioned before in this book, if the boss looks good, then each individual staff member also looks good. The converse is also true; if the individual members of the office staff look good, then the boss also looks good.

CONCLUDING REMINDER

There is undoubtedly no other single chapter in this textbook that has been assigned by more dentists and employers than Chapter 15. This chapter has been assigned as required reading by many dentists who have wanted their secretaries and receptionists to learn some new ways of doing things. Deans, personnel managers, and dental dealers have considered the suggestions and ideas in this chapter worthy of their own office staff's studying.

The reports that have come back from these dentists and the other employers have indicated that in every different type of office, secretaries and receptionists have some of the same abilities and shortcomings. For example, there are a large number who read a chapter like this and proceed immediately to put the ideas into action. There are a few, however, who scan over the chapter but find nothing in it that they want to take the trouble to put into operation.

Some students and some secretaries read an assignment with the notion that it is probably interesting and important for someone else, but that their own boss or employer does not really mean for them to profit from it. As suggested earlier in this chapter, the dentists and other employers need to test their secretaries and receptionists from time to time to see if they have profited from the assignments and suggestions that have been made. Obtaining a job or a position is one thing; holding on to it is another. Similarly, one may expect that salary increments will come to depend upon one's ability to demonstrate improvement and growth. Certainly an employer can expect his employee to learn from the assignments that he takes the time to give her. He will also be giving raises based upon the improvements that she can invent for herself.

CHAPTER 16 UNDERSTANDING THE PATIENT

JACK C. MILLER, B.A., M.S.W.

EDITOR'S INTRODUCTION

It is not enough for the dentist to understand the patient. Everyone who comes in contact with the patient in the dental office must be well enough acquainted with the patient that he can be an efficient member of the dental team and provide the help and the treatment that this patient seeks and needs. The dental assistant, as receptionist and secretary, will come in contact with all patients; hence, she will need to know something of their background and their individual needs when helping to introduce and orient them to the dental office and the dental operatory.

The dental assistant who works at the chairside also has an important role to play in helping her dentist provide dental care to the patient. She, too, must realize that she has an important role to play, not only in assisting her dentist, but also in allaying the possible fears and apprehensions of the patient.

The same person who enters a movie, enters a supermarket, drives into a filling station, goes to a sale on dresses, attends a church social, and goes to the physician's or dentist's office, goes to these places with different objectives and different frames of mind. The salesman who welcomes a potential customer knows his objectives and quickly tries to find out something about the person, so that he may properly orient the would-be customer. However, the salesman knows that the customer enters his business establishment with a different frame of mind than the customer does when he goes to his dentist or his physician.

It is important for the success of the dental office that the dental receptionist and the chairside assistant both recognize that the person coming to them for treatment may be apprehensive for any of many reasons and may have real fears. The reasons for the fears and apprehensions are not always easily understood, and they are not always obvious.

When the dental assistant chose the health profession as a career, she knew that this profession was not going to be as simple and mundane as being a saleswoman. Meeting the patient and trying to understand him should be her reward for selecting the health profession as a responsibility. Learning to know the patient, discovering the patient's special worries, and discovering ways of making the patient feel at ease in the office and in the operatory require some special talents and expertise that not everyone possesses and not everyone can develop. Being an excellent receptionist and an exceptional chairside assistant is not something that everyone can accomplish—it is a real challenge.

• • •

JUDGMENT AND DECISION-MAKING

As a person goes about his daily activities, he makes countless judgments and decisions; some are automatic, habitual, and formed with little or no awareness, while others require varying degrees of conscious thought, analysis, and evaluation. A significant element in the processes of judging and decision-making is one's set of beliefs and values;* that is, his estimate of the relative worth, importance, or excellence of things. Values are standards or measures of goodness and badness, pleasantness and unpleasantness, desirability or undesirability, effectiveness or ineffectiveness, degrees of good and bad. Some values are utilitarian, or of value because of what they will do. Other values are intrinsic, or valued for themselves, aside from what they will do.

Interwoven with norms or standards, values and disvalues (lack of values) become guides for deciding what is right or wrong, what is appropriate or inappropriate behavior, what is ethical or unethical action. Dental practitioners are continually helping people change their disvalues regarding their mouths into healthful values. If mouth care is not perceived as being valuable, a patient is not apt to take care of his mouth, or to take care of his mouth as adequately as the person who has strong convictions regarding the desirability and effectiveness of preventive home care.

To say a person's teeth are straight or crooked may be an objective fact, but to say they are beautiful or unattractive is to express a value judgment. Other people may not agree with this judgment, because their concepts of beauty, attractiveness, or normality are different. A value judgment, then, is an estimate of value, rather than an assessment of the objective characteristics of a person, people, situations, or actions. Value judgments can create misunderstanding, when they are interpreted as an objective appraisal. To say a patient is a trying or difficult person may be an objective assertion, but it usually means the patient's behavior is censored by some system of personal values.

Another determinant in the processes of judging and decision-making is the knowledge of facts gained through investigation, observation, and study. However, if one examines the process of decision-making, he will observe situations in which judgment and decisions are made on the basis of inaccurate information or information that is believed to be true but is not really in accord with established fact. At one time, it was considered common knowledge that the world was flat, and this belief influenced the theory and practice of navigating the oceans. Professions that deal with the lives of people place great value on accuracy and completeness of knowledge, because human life is precious.

A third factor in making judgment is drawing inferences, a process not based on direct observation. Since one cannot possibly know all there is to know, inference is a useful process in reasoning or problem-solving. In this process, a conclusion is based on other facts, premises, or indications. A patient's teeth are dirty—an observable fact. One may infer that the patient's home care of his mouth is not adequate. Inferences may be valid or invalid. It is common knowledge that children's deciduous teeth are replaced by permanent dentition. Some parents infer that since the "baby" teeth will be lost in a relatively short time, they do not need as much care as the permanent teeth. There is also a value judgment here—the deciduous teeth are not considered as important as permanent teeth by these parents.

*For futher examination of this subject, see Rokeach, M.: Beliefs, attitudes, and values, San Francisco, 1969, Jossey-Bass, Inc., Publishers.

A patient comes to a dental office for help with a problem, and he expresses a desire for relief of pain or restoration of a decayed tooth, for example. Implied in his purpose is his dependence on and expectation of others for professional judgment, based upon ethical values relative to his needs, a solid body of knowledge as a basis for decision-making, and sound reasoning in the problem-solving process. These 3 qualities are extremely important in diagnosis, in treatment-planning, in treatment including the fabrication of appliances, and in the working relationship.

One might infer from the foregoing that judgment regarding a patient's well-being is exclusively the function of the doctor-member of the dental team. The exercise of judgment in the performance of his roles and tasks is a function of each member of the team. There are differences in the kinds of judgments required of each team member.

The dental team is a social system, in that it is a group of people engaged in organized activities that are interrelated and interdependent. They are united by common goals and values relating to the care of people who have dental problems. Members of the team occupy positions that exist in terms of relationships with other positions—dentist, chairside assistant, hygienist, receptionist, technician, accountant, janitor. There may be other positions, or several positions may be combined into one.

Attached to each position are activities, functions, or duties (roles), which the occupant of a position is expected to carry out. Thus, the dentist's roles in relation to the patient are history-taking, examination, diagnosis, treatment-planning, patient counseling in some areas, patient education, treatment, and evaluation. The dentist may have other roles in addition to his patient-caring roles, such as consultation with other professionals, administration, supervision of his staff.

A role is accompanied by tasks or physical operations that perform some function in relation to the role. For instance, patient examination is a role that usually includes the tasks of taking, developing, and mounting x-rays, and reading or interpreting them. The act of taking x-rays requires careful judgment by the person performing the task, whether it be the dentist or other member of the team. Roles and tasks, then, may be delegated to or shared with other team members. The specific roles and tasks of an assistant are examined elsewhere in this book.

Roles are important, because they are related to specific responsibilities—who will be responsible for what, and when. They may suggest how each member acts in relation to the others, and these actions may involve decision-making. One needs to understand and accept the roles and tasks that accompany his position, as well as their limitations, as the basis for his judgment and decision-making. Lastly, one needs to understand and accept the other persons' positions, roles, and tasks, and their relation to his own.

If one is not aware of his personal limitations, or if he does not regard and respect the rights and responsibilities of his colleagues, he might assume responsibilities outside the scope of his position. Such action may create tension or even conflict, because he has usurped the role of another person, or because he has disrupted the organizational pattern of the team. One may also create ill feelings among others whose roles are interdependent by incompetent performance or by inappropriate decisions, leading to inadequate performance or behavior.

Judgment—the mental ability to perceive, discern, and distinguish relationships and alternatives, and make reasonable decisions—is inherent in the performance of roles and tasks at all levels of responsibility. There are differences and variables in the positions and roles of a team in relation to the patient. Some are of primary value and significance to the patient, such as the surgical role of the dentist. Other positions and roles are supportive, facilitative, or enabling.

Since the dental team exists for the benefit of people who seek dental care, understanding patients is of great value in the working relationship, especially for those who are in contact with the patient. The study of people and their behavior is so vast and complex that a chapter such as this can only present some views that seem relevant and useful. This chapter is not intended to prepare the team to become therapists, such as psychiatrists or clinical psychologists; its purpose is to present some ideas that may make one's performance more effective and rewarding. This chapter will enhance one's awareness that a patient is a person, like oneself, who feels, thinks, and acts not at all ideally, and that patient behavior does not just happen capriciously, but is the product of identifiable forces and processes. What may seem to be senseless behavior appears that way because the observer does not know and understand the nature of the behavior, the forces and processes that are components of the behavior. If one can sense some of the components of the patient's behavior and can be aware of his own part in the situation, he is more apt to carry out his roles with better judgment than if he were unaware of these behavioral elements.

DIMENSIONS OF BEHAVIOR

To understand patients is to consider their behavior, for it is through behavior that one discloses himself to others. Behavior is often defined as anything a person does. The act of reading this book or discussing it is a form of behavior. A patient behaves when he telephones the dental office to make an appointment; the person who answers the call is behaving. Other forms of behavior in a dental situation are history-taking, taking and developing x-rays, discussing diagnosis with a patient, giving an injection, filling a cavity, extracting a tooth, handing the dentist an instrument, removing sutures, teaching a patient how to keep his teeth clean, typing a letter, and keeping books. Different people in a given situation may behave differently. Thus, a patient who meets appointments regularly and promptly is behaving, as is the patient who is frequently tardy or uncooperative in the chair.

Behavior has dimensions other than acts of doing something. For example, one might read this chapter with little or no enjoyment, perhaps with boredom and dissatisfaction. Another might read it with enjoyment, gratification, or satisfaction. A member of a dental team may derive a sense of achievement, security, and self-fulfillment while working with other members, but another may feel frustration, anger, and depression while working in a dental office. A patient, likewise, may feel varying degrees of comfort or discomfort, satisfaction or dissatisfaction, with the dental operations or the behaviors of the various members of the team. Feelings, then, comprise a dimension of behavior.

The third dimension of behavior is thinking. One might read this book with only casual thought given to the content, perhaps merely pronouncing words, with no comprehension of what is being read. Another person might pause upon reading an idea to contemplate its meaning and implications. He might turn to a dictionary or another person for further clarification. The acts of making an appointment, answering the telephone, or interviewing involve thinking, as do such activities as cavity preparation, surgery, selecting an instrument, and cleaning the operatory. There are various levels of thinking, ranging from the simplest sensation and perception to reasoning and creation.

Two other dimensions that are intertwined with the action, feeling, and thinking components of behavior are cause and consequence. One may read this book in response to an assignment by an instructor, who, no doubt, has reasons or purposes for his action in designating this book for study. There may be other reasons or motivations than the fact it was assigned, such as intent to discover the knowledge, the talents, attitudes, and skills that one needs in order to be competent in performing the behaviors that characterize the work of an auxiliary.

Behavior is frequently the product of multiple and changing causes. While causes are often known and identifiable, some motivations are obscure and may not be understood, even to the actor himself. A patient may talk incessantly and repetitiously, out of anxiety. A person may giggle or laugh, out of nervousness or embarrassment that is more or less consciously recognized. A law-enforcement officer, widely recognized for his ability and courage in facing desperate criminals and bringing them to trial, had a toothache. In the dental chair, he became pale and visibly trembled. In explanation of this behavior, he said this situation was one in which he felt he was not in control. One wonders if he could explain why he had a need always to be in control. A 4-year-old child who continually and vigorously sucks his thumb is not apt to be able to explain his motivations for this behavior.

Some behaviors yield productive and constructive responses and results. Preventive home care, when consistently and adequately performed, tends to preserve the teeth, minimize dental caries, and contribute to one's sense of well-being. Other behaviors are frustrating and sometimes destructive, not only to other persons, but also to the individual himself. Some adults, for example, have only nominal anxiety and fear in the daily process of living; however, in a dental chair, they experience great difficulty in cooperating, because of intense feelings of fear and anxiety they are unable to explain, and they are annoyed with themselves.

To recapitulate, behavior includes not only what one does, but also one's feelings, or emotions, and thoughts. All behavior has cause, reason, purpose, or motivation. People are individuals who are not patterned from the same mold; individuals in a similar situation behave differently, because their thoughts, values, feelings, and motivations differ.

PERSON OF THE PATIENT

It can be said that a patient is a person who has a health problem. What is this person who is the concern of the health professions? One approach to this question is the concept of man as a *somato-* (*bio-*, or *physio-*) *psycho-social* being, who is in continual interaction with his physical and social environment.* According to one current concept, every disease in every patient has a somatic component, a psychologic component, and a sociocultural component. Health is also seen as the ability to function effectively in a given environment, and disease is the lack of ease in such functioning.

Derived from the Greek term *soma,* meaning body, *somato-* signifies the physical nature and characteristics of man. As a somatic being, man is a complex network of intricately designed parts, which, under normal conditions, are constantly working in coordination. Thus, the study of anatomy pertains to the shape and structure of the body and its organs and systems, such as the digestive system, cardiovascular system, and central nervous system. A structural defect of the mouth is the cleft palate, which affects chewing, swallowing, and speech. Physiology is concerned with function—how the organs do their various jobs and how the systems of the body work. Biochemistry pertains to the chemical reactions involved in the functioning of cells, tissues, organs, and systems.

Physiologic conditions, such as hunger,

*For further elaboration of this concept, see Kaluger, G., and Unkovic, C. M.: Psychology and sociology, St. Louis, 1969, The C. V. Mosby Co., and Dubos, R.: Man adapting, New Haven, Connecticut, 1965, Yale University Press.

thirst, bladder and colon pressure, temperature, sexual desire, restlessness, fatigue, and drowsiness represent needs and stimulate the individual to take in food and liquid, to eliminate, to dress, to copulate, to be active, to rest, or to sleep. These needs stimulate action; hence, how a person copes with these needs is his behavior.

These behaviors occur not only in man, but also in other forms of animal life, so that we might contemplate the characteristics that distinguish human life from other forms of life. The body is the cornerstone of personality, but a person is more than a collection of physical matter. When we look about us, we see people engaged in activities beyond those of meeting somatic needs. Man has a wider range of freedom in deciding to act and in the choice of action. He becomes aware of his existence, develops consciousness of self, becomes aware of his future, and determines a course of action accordingly. Man could not develop these characteristics without learning, together with a process of storing information (memory). An astonishing human characteristic is the faculty of forgetting and conscious remembering of past experience. These are workings of the mind.

The words psychologic and psychic are derived from the Greek *psyche,* meaning *spirit, soul, mind.* The American Heritage Dictionary of the English Language defines *psyche* as the mind, functioning as the center of thought, feeling, and behavior, and consciously or unconsciously adjusting and relating the body to its social and physical environment. It has been previously indicated that a person is recognized by what he does, which is influenced by his powers of thinking and emotions.

The intellect is the mental faculty involved in knowing and thinking, learning, memory, and consciousness. Other mental operations include the power of perception, the ability to perçeive differences and relationships, and such higher mental functions as the use of logic, the ability to reason in exercising judgment and solving problems. Intellectual functioning ranges from a lower level of sensation, perception, and memory, through higher levels of imagination and comparison, to conception, reasoning, and creation. In other words, there are differences in intellectual powers among individuals; thus, some are mentally retarded, while others have superior intelligence, and most are in-between.

Some persons have heard about the bacterial theory of tooth decay with more or less comprehension, but do not remember it; others remember it and apply it in their preventive maintenance behavior. Still others remember, but do not apply the theory. The intellect functions when a member of the dental team analyzes the patient's problems and formulates a diagnosis or, through his teaching activities, enables a patient to learn. These, as well as other dental operations, involve problem-solving thinking processes. Some people solve problems by careful analysis and reasoning; other make impulsive decisions, based largely upon emotional processes.

The emotions comprise an element of the human mind distinct from the intellect. Emotions are the feelings one experiences, such as joy, sorrow, happiness, depression, love, anger, fear, and guilt. Other feelings are senses of frustration, failure, success, achievement or accomplishment, security, self-confidence, safety, inadequacy, inferiority, apprehension, anxiety, and so on.

While distinct from the intellect, the emotions are linked to the thought processes. Feelings accompany thoughts. It may seem strange that a person can have mixed feelings and thoughts, that he can simultaneously want and not want, or that he can love and hate at the same time. An individual knows his teeth are diseased, and he earnestly wants to have them restored to a normal condition; yet he does not want to go through the processes of restoration because of fear of pain. One does not like pain and sometimes tries to avoid it by actions that are not really helpful. Thus, an individual may avoid thinking about his diseased teeth, or he may procrastinate excessively.

Sometimes the emotions are aroused so strongly that the intellect does not adequately function. Tension, worry, anger, and fear can affect the ability to think straight. Fear can be so great that one becomes panic-stricken. Witness in the dental chair a child whose fears overpower his ability to listen, much less reason. The child's immaturity and relative helplessness make him particularly susceptible to fears of people or things in his environment that he perceives as dangerous.

A person may acquire fears from earlier painful or disturbing medical or dental experiences. A tonsillectomy may be very stressful to a patient, evoking painful associations, so that he is afraid of any treatment of any kind. Earlier experiences, in some instances, have a special meaning for the patient, and the fear is not really associated with pain, but rather with bodily mutilation or even death. He may be aware of the real concerns, but frequently he is not conscious of them, or only partially aware of them. The patient's inferences or interpretations that lead to fear may seem irrational to others, but to the individual they are real. It is better to treat him with respect and understanding than to ridicule or talk down to him for having such unreal thoughts.

A boy refused to permit a model to be made of his teeth. He was led to express his ideas associated with the procedure. Through listening to him rather than lecturing to him, it was learned that he was afraid the "white stuff" for taking impressions would harden in his mouth and could not be taken out. His inference was that if he could not chew food and swallow, he would die. He was helped to cope with his fears by being permitted to see and handle the impression material. In this process, the qualities of the material were discussed. Then he placed the material in a tray himself. His fear diminished, and he was able to carry out his role as a patient.

A 7-year-old girl was extremely fearful of dental treatment, especially the injection procedure. Through counseling, she was helped to express her concerns and to recall earlier experiences. It was learned that, more unconsciously than consciously, she was afraid the needle would cause her mouth to die. The origins of this strange fear were traced to earlier experiences and the meanings they had for her. At age five, she suffered a broken arm below the elbow, and she wore a cast. This was her dominant arm, and it was difficult for her to eat or to play, and she wondered if the arm would ever get well. It was temporarily like the arm of one who has suffered infantile paralysis. Functionally, a paralyzed arm is, in effect, dead. At 3 years of age, a stomach pump was used to remove food; this process made her sick. She worried that it would "suck out" her stomach, remove her stomach as well as clean it out. The arm healed perfectly; she did not lose her stomach, and she was able to eat all kinds of food. Several years had elapsed since she had had these experiences, yet she was fearful.

These earlier experiences left an imprint upon the girl's mind that became a largely unconscious frame of reference, by which she considered the use of the needle in injections. The counseling process enabled her to recall half-forgotten material and to distinguish between fact and fantasy. She was freed of her fears and became a most cooperative patient, even eager to come to the dental clinic. When her treatment was concluded, it appeared likely that she had been freed from her fears for the rest of her life. One might speculate that when this girl becomes an adult and a mother, perhaps she will help her children develop suitable attitudes, values, and knowledge about their mouths, dental disease, and treatment.

Origins of fears are not limited to specific earlier medical or dental experiences. There are individuals who have had favorable medical or dental experiences, and yet they are afraid in a dental situation. Their fears may stem from the vicissitudes or changes of fortune, as illustrated in the following situation.*

A 12-year-old girl with no significant medical or dental experiences was extremely fearful in the dental chair. Interviews with her paternal grandmother disclosed that the child had had 3 mothers, and her father was unstable, both emotionally and occupationally. From the first year of life, she had moved many times. During the year preceding dental care, she lived with her grandparents, and her grandmother became the first person in whom she experienced confidence, faith, and trust. She felt deprived and was angry with the world for being deprived.

Her student-dentist and an instructor guided the girl through an intellectual experience of discovery, through examination of the "gunk" on her teeth by means of a microscope. The preparation of a model of her mouth, which was given her to keep, helped her acquire a realistic image of her mouth (body image). She participated in various steps of filling a cavity in an extracted tooth, thereby substituting the known for the unknown. Lastly, she put plastic clay on a model of teeth to simulate the gums; then she practiced giving shots with a syringe used in dental practice. In this process, she learned that the needle only went a short distance into the soft tissues, and that it was flexible and did not break. She learned to give the shot very slowly, so that the medicine could be absorbed. These experiences broadened her knowledge, and she found them interesting, exciting, and satisfying. Of particular significance, she learned that there are people who care and can be trusted.

Sometimes a person does not need explanations as much as experience. Put into words, the girl's behavior said, "People are interested in me. I am no longer nothing. I am a somebody." She became highly motivated in learning preventive maintenance, even requesting reading material. Although she did not like to have an injection in subsequent treatment, she was able to effectively cope with it, as well as other fear-arousing procedures. These other procedures included the application of a rubber dam, which may be perceived as a threat to breathing, and cavity preparation, filling cavities, and periodontal surgery, all of which may be perceived as pain-inducing.

This patient's behavior with people at home, in the classroom, at play, and in the clinic are examples of social behavior, or interaction between persons. Social behavior is behavior that occurs in response to the presence and/or activity of another person (or persons), even if the latter is not physically present.

The term "social" is derived from the Latin *socius,* meaning *assembly,* ally, partner, companion, fellowship, sharing. Sociology, concerned as it is with man's life in groups, is the study of the behavior of human beings with, to, against, and for one another, and of the resulting arrangements of relationships and activities that comprise society. The term "society" connotes a large grouping of human beings who share a more or less common way of life. Smaller groupings of people are the community, neighborhood, family, couple, and doctor and patient.

Beyond the notion of an aggregate or collection of individuals, "social" denotes a reciprocating or alternating process between 2 or more individuals (or groups). Meanings are exchanged by communication through language (verbal or written), symbols, nonverbal sounds, gestures, body movement, and, indeed, behavior.

Individuals are interacting when they converse, exchange goods and services, attend religious services, play together, fall in love, marry, and procreate. Not only sociologists, but also teachers and students, healers and patients, buyers and sellers, em-

*See Erikson, E. H.: Eight ages of man. In Childhood and society, New York, 1963, W. W. Norton & Co., Inc.

ployers and employees, parents and children, and many other persons are concerned with and give varying degrees of attention to the processes or types of human interaction, such as competition, conflict, arbitration, mediation, compromise, conciliation, accommodation, cooperation, and assimulation.

One has only to examine his own processes of daily living to see that, as a social being, he interacts with or is dependent upon other human beings for meeting his physiologic needs and for his intellectual and emotional satisfactions. One could not manage in a community nowadays without stores to purchase food, clothing, and other necessary goods and luxuries, without firms or agencies to provide utilities, without water, sewage, or educational facilities for himself and his children, without recreational facilities, without health practitioners, clinics, and hospitals, or without lawmaking and law-enforcing agencies.

SITUATION OF PATIENT IN DENTAL OFFICE

A patient is a person with a health problem that he cannot resolve without help and who comes to a place where a professional person helps him by performing certain procedures or engaging in a series of activities. These individuals, along with the doctor's staff (team), and sometimes the patient's family, comprise a social group in which there is interaction, or interpersonal behavior of some kind, among the members of the group. That is, each person in some manner acts upon, or influences, and reacts, or responds, to each of the others in the group and to the group as a whole.

Some kind of social behavior exists in the group. A curt, impatient receptionist may arouse feelings of resentment in a patient, who then carries over these feelings to the doctor or other members of the team. A patient may be enabled to endure dental operations by being permitted to hold an assistant's hand while the dentist is performing some operation upon the patient. Patients want their desires known: they want to be understood, and they feel frustrated if, during the history-taking process or some other operation, they are not given the opportunity to communicate their feelings and wants. Frustration breeds anger. Anger is equated with energy, which needs to be discharged, and how this energy is discharged often becomes a problem.

One may not comprehend the meaning of a patient's behavior; that is, he may not understand the cause. Yet, by his own accepting, nonjudgmental behavior (as opposed to rejecting, critical, ridiculing, condescending behavior), he can help the patient cope more effectively with the situation. Perhaps one can be receptive of another's behavior, because he is aware he does not understand, and because he can be accepting of his own limitations.

When the relationship among the members of a group is sympathetic and harmonious, rapport is achieved, and the group functions effectively in resolving the patient's problem. There are, however, situations in which rapport is disturbed, or never attained, and this condition becomes an obstacle or impediment to the accomplishment of the treatment goals. These unfortunate situations may be minimized, even prevented, if the patient is seen as a person, a human being, who somehow has acquired information and misinformation, who has partial understandings, who experiences varying degrees of tension, anxiety, fear, and anger, and who is capable of mixed feelings of wanting and not wanting at the same time. These are all associated with his health problem and/or the treatment, as he perceives them. It is probable that he perceives them differently than the other members of the group, since they have not had his life experiences, and he has not had theirs.

From the operator's standpoint, it would be preferable if a person could leave his unproductive thoughts and emotions at home when he comes to the doctor's office, clinic, or hospital, but the mind and body in combination make up the whole person. Therefore, he brings his thoughts and feelings along with his dental problem. A dental assistant might want to avoid knowing about the gaps in the patient's store of information, or his tensions and fears, but to do so can create or worsen behavioral problems, since one's expectations of the patient will probably be inappropriate.

Emotional distrubances may be causative factors in a disease; they may be by-products of the disease and aggravate the condition; and they may be an impediment in the treatment processes. A student-dentist had had little experience with small children, and he did not understand them. He spoke in words far above their ability to comprehend, and there were long silences during which he wished he could say something. He became unusually anxious when he was assigned a 5-year-old child, his youngest patient. She came to the clinic with very little apprehension, but she soon sensed his anxiety, and she became tense and uncooperative. When he was helped to understand the child's level of development, her needs for understanding and security, and how to guide her thoughts and the expression of her thoughts and feelings, he became more comfortable in her presence. She quickly responded to the change in his feelings by relaxing her own tensions, and she easily carried out her role as a patient.

Man has evolved codes of behavior, called ethics, which are guides to the determination of right or wrong behavior of individuals or groups in relation to other individuals. Professions that attend to the well-being of clients or patients have developed codes of behavior that are based on general ethics. Professional ethics are principles of right and wrong conduct, as they pertain to the profession's unique role in society. These principles, in part, are concerned with the rights of the clients or patients, who, by virtue of their needs, are dependent upon the professional's judgment. Thus, information given the professional, called privileged communication, is considered confidential and is expected to be treated with respect. Ethical implications in the processes of diagnosis, treatment-planning, and treatment can be explored by such questions as the following: What is best for this particular patient, a somatopsychosocial being? Who will do what in the treatment of this person's disease? Is he qualified to do so? How can each team member best carry out his functions in the best interests of the patient?

In summary, the patient, the doctor, and his staff comprise a social group, in which each member behaves in response to the presence and actions of the others. The more adequately the members are adjusted to their roles in the group, the more smoothly will the group function in achieving its goals of resolving the dental problems of the patient-members. A working knowledge of human behavior, empathy, ability to feel with compassion and to think with dispassion, awareness and acceptance of one's own behavior, and skills in relating to others are desirable attributes for persons who comprise the dental team.

Suggested readings

Bloom, S. W.: The doctor and his patient, New York, 1963, Russell Sage Foundation.

Dubos, R.: Man adapting, New Haven, Connecticut, 1965, Yale University Press.

Erikson, E. H.: Childhood and society, New York, 1963, W. W. Norton & Co., Inc.

Horton, P. B.: Sociology and the health sciences, New York, 1965, McGraw-Hill Book Co.

Kaluger, G., and Unkovic, C. M.: Psychology and sociology, St. Louis, 1969, The C. V. Mosby Co.

Krech, D., and Crutchfield, R.: Elements of psychology, New York, 1969, Alfred A. Knopf, Inc.

Overstreet, B. W.: Understanding fear in ourselves and others, New York, 1951, Harper & Row, Publishers.

Rokeach, M.: Beliefs, attitudes, and values, San Francisco, 1969, Jossey-Bass, Inc., Publishers.

Strecker, E. A., and Appel, K. E.: Discovering ourselves, New York, 1962, The Macmillan Co.

CHAPTER 17 MAINTAINING DENTAL EQUIPMENT

CHARLES O. CRANFORD, D.D.S.
ROGER E. BARTON, D.D.S.

The dream of every equipment manufacturer is the eventual development of all equipment to the point where no maintenance procedures need to be performed by the purchaser. Engineering research in recent years has led to a definite reduction in the frequency of maintenance and has, in some instances, completely eliminated some of the previously required care by the operator. For example, some new bearings are completely sealed and lubricated at the factory, and many electric motors require no maintenance by the operator. Also, much equipment is being miniaturized, and the use of sealed components is becoming increasingly popular. In spite of these improvements in engineering technology, the widespread development of maintenance-free equipment is still some distance in the future.

The assistant who has had the experience of owning and taking care of an automobile will understand the principle of periodic maintenance. Regular maintenance is regarded so highly by some auto manufacturers that they prescribe a definite schedule and checklist of maintenance procedures for the owner to follow, and, in some instances, the manufacturer's warranty is voided, if the maintenance program is not carried out as instructed.

Although most of these prescribed requirements are basic maintenance procedures that must be done at a service center, there are additional procedures that improve the function and the life of the automobile. These include regular lubrication of doors and latches, servicing of the battery and tires, and cleaning and polishing of exposed surfaces. Not only do these procedures improve the efficiency of the machine, but they enhance the pride of ownership that is felt when operating a clean, well-maintained automobile.

Similarly, the dental assistant will recognize the importance of maintaining the equipment with which she works from day to day. Modern and well-constructed equipment used in the dental office should give many years of useful service. However, it will not perform satisfactorily over a long period of time without proper and regular care. It is obvious that the dental team must have properly functioning equipment, if an efficient and profitable practice is to be conducted. The assistant performs a great service by organizing and carrying out a thorough maintenance program in the dental office.

Just as the auto manufacturer has prescribed a regular maintenance program for the vehicles he produces, the dental equipment manufacturer has designed a maintenance program for the dental office. Instructions regarding this prescribed maintenance program are usually delivered at the time the equipment is delivered or installed. The assistant should file these instructions and refer to them for guidance in caring for the equipment. If these instructions are not available in the dental office, the dealer or manufacturer will be willing to supply them upon request. A few minutes spent in studying this material may save the dental team hours of unnecesary delay and the frustration of having to cope with malfunctioning equipment.

Since the maintenance of equipment is so important to the operation of the dental office, it should not be approached carelessly by the dental assistant. In order to be sure that preventive maintenance is carried out correctly and at the proper time, the assistant should devise a schedule for systematically performing the necessary procedures.

Some maintenance must be done daily, whereas other functions are done weekly, monthly, or bimonthly. A good way to be sure that preventive maintenance is performed when needed is to make up a schedule listing the various tasks and the dates on which they are to be performed. A notebook, card file, or special calendar may be used for this purpose. Although the list may be long, each task performed as scheduled will actually take very little time.

The assistant is not expected to perform major repairs on equipment. Her role is in preventive maintenance, and she should not attempt to be a dental repairman. Repair of equipment should be left to those who are specially trained for that purpose. The role of the assistant in the equipment maintenance program, like that of the effective dental practice, primarily concerns prevention rather than repair.

DENTAL UNIT

The first concern in the care and maintenance of the *dental unit* is turning off the master electric switch and the main water valve at the end of the working day. This will eliminate a fire hazard, prolong the life of the heating elements in the unit, prevent the overheating of motors in case the rheostat is pressed against an object, and prevent any damage that might occur as a result of a water leak. The following are guidelines for care of the dental unit:

1. Dust and dirt must be removed daily from the engine pulley and the cord arm pulleys.
2. The air and water syringes should be checked daily for leaks.
3. Wax accumulations should be removed from the gas burner daily.
4. A pint of water should be flushed through the saliva ejector daily.
5. The cuspidor bowl should be cleaned daily to prevent staining.
6. The saliva ejector screen and the cuspidor trap should be removed and cleaned twice a week.
7. If the operating light fixture has vents for air circulation, the inside of the lens must be washed weekly.
8. The manufacturer's instructions for oiling the dental engine should be followed. Oiling requirements depend upon the type of dental engine; some engines require 2 drops of oil once a month.
9. The engine arm pulleys should be oiled every 2 months. Excess oil should be removed immediately, so that it will not spatter when the engine is run.
10. The water-supply screen should be cleaned twice a year.
11. A light coat of petroleum jelly should be placed on the contacts of the foot rheostat twice a year.
12. The assistant should report any signs of excessive wear or malfunction to the dentist when she first detects them.

The preceding guidelines for care of the dental unit apply primarily to the standard model. The dental unit is passing through an era of major changes in appearance and functional components, as are other major

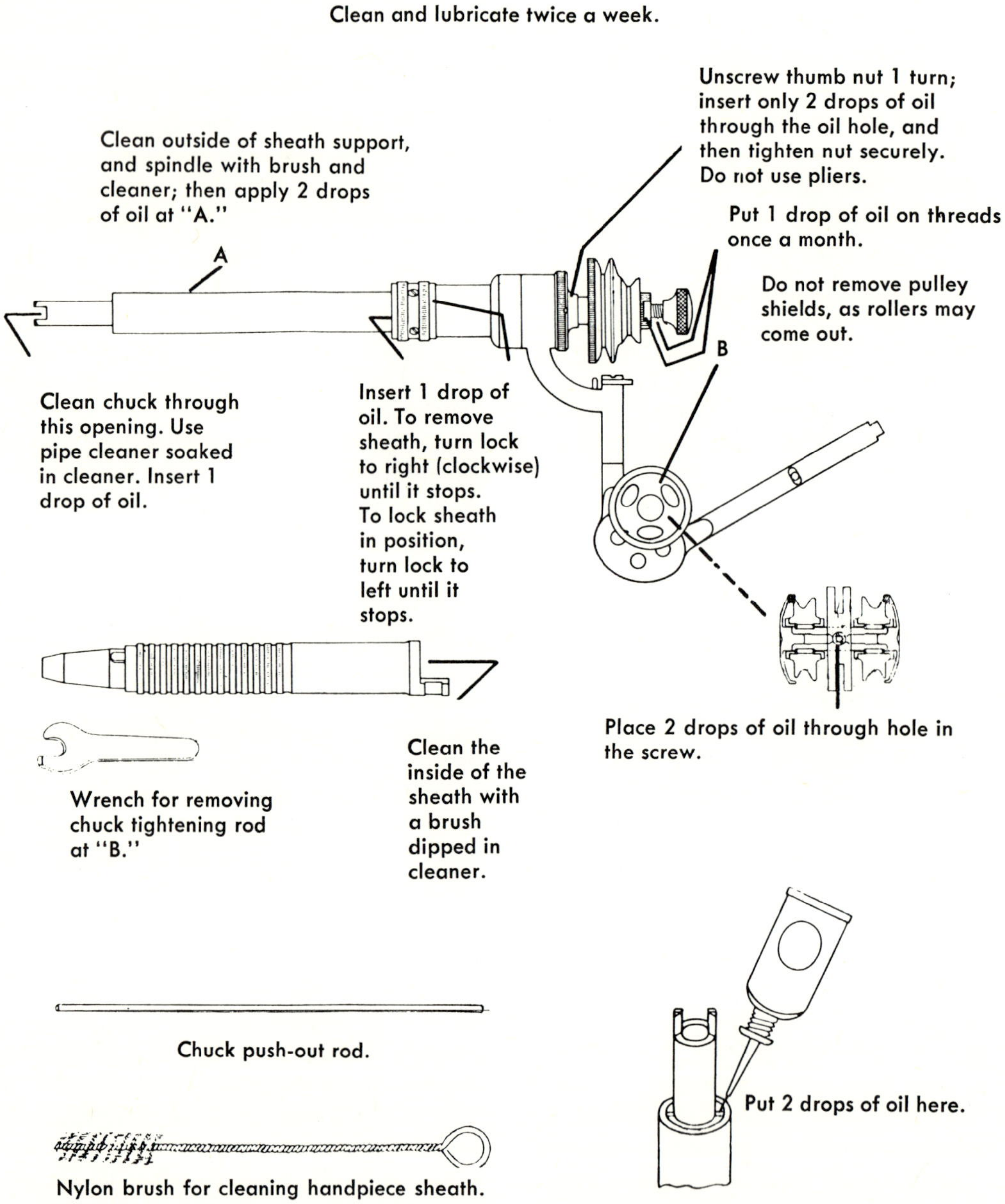

Fig. 17-1. Page from an instruction pamphlet depicting the procedure for lubricating an ordinary handpiece. (Courtesy Midwest Dental Manufacturing Company.)

pieces of equipment in the operating room. Some of the newer models are less complicated to maintain than the standard model, while others, having incorporated additional components, may require more steps in preventive maintenance.

HANDPIECES AND ANGLES

Special care must be given to the various kinds of handpieces. The methods of cleaning, sterilizing, and lubricating differ with the type of handpiece and contra-angle. Manufactures enclose specific maintenance instructions with all handpieces and contra-angles, and these should be explicitly followed. If a set of instructions is not available for the handpiece being used in the office, the manufacturer will furnish copies on request. General instruction for the care of a variety of handpieces and angles follow.

Ordinary straight handpiece

Twice a day, the sheath should be removed from the spindle; two drops of oil are placed on the front and rear bearings, plus 1 drop of oil on the surface of the spindle, where the end of the sheath revolves against it (Fig. 17-1).

Once a day, 1 drop of oil is placed in the oil hole on the shaft carrying the idler pulleys of the wrist joint. At the same time the sheath is removed from the spindle, the inside of the sheath is cleaned with a handpiece brush dipped in cleaner. A pipe cleaner is dipped in cleaning solution, and the chuck is cleaned out at the bur hole. The spindle is oiled, and the handpiece is reassembled. It is recommended that this procedure be the last thing done at the end of the day.

Once a week, the entire spindle should be removed for complete cleaning and lubrication.

Sterilization is best accomplished in a hot-oil sterilizer, although alcohol swabs can be used.

Ball-bearing, high-speed handpiece

Twice a week, the sheath is removed. The outside of the spindle is cleaned with a brush that has been dipped in cleaner, and the chuck is cleaned with a pipe cleaner that has been dipped in cleaner. Two drops of oil are placed in the center of the spindle, and 1 drop is placed in the chuck. One drop of oil should be placed at the top and bottom of the spindle. The thumbscrew over the top bearing should be unscrewed 1 turn, and 1 drop of oil should be placed before it is tightened. Two drops of oil should be placed in the oil hole at the wrist joint of the pulley.

Belt-driven, high-speed handpiece

The belt-driven, high-speed handpiece needs no lubrication. It is cleaned and cold-sterilized by wiping with a gauze sponge saturated with alcohol or a germicidal solution. The handpiece should be returned to the manufacturer when the belt needs changing or when repairs are necessary.

Standard-speed contra-angle

The standard-speed contra-angle should be lubricated between treatment sessions. This is accomplished by opening the bur latch and placing 1 drop of oil in the oil hole.

Failure to clean angles properly causes more breakdowns than lack of lubrication, because improper cleaning causes the lubricant to become contaminated with foreign materials. Once a day, the head of the contra-angle is removed and cleaned with a brush and cleaner, and the elbow gears and head are lubricated. When the angle is reassembled, it is important to see that the gears are properly meshed, before the lock nut on the head is tightened.

Ball-bearing angle, long-sleeve type

After each 10 minutes of running time, the angle should be run forward and in reverse in cleaner and lubricant for 5 seconds. A drop of oil should be placed in the oil hole once a day, and the inside of the sheath should be cleaned once a week with a brush that has been dipped in cleaner.

No attempt should be made to take apart a ball-bearing angle for cleaning and lubrication.

The angle is sterilized with an alcohol swab.

Prophylaxis right angle

The angles used for prophylaxis and polishing must be cleaned and lubricated after each use. The bearing and gear barrel are removed from the head, run in a cleaner, and blown dry. The inside of the head is also cleaned with a cleaner; then the back of the head is filled with a recommended grease, and the angle is reassembled.

If an oil sterilizer is used, the head should be removed before sterilizing and repacked with grease before assembling.

Airotor handpiece

Although the same principle of motivation applies to all air-turbine handpieces, the care and maintenance requirements of these instruments differ. In general, the handpiece itself needs very little, if any, maintenance. The assistant should check the air pressure daily, before the handpiece is used. She should also check the flow of the water coolant and clean the small opening, if it has become clogged. In some instances, it is recommended that the turbine bearings be lubricated once a day with 2 drops of the recommended oil.

Special attention should be paid to the manufacturer's instructions pertaining to conditioning of the handpiece after parts are changed and before or after long storage.

In many instances, the control panel contains an air filter and a water filter. These filters must be cleaned or changed as conditions warrant, and the assistant should not allow them to clog to the extent of impairing the function of the handpiece.

The automatic oiler in the system should be checked several times a day to make certain that oil is being used and that the oiler does not run dry. It is very important that the lubrication system be functioning properly at all times.

The turbines in most instruments can be changed in the office, if necessary. Whether or not this is done is up to the discretion of the dentist.

The assistant should replace the bur chuck, when the bur is not gripped tightly by the handpiece.

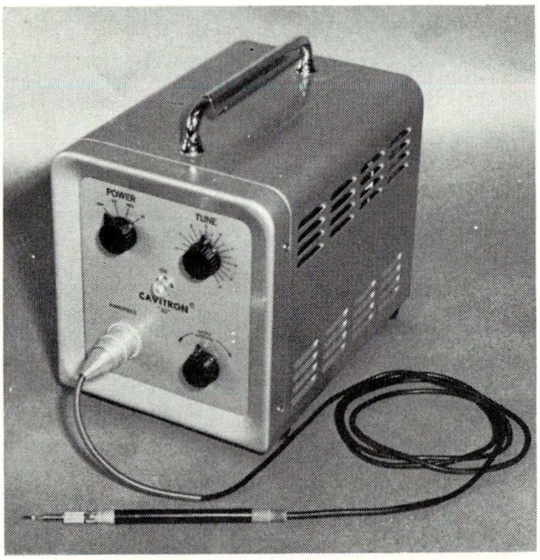

Fig. 17-2. Ultrasonic portable unit with handpiece and attached tip in foreground. This unit is used for prophylaxis, curettage, and gingivectomy procedures rather than for cutting tooth structure. The size and shape of the tips help give access to all areas. (Courtesy Cavitron Equipment Corporation.)

The turbine handpiece should not be sterilized in hot oil. They may be cold-sterilized by wiping with a germicide-saturated sponge or by immersion in the solution. If the handpiece is immersed, it should be lubricated before use.

Cavitron prophylaxis unit

When the Cavitron prophylaxis unit is in use, it should be located so that air is free to circulate on all sides of the cabinet.

At the close of the day, the power selector, should be turned off, the water valve should be shut off, and the prophylaxis insert should be removed from the handpiece and replaced with the steel rod provided to maintain the proper form of the handpiece (Fig. 17-2).

DENTAL CHAIR

The dental chair, like any piece of furniture, should receive proper monthly care. The various finishes, including the seat, the backrest coverings, and the enamel finish, should be cared for with the appropriate agents.

Some manufacturers advise that for maintenance of the hydraulic mechanism, the chair be left at the lowest level overnight and raised to its highest level once a week.

The vertical roller or slide paths should be lubricated every 2 months to maintain easy action. One drop of oil should be added every 6 months to any bearing surfaces of the motor chair.

The oil reservoir should be checked and brought to the proper level every 6 months.

OPERATING STOOLS

Seat coverings on the operating stools should be kept clean and should be treated with the appropriate agents for the type of covering. All moving parts should be lubricated once every 2 months.

ORAL EVACUATING UNITS

It is absolutely essential that oral evacuating units be kept clean throughout, in order to prevent unpleasant odors in the operatory. Typical illustrated cleaning instructions from a manufacturer's manual are shown in Fig. 17-3.

The motor should be shut off when the machine is not in use. When a unit has 2 mouthpieces (Fig. 17-4, *A* and *B*), both must be open when the unit is in operation; otherwise, the motor will be overloaded.

If the machine has a filter bag, it is changed at least twice a week while the unit is in daily use. The filter pan should be cleaned weekly.

The collection tank should be emptied twice daily, and a small amount of water with some germicidal solution added, before the tank in replaced.

Once a day a germicidal solution should be sprayed in the mouthpiece hoses, while the motor is running.

After each patient has been dismissed, a glass of water should be flushed through the hose that has been used.

The collection tank is always removed and scrubbed with soapy, lukewarm water once a week. Before the tank is replaced, petroleum jelly should be applied to the fittings to help prevent air leakage.

Once a month the motor should be checked for dirt and moisture, and the motor filter should be changed, if necessary.

Some of the preceding maintenance duties are not necessary when a central system is used in the office. When such a system is being utilized, the assistant must learn the maintenance procedures advocated by the manufacturer.

DENTAL CABINET

The working surface should not be waxed, but it should be cleaned with a damp cloth. The rest of the external finish should be waxed along with other furniture. The drawers should be emptied and thoroughly cleaned every 6 months. All medicament bottles should be clearly labeled, and new labels applied when necesary. In areas used for storage of surgical instruments or special surgical cabinets, autoclaved towels should be kept over and under the instruments. Care must be exercised to keep these towels and instruments sterile. Fresh towels should be placed weekly.

In offices utilizing the built-in cabinet arrangement, the single dental cabinet may be absent. Drawers for storing instruments and supplies appear in fixed cabinets, away from the immediate operating area. However, the same principles of care should be followed in maintaining clean and neat drawer arrangements. In offices where tray setups are stored in cabinets, the individual trays should always be covered while in storage.

STERILIZERS

Cold-sterilization containers should be emptied, scrubbed, rinsed, and filled with new solution twice a week. All soap must be removed from instruments, before the

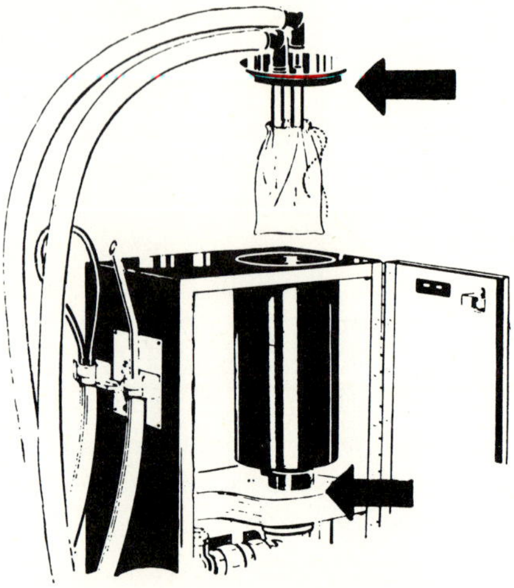

Filter tank lid removed—when replaced should be in original position with vaseline applied around edges (at arrows).

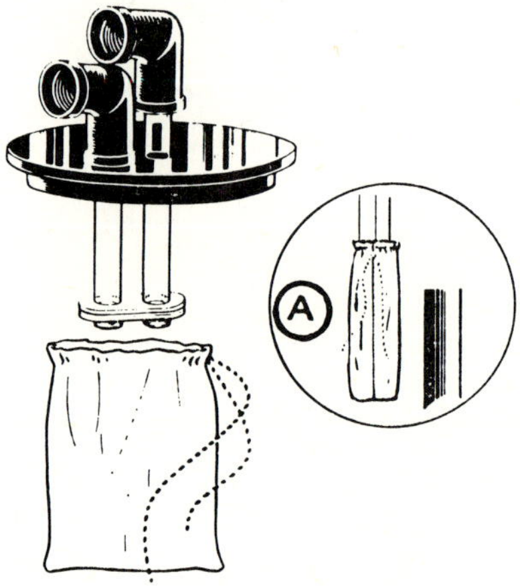

Replacing filter bag. Draw string should fit in groove with bag positioned parallel to air line tube, as in (A).

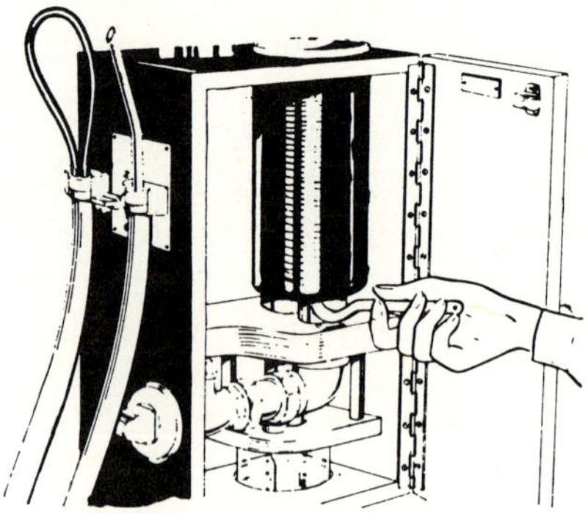

Remove filter tank by prying up with long jaw of special wrench.

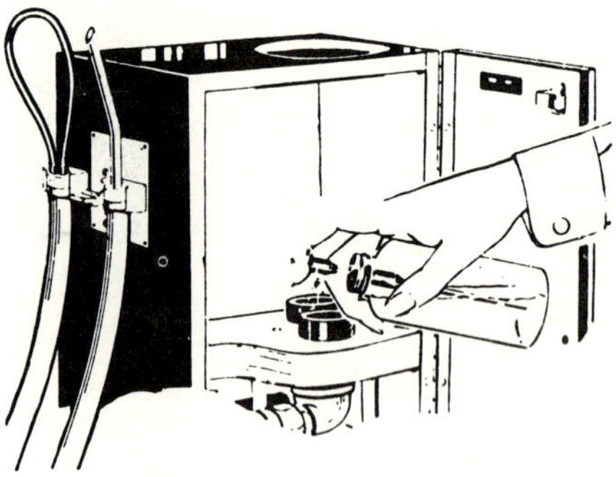

Spray filter tank connections with Vacudent Germicidal solution.

Fig. 17-3. Manufacturer's illustrations of a portion of the maintenance on an oral evacuating machine. (Courtesy Densco, Incorporated.)

instruments are placed in the cold-sterilizing solution (Fig. 17-5).

The oil level must be kept at the proper height in the hot-oil sterilizers, with only the recommended oil used. When the oil becomes dirty, the inside of the sterilizer should be drained, scoured, and refilled with oil (Fig. 17-6).

The assistant should check the reservoir of the autoclave before each use to be sure that it is two-thirds full of distilled water. Once a month, the water should be drained, and the reservoir and chamber scrubbed, rinsed, dried, and refilled. A thorough cleaning with mild soap at 6-month intervals is advocated. Complete rinsing to remove all soap is necessary, before distilled water is again added. Worn rubber gaskets

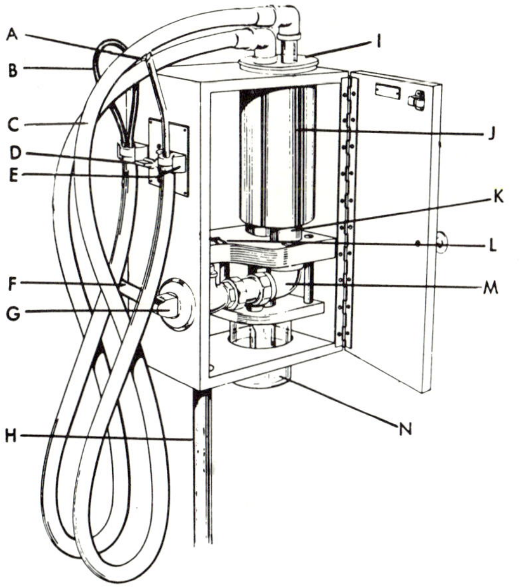

PARTS

A—Standard Mouthpiece
B—Hydroceptor Mouthpiece
C—Mouthpiece Hose
D—Manual on and off switch
E—Magnetic hose clip
F—Drain pipe for waste line
G—Cabinet outlet fitting for waste line
H—Main air line connecting power unit with cabinet
I—Dual outlet top for filter tank
J—Filter tank
K—Outlet fitting from filter tank to swing-check valve assembly
L—Cabinet electrical panel
M—Swing-check valve assembly
N—Automatic cutoff jar containing electrical contacts

Fig. 17-4. Office portion of a central oral excavating system. The motor for operating the suction is located in some other area. The cabinet is attached to the wall, and the drain is fitted directly to the office plumbing system. (Courtesy Densco, Incorporated.)

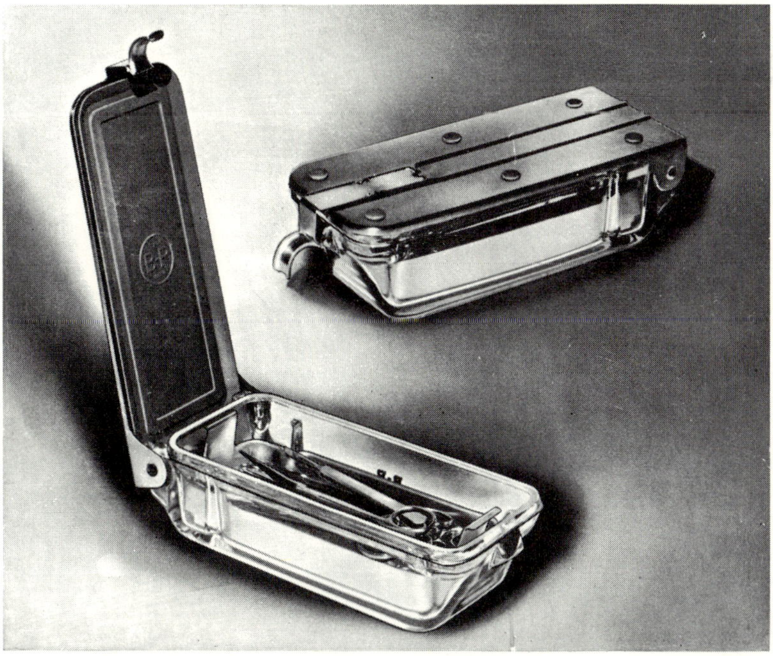

Fig. 17-5. Bard-Parker sterilizing container. (Courtesy American Hospital Supply Corp.)

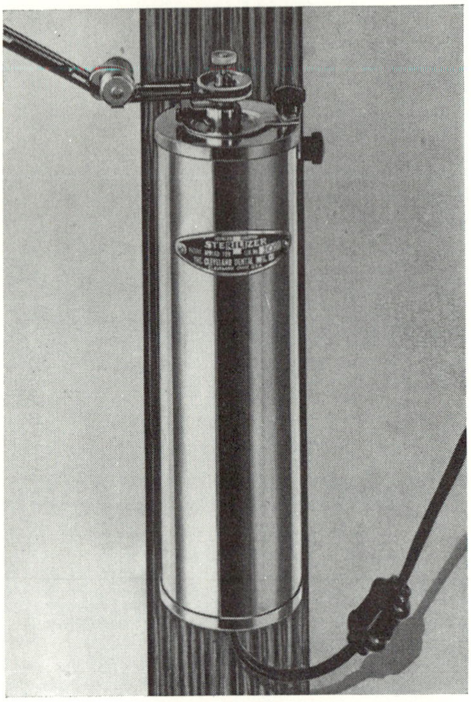

Fig. 17-6. Hot-oil sterilizer for nonprecision handpieces. Handpiece is in position in sterilizer. (Courtesy The Cleveland Dental Manufacturing Company.)

should be replaced, when necessary (Fig. 17-7).

In molten-metal sterilizers, the metal must be cleaned when in the molten state. This is done by simply gathering up the debris with a cotton roll. A sufficient amount of metal must be kept in the well to completely cover the working ends of the instruments to be sterilized.

X-RAY UNIT

The finish on the x-ray unit should be cleaned and polished periodically, along with the other items in the operating room.

The pilot light should be checked daily. If the light does not work, it is advisable to check power plugs and fuses, move the voltage compensator to the right or left, or replace the lamp, if it is found to be burnt out.

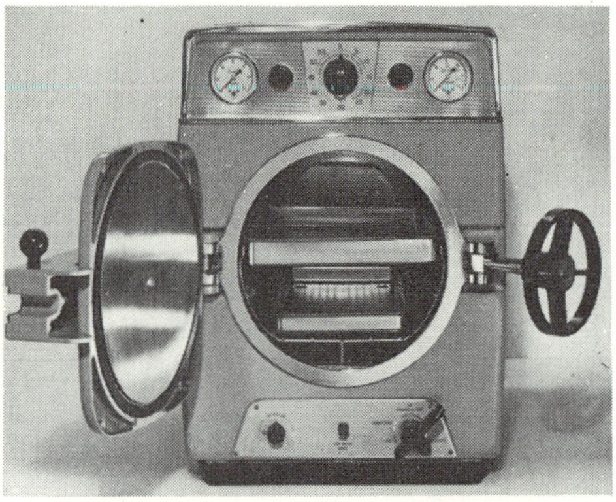

Fig. 17-7. Autoclave. The manufacturer's instructions must be carefully followed when operating this type of sterilizer. (Courtesy Wilmot Castle Company.)

The voltage compensator should always be adjusted so that the voltmeter reads within the limits shown during the x-ray exposure. If this reading cannot be obtained, the repairman should be notified.

If an overload causes the circuit-breaker to open, the assistant should wait 2 minutes before trying to set the breaker.

Accuracy of the timer should be checked periodically.

The vertical movement of the head is controlled by friction and can be adjusted by tightening or loosening the friction knob. No lubrication at these areas is required.

The assistant must not attempt any repair on the x-ray unit, but should report any difficulty to the dealer from whom the unit was purchased (Fig. 17-8).

MECHANICAL AMALGAMATOR

The amalgamator capsule and pestle must be kept free of all set amalgam. A small, stiff brush will remove any fresh amalgam from the capsule and lid immediately after the mix is made (Fig. 17-9).

The timer should be checked for accuracy every 6 months.

The actuating mechanism should be lubricated with a drop of oil each month.

A

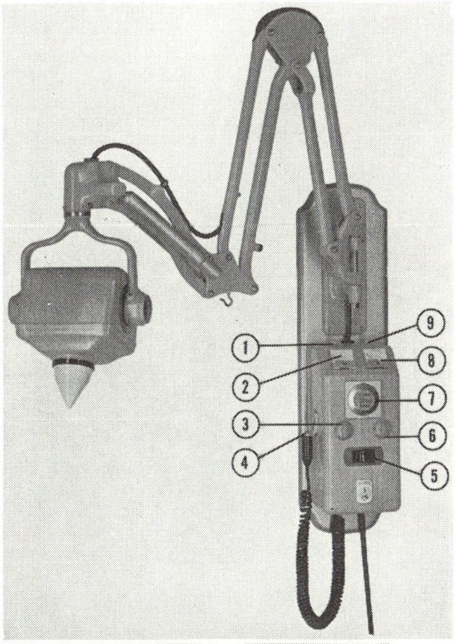

B

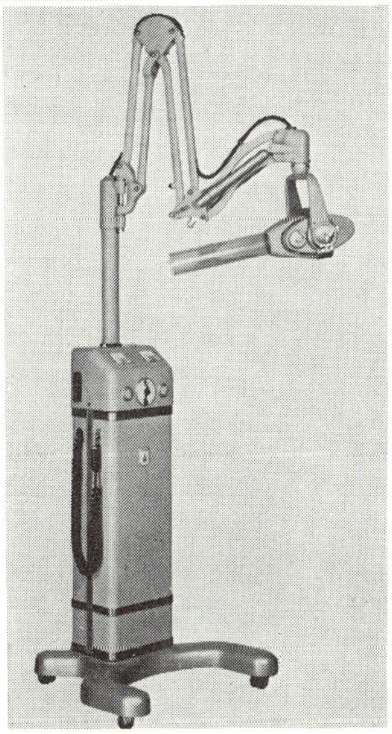

Fig. 17-8. A, Wall-mounted x-ray unit. The 3-unit extension arm permits adequate movement for exposures and compact retraction for out-of-the-way storage. **1,** Emission pilot light; **2,** milliammeter; **3,** filament resistor knob; **4,** time switch button; **5,** circuit breaker; **6,** penetration control; **7,** timer; **8,** kilovoltameter; **9,** pilot light. **B,** Mobile x-ray unit with attached long cone. Without the caster stand, this same type of unit becomes a fixed floor model. (Courtesy The Weber Dental Manufacturing Company.)

MECHANICAL SHARPENER

No motor lubrication is necessary in the maintenance of a mechanical sharpener. When the abrasive wheel becomes dark from accumulation of metal, about 6 drops of oil on a cotton roll held against the revolving wheel will clean it. Excessive pressure should not be used against the abrasive wheel, as this will reduce the blade of the instrument too fast and will groove the wheel (Fig. 17-10).

AIR COMPRESSOR

Although this piece of equipment is not generally located in the operatory, it is considered part of the equipment. This machine is not to be left running overnight or when the office is closed for a day or more at a time. Once a month, the condensed moisture should be drawn off through the drainage valve. The motors are usually factory sealed and, therefore, need no lubrication.

MODEL TRIMMER

It is necessary to use a sufficient amount of water to keep the grinding wheel moist when the model trimmer is in use; light pressure should be exerted on the model as it is held against the wheel.

After the model has been trimmed, the water and motor are never shut off, until clean water is flowing from the evacuating line.

The abrasive wheel should not be used dry, and metal objects should not be cut on the wheel. When the abrasive wheel becomes worn on one side, it can be removed and reversed (Fig. 17-11).

BALANCE

No oil or other lubricant should ever be applied to bearings. These bearings are kept in proper working condition by cleaning with a blast of air.

VACUUM INVESTOR

Only the designated equipment should be used with vacuum investors. The bowl,

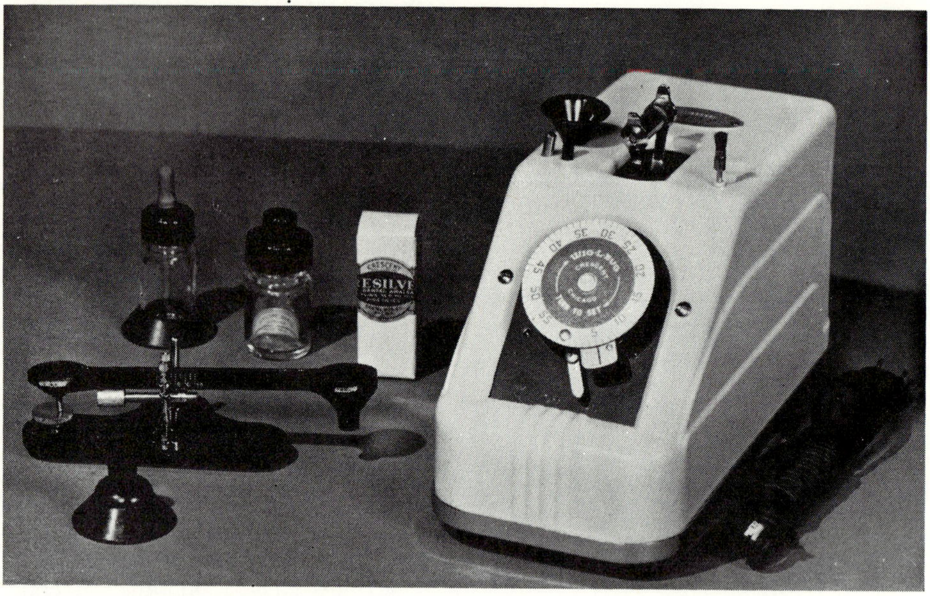

Fig. 17-9. Mechanical amalgamator and accessories, including plastic capsule and pestle in stand, alloy-mercury balance, and alloy and mercury dispensers. (Courtesy Crescent Dental Manufacturing Company.)

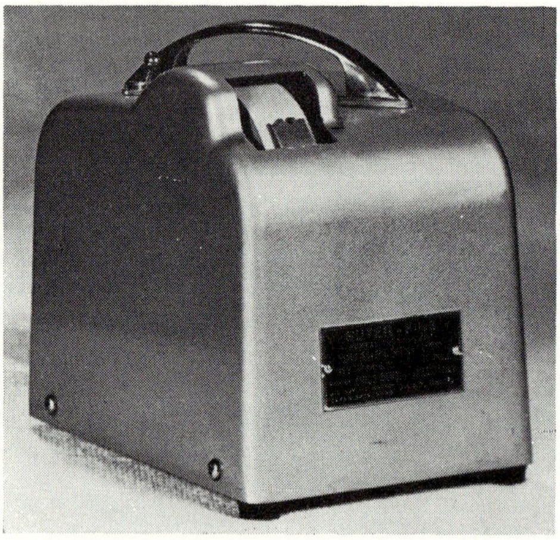

Fig. 17-10. Mechanical instrument sharpener. Note guide in front of wheel for use in placing the instrument blade to obtain the correct angle and bevel. (Courtesy Chico Dental Specialties.)

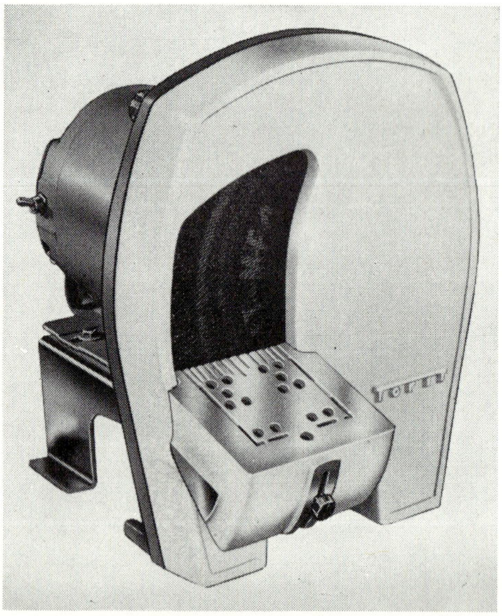

Fig. 17-11. Model trimmer. The model to be trimmed is placed on the platform attached to the disk guard and moved firmly against the revolving disk. The platform is adjustable to allow for angle variations during trimming. (Courtesy Torit Manufacturing Company.)

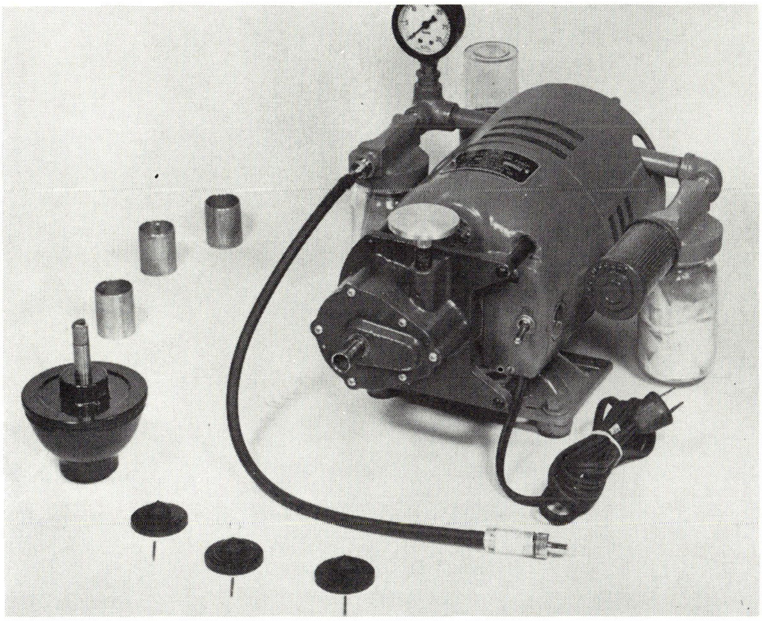

Fig. 17-12. Motorized vacuum investing unit. Accessories shown for investing are steel inlay rings, rubber bowl with mechanical mixer, rubber crucible formers, and metal sprue pins. Features of this type of machine include a vacuum pump, a vibrator table, a drive chuck for the mechanical mixer, and a filter on the vacuum hose connection. (Courtesy Kerr Manufacturing Company.)

plug, and spatulator should be washed free of investment immediately after use.

The filter should be checked before investing and changed, if investment has been drawn into it.

The drive shaft and spatulator should be lubricated monthly.

The oil level should be checked periodically; if oil is needed, only that recommended by the manufacturer should be used.

If the mixing bowl becomes badly scratched, it should be discarded and replaced by a new one (Fig. 17-12).

CENTRIFUGAL CASTING MACHINE

The tension spring should be placed under stress only before the centrifugal casting machine is to be used; the machine should not be left "wound" for long periods of time. The machine should be kept secured to prevent damage when in use. The manufacturer's instructions should be followed in keeping it properly balanced.

The shaft should be oiled lightly every 6 months.

The assistant must exercise caution when operating this type of casting machine to prevent personal injury, damage to the equipment, and loss of casting alloy (Fig. 17-13).

BENCH DENTAL ENGINE

The bench dental engine and engine arm pulleys should be oiled once every 2 months.

Ordinarily, the conventional or ordinary handpiece is used with the laboratory bench engine and is cleaned and lubricated in the same manner as the ordinary handpiece used in the operatory. The frequency with which it is cleaned and lubri-

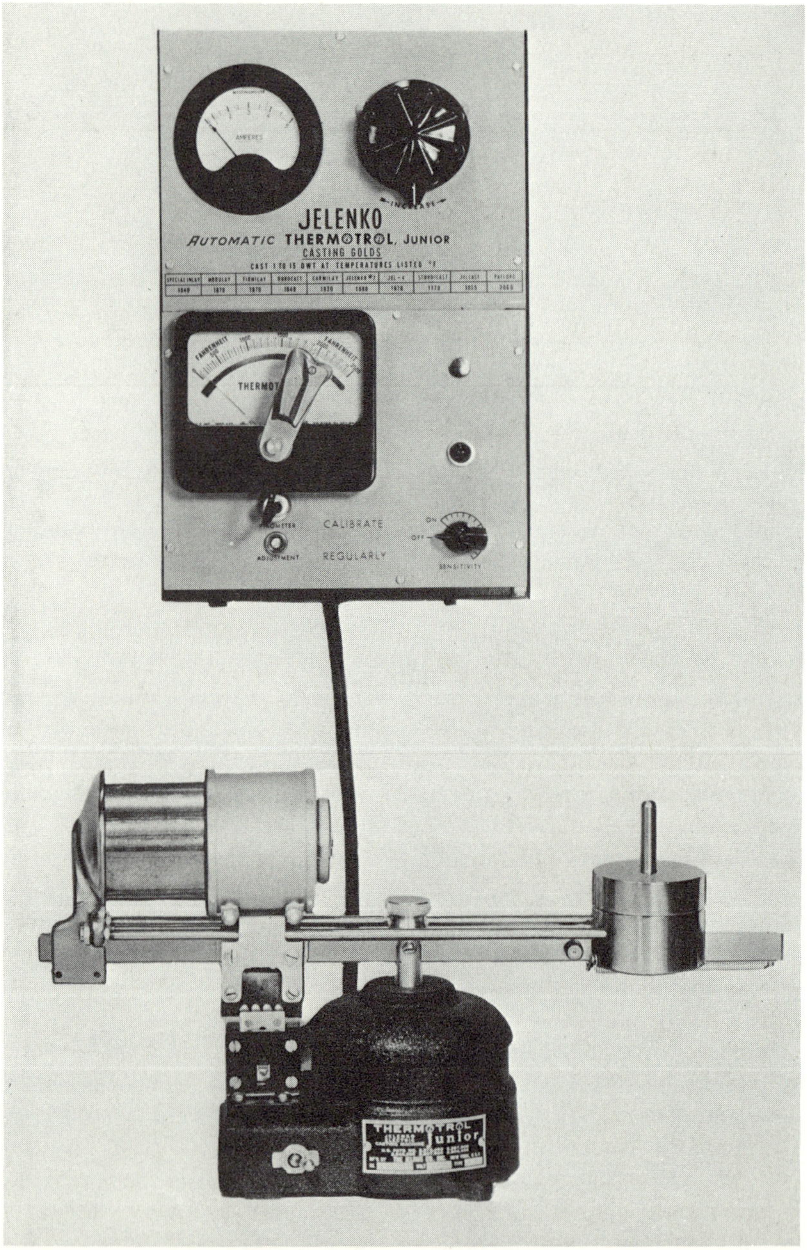

Fig. 17-13. Centrifugal casting machine with attached electric metal-melting unit. Temperature control and dials are located on adjacent wall. Uniform melting of metal is achieved in this nonoxidizing atmosphere. (Courtesy J. F. Jelenko & Company, Inc.)

cated depends upon the amount of use it is given.

Any electric motor in the laboratory should be lubricated only according to manufacturer's instructions.

HEATING EQUIPMENT

Inlay ovens (Fig. 17-14), processing tanks, and water baths should be checked periodically for accuracy of heating elements and gauges or pyrometers. Metals of specific low-fusing temperatures are used to check dry-heat ovens, and thermometers are used to check water-bath temperatures. The operation of heating appliances at very high temperatures for long, continuous periods of time should be avoided.

Collections of investment should not be allowed to accumulate on the sides or bottom of water baths. A mild scouring agent may be used to remove debris and film from water baths.

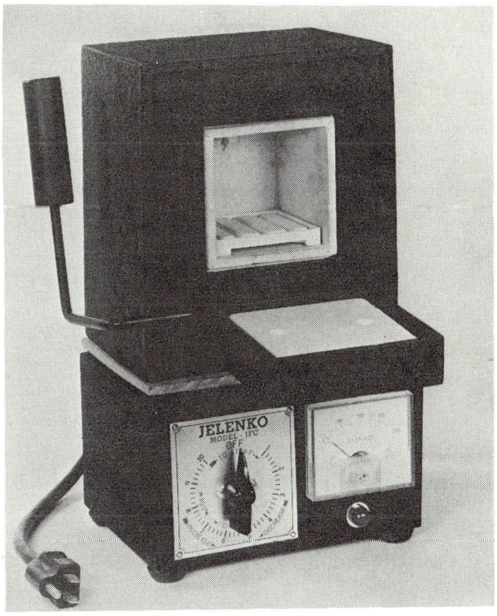

Fig. 17-14. Electric burn-out furnace. (Courtesy J. F. Jelenko & Company, Inc.)

VIBRATOR

The vibrator has a flat table that vibrates at a rapid rate with various intensities, according to the setting. When the unset gypsum product is placed on this table, the trapped air is forced out of the mix. All models should be poured over vibration to minimize air incorporation. When this equipment is in use, a towel should be placed over it to prevent the accumulation of excess plaster or stone on the table and on the sides of the motor housing (Fig. 17-15).

LIGHT LABORATORY EQUIPMENT

Most items classified as light laboratory equipment are simple in design, and their care is of a practical nature. The chief problems are dirt and rust. Items kept free of laboratory debris not only have a better appearance, but are also easier to work with.

Those items with moving parts should be lubricated, when necessary. It is impractical to set a time schedule because of the variation in utilization of the various items.

Knives used in the laboratory should be maintained with sharp edges (Fig. 17-16).

Gas burners should be kept free of wax accumulations (Fig. 17-17).

Plaster bowls and spatulas are always cleaned immediately after use, and badly scratched bowls are replaced (Fig. 17-18).

Every precision instrument should be covered when stored.

It is extremely important that articulators, especially the more complex models, be kept clean (Fig. 17-19). When a cast has been completed and removed, the articulator should be thoroughly cleaned, and all moving parts should be lubricated with a light oil.

A thin covering of petroleum jelly should be applied to the surfaces of metal items that are to be stored for a long period of time.

Gypsum products may be cleaned of metal or acrylic objects by soaking in a potassium citrate solution.

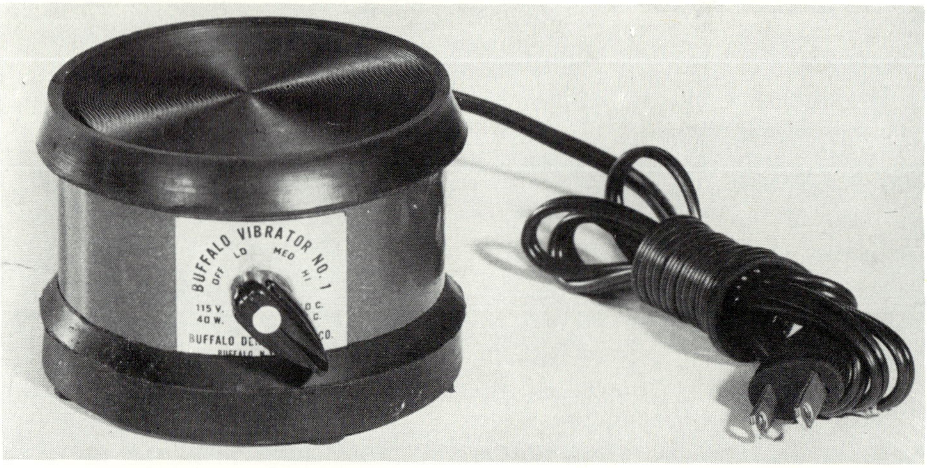

Fig. 17-15. Three-speed vibrator. The rubber covering on the vibrating table prevents a too violent vibration or sliding on the table, and it protects against chipping or cracking of any material placed against it. (Courtesy Buffalo Dental Manufacturing Company.)

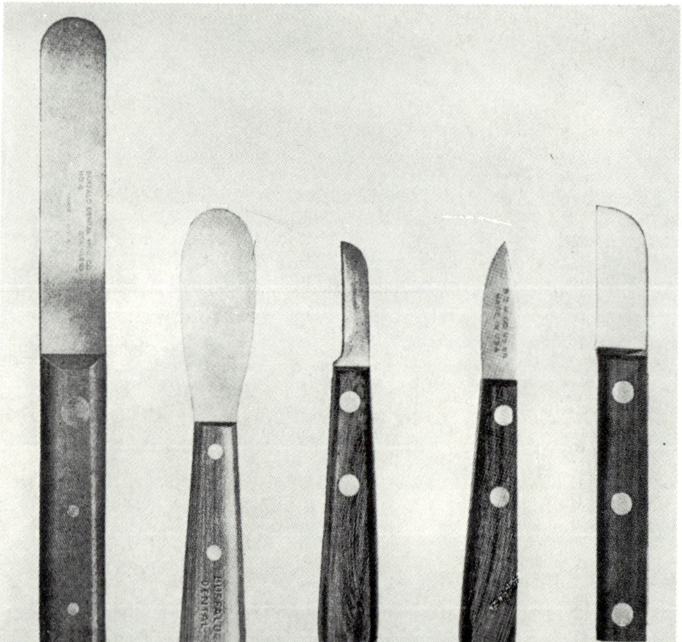

Fig. 17-16. Knives and spatulas. **No. 4R,** Spatula for large mixes of gypsum products; **No. 11R,** spatula contoured to fit sides of a plaster bowl and used for mixing gypsum products, as well as for impression compound work; **No. 6R,** plaster knife; **No. 7R,** compound knife; **No. 12,** heavy-duty knife with chisel-shaped end opposite the blade. (Courtesy Buffalo Dental Manufacturing Company.)

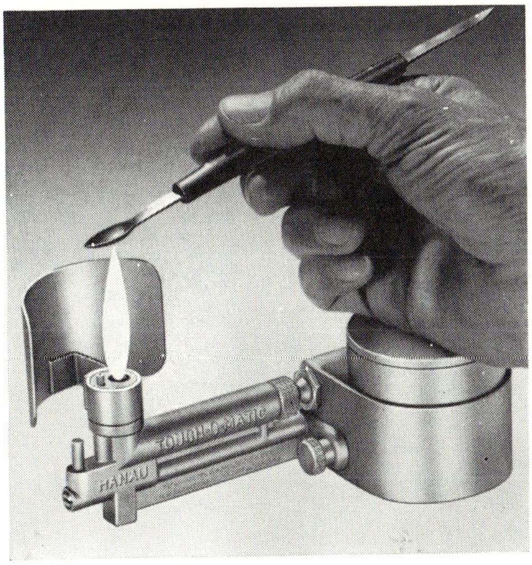

Fig. 17-17. Bunsen burner of advanced design that produces flame when platform is touched. It may also be regulated for constant flame. Attached shield protects flame from draft. (Courtesy Hanau Engineering Company, Inc.)

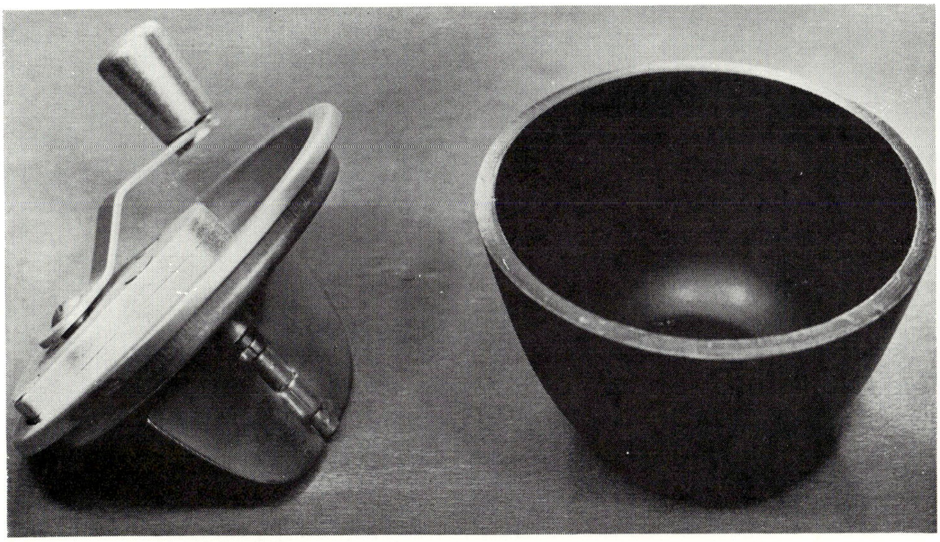

Fig. 17-18. Mechanical spatulator and rubber plaster bowl.

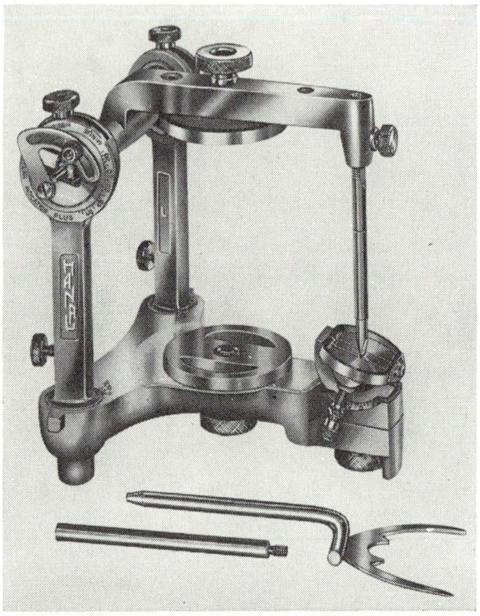

Fig. 17-19. Articulator with adjustable condylar guides and an adjustable incisal guide. Note bitefork and pin extension in foreground. (Courtesy Hanau Engineering Company, Inc.)

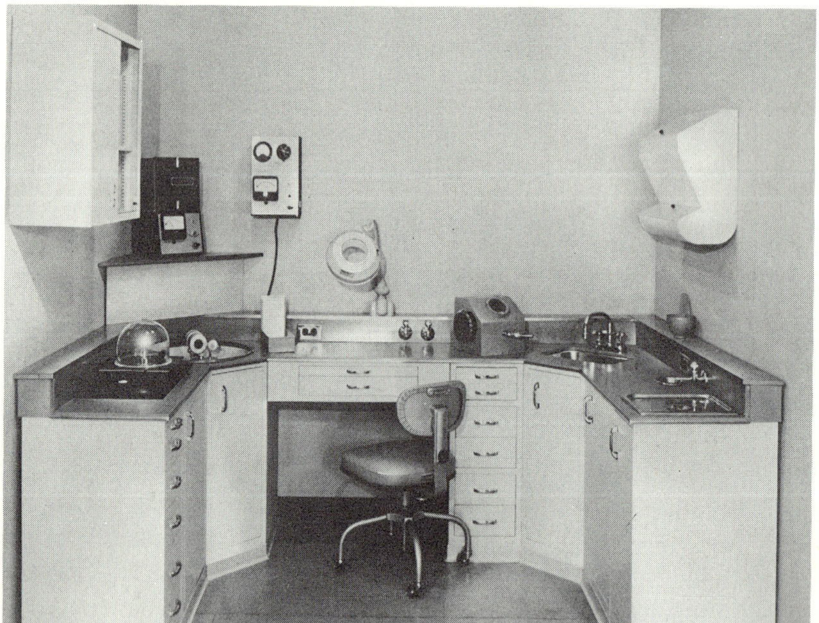

Fig. 17-20. A well-arranged dental laboratory. (Courtesy J. F. Jelenko & Company, Inc.)

DARKROOM

The dental assistant should take the responsibility of maintaining the developing room and its facilities. This responsibility includes keeping out all outside light; light other than the film safety light will decrease the effectiveness of the x-ray films.

The timer should be checked periodically for accuracy.

An adequate number of film hangers should be maintained at all times.

The temperature of the solutions should be checked daily and brought within a convenient and proper range. The solutions must be discarded and replaced once a month.

The tanks containing developer and fixer should be thoroughly cleaned every other month. The same tanks should be used for the refill each time, and the developer and fixer should not be switched from one tank to another.

LABORATORY

Depending upon the type of practice and the equipment used in the office, the dental assistant may find other items that require her attention. The dental assistant may or may not be required to perform laboratory procedures in the dental office with which she is associated. Whether she performs these procedures, or to what extent they are performed, depends on several factors. Among these factors are the type of practice in which she is employed, whether or not a laboratory technician is also employed, the number and types of other auxiliaries in the office, the extent to which a commercial dental laboratory is utilized, and the philosophy of the dentist regarding utilization of dental assistants.

When performing laboratory procedures, the assistant should be thoroughly familiar with the operation of each piece of laboratory equipment and the procedures necessary for its maintenance. In addition, the laboratory should be kept very clean. The assistant should constantly be reminded that much of the work produced in the laboratory will later be placed in contact with the patient in the operatory. A well-arranged dental office laboratory is illustrated in Fig. 17-20.

CONCLUSION

To be certain that dental equipment receives the proper attention, it is important to follow the manufacturer's instructions and to not rely on hearsay. At times, it may appear quite difficult to provide the care and maintenance of all furnishings and equipment used in the dental office. However, the assistant should realize that the dentist has placed his confidence in her ability to help him operate his practice at maximum efficiency, and this cannot be accomplished in untidy surroundings or with malfunctioning equipment.

Adequate cleaning and lubrication of mechanical equipment in the office will preserve the useful life of such apparatus. In addition, following the manufacturer's instructions in the use and maintenance of equipment will promote long mechanical endurance.

The dental assistant is not expected to be a repairman. Her role is in preventive maintenance, and a very important role it is, for without preventive maintenance, the daily operation of the office may be interrupted by costly and unnecessary delay due to equipment failure. This delay can more than offset any efficiency gained through improved operating techniques and organization in other aspects of the dental practice.

CHAPTER 18 MODERN OFFICE METHODS*

TILLIE D. GINSBURG, R.D.H., B.A., M.Ed.
MARILYN MOSS BECK, B.S., R.D.H.

It is customary in all offices to maintain records, financial reports, and correspondence files that reflect the daily activities of the office. These records are pertinent to the efficient management of the office and are necessary for tax and legal purposes. In the professional offices of dentists and physicians, however, it is also necessary to maintain detailed records for every patient who has been examined or given treatment. Not only will every dental assistant want to be familiar with the various records and filing systems, but her dentist-employer will also expect her to assume the responsibility of maintaining these records and to regard any information as confidential.

There are several ways in which these records may be classified, but in this discussion, they will be divided into 4 areas: (1) appointment records, (2) patients' clinical records, (3) financial and bookkeeping records, and (4) communication records.

APPOINTMENT RECORDS

The efficient flow of patients through a dental office largely depends upon systematic scheduling of appointments to provide the maximum amount of dental care with minimum strain to the dentist, the patient, and the other office personnel. The long-range health service that should be provided for the patient depends upon an efficient system of recall. The public has learned that appointments must be made for dental care, except when emergency treatment is needed. The dentist knows that he must schedule his time wisely. For the efficient management of appointment control, it is essential that this responsibility be delegated to 1 person. Patients will need to be taught that this responsibility has been given to the dental assistant, and that it is not necessary to speak to the doctor when making an appointment. The dentist and the other office personnel will need to respect this delegation of responsibility and take over only in emergency situations.

The dental assistant will probably find that her dentist-employer has a system of making appointments, and she will need to acquaint herself with this system. The present discussion offers some suggestions that may help her improve her ability to use the existing plan. It may also provide her with ideas that she will wish to diplomatically present to her dentist-employer.

The dentist looks to his staff to keep much of his office routine operating smoothly, without his constant supervision. The dental assistant who can maintain ac-

*This chapter is dedicated to the late Beth Linn, a contributor on a similar chapter to this in an earlier edition, and contributor of some material and explanations used in this chapter.

curate and effiicient appointment schedules is helping to guarantee successful office operation.

Making appointments requires many skills and good judgment and diplomacy. The dental assistant must understand human behavior, particularly as it is related to the dental office atmosphere.

Appointment books

There are several types of appointment books available to members of the dental profession. The type of book selected will depend upon the policies of the particular dental office and the number of members of the dental health team who provide a dental health service.

Appointment books are usually organized on a yearly basis and may be bound or loose-leaf. The advantages of the loose-leaf type of appointment book are that pages can be added as needed (eliminating handling 2 appointment books at the end of the year) and pages can be easily removed for making changes.

Appointment books are usually arranged so that the entire week is shown at a glance (Fig. 18-1, *A* and *B*). The daily division of time in an appointment schedule book is arranged on an hourly basis and subdivided into 15- or 30-minute intervals. The 15-minute arrangement is very satisfactory, as each 15 minutes can be considered a unit of time. Appointments are reserved according to the number of units required, rather than the number of minutes.

Blocking off the appointment book

The dental assistant is responsible for indicating clearly in advance the time not available for the routine scheduling of patients. A brightly colored pen or pencil may be used to block off lunch hours, buffer time, staff meetings, professional meetings, legal holidays, and vacations (Fig. 18-1, *A*). Buffer time can be that period during the working day that is reserved for emergency situations and appointments that may run beyond the scheduled time. Buffer time may be arranged in various ways. Ideally, it would consist of 2 units of time, in the morning and in the afternoon, preferably at the end of each scheduling session. If there is only 1 buffer period per day, it should be scheduled immediately before or after lunch.

Recording appointments

When recording reservation time for the patient, certain pertinent information should be considered. All appointments should be printed in pencil to permit erasure and rescheduling. The patient's full name is recorded on the appointment schedule, preferably with last name first to facilitate reading the schedule and removing filed records. The patient's telephone number should always be indicated. If the time reserved is for a new patient, the address and the name of the individual who referred the patient to the office should also be recorded. There are some appointment schedules that allow space for the service rendered next to the patient's name. When such an arrangement is not provided, this information may be entered immediately below the patient's name. The length of the appointment is indicated by drawing a vertical arrow through the appropriate number of units of time. If there are a series of appointments, the dates of the next reservations should be recorded opposite each previous appointment for quick reference (Fig. 18-1, *B*).

Considerations in making appointments

There are several important factors to be kept in mind in maintaining appointment control.

1. Morning appointments should be reserved for those procedures for which the operator and the patient need to be at their best. This time is especially good for the child patient.

2. Longer appointments should be

A

B

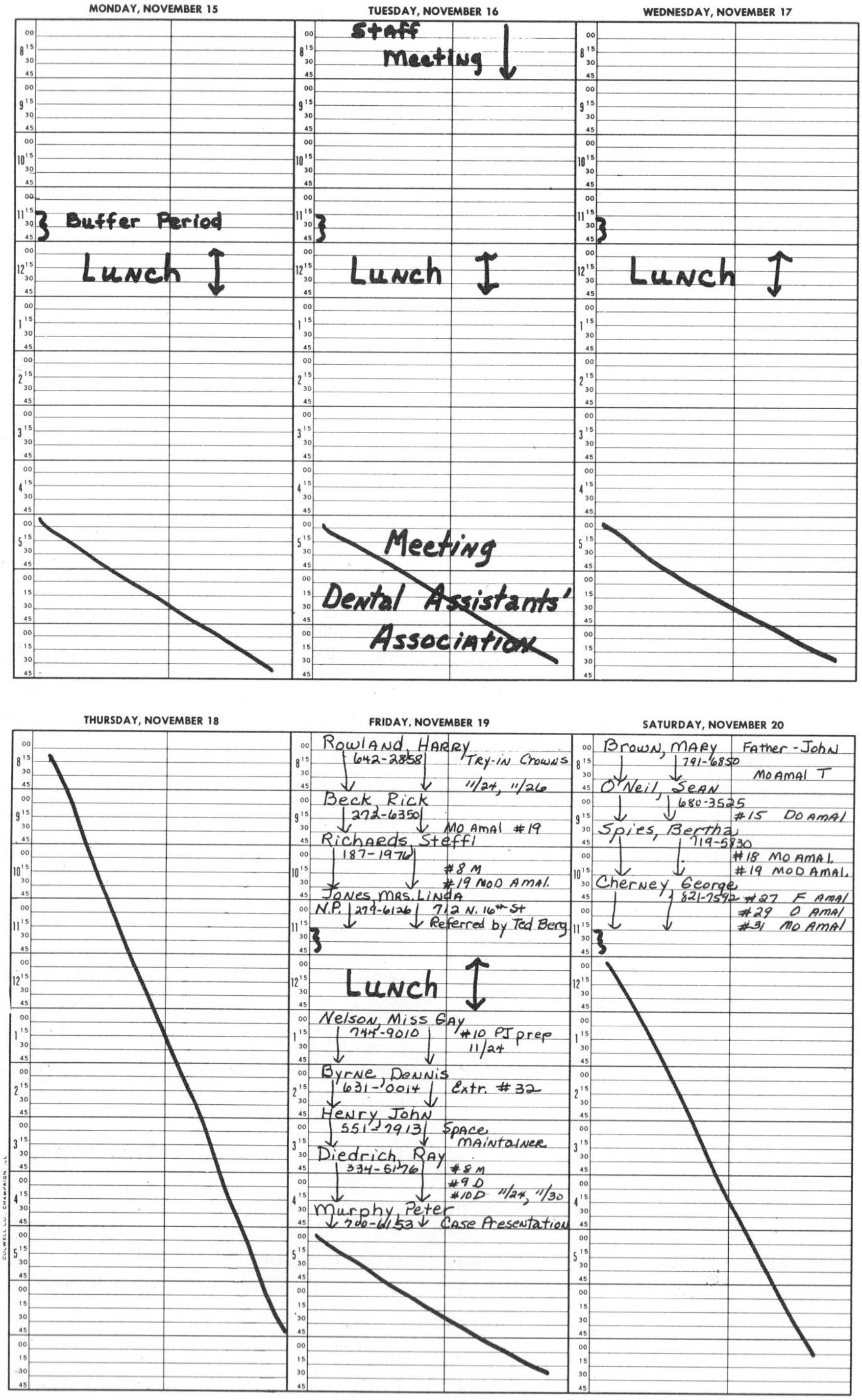

Fig. 18-1. A, Appointment book blocked off; **B,** record of appointments. (Courtesy Colwell Co.)

scheduled for those patients who will need extensive dental treatment.

3. If possible, the appointment should be scheduled on the most convenient day and at the best time for the patient.

4. When it is necessary to schedule a series of appointments, an effort should be made to schedule these appointments on the same day and at the same time for consecutive weeks.

5. Patients who need only a few minutes of chair time (for postoperative treatment, such as suture removal) may be scheduled at the same time as another patient, either at the beginning or end of that appointment.

6. The dental assistant will be far more efficient if she knows the length of time to be reserved before the patient comes to the desk or calls to reserve time.

a. There should be a standard office policy regarding units of time reserved for new patients.
b. Time analysis of the dental practice should yield an average time for operative procedures. For example, a 2-surface alloy restoration requires 2 units of time.
c. The time allotted for periodic examination can be recorded on the patient's recall records for quick reference.
d. For those patients needing more extensive dental work, appointment planning will be included in the treatment plan (Fig. 18-2).
e. If the patient needs only 1 or 2 appointments, the dentist could indicate this to the assistant before the patient leaves the chair. In each operatory, routing slips may be kept; it is then the assistant's duty to ascertain the information before each patient leaves the chair (Fig. 18-3). This slip is taken to the appointment control desk before the patient arrives there.

Appointment reminders

The efficient dental assistant who handles the details of making appointments will also assume the responsibility of seeing that a system is devised for reminding patients of their appointments and keeping the flow of patients on schedule. Various reminders will be needed for an effective system, and the dental assistant should have some understanding of the individual patient, in order to determine the method or combination of methods that will be most effective.

Appointment card

In many offices, it is customary to give the patient an appointment card at the time a schedule of appointments is arranged. An appointment card that records for the patient the day, date, and time of future appointments, as well as the dentist's name, telephone number, and address, is illustrated in Fig. 18-4. In some offices, appointment cards are bought in pads, and a carbon copy of each appointment card is retained in the office. This is particularly useful if another member of the staff may need to take over for the person making the original appointment, since the duplicate will show the exact information that has been given to the patient.

Colored appointment cards have proved effective, because the color helps the patient identify the card with the dental office. This is particularly true if statements and letterheads used by the office are in the same color.

In some offices, the appointment card will also be used to state some of the office policies regarding notices of cancellation or fees for broken appointments. In some offices, the appointment card is worded so that the patient reserves time with the dentist, rather than the dentist making an appointment with the patient.

Telephone reminders

Some patients prefer to be reminded of their appointments by telephone. On their

TREATMENT PLANNING FORM

Patient Jones, James E. Date May 10, 1967

Preferred day Tuesday Preferred time Mornings

TREATMENT PLANNED	UNITS REQUIRED	APPOINTMENT DATE	
Pt. Counseling, Prophylaxis	5	5/17/67	9:00 AM.
M.O.D. Amalgam #5	3	5/24/67	9:00 AM.
D. Synthetic # 8	2	6/1/67	9:00 AM
M. Synthetic # 9	2	6/7/67	9:00 AM.

Fig. 18-2. The treatment planning form is used for describing the patient's entire dental treatment.

35.–	Jones Candy
PREVIOUS BALANCE	NAME

Please present this slip to receptionist before leaving office.

SERVICES RENDERED

EXAMINATION			
X-RAY	✓	15	00
EXTRACTION			
CLEANING			
FILLING			
BRIDGE			
DENTURE			
TOTAL	$		

№ 06242 NEXT APPOINTMENT 3 units

Fig. 18-3. A routing slip indicating length of time for next appointment. (Courtesy Control-O-Fax.)

HUGH G. MURDOCH, D. D. S.
4160 N. OAKLAND AVENUE SHOREWOOD, WISCONSIN
THE TIME NOTED ON THIS CARD IS RESERVED FOR YOU
MONDAY________________________AT__________
TUESDAY________________________AT__________
WEDNESDAY________________________AT__________
THURSDAY________________________AT__________
FRIDAY________________________AT__________
SATURDAY________________________AT__________
IF APPOINTMENT CANNOT BE KEPT, PLEASE GIVE 24 HR. NOTICE
OFFICE PHONE: WOODRUFF 4-4780

Fig. 18-4. Appointment card for confirmation.

records, the assistant will indicate the individual preferences of these patients regarding telephone contact. These notations might include length of time prior to appointment that the call should be made (that is, 1 week, 24 hours, or same day), whether the contact must be directly with the patient or whether a message may be left, and whether the call is to be made only to the patient's residence or whether he may be called at his place of business.

In the case of patients who have had appointments several weeks or months in advance, the telephone call makes it possible for the assistant to confirm the appointment immediately or to make alternate arrangements. On the other hand, the telephone reminder is time-consuming, particularly if patients are difficult to reach, and and there is always the risk of irritating a patient by calling at an inopportune time.

If the telephone reminder is used, and the call is made more than 24 hours in advance of the appointment, a postcard confirming the telephone call is sent to eliminate possible misunderstanding.

Daily schedules

Effective appointment control requires that the reception desk, office, laboratory, and every operatory have a complete record of the appointments for that particular day. Each member of the dental health team should be aware of the schedules of the other members. If a loose-leaf type of appointment book is used, and the office has a copying machine, the daily schedules may be quickly made, or the schedules may be typed with the necessary carbons. These daily schedules will be posted in all the working areas (Fig. 18-5).

Call lists

For efficient use of time, appointments that are cancelled on very short notice should be filled when possible from an emergency call list. On this list are included the name, address, and telephone number of each patient, as well as necessary treatment of patients who can come to the office on short notice. The amount of time available will determine which patient is called. For the dentist located in a downtown area, the emergency call list may be made up of persons who work in offices in the same vicinity; if the dentist is located in a residential area, housewives and children will make up the bulk of the emergency call list. Some patients may prefer to be scheduled on short notice and are very willing to have their names on the emergency call list.

DAYS PLAN DATE Friday, September 17

	Dr.'s Patient	Procedure	Hygienist's Patient
8	Rowland, Harry	Bridge prep. #6	Moore, Mrs. Kaaren
			Proph., x-rays
9	Hanson, Mrs. Ted	#14 MOD	Hanson, Mr. Ted
		#19 MOD	Proph., x-rays
10			Berger, Lynn
			Proph., S Fl_2
30	Simon, Judy	Extr. #32 imp.	
11			Curtis, Mr. Ed.
	Ed Smith	PO-suture removal	Proph., Full
	Norris, Dave Tooth Ache		mouth radiographs
1	Jones, Mrs. Marilyn	New patient	Jones, Cindy N.P.
		Ref. Mary Brahm	5 yrs. old
			Jones, Terri N.P.
2	Stein, Michael	Inlay #5 LAB.	7 yrs. old
			Adams, John
	Richards, Mr. John	#8 M	Proph., study
3		#9 D	impressions
			Mueller, Sam
	Smith, Patricia	Extr. # 3	Proph., x-rays
4			
			Schneider, Marie
	George, Mrs. Pam	Case Presentation	Proph.,
			No x-rays

CALLS:

Fig. 18-5. Daily schedule.

Waiting lists

The dental assistant may also maintain a list of patients who are not in need of immediate dental service, but who wish an appointment as soon as one is available. The assistant may call patients from this list to fill cancelled appointments.

Special situations

Although most offices have established general policies and rules that the dental assistant will follow, there are some special situations in which the assistant may be called upon to exercise judgment and tact.

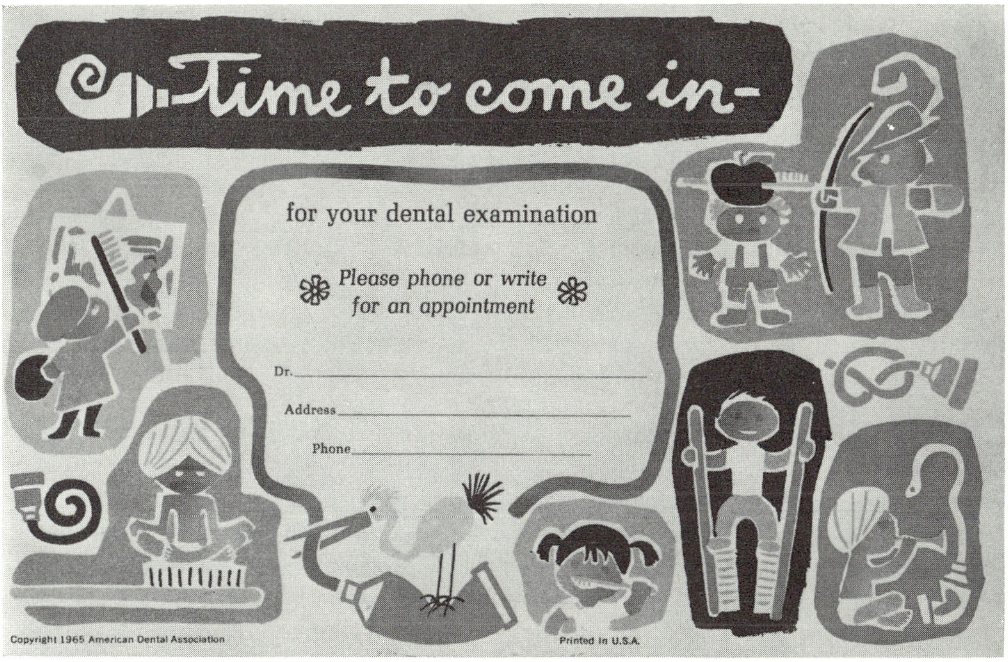

Our records show that it is now time for your dental examination. Please call or write our office for an appointment.

Sincerely yours,

*Dr.*____________________

MEMBER OF THE AMERICAN DENTAL ASSOCIATION

ADDRESS TELEPHONE

Fig. 18-6. Two types of recall cards.

"Drop-in"

If a new patient drops in, the dental assistant should explain that the dentist works by appointment only, and she should make an appointment for a later date or place the patient's name on the waiting list.

When a patient comes to the office in need of emergency care, the dental assistant should explain the situation to the person who had that time reserved, so that the dentist can render emergency care immediately.

Another type of drop-in may be a patient whom the dentist has decided he can no longer treat. If such a patient comes to the office, the assistant will have to refuse to make an appointment. She might suggest that the patient would be happier with another dentist, or she might tell him that, because he has failed to cooperate, the dentist does not want to take the responsibility for the dental treatment that is needed.

Business representatives

Detail men and salesmen for dental equipment and supply firms constitute another group that the dental assistant will confront in keeping control over appointment time. It may be possible to arrange a specific time for these business representatives to call, or the dental assistant may have to use buffer time for unscheduled visits. If the dental assistant has been given the responsibility of ordering supplies and equipment, she will want to schedule time for this duty.

Personal visitors

Personal visitors present a problem for which the dentist and dental assistant will want to establish a policy. If the visitor asks to talk with the dentist, the assistant may handle the situation with a stock answer, such as: "The doctor is with a patient and cannot be disturbed. May I take a message to him?" Personal friends of the dental assistant should never be permitted to visit her at the office during working hours.

Recall programs

When the dentist accepts a patient, it becomes his responsibility to provide that patient with dental care and preventive measures that will ensure optimum dental health. This is done by providing dental treatment and then recalling the patient periodically and systematically. The recall system is a methodical means of scheduling patients for future periodic appointments, according to the individual needs determined by the dentist. Recall of a denture patient will be quite different from that of a patient receiving periodic prophylaxes. The dental assistant responsible for appointment control will also be responsible for maintaining an effective recall system as part of the appointment control. She will want to be certain that the patient understands the necessity of these periodic visits and the manner in which the recall system operates.

Types of recall programs

It is difficult to say which type of recall program will be the most effective for any one office, as this will depend upon the type of practice, the personnel in the office, and the accuracy of the recall records maintained.

Letters or postal card recall

In the letter type of recall program, patients are notified either by form letter or postal card that it is time for them to make an appointment for evaluation of their oral health (Fig. 18-6). This puts the responsibility of arranging for the appointment on the patient. This method is the least effective in terms of response, but it is also the least time-consuming for the office personnel. A definite appointment could be included with the recall message to avoid placing all the responsibility of the reservation on the patient. The reservation would be determined from the patient's recall record, in which the patient has indicated his preference of day and time. A double postal card may be used. One card will relay the recall message with a given reservation; the other card will indicate the patient's confirmation of the appointment and will be mailed to the dental office by the patient (Fig. 18-7).

Telephone recall

In the telephone recall method, the patient is contacted by telephone, and a definite appointment is arranged. This method can be very effective for the following reasons:

1. Verbal comunication is more immediate.

2. It gives the dental office an opportunity for further reinforcement of the bene-

DR. PAUL F. NEVIN
300 E. First St.
Shakopee, Minn.

I do........, I do not........, accept Dr. Nevin's

Preventive Reservation for:

Day .... Date .... Time ....

Signed ....

Fig. 18-7. Double postal card used for reminding patients of their recall reservation or sending a definite recall appointment. The patient returns one card for confirmation of the reservation.

Postage Will Be Paid by Addressee

No Postage Stamp Necessary If Mailed in the United States

BUSINESS REPLY CARD

First Class Permit No. 2 Shakopee, Minn.

Dr. Paul F. Nevin

300 E. First St.

Shakopee, Minnesota

DR. PAUL F. NEVIN

This is a reminder that it is now due time for you to return to our office for your Preventive service and Dental Checkup.

For your convenience the following time has been reserved:

Day__________ Date __________ Time __________

Please return the attached card indicating your intention. Thank you.

Fig. 18-7, cont'd. For legend see p. 361.

fits the patient will receive in following the program.

3. Misunderstandings can be handled at this time.

4. The patient may find it difficult to refuse an appointment.

For this method to function with maximum efficiency, ample time and personnel must be available.

Advanced scheduling

At the time of the completion of the dental work or recall appointment, the patient is given a definite reservation for the next evaluation. In this program, the patients must be reminded of their appointments by either postal card or telephone, depending upon the office's policy of notification. A double postal card may be used as a reminder. In some offices, the patient addresses the card to himself. The card is then placed with the patient's recall record until 3 to 5 days before the appointment and is then mailed. The patient will be quite surprised to receive his recall reservation addressed in his own handwriting.

Advanced scheduling could prove to be the most effective recall program. However, the appointment schedule may tend to become solidly booked as far as 6 months in advance; this presents a problem in case of any change or illness in the office personnel, especially in case of absence of the dental hygienist.

Recall records

No matter what type of recall program is established, its success will depend upon the orderliness and accuracy of the office personnel who maintain the recall records.

Double-file, or cross-reference, recall records

The double-file, or cross-reference, system has been found to be one of the most efficient record systems and can be used for all types of recall programs. The double-file system includes 1 card filed alphabetically by the patient's name and a second card filed under the month in which the patient is to be recalled.

The card in the alphabetical file should have the following information on it: patient's name, home and business addresses and telephone numbers, and remarks concerning the day of the week and the time of day most suitable for dental appointments, the type of reminder desired (card, telephone call, or both), a record of previous recall appointments, reasons for recall, and desirable recall time.

The other card, filed according to the month in which the patient is to be recalled, contains the patient's name, the way he is to be notified, and the exact appointments that have been given previously. Depending on the policy of the office, but usually a month in advance, the dental assistant will review the recall records for the next month from the chronologic file. Recall form letters are prepared for each patient when this method is being used. If definite appointments are to be scheduled, they are recorded in the appointment book at this time, and a double postal card is prepared for mailing. When recall appointments have been recorded at the time of the previous visit, double postal cards are mailed. For those recalls requiring telephone calls, the card will be pulled at the time of the call.

No matter what type of recall program is used, a note is made on the recall record, giving the date of notification of recall or reminder and/or appointment.

At the time of the recall appointment, both the alphabetical and chronologic cards are removed from the file. On the alphabetical card, the date, service, and any pertinent information regarding the evaluation is recorded. The date of the next recall is indicated on the chronologic card and refiled. This card is refiled according to the month in which the patient will again be recalled.

Periodically, the recall records that have not been removed from the present month's file must be examined to determine the patient's recall status. If the patient has a definite appointment at a later date, the recall card can be tagged to indicate this. For those people who have failed to respond or keep their appointment, postal cards may be used to determine the patient's intentions regarding the preventive program. A postal card, which is to be completed by the patient and returned to the dental office, can be used. Its message could read as follows:

> I understand the benefits of the preventive program in Dr. Smith's office.
> I do
> wish to continue this program.
> I do not
> Name________________ Date_____

If time permits, a telephone call might be preferred, as telephone response is more immediate.

PATIENT CLINICAL RECORDS

It is extremely important that accurate clinical records be maintained for each patient who comes to the office for treatment or consultation. These will include pertinent information of the patient's past and present health status, a record of past oral conditions or treatment, a record of the treatment planned by the dentist for the patient, and a record of the treatment rendered by the dentist. Some additional materials that are part of the clinical record are study models, radiographs, photographs, and cephalometric tracings, where indicated. Forms used for keeping these records will vary from office to office, but the basic information that must be recorded will probably come under the headings that follow.

Office policies

Many dental offices have established policies concerning fees for broken appointments, the use and need of roentgenograms and study models, payment plans, rendering of statements, and so on. These may be printed on a special form that is given to the patient to read (Fig. 18-8), or the dental assistant responsible for records may go over these policies with the patient. The latter method allows the assistant to clarify any questions and permits her to inform the patient more fully regarding the reasons behind such policies. Because office policies are a part of the office procedures, the assistant should see that a patient is fully aware of these policies at the first visit, in order to prevent misunderstandings after treatment has been started.

Acquaintance forms

For each new patient who comes to the dental office, certain basic information is needed. This information includes the patient's name, address, telephone number, birth date, physician's name, and the name of the person who is responsible for finances. Frequently, this information is compiled on a registration form (Fig. 18-9) that the patient is asked to complete. In some offices, the dental assistant may complete the card and ask the patient the pertinent questions. This form is a "get acquainted card," because it permits the assistant to learn something more about the patient as she gathers the information needed for completion of the card. In some offices, this information is included on the patient's individual record, instead of being kept on a separate card.

Health status forms

The past history of the patient's health is an important part of the record of each individual patient. A health status form (Fig. 18-10) should be completed before any extensive treatment is given, for there may be some factors in a patient's health record that would prevent the dentist from following his usual operative procedures. A patient may be allergic to certain medications, or the dentist may wish to consult with the family physician concerning the patient's general physical condition before

POLICIES OF THIS OFFICE

We believe that service to our patients is at its best when there is complete mutual understanding and cooperation.

In our operation relationships, the patients expect certain ethical and professional standards of us.

In the establishment of fees and necessary arrangement for payment thereof, we expect your cooperation, to the end that this be done in accordance with sound business principles and standards.

We believe that our patients should expect from us:—

1. A high degree of professional skill and ability.
2. That we studiously keep abreast of progress in dental science.
3. The integrity to perform all services to the best of our knowledge and ability.
4. An explanation of our findings resulting from a thorough diagnosis, and the establishment of an estimated fee for work to be done.

In return, we believe we must expect from our patients:—

1. Complete cooperation in making and keeping appointments.
2. A conscientious effort to follow our instructions on home care and mouth hygiene.
3. Recall visits at such time as is indicated, according to individual mouth conditions.
4. A definite arrangement for the payment of fees.

In order to avoid interruption in our work with patients, the secretary has been given responsibility for making appointments and the collections of fees and accounts.

Please consult her concerning these matters.

Your cooperation will be appreciated.

Printed in U.S.A.

Fig. 18-8. The office policy form for new patients, giving information on office policies.

ACQUAINTANCE FORM

Date__________

Patient's Name__________ Date of Birth__________

Person responsible for account__________

Residence Address__________

Business Address__________

Residence Telephone__________ Business Telephone__________

Employer__________ How Long?__________

Occupation or type of work__________

Physician__________ Referred by__________

Relative or close friend__________

Former Dentist__________

Convenient Time for Appointments__________

F204 REV. 4-63 SPILLANE'S, MINNEAPOLIS 4, MINN.

Fig. 18-9. Acquaintance or registration form can be used to obtain additional pertinent information.

For your welfare and our efficiency of diagnosis and treatment, please fill in the following confidential form **completely.**

HEALTH HISTORY

Date ____________

Name of Physician ____________ City ____________

1. Approximate date of last physical examination ____________
2. Please circle any of the following conditions you have or have had: Anemia, Arthritis, Asthma, Diabetes, Dizziness, Fainting, Heart Ailment, High or Low Blood pressure, Kidney or Liver involvement, Nervous disorders, Rheumatic Fever, Tuberculosis.

	Yes	No
3. Excepting childhood diseases, have you had any other disease NOT mentioned above?	___	___
4. Are you being treated by a physician now?	___	___
5. Do you take any drugs or medication?	___	___
6. Have you ever had X-Ray Therapy?	___	___
7. Are you subject to prolonged bleeding?	___	___
8. Have you ever had any ill effects from Novocain—Penicillin—or other Antibiotics, Sulfa or any other drugs or food?	___	___
9. Approximate date of last dental visit?	___	___

10. Approximate date when teeth were last cleaned? ____________
11. Approximate date of last full mouth X-Ray? ____________
12. How often do you have your teeth cleaned? ____________

	Yes	No
13. How often do you brush your teeth?		
14. Do your gums bleed while brushing?	___	___
15. Do you avoid any part of your mouth while brushing?	___	___
16. Does food catch between your teeth?	___	___
17. Do your gums feel tender or swollen?	___	___
18. Have you ever been treated for "Trench Mouth"?	___	___
19. Have you ever had Pyorrhea (Periodontal) treatments?	___	___
20. Do heat, cold, or sweets cause pain in your mouth?	___	___
21. Do you have any other pain in your mouth?	___	___
22. Do you clench your teeth during the day or night?	___	___
23. Do your jaws ever feel tired?	___	___
24. Have you ever had pain in or near your ears?	___	___
25. Do you bite fingernails, pencils, bobby pins, pipe stems, or thread?	___	___
26. Have you had any **difficult** extractions in the past?	___	___
27. Have you any teeth missing that were not replaced by bridgework, partial or full dentures?	___	___

If the answer is YES to any of the above questions, Please explain fully:

____

____

____

	Yes	No
28. Have you ever been instructed in the proper home care of your mouth?	___	___
29. Have you ever been instructed on a proper diet?	___	___
30. Have you ever had a local anesthetic (Novocain)?	___	___

31. I hereby authorize the release of my medical records to this office. ____________
32. What do you think of your teeth? ____________

____

____

Date of Birth ____________ Signature ____________

Fig. 18-10. The health history form provides necessary information on the patient's health status.

proceeding with treatment. A medical history that includes special conditions should be tagged to indicate at a glance the urgency for precautions. The dental assistant needs to be familiar with these health records, since it may be her responsibility to remind the dentist of certain conditions when the patient is scheduled for treatment.

The health history may be recorded on a separate form that the patient is asked to fill out at home. This method has disadvantages, in that the patient may fail to answer all the questions or may give inaccurate answers. Sometimes, the dental assistant is given the responsibility of completing a portion of the health history as she questions the patient. In other instances, the dentist will question the patient, and the assistant will record the answers as the patient gives them. By examination and questioning, the dentist may ascertain the present state of the patient's health, and the dental assistant will record this information.

Patient's chart of current findings

A complete dental clinical record is maintained for each patient. The assistant will enter on this clinical record the findings of the intraoral examination and the radiographs made by the dentist. The record will include the dental treatment that was previously rendered for the patient and the treatment now needed (Fig. 18-11, *A*). The assistant will record services that are completed as the dental treatment progresses.

The clinical record includes a chart of the teeth, showing the 5 surfaces of the teeth—mesial, distal, facial, lingual, and occlusal for the posterior teeth, and mesial, distal, facial, lingual, and incisal for the anterior teeth. The charts show the permanent teeth numbered in arabic numerals, from 1 to 32, beginning on the maxillary right; the primary teeth are indicated by letters A through T, beginning on the maxillary right. This is one of the many ways in which teeth are designated on a chart. Sometimes the teeth are designated by numbers 1 through 8 on either side of the median, upper and lower; in other instances, the primary teeth may be designated by Roman numerals I through V.

Each office will have a charting system that is the written and/or diagrammed interpretation of findings, but all systems will want to show the patient's treatment record graphically, in a way that requires a minimum amount of study.

The following are some examples of charting procedures shown on Fig. 18-11:

1. The dental treatment previously received by the patient may be recorded in a different colored ink to make it stand out from the current treatments.
2. The carious areas (dental decay) are outlined to cover the involved surface(s).
3. When the carious areas are restored, the outline is filled in.
4. An "X" over the diagram of the tooth is used to indicate removal of the tooth (extraction).

Included in the patient's clinical record is the plan of treatment that the dentist uses for case presentation. This will include an estimate of the type of dental care, the amount of time that will be required, and the fees that will be assessed.

In some offices, a work schedule for each appointment (Fig. 18-12) is used by the dentist and other office personnel. The data includes the dentist's plan for the operation, and this enables the person who assists him to know the area of the mouth to be treated and the type of materials to be used. In this way, the instruments that will be needed, the position of the patient, the kind of anesthetic needed, and the amount of materials needed can be anticipated and made ready for the dentist's use.

Record maintenance

Patient clinical records may be maintained in various ways—card systems, ledger books, or individual patient folders.

A

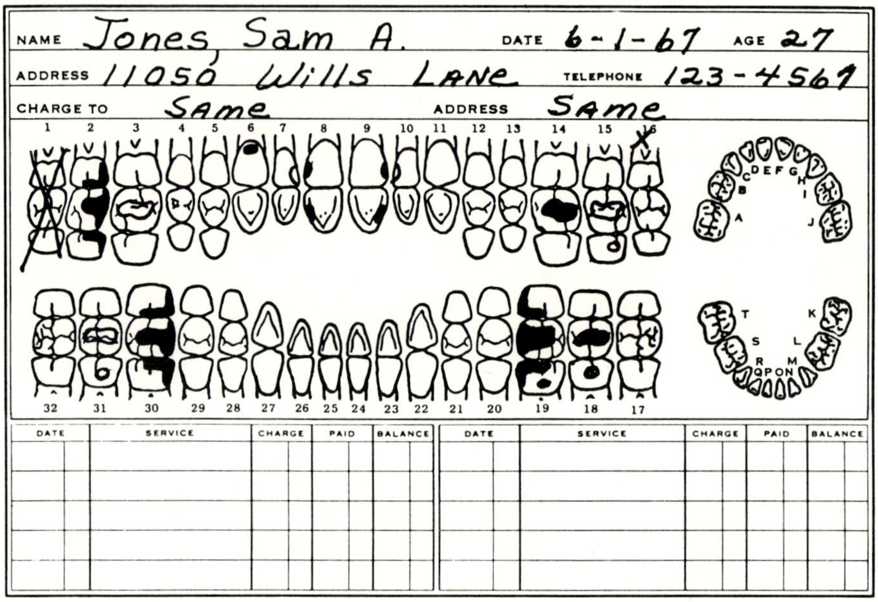

B

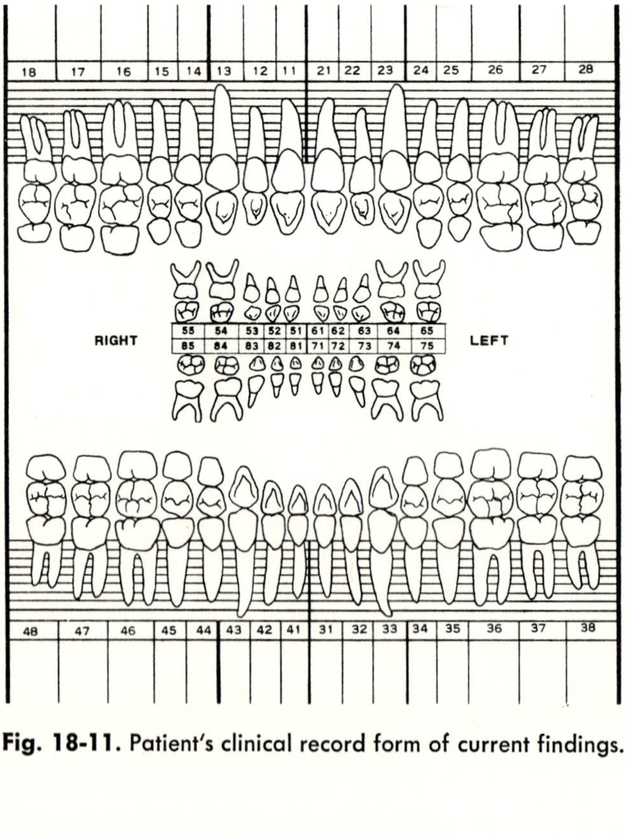

Fig. 18-11. Patient's clinical record form of current findings.

TREATMENT PLANNING FORM

To be completed by dentist:

Patient______________________; File No.________; Date_____

- -

TEETH & SURFACES: ____ ____ ____ ____ ____

RESTORATIVE MATERIAL: ____ ____ ____ ____ ____

- -

Information to be supplied by assistant:

INSTRUMENTS & MATERIALS:	BASIC	ROTARY	HAND	OTHER
	____	____	____	____
	____	____	____	____
	____	____	____	____

ANESTHESIA:______________________

POSITION - of patient:______________; -of foot control______________.

COMMENTS:____.

DENTIST______________: DENTAL ASSISTANT(S)__________________.

- -

Fig. 18-12. Work schedule form.

These records are often filed separating patients who are currently receiving treatment and patients who are not currently under treatment.

These records are taken from the file and made available to the dentist to review; they are then placed in the operatory when the patient is there for an appointment. The dental assistant's responsibility includes recording the date, services rendered, and fee for the treatment.

FINANCIAL AND BOOKKEEPING RECORDS

The bookkeeping involved in recording the financial records of the dental office must be accurate, complete, and current at all times. This is necessary for the protection of the dentist and the patient, for tax purposes, and for practice analysis. These records are written on permanent forms for present use and future reference. Although there are complete systems that may be used, many dentists have adapted forms or portions of these systems to meet their individual needs. The dental assistant who is responsible for the financial records will find that bookkeeping is involved in records concerning the individual patients, the operation of the office, and the personal accounts of the dentist-employer. She must recognize that these records are privileged information and are not to be divulged to anyone.

Patient financial records

Estimate record

It is customary for the dentist to make a treatment plan for each patient and to estimate in advance of any treatment the amount of time that will be required and the fees that will be involved. This plan is then presented to the patient, and an agreement is reached between the dentist and patient concerning how the patient will handle the payment of his account. The dental assistant will be responsible for recording the treatment plan and the estimate

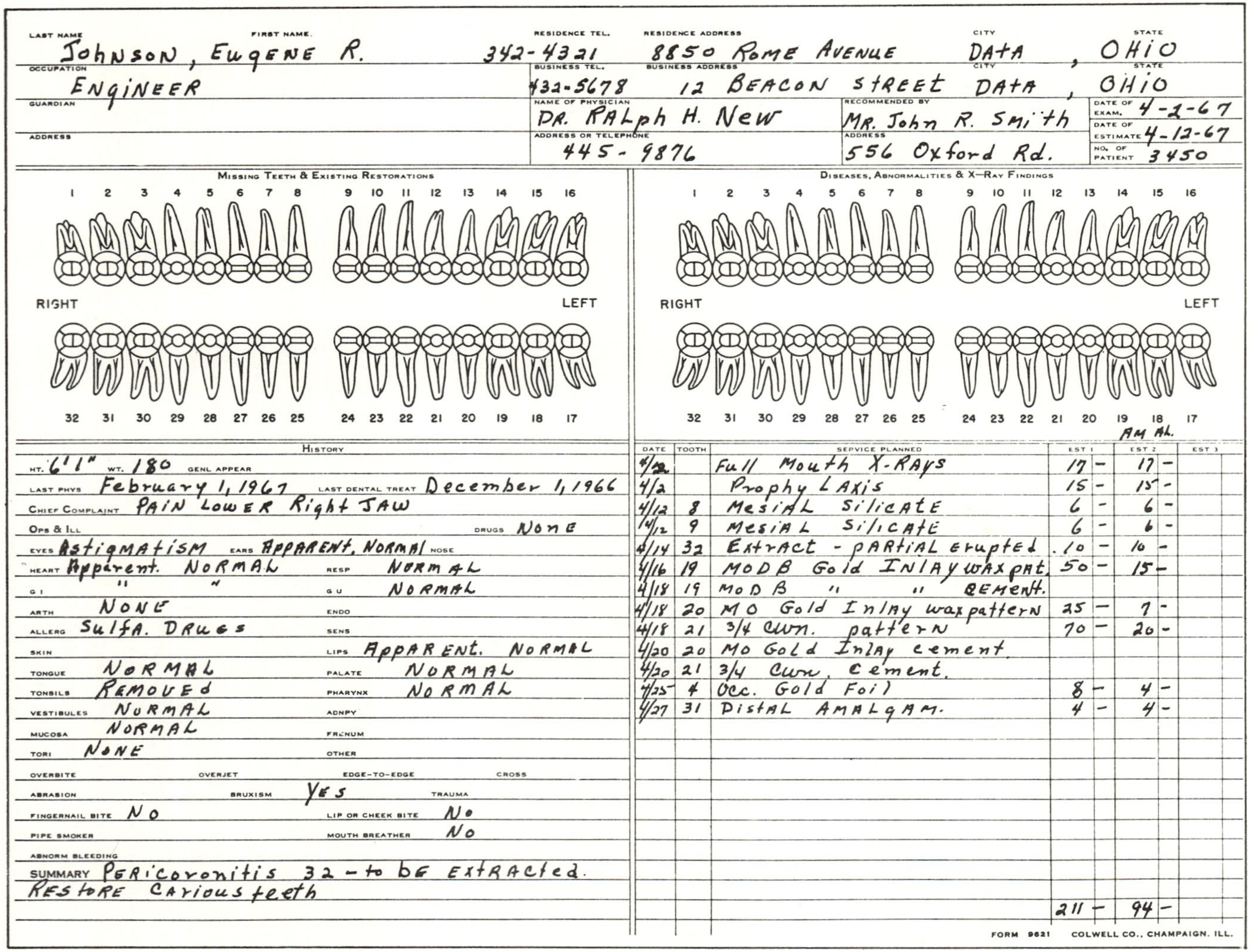

LAST NAME / FIRST NAME: Johnson, Eugene R. RESIDENCE TEL.: 342-4321 RESIDENCE ADDRESS: 8850 Rome Avenue CITY: Data, STATE: Ohio

OCCUPATION: Engineer BUSINESS TEL.: 432-5678 BUSINESS ADDRESS: 12 Beacon Street CITY: Data, STATE: Ohio

GUARDIAN NAME OF PHYSICIAN: Dr. Ralph H. New RECOMMENDED BY: Mr. John R. Smith DATE OF EXAM.: 4-2-67

ADDRESS ADDRESS OR TELEPHONE: 445-9876 ADDRESS: 556 Oxford Rd. DATE OF ESTIMATE: 4-12-67 NO. OF PATIENT: 3450

MISSING TEETH & EXISTING RESTORATIONS

1 2 3 4 5 6 7 8 9 10 11 12 13 14 15 16

RIGHT LEFT

32 31 30 29 28 27 26 25 24 23 22 21 20 19 18 17

DISEASES, ABNORMALITIES & X-RAY FINDINGS

1 2 3 4 5 6 7 8 9 10 11 12 13 14 15 16

RIGHT LEFT

32 31 30 29 28 27 26 25 24 23 22 21 20 19 18 17

Am Al.

HISTORY

HT. 6'1" WT. 180 GENL APPEAR

LAST PHYS February 1, 1967 LAST DENTAL TREAT December 1, 1966

CHIEF COMPLAINT Pain lower right jaw

OPS & ILL DRUGS None

EYES Astigmatism EARS Apparent, normal NOSE

HEART Apparent. Normal RESP Normal

G I " " G U Normal

ARTH None ENDO

ALLERG Sulfa. Drugs SENS

SKIN LIPS Apparent. Normal

TONGUE Normal PALATE Normal

TONSILS Removed PHARYNX Normal

VESTIBULES Normal ADNPY

MUCOSA Normal FRENUM

TORI None OTHER

OVERBITE OVERJET EDGE-TO-EDGE CROSS

ABRASION BRUXISM Yes TRAUMA

FINGERNAIL BITE No LIP OR CHEEK BITE No

PIPE SMOKER MOUTH BREATHER No

ABNORM BLEEDING

SUMMARY Pericoronitis 32 – to be extracted. Restore carious teeth

DATE	TOOTH	SERVICE PLANNED	EST 1	EST 2	EST 3
4/2		Full Mouth X-Rays	17 –	17 –	
4/2		Prophylaxis	15 –	15 –	
4/12	8	Mesial Silicate	6 –	6 –	
4/12	9	Mesial Silicate	6 –	6 –	
4/14	32	Extract - partial erupted	10 –	10 –	
4/16	19	MODB Gold Inlay wax pat.	50 –	15 –	
4/18	19	MODB " " cement.			
4/18	20	MO Gold Inlay wax pattern	25 –	7 –	
4/18	21	3/4 Crwn. pattern	70 –	20 –	
4/20	20	MO Gold Inlay cement.			
4/20	21	3/4 Crwn. cement.			
4/25	4	Occ. Gold Foil	8 –	4 –	
4/27	31	Distal Amalgam.	4 –	4 –	
			211 –	94 –	

FORM 9621 COLWELL CO., CHAMPAIGN, ILL.

Fig. 18-13. A dental clinical record, which includes an estimate form.

STATEMENT

JOHN H. JOHNSON, D. D. S.
GENERAL DENTISTRY
2800 FALLS AVENUE
ANY TOWN, U. S. A., ZIP CODE

Phone
233-3363

FAMILY NAME
HIS STREET ADDRESS
HIS CITY, STATE, ZIP CODE

A-1000-03L

NUMBER	DATE	DESCRIPTION SEE CODE BELOW		CHARGE	PAYMENT	CURRENT BALANCE
1456	5/1	Am	Mary	7 –		7 –
1541	5/10	EX	John	5 –		12 –
1564	5/11	FMS	John	15 –		27 –
1601	5/20	CR	John	200 –	50 00	177 –
1610	5/29	3Am	John	PCC		177 –
1615	6/10	PD	John	PCC		177 –
1650	6/20	ROA			50 00	127 –
2100	7/20	ROA			50 00	77 –

COPYRIGHTED FORM OF LATTA'S INC., WATERLOO, IOWA 12-59
CONTROL-O-FAX REG. U. S. PAT. OFFICE NO. 668323 FORM A-1000-03L

PLEASE PAY THE LAST FIGURE IN THIS COLUMN

AM–Amalgam Filling
BR–Bridge
CN–Crown
D–Denture
EX–Examination
EXT–Extraction
FA–Failed Appointment
NT–Nerve Treatment
PD–Partial Denture
PF–Porcelain Filling
PRO–Prophylaxis
RCT–Root Canal Treatment
X–X-Ray
GT–Gum Treatment
G–Gold Inlay
NC–No Charge
DR–Denture Repair
SF–Silver Filling
FMS–Full Mouth Survey
SFT–Stannous Fluoride Treatment
ROA–Received on Account
SM–Space Maintainer
CR–Complete Restoration
PCC–Previously Charged on Account

THIS IS A THERMO-FAX DRY COPY OF YOUR ACCOUNT AS IT APPEARS ON YOUR LEDGER CARD

Fig. 18-14. An example of a monthly itemized family statement. (Courtesy Control-O-Fax.)

of time and fees. This record may take the form of a contract signed by the patient and included in the patient's folder, or the estimate may be an entry on the patient's individual record.

Monthly statements

The monthly statement (Fig. 18-14) is the most commonly used method of reminding patients of payment due. The statement is sent to the person who was indicated as responsible for payment of the account. If several members of a family are currently receiving dental service, only 1 statement is generally sent to that family. Some professional offices do not itemize services rendered. The policy of the office will determine the time of the month that statements are issued. Some offices send all statements at a particular time of the month, while other offices prefer to issue statements throughout the month.

Receipts

A receipt (Fig. 18-15) is a written acknowledgement indicating that something has been obtained from another person. In the dental office, the receipt book is a necessary record in the bookkeeping system. The receipt is prepared in duplicate; one copy is presented or mailed to the patient, and the carbon copy is retained in the receipt book for the dental office records. A receipt should be made for every payment received, regardless of whether it is made by cash, by check or money order, in person, or by mail. The receipt should show the date, the amount paid, and the name of the person whose account is to be credited, if it is different from the payer. If a check made out to the dentist is for a sum larger than the payment and change is given to the payer, this information should be indicated on the receipt. All payments must be recorded on the patient's individual record and on the daily sheet.

Financing of dental care

Dental care may be financed in a number of ways. A relatively new concept in financing is the prepayment plan.

Prepayment

A prepayment plan involves a contract between a dental service corporation or insurance company and an individual to provide for the cost of dental care. The individual pays premiums, as he would for other types of health insurance. The contractor compensates or reimburses the subscriber for the cost of his dental care. Prepayment plans are becoming more widly used.

Postpayment

A postpayment plan involves a contract between an individual and a bank or cor-

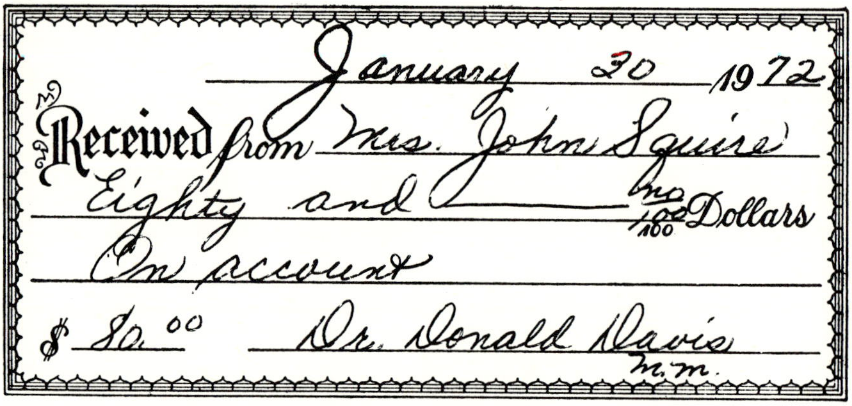
January 30 1972
Received from Mrs. John Squire
Eighty and no/100 Dollars
On account
$ 80.00 Dr. Donald Davis
m.m.

Fig. 18-15. Receipt.

poration to pay for the necesary dental services. The dental office receives the total fee before or at completion of the work. The individual arranges for regular payments with the bank or corporation.

Budget plan

A budget plan is a contract between the patient and the dental office to pay the total dental fee in prearranged amounts at regular intervals.

Government Assistance Program Title XIX

Title XIX, authorized by the Social Security Amendments of 1965, provides a medical assistance program in which both state and federal governments participate. Families who are receiving governmental assistance or who are unable to meet the cost of needed health services are eligible. These services include basic dental care. Preauthorization is needed only for those procedures considered as extended dental services, for example: orthodontics, dentures, and porcelain jacket crowns.

The Title XIX programs may vary from one state to another, as the programs involves both state and federal government participation.

The dental assistant will want to become familiar with the Title XIX program in the state in which she is employed. She should be able to complete the necessary records for the patient covered by insurance or under Title XIX.

Daily sheet

The daily sheet (Fig. 18-16) is a detailed record of each financial transaction of the day. This record is usually divided into labeled columns, in which the following are entered: patient's name, specific professional service rendered, time utilized, consultations, fees for each of the services, receipts, and disbursements. This daily sheet serves as the basis for the completion of other office record forms. The daily sheet is the most time-consuming part of the dental office bookkeeping system, and it requires the most accurate recording. Care must be taken to make sure that the fee for each service is recorded immediately after the service has been performed, and that funds that have been collected or disbursed are properly entered.

From this daily sheet, entries are transferred to the patient's clinical record and to the patient's financial record if a separate financial record card is maintained. This record will contain the specific date, professional service rendered, fee for each procedure, payments on account, and balance due on the account (Fig. 18-17).

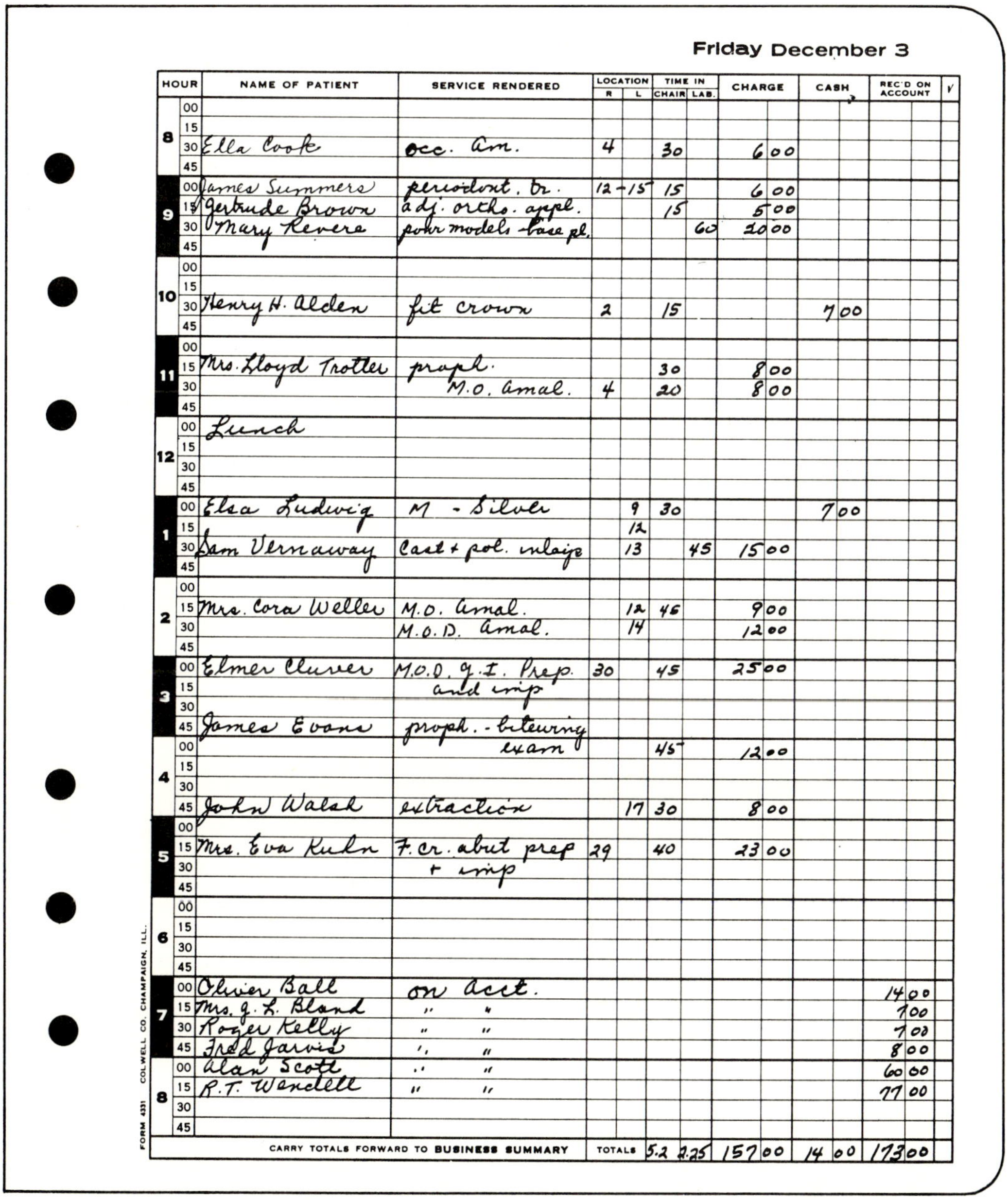

Friday December 3

HOUR		NAME OF PATIENT	SERVICE RENDERED	LOCATION R	LOCATION L	TIME IN CHAIR	TIME IN LAB.	CHARGE	CASH	REC'D ON ACCOUNT	✓
8	00										
	15										
	30	Ella Cook	occ. am.	4		30		6 00			
	45										
9	00	James Summers	periodont. tr.	12–15		15		6 00			
	15	Gertrude Brown	adj. ortho. appl.			15		5 00			
	30	Mary Revere	pour models base pl.				60	10 00			
	45										
10	00										
	15										
	30	Henry H. Alden	fit crown	2		15			7 00		
	45										
11	00										
	15	Mrs. Lloyd Trotter	proph.			30		8 00			
	30		M.O. amal.	4		20		8 00			
	45										
12	00	Lunch									
	15										
	30										
	45										
1	00	Elsa Ludwig	M - Silver		9	30			7 00		
	15				12						
	30	Sam Vernaway	Cast + pol. inlays		13		45	15 00			
	45										
2	00										
	15	Mrs. Cora Weller	M.O. amal.		12	46		9 00			
	30		M.O.D. amal.		14			12 00			
	45										
3	00	Elmer Cluver	M.O.D. G.I. Prep. and imp	30		45		25 00			
	15										
	30										
	45	James Evans	proph. - bitewing exam								
4	00					45		12 00			
	15										
	30										
	45	John Walsh	extraction		17	30		8 00			
5	00										
	15	Mrs. Eva Kuhn	F. cr. abut prep + imp	29		40		23 00			
	30										
	45										
6	00										
	15										
	30										
	45										
7	00	Oliver Ball	on Acct.							14 00	
	15	Mrs. J. L. Bland	" "							7 00	
	30	Roger Kelly	" "							7 00	
	45	Fred Jarvis	" "							8 00	
8	00	Alan Scott	" "							60 00	
	15	R.T. Wendell	" "							77 00	
	30										
	45										
CARRY TOTALS FORWARD TO **BUSINESS SUMMARY**				TOTALS		5.2	2.25	157 00	14 00	173 00	

FORM 4331 COLWELL CO. CHAMPAIGN, ILL.

Fig. 18-16. The daily sheet is a detailed record of patients treated, services rendered, fees, and receipts.

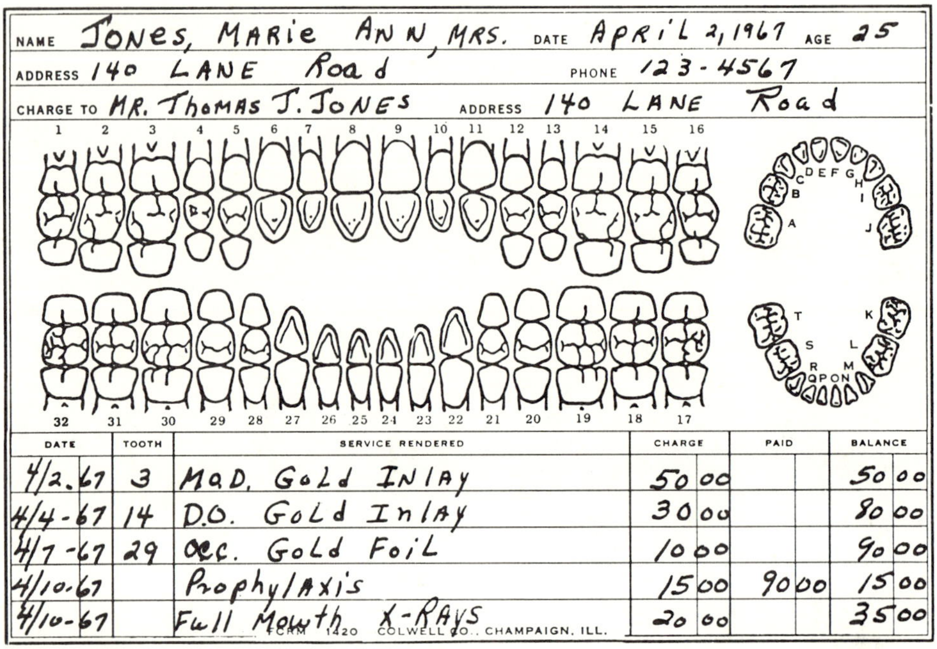
NAME JONES, MARIE ANN, MRS. DATE APRIL 2, 1967 AGE 25

ADDRESS 140 LANE Road PHONE 123-4567

CHARGE TO MR. Thomas J. JONES ADDRESS 140 LANE Road

1 2 3 4 5 6 7 8 9 10 11 12 13 14 15 16

C D E F G H B I A J

T K S L R M Q P O N

32 31 30 29 28 27 26 25 24 23 22 21 20 19 18 17

DATE	TOOTH	SERVICE RENDERED	CHARGE	PAID	BALANCE
4/2-67	3	MOD. Gold INLAY	50 00		50 00
4/4-67	14	D.O. Gold Inlay	30 00		80 00
4/7-67	29	Occ. Gold Foil	10 00		90 00
4/10-67		Prophylaxis	15 00	90 00	15 00
4/10-67		Full Mouth X-RAYS	20 00		35 00

FORM 1420 COLWELL CO., CHAMPAIGN, ILL.

Fig. 18-17. Patient's financial record, including date, services rendered, fees, payment on account, and balance due.

Monthly record

A summary of totals on all columns of the daily sheet is posted on the monthly record (Fig. 18-18, *A* and *B*). Additional information available on the monthly sheet is totaled for the month, and the totals from previous months and the grand total to date are calculated. These totals provide at a glance the difference between total business and total fees paid on account, indicating the dental load, fees collected, and accounts receivable. The record of the balance due on the accounts of each patient makes up the accounts receivable. The totals of accounts receivable are summarized on the daily, monthly, and yearly sheets.

Expense sheet

Another bookkeeping record that might be used is shown in Fig. 18-19, *A* and *B*, which illustrates a method of recording the overall expenses incurred in the operation of the dental office.

Annual records

A yearly recapitulation sheet maintained from the monthly records provides a monthly and yearly analysis that is very important to the economy of the office. The annual summary (Fig. 18-20) gives the overall totals for the business of the office, including charges, income, and disbursements. The annual summary of the expense sheet (Fig. 18-21) provides an itemized breakdown of office overhead expenditures on a monthly basis, with annual totals. This record provides information necessary in completing income tax returns. The nondeductible and deductible items for income tax returns are easily identified from this sheet.

Payroll

The payroll sheet (Fig. 18-22) is an accurate account of all gross salaries, federal withholding, Federal Insurance Contributions Act deductions, and net salaries paid.

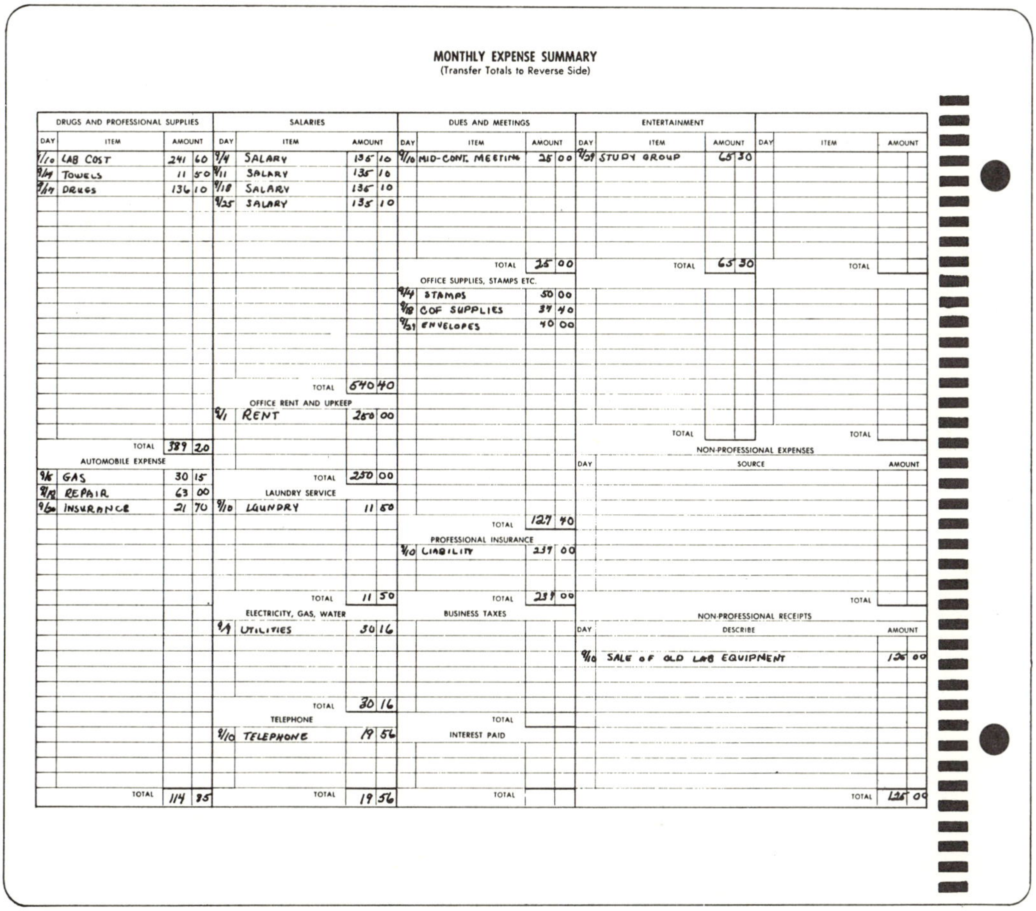
MONTHLY EXPENSE SUMMARY
(Transfer Totals to Reverse Side)

DRUGS AND PROFESSIONAL SUPPLIES

DAY	ITEM	AMOUNT	
9/10	LAB COST	241	60
9/14	TOWELS	11	50
9/17	DRUGS	136	10
	TOTAL	389	20

AUTOMOBILE EXPENSE

DAY	ITEM	AMOUNT	
9/5	GAS	30	15
9/12	REPAIR	63	00
9/20	INSURANCE	21	70
	TOTAL	114	85

SALARIES

DAY	ITEM	AMOUNT	
9/4	SALARY	135	10
9/11	SALARY	135	10
9/18	SALARY	135	10
9/25	SALARY	135	10
	TOTAL	540	40

OFFICE RENT AND UPKEEP

DAY	ITEM	AMOUNT	
9/1	RENT	250	00
	TOTAL	250	00

LAUNDRY SERVICE

DAY	ITEM	AMOUNT	
9/10	LAUNDRY	11	50
	TOTAL	11	50

ELECTRICITY, GAS, WATER

DAY	ITEM	AMOUNT	
9/9	UTILITIES	30	16
	TOTAL	30	16

TELEPHONE

DAY	ITEM	AMOUNT	
9/10	TELEPHONE	19	56
	TOTAL	19	56

DUES AND MEETINGS

DAY	ITEM	AMOUNT	
9/10	MID-CONT. MEETING	25	00
	TOTAL	25	00

OFFICE SUPPLIES, STAMPS ETC.

DAY	ITEM	AMOUNT	
9/4	STAMPS	50	00
9/18	COF SUPPLIES	37	40
9/21	ENVELOPES	40	00
	TOTAL	127	40

PROFESSIONAL INSURANCE

DAY	ITEM	AMOUNT	
9/10	LIABILITY	237	00
	TOTAL	237	00

BUSINESS TAXES

DAY	ITEM	AMOUNT	
	TOTAL		

INTEREST PAID

DAY	ITEM	AMOUNT	
	TOTAL		

ENTERTAINMENT

DAY	ITEM	AMOUNT	
9/29	STUDY GROUP	65	30
	TOTAL	65	30

DAY	ITEM	AMOUNT	
	TOTAL		

NON-PROFESSIONAL EXPENSES

DAY	SOURCE	AMOUNT	
	TOTAL		

NON-PROFESSIONAL RECEIPTS

DAY	DESCRIBE	AMOUNT	
9/10	SALE OF OLD LAB EQUIPMENT	125	00
	TOTAL	125	00

Fig. 18-18. Monthly record of office expenditures and receipts.

Also recorded on this sheet is the name of employees, the social security numbers, and the number of exemptions claimed by each person. In cases in which a state income tax is assessed, one column can be labeled for that withholding. This record is essential for accurate tax returns for the employee and employer.

Bank account

Checks

A check (Fig. 18-23) is an order to pay a specified sum of money to a person or party. The check contains the date issued, the name of the person or party to whom the money is paid, the amount, and the signature of the issuer.

Endorsement of checks

The endorsement (Fig 18-24) is a signature on the back of the check, usually on the top left-hand side, whereby the endorser transfers his rights in the check to another person or party.

Bank statement

The bank statement (Fig. 18-25) is an itemized report from the bank, indicating the balance brought forward from the previous month, the amount of each check pro-

Text continued on p. 385.

CONTROL-O-FAX® MONTHLY SUMMARY

FORM NO. A-1000-197J 4-64 LITHO IN U.S.A.
THIS IS A COPYRIGHTED FORM OF LATTA'S INC. WATERLOO, IOWA

CONTROL-O-FAX

DAY OF MONTH	CHARGES (COLUMN "A")		PAYMENTS (COLUMN "B")		MISC. SUMMARIES X-RAY			
1	175	00	200	00	30	00		
2	97	50	156	00	12	00		
3	200	00	185	00				
4	217	00	39	50	46	00		
5								
6								
7	155	50	275	50	50	00		
8	186	00	86	00	12	00		
9	205	00	173	00	40	00		
10	137	00	123	00	15	00		
11	163	50	177	00	8	00		
12								
13								
14	300	00	376	00	17	00		
15	79	50	123	00	6	00		
16	135	00	147	00				
17	179	00	183	00				
18	206	00	139	00	26	00		
19								
20								
21	196	00	279	00	16	00		
22	93	00	75	00				
23	156	00	146	00	20	00		
24	120	50	193	00	7	00		
25	136	50	121	00	9	00		
26								
27								
28	146	00	190	00				
29	170	00	188	00	27	00		
30	96	00	107	00				
31								
TOTAL FOR MONTH	3549	00	3,682	00	340	00		
BROUGHT FORWARD	27,394	00	24,993	00	2,107	00		
GRAND TOTAL	30,943	00	28,675	00	2,447	00		

SUMMARY OF EXPENSE (From Reverse Side)	AMOUNT	
DRUGS AND PROFESSIONAL SUPPLIES	389	20
AUTOMOBILE EXPENSE	114	85
SALARIES	540	40
OFFICE RENT AND UPKEEP	250	00
LAUNDRY SERVICE	11	50
ELECTRICITY, GAS, WATER	30	16
TELEPHONE	19	56
DUES AND MEETINGS	25	00
OFFICE SUPPLIES, STAMPS, ETC.	127	40
PROFESSIONAL INSURANCE	237	00
BUSINESS TAXES		
INTEREST PAID		
ENTERTAINMENT	65	30
TOTAL FOR PRESENT MONTH	1810	37
FORWARDED FROM PREVIOUS MONTH	12,463	19
GRAND TOTAL	14,273	56
MONTHLY BALANCES		
For The Present Month		
TOTAL RECEIPTS (COL. B)	3,682	00
TOTAL EXPENSE	1,810	37
NET EARNINGS	1,871	63
For The Year To Date		
GRAND TOTAL RECEIPTS	28,675	00
GRAND TOTAL EXPENSE	14,273	56
NET EARNINGS	14,401	44
ACCOUNTS RECEIVABLE (FROM LAST DAY SHEET OF THE MONTH) $ 9,344	00	CHECKED BY HCG

Month SEPTEMBER Year 1964

CONTROL-O-FAX® SUMMARY SHEET — MONTHLY INDEX

Fig. 18-18, cont'd. For legend see p. 375.

December Expense Sheet One

DENTAL SUPPLIES

DAY	ITEM	AMOUNT	
3	Circle Dental	45	65
3	J.S. Fischer Co.	99	15
3	Dentist Supply	112	80
18	West Drug Co	43	06
23	C. Miller Co.	92	50
	TOTAL	393	16

LABORATORY FEES

DAY	ITEM	AMOUNT	
3	Cox Lab.	85	12
3	Smith Lab.	126	63
18	Cox Lab.	72	25
	TOTAL	284	00

SALARIES

DAY	ITEM	AMOUNT	
2	Mary Wells	61	52
9	" "	61	52
16	" "	61	52
23	" "	61	52
30	" "	61	52
2	Ruth Freeland	82	83
9	" "	82	83
16	" "	82	83
23	" "	82	83
30	" "	82	83
	TOTAL	721	75

OFFICE RENT, UPKEEP

DAY	ITEM	AMOUNT	
3	Bldg. & Loan	180	00
5	Fall & Sons	98	00
	TOTAL	278	00

LAUNDRY SERVICE

DAY	ITEM	AMOUNT	
5	Towel Service	18	75
9	Gen'l. Ldy.	14	90
23	Towel Service	23	15
	TOTAL	56	80

ELECTRICITY, GAS, WATER

DAY	ITEM	AMOUNT	
14	State Power Co	45	75
	TOTAL	45	75

TELEPHONE, TOLLS

DAY	ITEM	AMOUNT	
14	State Bell	26	80
	TOTAL	26	80

DUES, MEETINGS

DAY	ITEM	AMOUNT	
22	State Dental Ass'n.	25	00
	TOTAL	25	00

OFFICE SUPPLIES, STAMPS ETC.

DAY	ITEM	AMOUNT	
6	Stamps	20	00
12	Life Magazine	7	00
15	Petty Cash	29	14
20	Colwell Co.	42	50
	TOTAL	98	64

PROFESSIONAL INSURANCE

DAY	ITEM	AMOUNT	
14	Mutual Ins. Co	38	20
	TOTAL	38	20

CARRY TOTALS FORWARD TO **SUMMARY OF EXPENSE**

DEC

Fig. 18-19. An example of an expense sheet.

Expense Sheet Two December

BUSINESS TAXES				ENTERTAINMENT				MISCELLANEOUS			
DAY	ITEM	AMOUNT		DAY	ITEM	AMOUNT		DAY	ITEM	AMOUNT	
15	Co Collector	38	06	4	Lunch-Dr. Boyd	2	50	3	C. Johns		
				12	Flowers				repair chair	14	50
					Mrs. Bell	7	50	4	W. J. Grum	10	70
				20	Elks Benefit	5	00				
	TOTAL	38	06		TOTAL	15	00				
INTEREST PAID											
	TOTAL				TOTAL				TOTAL	25	20

CARRY TOTALS FORWARD TO **SUMMARY OF EXPENSE**

SUMMARY OF EXPENSE

	AMOUNT	
DENTAL SUPPLIES	393	16
LABORATORY FEES	284	00
SALARIES	721	75
OFFICE RENT UPKEEP	278	00
LAUNDRY SERVICE	56	80
ELECTRICITY, GAS, WATER	45	75
TELEPHONES TOLLS	26	80
DUES MEETINGS	25	00
OFFICE SUPPLIES, STAMPS, ETC.	98	64
PROFESSIONAL INSURANCE	38	20
BUSINESS TAXES	38	06
INTEREST PAID		
ENTERTAINMENT	15	00
MISCELLANEOUS	25	20
TOTAL FOR PRESENT MONTH	2046	36
FORWARDED FROM PREVIOUS MONTH	2939	40
GRAND TOTAL	4985	76

FORM 4343 COLWELL CO. CHAMPAIGN, ILL.

MONTHLY BALANCES

FOR THE PRESENT MONTH

TOTAL CASH RECEIVED	3884	00
TOTAL EXPENSE	2064	36
NET EARNINGS	1837	64

FOR THE YEAR TO DATE

GRAND TOTAL CASH	12264	00
GRAND TOTAL EXPENSE	4985	76
NET EARNINGS	7278	24

EQUIPMENT (NONDEDUCTIBLE)

DAY	ITEM	AMOUNT	
20	X-Ray Supply Co.-on acct	160	00
22	Reliable Furn. Co.		
	rec. rm. chair	74	28
	*TOTAL	234	28

* ENTER THIS TOTAL DIRECT IN **ANNUAL SUMMARY**

DEC

Fig. 18-19, cont'd. For legend see p. 377.

Annual Summary

Section	Item	Amount	¢	Total	¢
VOLUME (FROM DECEMBER GRAND TOTALS)	TOTAL CHARGE BUSINESS	44,165	70		
	TOTAL CASH BUSINESS	3,415	20		
	TOTAL BUSINESS			47,580	90
RECEIPTS (FROM DECEMBER GRAND TOTALS)	TOTAL REC'D ON ACCOUNTS	40,361	40		
	TOTAL CASH BUSINESS	3,415	20		
	TOTAL CASH FROM PROFESSION			43,776	50
DISBURSEMENTS (FROM OPPOSITE PAGE)	DENTAL SUPPLIES	2,506	33		
	LABORATORY FEES	2,012	73		
	SALARIES	9,359	85		
	OFFICE RENT UPKEEP	2,904	00		
	LAUNDRY SERVICE	409	06		
	ELECTRICITY GAS WATER	495	89		
	TELEPHONE TOLLS	418	40		
	DUES MEETINGS	517	75		
	OFFICE SUPPLIES STAMPS ETC.	511	04		
	PROFESSIONAL INSURANCE	179	74		
	BUSINESS TAXES	330	24		
	INTEREST PAID	625	40		
	ENTERTAINMENT ETC.	257	23		
	DEPRECIATION	653	40		
	MISCELLANEOUS	325	79		
	TOTAL PROFESSIONAL EXPENSE			21,506	84
	NET FROM PROFESSION			22,269	66
	DIVIDENDS, INTEREST			1,240	00
	NET FROM OTHER SOURCES			2,216	40
	TOTAL INCOME			25,726	06

OTHER EXPENSE (NONDEDUCTIBLE)	TOTALS	¢	NON PROFESSIONAL DEDUCTIONS	TOTALS	¢
FEDERAL INCOME TAX (FROM OPPOSITE PAGE)	3827	15	CONTRIBUTIONS (FROM NEXT PAGE)	1150	00
OFFICE FURNISHINGS " "	211	60	REAL ESTATE TAX " " "	580	39
INSTRUMENTS " "	393	89	OTHER TAXES " " "	78	75
BOOKS " "	130	00	Sales "	320	00
PERSONAL EXPENSE (FROM DECEMBER GRAND TOTAL)	11,204	55			
INVESTMENTS " "	7,260	85	INTEREST EXPENSE " " "		
			BAD DEBTS " " "		
			LOSSES " " "	41	90
TOTAL	23,028	04	TOTAL	2171	04

FORM 4338 COLWELL CO. CHAMPAIGN, ILL.

Fig. 18-20. Example of an annual summary record.

Annual Summary of Expense

OFFICE OVERHEAD (DEDUCTIBLE FOR INCOME TAX)										
	DENTAL SUPPLIES	LAB FEES	SALARIES	OFFICE RENT UPKEEP	LAUNDRY SERVICE	ELEC GAS WATER	TELEPHONE TOLLS	DUES MEETINGS	OFFICE SUPPLIES	PROF INS
JAN	289 08	283 44	577 40	180 00	42 15	38 85	21 40	23 00	15 30	43 09
FEB	178 10	116 74	577 40	180 00	48 60	40 60	32 10	112 00	12 00	
MAR	393 16	284 00	721 75	275 00	56 80	45 75	26 80	25 00	98 64	38 20
APR	262 40	239 55	1040 80	180 00	32 90	37 00	24 40		29 00	16 40
MAY	192 45	94 60	577 40	180 00	26 40	41 25	32 55		44 25	
JUN	211 23	159 63	721 75	295 00	51 60	46 70	36 10	25 00	8 00	
JUL	160 30	147 88	1040 80	250 00	14 85	26 19	20 70		12 64	22 10
AUG	161 82	64 51	577 40	250 00	9 16	42 80	48 55	210 30		
SEP	158 69	101 90	721 75	361 60	19 60	41 60	56 40	35 00	108 75	50 00
OCT	283 26	292 40	1040 80	250 00	46 90	42 10	24 80		46 12	
NOV	103 40	86 28	577 40	250 00	22 00	48 65	41 65		117 64	
DEC	112 44	141 80	1185 20	250 00	38 10	44 40	52 95	87 75	18 70	9 95
TOT	2506 33	2012 73	9359 85	2904 00	409 06	495 89	418 40	517 75	511 04	179 74

OFFICE OVERHEAD CONTINUED							NONDEDUCTIBLE ITEMS			
	BUSINESS TAXES	INTEREST PAID	ENTER TAINMENT	MISCEL LANEOUS			FEDERAL INCOME TAX	OFFICE FURN	INSTRU MENTS	BOOKS
JAN			19 87	47 50				25 10	60 00	
FEB			18 66	42 12					60 00	
MAR	38 06		15 00	25 20			945 00	74 28	60 00	
APR	73 06		10 10	49 06					66 00	
MAY			6 00	9 42						
JUN		312 70	7 45	18 20			945 00		39 25	
JUL	73 06		18 25							
AUG				96 24					54 00	
SEP			108 00	22 05			945 00	112 22		
OCT	73 06		7 75	32 43					42 40	
NOV		312 70	34 15	119 97					12 24	
DEC			12 00	143 60			992 15			
TOT	330 24	625 40	257 23	325 79			3827 15	211 60	393 89	

OTHER EXPENSE (NONDEDUCTIBLE)			OTHER EXPENSE (NONDEDUCTIBLE)			OTHER EXPENSE (NONDEDUCTIBLE)		
DATE	ITEM	AMOUNT	DATE	ITEM	AMOUNT	DATE	ITEM	AMOUNT

Fig. 18-21. A sample annual summary expense sheet that provides detailed record of monthly expenditures.

Payroll December

NAME: Mary Wills SOC. SEC. NO. 347-28-9331 NUMBER OF EXEMPTIONS 1

DATE	HOURS	RATE	GROSS PAY		WITHHOLDING		F.I.C.A.						NET PAY	
Dec. 2			75	00	11	14	2	34					61	52
9			75	00	11	14	2	34					61	52
16			75	00	11	14	2	34					61	52
23			75	00	11	14	2	34					61	52
30			75	00	11	14	2	34					61	52
		TOTALS	375	00	55	70	11	70					307	60
QUARTER		BROUGHT FWD	600	00	89	12	18	72					492	16
		TO DATE	975	00	144	82	30	42					799	76
YEAR		BROUGHT FWD.												
		TO DATE												

NAME: Ruth Freeland SOC. SEC. NO. 395-17-1444 NUMBER OF EXEMPTIONS 0

DATE	HOURS	RATE	GROSS PAY		WITHHOLDING		F.I.C.A.						NET PAY	
Dec. 2			105	00	18	89	3	28					82	83
9			105	00	18	89	3	28					82	83
16			105	00	18	89	3	28					82	83
23			105	00	18	89	3	28					82	83
30			105	00	18	89	3	28					82	83
		TOTALS	525	—	94	45	16	40					414	15
QUARTER		BROUGHT FWD.	840	00	151	12	26	24					662	64
		TO DATE	1365	00	245	52	42	64					1076	79
YEAR		BROUGHT FWD.												
		TO DATE												

NAME: SOC. SEC. NO. NUMBER OF EXEMPTIONS

DATE	HOURS	RATE	GROSS PAY		WITHHOLDING		F.I.C.A.						NET PAY	
		TOTALS												
QUARTER		BROUGHT FWD.												
		TO DATE												
YEAR		BROUGHT FWD.												
		TO DATE												

NAME: SOC. SEC. NO. NUMBER OF EXEMPTIONS

DATE	HOURS	RATE	GROSS PAY		WITHHOLDING		F.I.C.A.						NET PAY	
		TOTALS												
QUARTER		BROUGHT FWD.												
		TO DATE												
YEAR		BROUGHT FWD.												
		TO DATE												

FORM 4213 COLWELL CO. CHAMPAIGN, ILL.

DEC

Fig. 18-22. An accurate recording of all salaries paid, with required deductions made on the payroll sheet.

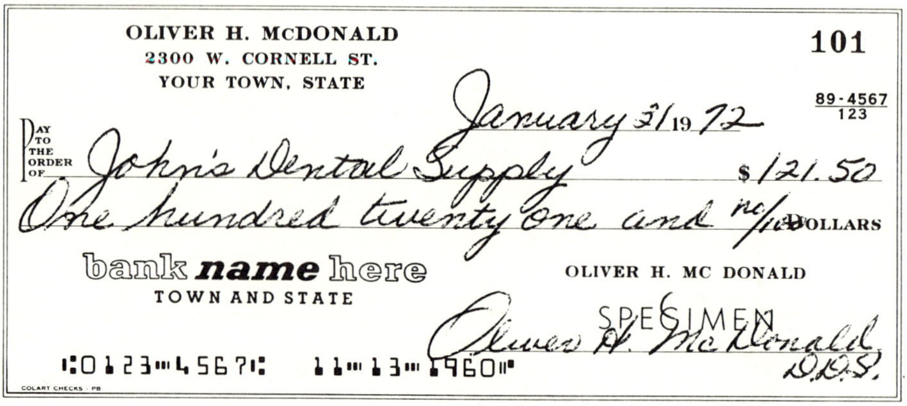

Fig. 18-23. A bank check.

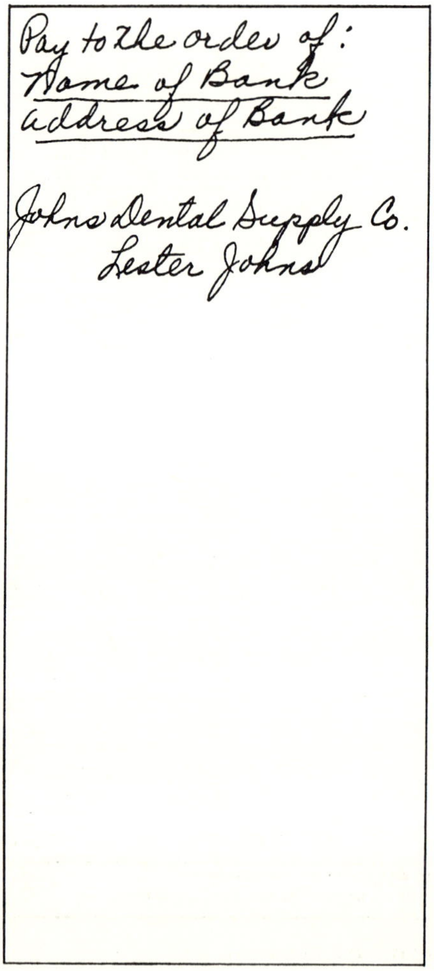

Fig. 18-24. Endorsement of a check.

STATEMENT

M&I BANK MARSHALL & ILSLEY BANK
MILWAUKEE, WISCONSIN 53201 • 276-7700

DATE – LAST STATEMENT	NUMBER OF DEBITS	NUMBER OF CREDITS	DATE – THIS STATEMENT	PAGE
5-6-65	4	1	6-7-65	1

BALANCE – LAST STATEMENT		TOTAL AMOUNT – DEBITS		TOTAL AMOUNT – CREDITS		SERVICE CHARGE		BALANCE – THIS STATEMENT
$375.00	−	$120.00	+	$200.00	−	$1.00	=	$454.00

Mr. Oliver McDonald
1111 West South Street
Milwaukee, Wisconsin

00-00 0000
ACCOUNT NUMBER

CODE
C – CERTIFIED CHECKS
L – LIST OF CHECKS
M – MISCELLANEOUS DEBIT OR CREDIT
OD – OVERDRAFT
R – RETURNED CHECK
S – SERVICE CHARGE FOR PREVIOUS PERIOD UNLESS OTHERWISE NOTED
X – CHARGE FOR OVERDRAFT OR RETURNED CHECK

CHECKS AND OTHER DEBITS			DEPOSITS AND OTHER CREDITS	DATE	BALANCE
				5-6	$375.00
$20.00				5-10	355.00
$60.00				5-12	295.00
			$200.00	5-17	495.00
$15.00				5-19	480.00
$ 1.00 S				5-31	479.00
$25.00				6-2	454.00

S A M P L E

PLEASE EXAMINE AT ONCE AND REPORT ANY DIFFERENCES TO OUR AUDITING DEPARTMENT.
ITEMS CODED WITH THE SYMBOL "R" WERE POSTED ON THE DAY SUBSEQUENT TO THE ORIGINAL POSTING ENTRY

Fig. 18-25. Example of a bank statement.

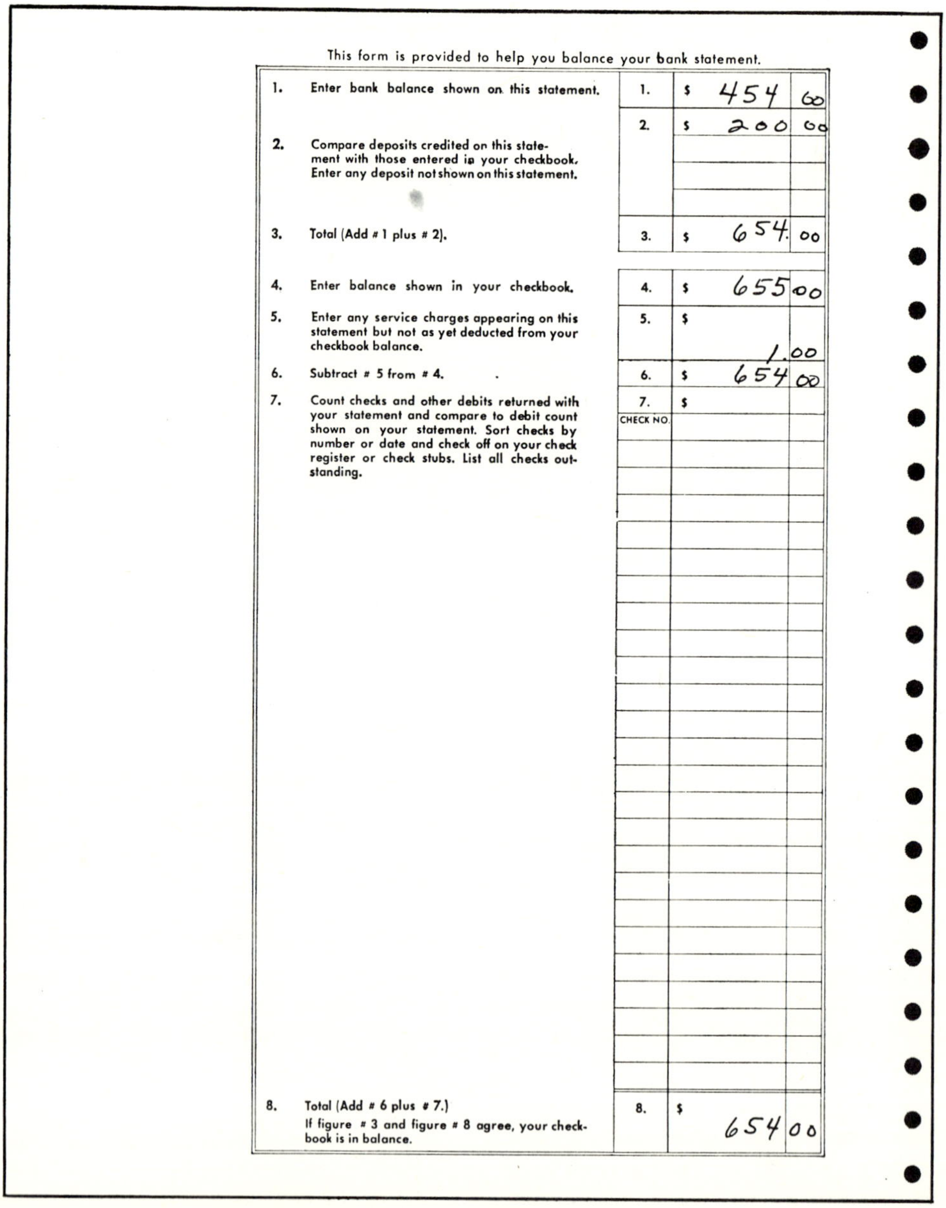

This form is provided to help you balance your bank statement.

1.	Enter bank balance shown on this statement.	1.	$ 454	60
2.	Compare deposits credited on this statement with those entered in your checkbook. Enter any deposit not shown on this statement.	2.	$ 200	00
3.	Total (Add # 1 plus # 2).	3.	$ 654.	00
4.	Enter balance shown in your checkbook.	4.	$ 655	00
5.	Enter any service charges appearing on this statement but not as yet deducted from your checkbook balance.	5.	$ 1.	00
6.	Subtract # 5 from # 4.	6.	$ 654	00
7.	Count checks and other debits returned with your statement and compare to debit count shown on your statement. Sort checks by number or date and check off on your check register or check stubs. List all checks outstanding.	7. CHECK NO.	$	
8.	Total (Add # 6 plus # 7.) If figure # 3 and figure # 8 agree, your checkbook is in balance.	8.	$ 654	00

Fig. 18-26. Reconciliation of the bank statement.

CHECK NO.	DATE	CHECKS ISSUED TO OR DESCRIPTION OF DEPOSIT		√	BALANCE FORWARD	
					1753	80
1766	9/1	TO Chybowski Dental Supply	CHECK OR DEPOSIT AMOUNT	✓	320	00
		FOR Dental Supplies	NEW BALANCE		1433	80
	9/1	TO Deposit	CHECK OR DEPOSIT AMOUNT		300	00
		FOR	NEW BALANCE		1733	80
1767	9/2	TO Radiographs, Inc.	CHECK OR DEPOSIT AMOUNT	✓	150	00
		FOR X-ray film	NEW BALANCE		1583	80
1768	9/2	TO Wallace, Inc.	CHECK OR DEPOSIT AMOUNT	✓	75	00
		FOR Office Record Supplies	NEW BALANCE		1508	80
1769	9/2	TO Mrs. Jane Rowland	CHECK OR DEPOSIT AMOUNT	✓	100	00
		FOR Salary 8/15-9/1	NEW BALANCE		1408	80

Fig. 18-27. Cancelled checks marked off in the checkbook.

cessed by the bank, the deposits for the month, and the total amount of the balance in the checking account.

Reconciliation of bank account

Reconciliation (Fig. 18-26) is generally a monthly procedure. All canceled checks are arranged in numerical order; each check is marked off on the stubs in the checkbook (Fig. 18-27); the deposits are tallied; and outstanding checks are recorded. The bank statement balance should agree with the checkbook balance.

Deposit slips

Deposit slips (Fig. 18-28) are itemized memoranda of cash, checks, and money orders that the depositor presents to the bank with the money to be credited to his account. A deposit slip should be prepared for each deposit, with a duplicate copy to be retained in the office. Coins, currency, checks, and money orders are itemized individually and then totaled. Bank deposits should be made daily to avoid delay in processing checks, confusion in preparing lengthy deposits tickets, and possible loss of large sums of money by theft. If making deposits by mail, currency and coins should not be included. A postal money order should be purchased with the currency and coins mailed in or personally deposited at the bank.

Credit ratings

In our society, credit ratings are established on the basis of a person's earnings, bank accounts, and the manner in which he pays his bills (for example, prompt, often delinquent, or slow). As a part of the business procedures in a dental office, it may be necessary to secure a patient's credit rating before the dentist begins extensive treatment. This rating is obtained from a credit bureau of which the dentist is a member.

A good credit rating is as necessary for the dentist as it is for others. To ensure this credit rating, prompt payment of dental office bills is very important; credit ratings are influenced by the promptness with which a person's debts are paid. Special attention should be given to due dates on bills and expiration of discount rates, in order to benefit from lower costs.

Collection agencies

In the collection of fees the dentist may find that some patients fail to respond to the monthly statement or other collection measures, such as follow-up letters (Fig. 18-29) and telephone calls, used by the office personnel. In such cases, many dentists will turn the delinquent accounts over to commercial agencies that collect accounts. The collection agencies charge a fee which is usually a percentage of the amount collected.

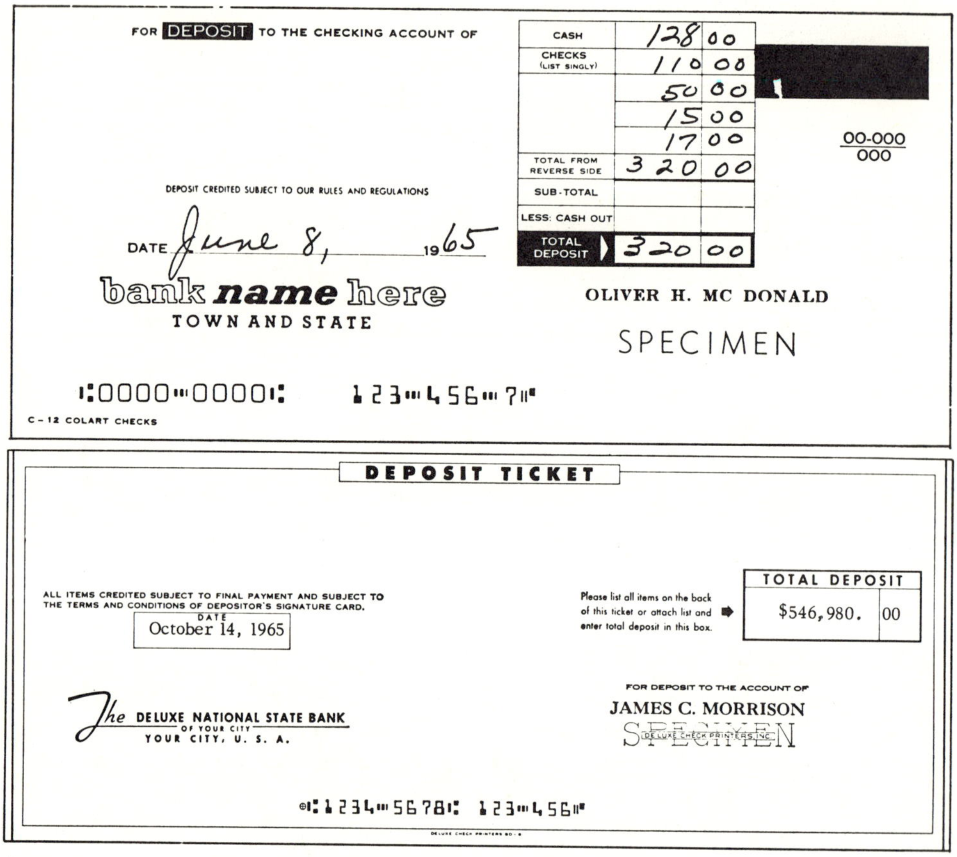
FOR DEPOSIT TO THE CHECKING ACCOUNT OF

CASH	128	00
CHECKS (LIST SINGLY)	110	00
	50	00
	15	00
	17	00
TOTAL FROM REVERSE SIDE	320	00
SUB-TOTAL		
LESS: CASH OUT		
TOTAL DEPOSIT	320	00

[redacted]

00-000
000

DEPOSIT CREDITED SUBJECT TO OUR RULES AND REGULATIONS

DATE June 8, 1965

bank name here
TOWN AND STATE

OLIVER H. MC DONALD
SPECIMEN

⑆0000⑈0000⑆ 123⑈456⑈7⑉

C-12 COLART CHECKS

DEPOSIT TICKET

ALL ITEMS CREDITED SUBJECT TO FINAL PAYMENT AND SUBJECT TO THE TERMS AND CONDITIONS OF DEPOSITOR'S SIGNATURE CARD.

DATE October 14, 1965

Please list all items on the back of this ticket or attach list and enter total deposit in this box.

TOTAL DEPOSIT $546,980. 00

FOR DEPOSIT TO THE ACCOUNT OF
JAMES C. MORRISON
SPECIMEN

The DELUXE NATIONAL STATE BANK
OF YOUR CITY
YOUR CITY, U. S. A.

⑆1234⑈5678⑆ 123⑈456⑉

Fig. 18-28. Examples of deposit slips.

Multiple recording systems

One of the most recent and successful innovations to simplify the financial and bookkeeping records is the "write-it-once" or "pegboard" system. A master board with pegs on the left-hand side for attachment of the necessary forms is provided. Carbon-backed forms are used to post the patient's financial statement, receipt, service slip, appointment slip, and day sheet with 1 writing (Figs. 18-30 and 18-31). Cumulative records for the day, month, and year are available from these forms. A check-writing system to provide a record of office disbursements and banking activities is also available. The advantage of this system is the elimination of transpositional errors and the immediate availability of current bookkeeping records.

Electronic data processing

The use of computers is bringing the electronic age to the professional office. Computers may have the advantage of providing the dental office personnel with more time to devote to the patient. Data reflecting the daily transactions of the dental office are sent to a centralized computer center. The information is transfered to cards processed through the computer, and printed reports containing this information are available upon request. Electronic data processing may be used for various types of records that report the activities of the

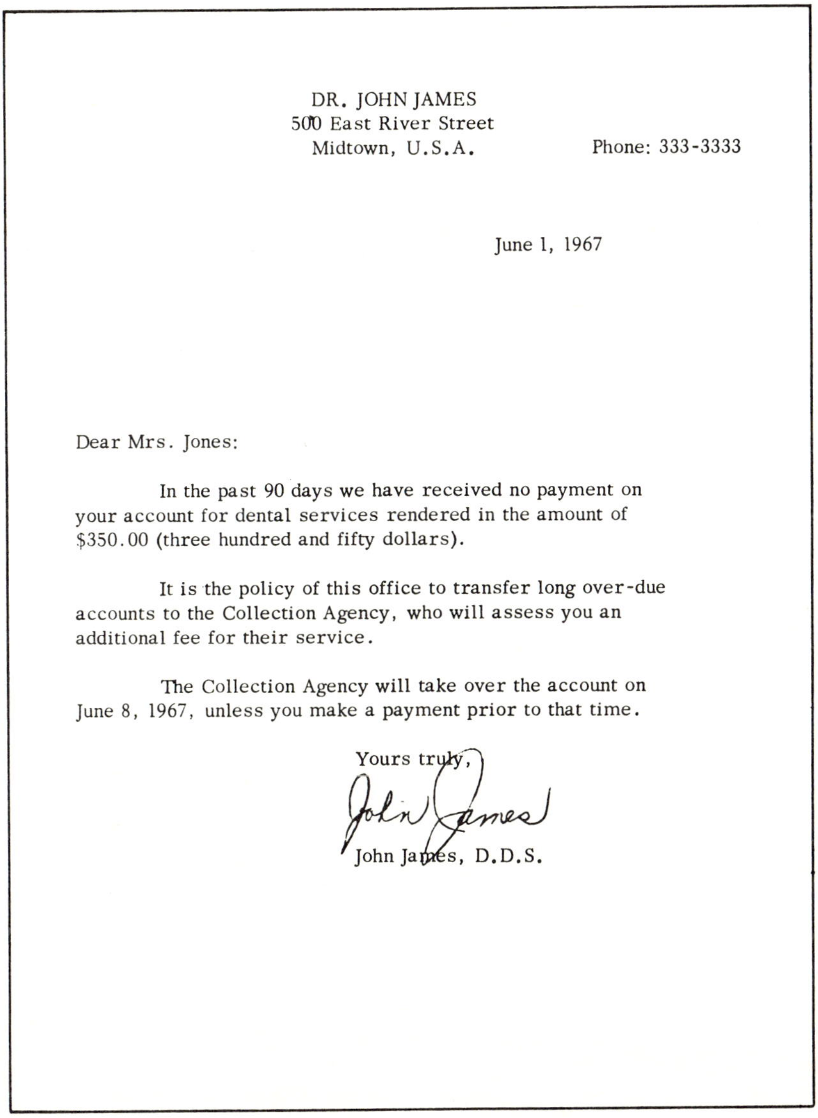

DR. JOHN JAMES
500 East River Street
Midtown, U.S.A. Phone: 333-3333

June 1, 1967

Dear Mrs. Jones:

In the past 90 days we have received no payment on your account for dental services rendered in the amount of $350.00 (three hundred and fifty dollars).

It is the policy of this office to transfer long over-due accounts to the Collection Agency, who will assess you an additional fee for their service.

The Collection Agency will take over the account on June 8, 1967, unless you make a payment prior to that time.

Yours truly,

John James

John James, D.D.S.

Fig. 18-29. A follow-up letter.

office, such as monthly statements and bookkeeping summaries.

Depersonalization and expense of operation may be a disadvantage of these systems.

COMMUNICATION RECORDS

There are 3 ways in which the dental assistant communicates with the public as a representative of the dental office with which she is associated—face to face, in writing, and by telephone. In all situations, the dental assistant must learn to use all her professional knowledge, her personal qualities, and her understanding of human relations involved in communication to prove herself an asset to the dental office. She must be alert to communicate so effec-

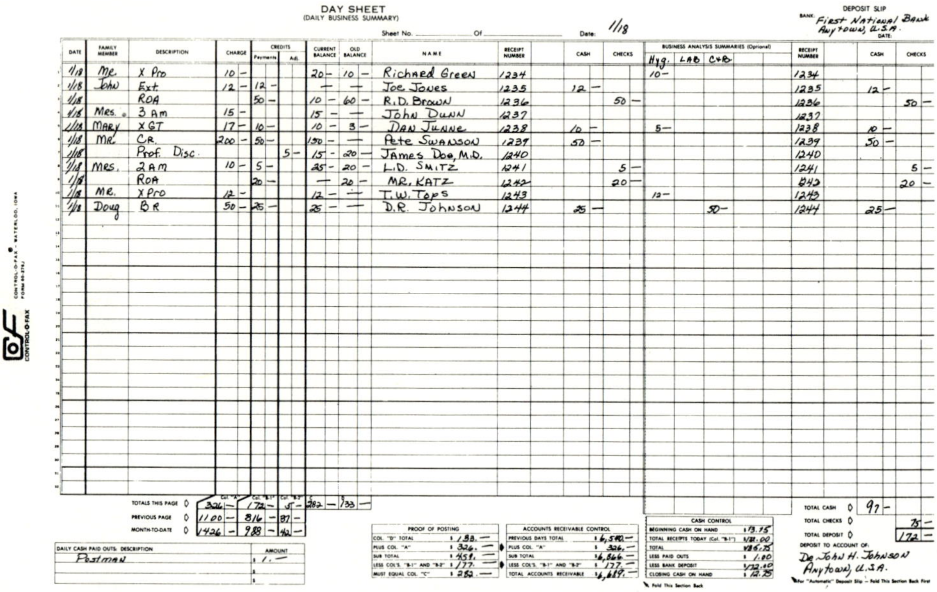

DAY SHEET
(DAILY BUSINESS SUMMARY)

Sheet No. ______ Of ______ Date: 1/18

DEPOSIT SLIP
BANK: First National Bank Anytown, U.S.A.
DATE:

DATE	FAMILY MEMBER	DESCRIPTION	CHARGE	CREDITS Payments	CREDITS Adj.	CURRENT BALANCE	OLD BALANCE	NAME	RECEIPT NUMBER	CASH	CHECKS	BUSINESS ANALYSIS SUMMARIES (Optional) Hyg.	LAB	C+B	RECEIPT NUMBER	CASH	CHECKS
1/18	Me.	X Pro	10 –			20 –	10 –	Richard Green	1234			10 –			1234		
1/18	John	Ext.	12 –	12 –		—	—	Joe Jones	1235	12 –					1235	12 –	
1/18		ROA		50 –		10 –	60 –	R.D. Brown	1236		50 –				1236		50 –
1/18	Mrs.	3 Am	15 –			15 –	—	John Dunn	1237						1237		
1/18	Mary	X GT	17 –	10 –		10 –	3 –	Dan Junne	1238	10 –		5 –			1238	10 –	
1/18	Mr.	CR.	200 –	50 –		150 –	—	Pete Swanson	1239	50 –					1239	50 –	
1/18		Prof. Disc.			5 –	15 –	20 –	James Doe, M.D.	1240						1240		
1/18	Mrs.	2 AM	10 –	5 –		25 –	20 –	L.D. Smitz	1241		5 –				1241		5 –
1/18		ROA		20 –		—	20 –	Mr. Katz	1242		20 –				1242		20 –
1/18	Mr.	X Pro	12 –			12 –	—	T.W. Tops	1243			12 –			1243		
1/18	Doug	BR	50 –	25 –		25 –	—	D.R. Johnson	1244	25 –				50 –	1244	25 –	

	Col. "A"	Col. "B-1"	Col. "B-2"	C	D
TOTALS THIS PAGE	326 –	172 –	5 –	282 –	133 –
PREVIOUS PAGE	1100 –	816 –	37 –		
MONTH-TO-DATE	1426 –	988 –	42 –		

DAILY CASH PAID OUTS: DESCRIPTION	AMOUNT
Postman	$ 1.–
	$
	$

PROOF OF POSTING	
COL. "D" TOTAL	$ 133.–
PLUS COL. "A"	$ 326.–
SUB TOTAL	$ 459.–
LESS COL'S. "B-1" AND "B-2"	$ 177.–
MUST EQUAL COL. "C"	$ 282.–

ACCOUNTS RECEIVABLE CONTROL	
PREVIOUS DAYS TOTAL	$ 6,540.–
PLUS COL. "A"	$ 326.–
SUB TOTAL	$ 6,866.–
LESS COL'S. "B-1" AND "B-2"	$ 177.–
TOTAL ACCOUNTS RECEIVABLE	$ 6,689.–

CASH CONTROL	
BEGINNING CASH ON HAND	$ 13.75
TOTAL RECEIPTS TODAY (Col. "B-1")	$ 172.00
TOTAL	$ 186.75
LESS PAID OUTS	$ 1.00
LESS BANK DEPOSIT	$ 172.00
CLOSING CASH ON HAND	$ 12.75

Fold This Section Back

TOTAL CASH 97 –
TOTAL CHECKS 75 –
TOTAL DEPOSIT 172 –
DEPOSIT TO ACCOUNT OF: Dr. John H. Johnson Anytown, U.S.A.
For "Automatic" Deposit Slip – Fold This Section Back First

CONTROL-O-FAX

Fig. 18-30. An example of a daily sheet of a multiple recording system. (Courtesy Control-O-Fax.)

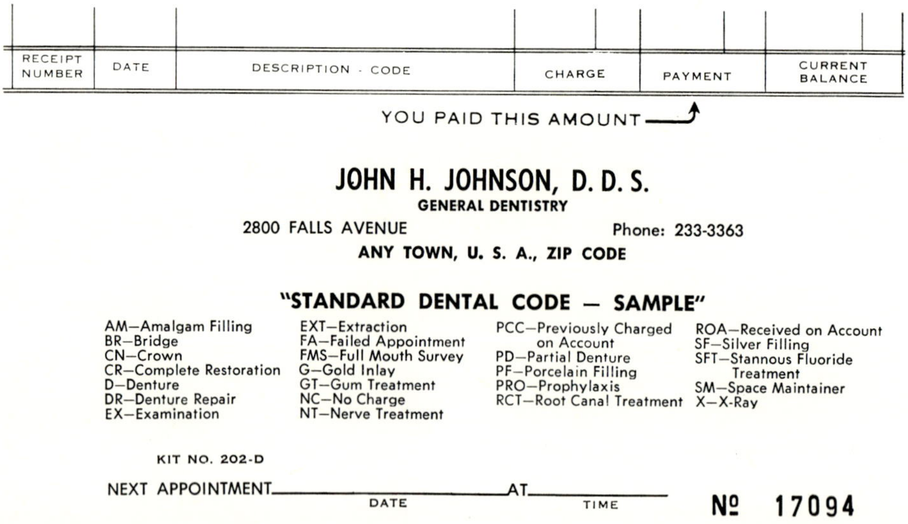

RECEIPT NUMBER	DATE	DESCRIPTION - CODE	CHARGE	PAYMENT	CURRENT BALANCE

YOU PAID THIS AMOUNT

JOHN H. JOHNSON, D. D. S.
GENERAL DENTISTRY
2800 FALLS AVENUE Phone: 233-3363
ANY TOWN, U. S. A., ZIP CODE

"STANDARD DENTAL CODE — SAMPLE"

AM—Amalgam Filling
BR—Bridge
CN—Crown
CR—Complete Restoration
D—Denture
DR—Denture Repair
EX—Examination
EXT—Extraction
FA—Failed Appointment
FMS—Full Mouth Survey
G—Gold Inlay
GT—Gum Treatment
NC—No Charge
NT—Nerve Treatment
PCC—Previously Charged on Account
PD—Partial Denture
PF—Porcelain Filling
PRO—Prophylaxis
RCT—Root Canal Treatment
ROA—Received on Account
SF—Silver Filling
SFT—Stannous Fluoride Treatment
SM—Space Maintainer
X—X-Ray

KIT NO. 202-D

NEXT APPOINTMENT ______ AT ______
DATE TIME

№ 17094

Fig. 18-31. A form used in the multiple recording system to post the patient's financial statement, receipt, service slip, appointment slip, and day sheet with one writing. (Courtesy Control-O-Fax.)

tively in person, in writing, and by telephone that there is no misunderstanding or misinterpretation.

Written communication

The written communications that are used to carry on the business of the dental office are usually in the form of cards or letters. The manner in which these communications are written and the correctness and clarity of the message will reflect the nature of the office and the person responsible for sending the communications. Neatness, correct spelling, and good grammar are essential, and the dental assistant who is responsible for preparing and sending written material from the office should provide herself with a reliable dictionary and a book of simple rules of grammar.

The most common communications are those written to thank someone for referring a patient, to refer a patient to another professional person, to request information, to request payment of accounts, or to send courtesy messages on birthdays and other special occasions. The dentist will also require the assistant to handle some of his personal correspondence, and many dentists expect their assistants to help them in the preparation of formal papers for publication or oral presentation.

Letters

The letter is a written form of communication that conveys a special message. It may be handwritten or typewritten, but in the business office typewritten letters are preferable, since they are legible to all who read them. There are many manuals and books on letter writing, but there are some general rules and suggestions concerning the format of a business letter with which each dental assistant should be familiar (Fig. 18-32).

Heading and date

If the printed letterhead is centered on the stationery, the date is centered below it. If the letterhead is printed across the top, the date is placed below it and may be either in the center or the right-hand side of the sheet of paper. In general, the date is placed halfway between the letterhead and first line of the inside address. The date should be written out in full.

Inside address

The block style of address, as follows, is recommended.

Name		Name
Address	or	City
City and state		State

Salutation

The salutation is placed directly below the inside address and 2 spaces below the last line of the address.

Text of the letter

Block style is recommended, with the left-hand margin kept even. A letter should always be single spaced, unless it consists of 5 lines or less.

Three spaces should be allowed between the heading on the second page and the continuation of the letter. One should try to avoid carrying only 2 or 3 lines to the second page of the letter. It is never permissible to carry only the signature to the second page.

Complimentary close

The complimentary close is placed 2 spaces below the body of the letter and aligned in block style with the date. On 2-page letters, it should be aligned with the page number, which is always centered.

Signature

Four spaces should be left between the complimentary close and the signature. The writer's name and degrees are typed in block style on the first line. His title or the name of his department is typed on the second line.

DOCTOR SAUL D. SIMS, D.D.S.
196 West Grand Avenue
Milwaukee 80, Wisconsin

Current Date

Miss Dental Assistant
American Dental Office
Everytown, U.S.A.

Dear Madam:

The format of the business letter includes the size, shape and general arrangement of the letter. The letter should be carefully spaced and arranged. It should have a well-balanced look. Plan your margins according to the length of the letter.

Each business letter is made up of the following parts:

1. Heading. The date only, as the address is in the letterhead.

2. Inside address. The name and address of the person to whom the letter is written.

3. Salutation. The complimentary greeting, examples: Dear Sir, My Dear Sir, Gentlemen.

4. Body of the letter. The subject matter or message.

5. Closing. The complimentary conclusion, example: Yours truly, Sincerely yours.

6. Signature. The name of the person sending the message.

Sincerely yours,

Mary Jones
Your Helpful Dental Assistant

MJ:ks

Fig. 18-32. Format of business letter.

Initials and carbon copy notation

The initials of the person signing the letter and those of the secretary typing the letter are usually placed 2 single spaces below the last line of the signature, flush with the left-hand margin. The 2 initials may be separated by a colon or a diagonal mark. Any notations regarding enclosures are made below these initials. If a carbon copy of the letter is prepared for someone other than the addressee, "cc," followed by the name of that person, is typed at the left-hand margin, 2 spaces below the initials of the person writing the letter.

Envelope

Open punctuation and block style should be used on envelopes. The first line should be slightly to the right of the center of the envelope.

Carbon copies of correspondence relative to all activities in the dental office should be retained in the appropriate file.

Telephone communication

Correct telephone communication should be studied and cultivated by the dental assistant. The telephone, if used properly, is one of the most valuable means of communication in the dental office. Because only auditory impressions are given, the dental assistant must be careful of voice quality, choice of words, and the manner in which the words are spoken. The voice alone must convey intelligence, understanding, authority, sympathy, courtesy, and helpfulness. The telephone company in any locality is willing to help persons to improve their telephone techniques and personalities by means of tape recordings, dual telephone practice, and films. The following are some general suggestions that the dental assistant might use as a check on her own telephone technique.

1. Answer the telephone promptly.
2. Identify the office.
3. Identify yourself.
4. Inquire who is calling. Use the individual's name at least once in the following conversation.
5. Determine the nature of the call.
6. Handle the call efficiently.
   a. Record all pertinent information.
   b. Keep a tabulation of all telephone calls. This may be done by using a stenographic notebook and recording the date, name of caller, and reason for and handling of the call.
   c. Screen those callers who insist on speaking directly with the dentist. If the call cannot be handled, a written message is prepared and handed or shown to the dentist. He can then direct the proper action. There are prepared pads available for telephone messages.
   d. Thank the person for calling, and let the caller hang up first.

CONCLUSION

Clinical and financial reports, appointment records, and correspondence files reflect the activities of the dental office and are important for efficient management and practice. It is essential that detailed records be maintained, to insure that the patient receives the individual attention his medical and dental record dictates. Legal protection, favorable practice analysis, and correct tax records are contingent upon detailed, accurate office records.

CHAPTER 19 THE DENTAL OPERATORY OF THE FUTURE

GERTRUDE M. SINNETT, B.S., R.D.H.
ARTHUR H. WUEHRMANN, A.B., D.M.D.

The modern dentist takes great pride in the quality of his work, the comfort of his patients, the efficiency with which he can provide service to an increasing number of patients, and the overall organization of his practice. The progressive dentist and the graduate entering practice usually acquire the newest and most modern equipment, so that they and their auxiliary personnel can provide the best possible dental health care. At present, many enterprising and resourceful dentists are not satisfied with standard equipment. Such dentists are designing and locating basic equipment items to suit the needs of their individual practices. Thus, the modern dentist often becomes his own architect and design engineer.

Original designs and custom-made offices make it difficult for manufacturers to meet requests. Dentists find they must use compromise equipment that does not totally meet their requirements. Some manufacturers are gradually responding to the profession's needs, but confusion continues to exist, because no clearly defined equipment criteria have been accepted. Dental manufacturers have previously provided the profession with durable equipment, designed to last a lifetime. Durability is of utmost importance; equipment breakdown seriously impairs practice. Even the multiple-chair office is seriously handicapped if one piece of equipment fails to operate smoothly and efficiently. Equipment, though new and different, must be durable.

Since it is evident that national dental manpower requirements will increase as the population expands and as socioeconomic changes occur, more effective and efficient ways of providing dental care must be found. Improvements will center around the dentist and the proper utilization of his time and energy, but auxiliary personnel and equipment will become increasingly important. Carefully designed procedures, performed with the assistance of necessary auxiliary personnel and functional equipment, will result in greater productivity and, quite possibly, in increased quality of service.

Traditionally, the dentist works alone and in a standing position. His assistant, if he uses one, often functions on an on-call basis. The dentist in the future will be highly dependent upon a full-time chairside assistant and other auxiliaries. He will operate in a sitting position and will depend upon auxiliary personnel to perform all procedures that auxiliaries can legally do. He will perform those operations that must, by law, be done by the licensed practitioner.

Some people have a mistaken belief that increased efficiency and acceleration of dental service is primarily designed to automate the professional man in order to increase the number of people he can see and multiply the number of dollars he can earn. Actually, modern dentistry recognizes the need for the dentist to devote an increasing amount of time to continuing dental education; he must continually update his professional knowledge. In addition, he should be more active in civic affairs and professional societies; he must be a leader in his community. Efficient use of office time and auxiliaries will provide more opportunity for such service.

It is impossible to predict the future of the dental operatory, but by carefully observing the modern dental office, one can gain some insight into future trends. Many aspects of dental practice are likely to change. This discussion is limited to current thinking about the dental operatory and trends that are likely to effect the future. Major topics covered are minimization of body movements, operating zones, basic operatory equipment, and equipment location for effective assistant utilization.

MINIMIZATION OF MOVEMENTS

All suggestions presented in this chapter are designed to minimize body motion. Successful accomplishment of objectives, therefore, is evidenced by a reduction in body movement. Recognition of time and motion phenomena is not new. However, interested members of the dental profession have only recently gained an insight into work simplification procedures long used successfully in industry.

Body motions are divided into 5 classes. Class I includes movement of the fingers only. Class II movement involves the fingers and wrist. Class III movement includes the fingers, wrist, and forearm. Class IV movement is movement of the fingers, wrist, forearm, and shoulders, and a Class V movement involves turning the entire body. In order to minimize time consumption, fatigue, and stress, every effort is made in industry to provide working conditions that allow Classes I and II movements to predominate. The same should be true for modern dentistry. As much as possible, all common, frequently made movements should be of Classes I and II. Routine Class III, Class IV, and Class V motions must be critically examined to see why they exist, to determine if they are essential, and to eliminate them, if possible. Infrequent Classes III, IV, and V movements can, of course, be tolerated.

The dentist and his auxiliaries must continually be alert to the need for eliminating, combining, rearranging, and simplifying methods and procedures. All personnel should utilize body motions requiring the least amount of time and a minimum number of motions. Every effort should be made to reduce the length of motions and to make them as smooth as possible. All instruments and materials should be positioned in a predetermined place and used in sequence; they should be located as close to the treatment area as possible. Work surfaces should be approximately 2 inches lower than the user's elbow, and stool height should permit good posture while absorbing the worker's full weight. These practices contribute to motion minimization. Long-standing practice habits are not easy to eliminate, but corrections must be instituted if operatory efficiency is to be attained.

OPERATING ZONES

Dental treatment planning involves consideration of the entire patient; however, treatment aspects of dentistry are largely carried out directly in the mouth. Since all dental operations take place in the mouth, it is logical that the flow of supplies and

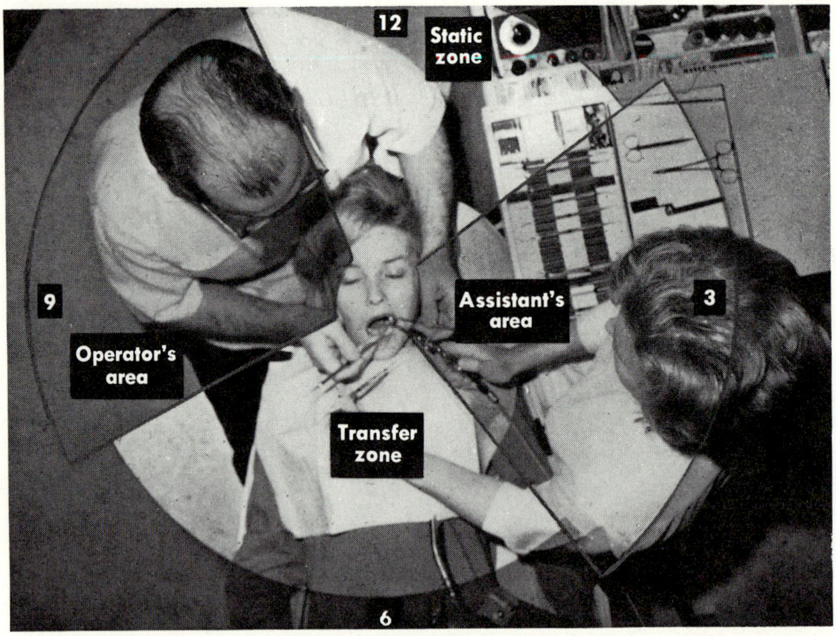

Fig. 19-1. Operating zones.

equipment should be toward the mouth. Everything concerned with any given operation should be located in a position that is easily accessible to the treatment area.

Regardless of the type of operation, some actions are done repeatedly, and others are done less frequently. Instruments and supplies used in repetitive operations should be located closest to the treatment area. Equipment and supplies used infrequently can be located some distance away from the mouth because the relative time consumption involved in getting such items is negligible. Equipment and/or supplies used very infrequently should not be located in the dental operatory; they should be stored in a suitable, accessible storage area elsewhere in the dental office.

In considering operating zones, first consider the dentist as he operates with an assistant. Fig. 19-1 illustrates a patient reclining in a contour chair. Superimposed is a circle, with the patient's mouth at its center. Zones within this circle are oriented to the face of a clock, wherein 6 o'clock is toward the patient's feet, and 12 o'clock is above the patient's head. The dentist operating with the aid of a full-time chairside assistant ordinarily functions in the zone from 8 to 11 o'clock. The assistant functions primarily in the zone from 2 to 5 o'clock. The zone in the vicinity of 12 o'clock (static zone) is largely unused. Equipment used infrequently is moved into this area as needed. The zone directly in contact with the patient's face, extending from approximately 5 to 8 o'clock, is the zone of instrument transfer. Instrument transfers should take place literally at the mouth, not elsewhere in the transfer zone.

The operator's position is identical for the dental hygienist or the expanded-function auxiliary operating with a chairside assistant. When operating with a dental assistant, the dentist or auxiliary should perform operating procedures on the basis that the eyes not be removed from the field of operation and the hands remain in contact with the patient's mouth and in operating position during the entire course of the operation. When operating without an assistant, the cabinet and instruments normally used by the assistant are relocated in front of the operator. The handpiece and evacuating system, together with the air-water-spray syringe, must be located in a position convenient to the operator and as close to the oral cavity as possible.

BASIC OPERATORY EQUIPMENT

Present-day dental operatories, whether they are equipped for the dentist or the dental hygienist, are becoming outmoded. Industry designs products to meet demands. Until recently, the profession had failed to give the manufacturer direction in terms of equipment needs, and, as a result, the dental operatory has remained essentially static during the past several decades. The appearance of the equipment has changed, but its function and placement have remained constant. Dental operatories are stereotyped because the profession has not undertaken clinical research designed to encourage change, and industry has failed to evaluate its equipment objectively in terms of dental profession needs.

At present, the dental operatory and its equipment are such that the dentist, the assistant, and the hygienist must accommodate their procedures to available equipment. The reverse should be true. Everything in the operatory should be oriented to the patient's mouth and to the comfort of the operator and his assistant. Every effort should be made to simplify, rather than complicate, dental procedures.

If the dentist is to use an assistant effectively, he must replace his dental unit and include in his operatory a contour dental chair, operating stools for the dentist and his assistant, modern cutting equipment, oral evacuation equipment, combined air-water-spray syringe, mobile cabinet, preprepared instrument trays, artificial light, sinks, adequate storage space, and x-ray equipment.

Dental unit replacement

The traditional, space-consuming dental unit is nothing more than a mechanism for holding or supporting cutting devices, oral evacuation mechanisms, air-water spray syringes, instruments, and, in some cases, the operating light. In other words, the unit gives the operator a bracket table, light, power, and waste disposal. It also occupies valuable space needed by the dental assistant. Modern concepts of dental office equipment involve a radical departure from the conventional unit. Fortunately, modern cutting and oral evacuating equipment is connected to flexible hosing, as is the combination air-water-spray syringe. The principal problem in unit replacement is placing these various equipment items in the transfer zone for easy use by the assistant or the operator.

Unit replacement can be accomplished through the use of a "Dentassist"* (see Fig. 19-2), which is merely a hinged arm that can be lowered across and over the patient's abdomen and chest without contacting the patient. The power supply for all tubing on the Dentassist is contained within it. Other commercial equipment that accomplishes essentially the same purpose for which the Dentassist was designed is available, but care must be used in selection. Some new developments in unit replacement impede, rather than enhance, operating efficiency.

It is obvious that the substitution of the Dentassist for the dental unit substantially increases the available space at the left of the dental chair and makes dental assisting considerably more effective. Hose-attached instruments are readily accessible, should the operator have to work unassisted. In the absence of a dental assistant, the space previously occupied by the dental unit is unoccupied, but the room appearance is improved by the absence of heavy equipment.

*Marketed by Health Science Products Company, Pinson, Alabama; developed at University of Alabama in Birmingham School of Dentistry.

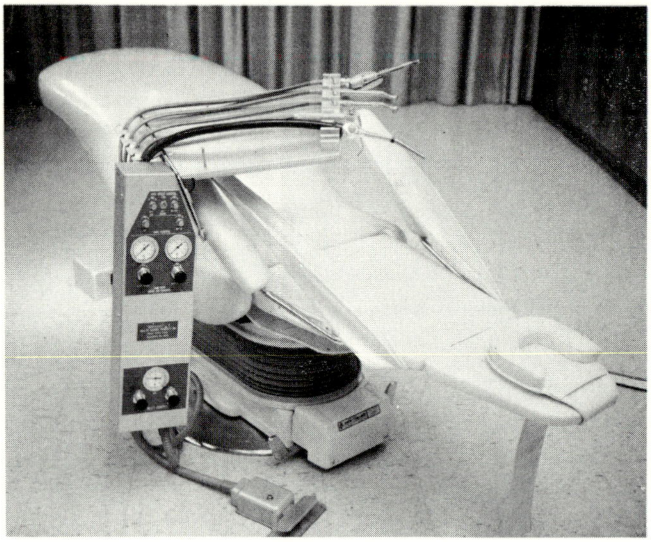

Fig. 19-2. The Dentassist. (Courtesy the University of Alabama in Birmingham School of Dentistry.)

Dental chair

The conventional chair with its footrest, hard seat, uncomfortable back, and head stabilizer is obsolete. The patient must have complete body support, including arm slings, if he is to be positioned horizontally. To provide flexibility for patient positioning, the chair should be contoured, with back and leg segments independently movable. The mechanism for moving the chair vertically, as well as for adjusting the back and leg sections, must be operable by both the dentist and assistant. Power operation of the chair adds to office efficiency and reduces fatigue. The chair must rotate on its base. There is a need for a chair base that will permit maximum lowering of the chair. A thin-back chair with no protruding adjusting devices is essential. The operator performs dental procedures with the patient's head literally in his lap, separated only by the back of the chair. Protruding devices impinge on the operator's thighs. All work should be done at the level of the operator's elbows. Chair backs that are excessively thick automatically raise the height of the patient's head to an undesirable level.

Operating stools

Operating stools on which the dentist and his assistant sit have specific requirements. They must have a broad, heavy base for stability and must be completely mobile. Operating stools attached to the chair and those of a pedestal type limit the movement of the operator and/or assistant and make it difficult for them to function efficiently. The seats of the operating stools must be relatively large and padded for complete body support and comfort; they are used continuously. The operator's stool should be adjustable in height, but need not be freely adjustable. Once adjusted, the operator rarely changes his stool height. The assistant's stool height must be freely adjustable. The patient will be positioned for the convenience of the operator, and the assistant will want to alter her stool height to view the operation and to assist effectively.

When she is seated correctly, the assistant's eye level will be 3 to 6 inches higher than that of the person she is assisting; she must lean forward for visual purposes. The base of the assistant's stool is used as a footrest. A heavy stool base and weight distribution on at least five casters is required. Operating stools should provide body support alternately for the side, back, and abdomen. This diversity of support can be accomplished by a rotating arm that can be used interchangeably. Many operators prefer a positive back support rather than a rotating arm, but the assistant needs a body support.

Modern cutting equipment

High-speed cutting equipment is essential to modern dentistry, but there is also a need for slower-speed cutting instruments. Both types must be controlled with a variable-speed foot control. The control pedal should move vertically, rather than horizontally, for the seated operator. Many varieties of handpieces, burs, and stones that fullfill the present needs of dentistry are available. Handpiece accessibility is of considerable importance. (For optimum positioning see p. 400.)

Oral evacuation equipment

The cuspidor has been eliminated from the modern dental operatory, making it necessary to mechanically evacuate fluids and debris from the patient's mouth. Oral evacuation is done through the use of high-velocity, low-pressure evacuating systems, which should drain and exhaust directly into the waste line after passing through a strainer. Some oral evacuation equipment is designed to drain into a waste bottle within the operatory. This equipment may function satisfactorily, but it requires frequent emptying of the container and has greater potential for recirculating pathogenic bacteria into the room. Conventional saliva ejectors use low-velocity, high-pressure systems and are not satisfactory for the modern dental office. The conventional saliva ejector does not have the capacity to withdraw the volume of water that collects in the mouth from the use of high-speed cutting equipment and from salivary secretions. Oral evacuating equipment must be literally able to lift liquids and debris through air to be effective. The power source for oral evacuating equipment should be placed in a remote area to eliminate noise. It is essential that the oral evacuating equipment be easily cleaned and serviced.

Air-water-spray syringe

The air-water-spray syringe must be light in weight and easily operated. It should be combined in 1 element. There may be a need for 2 such syringes, one to be used by the operator and the other by the assistant.

Operatory cabinets

With the exception of cabinets that house plumbing, all cabinets in the dental operatory should be movable. This is true even though certain cabinets may not be moved under ordinary operating conditions. The number of cabinets should be kept to the minimum required for the storage of essential, routinely used items.

The instrument cabinet should be freely movable and preferably adjustable for height. It should have a working area top that can be pulled horizontally toward the assistant (Fig. 19-3).

The space under the sliding top (the "well") holds the amalgamator and serves as a source for supplies. The drawers in the cabinet contain off-tray additions, instruments and supplies not ordinarily included on a preset tray. The ability of the cabinet top to move forward over the assistant's knees makes various instruments on the preset tray and in the well readily accessible.

The cabinet height should be below the level of the assistant's elbows as she works seated. If the dentist is unassisted, the cabinet can be repositioned in front of him.

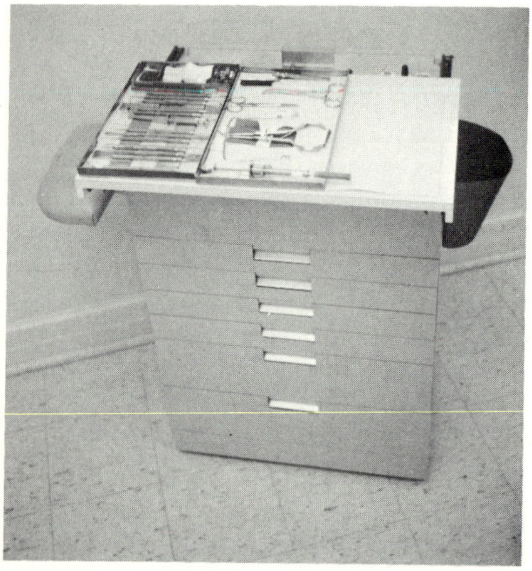

Fig. 19-3. Instrument cabinet. (Developed at the University of Alabama School of Dentistry.)

In this case, the height of the cabinet should be somewhat lower than the cabinet height used by the assistant. This is because the assistant's position is 3 to 6 inches higher than that of the dentist. It is for this reason that the cabinet should be height adjustable.

Preprepared instrument trays

Preprepared instrument trays should be located on top of the mobile cabinet. The tray should include a minimum number of double-ended instruments and supporting materials essential for the planned operation. The preprepared tray is one on which instruments are placed and sterilized as a unit. To effectively use preprepared trays, the operator and his assistant must give considerable thought to the instruments they plan to use and the sequence in which they plan to use them. It should be emphasized that preprepared trays eliminate the process of placing sterilized instruments in a cabinet and removing them when needed. This procedure is both time-consuming and unclean. The preprepared tray, as a unit, is stored in a readily accessible area.

Artificial light

The modern dental office no longer depends on natural light. It is not necessary for the operatory to face in any particular direction. Room light must be of sufficient intensity to avoid shadows and distinct contrasts between the room light and the operating light. The ratio of room to operating light should be one to four. A minimum of 250 footcandles is recommended for room light. Alterations in this ratio will cause eye fatigue. Operating light(s) supplying 1000 footcandles should be mounted overhead and easily adjustable by either the assistant or the dentist, preferably by the assistant. Operating lights should be freely adjustable for any chair position. In general, ceiling-mounted track lights seem to be more adaptable than operating lights mounted in some other fashion.

Under optimal conditions, the operating light should be manipulated by a remote control; no such light is currently available. At present, the assistant or operator must handle the light in order to direct the beam into the field of operation. Obviously, this is unsatisfactory from the standpoint of asepsis. More sophisticated equipment no doubt will be manufactured in the future.

Operatory sinks

Although only one sink in an operatory is adequate, it is more efficient for the dentist and the assistant to have separate sinks because they frequently use them concurrently. Water should be activated by either knee or foot controls. Faucets should be eliminated for sanitary reasons. Sinks must be of adequate size, stain resistant, and easily cleanable. Disposable paper towels and a soap dispenser should be used. A convenient and easily emptied waste drop for used towels should be provided. It is realistic to think of activating the water supply by a photoelectric beam that, when interrupted, causes the water to flow. This type of control is commercially available, but usually activates water of only one temperature.

Consideration should be given to sink height. The assistant usually uses the sink while standing, but a sink of sit-down height may be preferable for the operator.

X-ray equipment

Conventional dental x-ray equipment has proved to be satisfactory for use with the equipment changes suggested in this chapter. The extended-cone parelleling technique permits radiographic procedures with the patient in a horizontal position. However, if the bisecting technique is employed, it may be necessary to adjust the contour chair to a more upright position.

The location of the dental x-ray machine must be decided on the basis of use priority. Some offices require more than one x-ray machine. It is suggested that the machine be wall-mounted at the left of the chair slightly back of the chair base center. The control panel should be placed behind suitable shielding. The panel is often located in the corridor adjoining the operatory.

The height at which the machine is installed on the wall will depend on the manner in which the machine is to be used. If the conventional bisecting technique is the procedure of choice, the patient ordinarily will be seated in an upright position, and the machine should be located at a height designed for use with the patient in this position. If the long-cone parelleling technique is employed, all exposures can be made with the patient in a fully supine position. It must be recognized that the chair can be moved horizontally and vertically on its base, and that the patient's head can be rotated from left to right for film placement and exposure.

EQUIPMENT LOCATION FOR EFFECTIVE ASSISTANT UTILIZATION

The dental chair and unit have been traditionally fixed in a predesignated position, and the location of all remaining supporting operatory equipment has been dictated by the fixed position of the chair and unit. It might be added that not a great deal of thought was given to efficient arrangement, and the operator forced himself to accommodate to major and minor inconveniences. When considering equipment location, one must simultaneously consider room dimensions, the necessity for minimizing excessive body motions, location priority based on equipment and instrument usage, and the degree of mobility available to the operating team through use of modern equipment. The location of cabinets and other pieces of equipment is dictated by the requirements of the operator in efficiently using auxiliary personnel and by the type of service he renders.

For discussion of body motions and operating room mobility see pp. 393 and 394.

Room size

The room size required for an operatory depends on the type of work to be done there. If cabinets are located in back of the chair and on only one side of the room, an operatory with a width of between 8 and 11 feet is desirable. The room length should be at least 10 feet. The patient's entrance should be near the foot of the chair and not through the work area.

Under ordinary circumstances, the chair is positioned diagonally (Fig. 19-4), with the foot of chair closer to the assistant's wall (left wall) and the head of the chair toward the operator's wall (assuming a right-handed operator). This arrangement makes it possible to use floor space more adequately (contour chairs require additional length, as compared to the conventional sit-up dental chair) and gives the assistant a maximum amount of functional space in her corner. The operator has ample room at the right of the chair. If cabinets are desired on both side walls, the width of the room must be 11 feet minimum (Fig. 19-4).

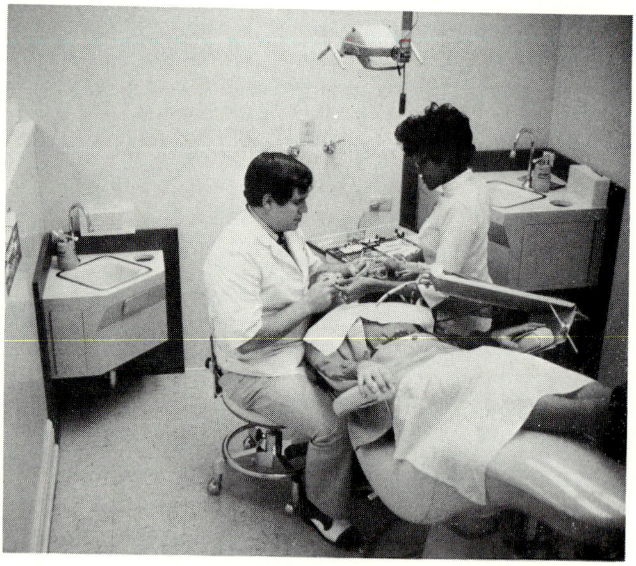

Fig. 19-4. Positioning of dental chair.

Location priorities

Dental practices are either of a generalized or a specialized nature. No attempt will be made to discuss equipment location in specialized practices. The average general practitioner spends the greatest portion of his time doing operative dentistry. Dentistry for children may be next most demanding of his time. The remainder of his efforts, in decreasing order of emphasis, is distributed between oral surgery, complete denture prosthesis, crown and bridge prosthesis, periodontics, partial denture prosthesis, oral diagnosis, endodontics, and orthodontics. The order will vary for specific practitioners. In any case, the most frequently used instruments and equipment must be located in the most convenient position for use by the assistant and/or operator.

Since the practitioner spends the greatest portion of his time performing operative dentistry, it is essential that items used by the operating team be readily accessible. Modern concepts of assistant utilization dictate that the operator not reach for anything. Instead, the correct instrument is placed in his hand at the right time. Thus, instruments and supplies must be strategically placed for the assistant, so that she can obtain and pass them to the operator with a minimum of effort. The mobile dental cabinet, designed to contain restorative materials, an amalgamator, and such items as mixing slabs, spatulas, and operating instruments not included in the preset tray, is rolled into an operating position convenient for the assistant. The sliding top surface of this cabinet is used as a work surface as well as an area for locating the preprepared instrument tray. This cabinet can also be used for pedodontics and prosthetics.

Supplies for special procedures should be made available by the assistant when the operatory is prepared for the patient. Additional movable cabinets may be necessary for other clinical operations. It is impossible to completely visualize the needs of all individual practitioners for cabinetry beyond the basic requirements. Each individual must envision his own practice habits, perhaps with some revisions, and equip additional cabinets for his use. Space in routinely used mobile cabinets should not be used for storage. Less accessible cabinets, perhaps wall-mounted, should store items less frequently used. Infrequently used equipment, supplies, and materials should not be found in the operatory.

It is obvious that equipment, materials, and supplies for all procedures cannot be located within reach of the assistant or the operator as they sit near the head of the chair. There will be an occasional need for one or the other to move bodily, but the frequency of this need should be minimized by the strategic placement of cabinets and equipment. Under ordinary circumstances, neither the dentist nor the assistant should leave the operating stool once the treatment has started.

SUMMARY

The operatory of the future is designed to allow an increased amount of dental service by each dentist without reducing the quality of care. The use of a full-time chairside dental assistant is mandatory. All clinical operations are performed with the operating team in a seated position and with the patient supported in a supine position by a contour-type chair. The location of equipment and supplies should be based on maximization of efficiency and minimization of fatigue.

Suggested readings

Andersen, J. A.: Dental office design and layout, J. Amer. Dent. Ass. **60**:344, 1960.

Golden, S. S.: Engineering comfort into dentistry, Mechanical Engineering **86**:39, Aug. 1964.

Kilpatrick, H. C.: Work simplification in dental practice, Philadelphia, 1964, W. B. Saunders Co.

McDevitt, E. J., and others: Four-handed dentistry: a practical approach to unit replacement, Alabama J. Med. Sci. **7**:72, Jan. 1970.

Miller, E. M., and Miller, J. S.: Oral lighting, J. Amer. Dent. Ass. **71**:856, 1965.

Robinson, G. E., and others: Four-handed dentistry: the whys and wherefores, J. Amer. Dent. Ass. **77**:573, Sept. 1968.

Sinnett, G. M., and others: Four-handed dentistry: a new mobile dental cabinet design, J. Amer. Dent. Ass. **78**:305, Feb. 1969.

Stinaff, R. K.: Dental practice administration, St. Louis, 1964, The C. V. Mosby Co.

Survey of dentistry, Washington, D. C., 1961, American Council on Education.

CHAPTER 20 DENTAL TERMINOLOGY AND GLOSSARY

KATHRYN S. GOLLER, C.D.A., R.D.H.

This chapter is not intended to be a complete dictionary of dental terms. It is an endeavor to make dental auxiliaries cognizant of their responsibility of learning dental terminology and to serve as a guide to word formation. In addition, it provides a glossary of terms frequently used in dentistry today.

When the student dental assistant begins training, she finds herself in a new world, surrounded by people speaking a new language. It is estimated that during the first few months of training, the dental auxiliary will increase her vocabulary by several thousand words.

Learning new words can be an interesting and rewarding challenge. Learning new words and being able to use them correctly in conversation has many rewards, but in this case, it is also essential for the success of the new dental assistant's career. It is necessary for her to acquire a thorough working knowledge of dental terminology to enable her to communicate effectively with (1) the dentist, (2) other members of the dental health team, (3) members of the dental and medical health professions, and (4) the patient.

The persons in the first 3 categories have been trained to use dental terminology; therefore, it is obvious why the new dental assistant needs to obtain a working knowledge of dental terminology to communicate with them effectively. It is the dental auxiliary who usually makes the initial contact with the patient, teaches dental health education during office visits, and has the final patient contact when the patient is dismissed. Her ability to understand and correctly use dental terms will have an important and lasting impact upon the patients and their attitude toward good dental health. Patients are duly impressed when they learn new words pertaining to their dental health. They learn this by conversing with the dentist and assistant who are knowledgeable about dental terminology.

Many medical and dental terms are derived from Latin or Greek words. Therefore, it is useful to concentrate on the roots or word parts. A root contains a specific idea that can usually be represented by a single English word. It may undergo considerable modification. To acquire a good working knowledge of dental terminology, the student should understand the following terms:

An *inflection* is a change in the form of a word to make a certain grammatical relation, such as the declension of nouns, the conjugation of verbs, and the comparison of adjectives. For example, adding "s" to a noun to form a plural or "ed" to a verb to form the past tense is an inflection.

The *stem* is the part of an inflected word that remains after the inflectional additions have been removed.

A *root* is the element common to all the words of a group of kindred meaning that remains after the formative additions (prefixes, suffixes, and inflections) have been removed.

A *prefix* is a syllable or group of syllables joined to the beginning of a word to change its meaning.

A *suffix* is a syllable or group of syllables joined to the ending of a word to change its meaning.

A *simple word* contains 1 stem.

A *compound word* contains more than 1 stem.

The student who sees the compound words used in dental textbooks for the first time may recoil with something of a shock. But if she knows the individual parts that make up these complex terms, what appears to be an unintelligible assortment of letters stands out with clarity. A word is much more easily remembered, spelled, and pronounced when its derivation is known.

As a further aid to understanding terminology, the student should know the frequently used prefixes and suffixes of words that are related to the healing arts. Often, by referring to either the prefix or suffix of a word, one can determine the definition of the word. For example, the word "leukocyte" is a combination of the prefix "leuko" and the suffix "cyte." "Leuko" is defined as "white," and the definition of "cyte" is "cell." Therefore, "leukocyte" means "white cell."

As the student examines the different word parts that are listed below, she will realize that many of these are not new, and that she has been using many of them for a long time. For example, all her life she has been using words with the word part or prefix "sub." She has learned to know what is meant by words such as "submarine," "subtract," "submerge," "subterranian," and a host of others. All of these words have 1 thing in common. This common element can be attributed to the prefix word part "sub," which means "under." Therefore, when one forgets what a prefix or a word part means, it is easy to think back to other, more common words containing that word or word part. Then one decides what all of these words have in common and figures out the word-part meaning.

Working with complex words that have been constructed from word parts is an interesting exercise that has many rewards. Following is a partial listing of frequently used roots, stems, prefixes, and suffixes to aid the student in word formation, and a glossary containing many dental terms to serve as a reference for the text.

WORD PARTS

a, an Negative.
ab, abs Away, from.
ac, acet Sharp, sour, pointed, as in acetabulum, acetone.
acou, acu, aco Hear, as in acoustic.
ad Toward.
aden Gland, as in adenitis, adenocarinoma.
adip, adep Fat, as in adipose.
aemia Blood.
aer Air.
aesthesia Sensation.
alb White, as in albino, materia alba.
alg Pain, as in odontalgia, analgesic.
aliment Food, as in alimentation.
all Other, foreign, as in allergy.
amb Both, on both sides.
ambl, ambul Walk, as in ambulatory, somnambulation.
amph Around, on both sides.
ana, an Up.
angi Vessel, as in angitis.
angio Relating to blood or lymph vessels.
ang, angul Sharp, bend, as in bi angle.
ante Before, as in anterior, antecedent, anteroom.
anti Against as in antibiotic, antifreeze, antiseptic.
apex, apic Top or pointed extremity of any conical part, as in apicoectomy, apical.
apo From, opposed.
aud Hear, as in audiometer, audiovisual.
aut, auto Self.

bi, bis Two, twice, or double, as in bicuspid, bifurcation, bicycle.
bio Life, as in biology, biochemistry, biography.
bucc Cheek, as in buccal.
cad, cas, cay, cid Fall, as in casualty, decay, accident, deciduous.
cal Heat, as in calor, calory.
card Heart, as in cardia, cardiovascular.
cari Rottenness, as in caries, carious.
cav Hollow, hole, or lesion, as in cavity, excavate.
cent Hundred.
cephal Relating to head.
cerebr, cereb Brain, as in cerebral, cerebellum.
cern, cret, cri Separate, as in excrete, secrete.
cervic, cervix Neck, as in cervical.
cheil, chil Lip, as in cheilosis.
chlor, chloas Green, as in chloride, chlorophyll.
chrom, chromo Color.
cide Causing death.
circum Around.
co, com, con Together.
contra Against.
cosm Order, beauty, as in cosmetic.
cran Skull, as in cranium, cranial.
cresc, crem, cret Grow, as in concrescence, increment.
cusp Point, as in bicuspid, cuspid.
cyan Blue, as in cyanosis.
cyst Bag, bladder.
cyte Cell.
de From, not.
deca Ten.
deci Tenth.
dent Relating to the teeth, as in dentist, dentin, dentition.
derma Relating to the skin.
di Separation or division, as in diatomic, diaphragm, diplococci.
dia Through, between, asunder.
digit Finger, as in digital.
dipla, diplo Double.
dynia Pain.
dys Difficult, bad.
ectomy Cutting out.
ed, esc, ex- Eat, as in edible.
edema Swelling, as in edematous, edema.
ef, es, ex, exo Out.
emes, emet Vomiting.
endo Within, as in endodontics, endoderm, endoskeleton.
epi Upon.
esthesia Sensation.
etio Cause, as in etiology.
ex Out, as in exodontics, excavate, exclude.
extra On the outside, beyond.
fac Face, as in facial, maxillofacial.
fore Before, in front of.
flag, flam Burn, flame, as in inflammation.
gastro Stomach, belly.
gen Beget, produce, as in genetics.
geni Chin, as in genial.
geus, gust Taste, as in gustation.
gloss, glot Tongue, as in glossitis, epiglottis.
gluc, gly Sweet, sugar, as in glucose, hyperglycemia.
gnath Jaw, as in gnathology, prognathia.
gno, gnos Know, as in pathognomy, diagnosis, prognosis.
gog To make flow.
gram Tracing, mark.
graphy Writing, record.
hem, hemato Relating to blood.
hemi Half.
hepa Liver.
homo, homeo Same, similar.
hydra, hydro Relating to water, as in hydrated.
hygie, hygei, hugi Health, as in hygiene.
hyper Over, above, beyond, abnormal, or excessive.
hypo Under, deficient, or beneath.
hypn Sleep, as in hypnotic.
iasis Condition, pathologic state.
ics Practice of dentistry, as in orthodontics, periodontics, pedodontics.
idio Peculiar to the individual or organ.
infra Beneath.
infer Low, as in inferior.
inter Between, as in interproximal.
intra, intro Within or inside.
ism Condition, theory.
itis Inflammation, as in pulpitis, bronchitis, arthritis.
ize To treat by a special method.
labi Lip, as in labial.
lamin, lamn, lamel Flat plate, as in lamina dura.
laryng, laryngo Larynx.
latero Side.
lepto Small, soft.
leuco, leuko White.
lig Bind, as in ligate, ligament.
lingu Tongue, as in lingual.
lip Fat, as in lipid, lipoma.
liqu Pour, as in liquid.
logia, logy Science or study of.
lysis Setting free, disintegration.
macro Large, long, big, as in macrodontia.
mal Bad, poor, evil, as in malaria.
marg Edge, as in margin.
med, mes, mid Middle, as in median, mesial, middle.
meta Beyond, over, between, change, or transposition.
meter Measure.
micro Small.
mio Less or smaller.
mono Single.
multi Many.

myo Muscle.
nas, nar Nose, as in nasal, nasopalatine.
neu, neuro Nerve, as in neuritis.
non Not, no.
nucleo Nucleus.
ob Against.
ocul Eye, as in oculist, oculomotor.
ode Old, form, shape, resemblance.
odont Pertaining to teeth, as in odontoma, odontogenic.
oma Tumor.
orific Opening, as in orifice.
ortho Straight, normal.
oss, ost, oste Bone, as in osseous, osteoid, ossification.
osis Condition, disease, intensive.
ostomosis To furnish with mouth or outlet.
oxy Sharp, acid.
pan All, entire.
para Alongside.
path, pathy Disease.
penia Lack of.
per Excessive, through.
phag Eat.
pharm Medicine, as in pharmacy.
phobia Fear.
phon Sound, voice, as in phonetics.
phylac, phylax, phylact To guard or protect.
plasm To mold.
plastic Molded, indicating restoration of lost or badly formed features.
plegia Stroke.
plur More.
pneu Relating to air or lungs.
poly Much, many.
post After, as in postoperative.
pre Before, as in preoperative.
pro Before, in behalf of.
prosop Face, as in prosopalgia.
prox Next, next to, as in proximal.
pseud, pseudo False.
psych Relating to the soul or mind.
pus, pur Liquid inflammatory product as in pus, suppurate, purulent.
py, pyo Pus.
retro Backward.
rhage, rhagia Hemorrhage, flow.
rhea To flow, indicating discharge.
sacro Sacrum.
saliva Spittle, as in salivation.
sclero Hard, relating to sclera.
sclerosis Dryness, hardness.
scopy To see.
semi Half.
sen Old, as in senile, senior.
sep Rot, decay.
sicc Dry, as in desiccate.
spor Seed.
stom, stomat Mouth, orifice, as in stomatology.
sub Under or below, as in subgingival, submaxillary.
sulc Groove, furrow, as in sulcus.
super, supra Above or over, as in supernumerary.
sutur Sewing together, as in sutural.
syn With, together.
syncop Fainting, as in syncope.
tele Distant, for.
therap Treatment, as in therapeutic.
therm Heat, as in thermal.
thromb Lump, clot.
tomy Cutting.
tox Poison, as in toxicology.
trans Across.
tri Three.
tropho Relating to nutrition.
tum Swelling, as in tumor.
ultra Beyond or excess, as in ultrasonic.
uni One.
uria Relating to urine.
vacu Empty, as in vacuole, vacuum.
vas, vaso Vessel.
venter, ventro Abdomen.
vir Poison, as in virulent.
vit Life, as in vital, vitamin.
zo Animal life, as in zoology.

TERMS

abrasion The wearing away or wearing down of teeth due to mastication, as in occlusal abrasion.
abscess Puss formation that is localized and limited in extent in any part of the body.
abutment Tooth that provides the point of anchorage and support for a bridge or other prosthodonic appliance.
accelerator Agent that speeds up a chemical reaction.
acrylic resins Plastic materials that are used in the fabrication of dentures and crowns and occasionally as a restorative filling material.
acute Having severe and pronounced symptoms, but of short course or duration; the opposite of *chronic*, which means of long duration.
A.D.A. Abbreviation for American Dental Association.
A.D.A.A. Abreviation for American Dental Assistants Association.
A.D.H.A. Abbreviation for American Dental Hygienists Association.
adhesive Sticky. Wax is adhesive.
aerobic Requiring oxygen to live; aerobic microorganisms, for example.
A.H.A. Abbreviation for American Hospital Association.
alcohol An organic compound that is volatile, colorless, and nearly odorless and tasteless. In

high concentrations, it may be used as a disinfectant. It is nontoxic and readily evaporates without residue. It acts by denaturation of protein and may precipitate a protective coat around bacteria contained in blood, pus, and mucus; should not be used on instruments, unless they have been cleaned.

allergy The sensitiveness of a person to a specific substance that, in turn, causes no reaction in a person who is not sensitive to it.

alloy The product (not chemical compound) formed as a result of combining or fusing 2 or more metals; a mixture of 2 or more metals, mutually soluble when in a molten state (see *amalgam*).

alveolar process The projection of the maxillary and mandibular bones, which envelops the roots of the teeth and forms their alveoli. The alveolus is the cavity or socket in the process of the maxillary and mandibular bones in which the root of the tooth is fixed.

alveolus (pl., alveoli) The tooth socket in the alveolar process.

alveolectomy (alveoloplasty) The shaping of the alveolar ridge by surgical procedures for the removal of bony prominences, usually in preparation for the construction of a prosthetic appliance.

amalgam An alloy composed of 2 or more metals, one of which is mercury. An amalgam composed of silver, tin, copper, zinc, and mercury is used extensively in dentistry for restorations. A.D.A. Specification #1 for dental amalgam alloys requires the chemical composition to be within the following limits: silver; 65% minimum; copper, 6% maximum; zinc; 2% maximum; and tin, 25% minimum.

ambeloblast A dental enamel-forming cell. One of a group of cells from which the enamel on teeth is formed.

ammeter An electrical instrument, commonly found on x-ray machines and other equipment, which registers the flow of electrical current through a circuit. In the case of an x-ray machine, it registers the current flowing through the x-ray tube; the greater this current is, the greater is the production of penetrating radiation. Therefore the high current permits exposures to be made in a shorter time because of the increased power of the rays.

amorphous Not having a definite crystalline structure. Some dental waxes are amorphous.

ampere A unit that describes the rate at which current is flowing through a circuit. One ampere is the rate at which current will be pushed through a circuit having 1 ohm of resistance, if it is pushed through by a pressure of 1 volt. The current flowing through an x-ray tube is usually measured in milliamperes, which is 1/1,000 of 1 ampere (see *ammeter*).

ampule (ampul) A hermetically sealed container such as used for storing measured doses of hypodermic solutions.

anaerobic Term applied to microorganisms that cannot exist in the presence of oxygen.

ancillary Little-used term that has been replaced by "auxiliary" to refer to personnel who assist the dentist by working under his direction, and for whose work and service the dentist assumes the responsibility.

anemia A condition in which there is a significant reduction in the number of red blood cells, which, in turn, results in reduction in the oxygen-carrying capacity of the blood.

anesthesia A loss of sensation or feeling.

anesthetic A drug that produces anesthesia, or a loss of sensation (see *general anesthetic* and *local anesthetic*).

Angström A unit of measure that describes the wavelength of certain very high-frequency radiations. The behavior and the penetrating power of radiations vary with their frequency, which is related to their wavelength. Broadcast radio stations have wavelengths of from 200 to 600 meters, and x-rays have a wavelength of less than 1 Angström unit, or less than one billionth of a meter.

anneal To temper glass or metal by alternate heating and cooling.

anode The positive terminal in an electric circuit. In the case of an x-ray tube, the target is the anode, for it has a positive charge and is bombarded by electrons that are negatively charged.

anodontia Absence of teeth.

anomaly A deviation from a normal standard; may be a congenital structural defect.

anterior Indicating a forward position, or a position in the front part of the mouth; a term commonly used to denote the incisor teeth.

anteroposterior From the front to the rear.

antibiotic The product of an organism that may be used to destroy other organisms that are disease-producing.

antidote An agent that counteracts or prevents the action of a poison.

antisepsis The destruction of germs that cause disease, fermentation, or putefaction.

antiseptic A substance that stops or inhibits the growth of bacteria but does not necessarily kill them.

antrum A cavity or chamber, especially one within checkbones.

apex The point or extremity of a conical object, such as the terminal end of the root of a tooth, which is called the apical end of the tooth.

A.P.H.A. Abbreviation for American Public Health Association.

apical curettement Surgical removal of infectious material surrounding the apex of a tooth root, not involving removal of the root tip.

apicoectomy The surgical removal of the apex of the tooth root. Most often done in conjunction with, or as an adjunct to, root canal therapy.

apical foramen The tiny opening of the pulp canal at the tip end of the root of the tooth. The vessels and nerves of the dental pulp pass through the apical foramen.

apoplexy Sudden loss of consciousness, voluntary motion, and: sensation, caused by rupture or obstruction of an artery of the brain. Commonly called a stroke.

appliance A device worn by a dental patient during a course of treatment, but not used as a substitute or reconstruction of oral or facial structures, such as space maintainer, periodontal splints.

arch, dental The curved composite structure of the natural dentition, and the residual ridge or the remains thereof after the loss of some or all of the natural teeth.

armamentarium Technically, all the instruments, equipment, medicines, books, and journals needed by the dentist, dental hygienist, or physician in his or her profession. Practically, the term as used refers only to the instruments that are used.

artifact (artefact) A structure that is not natural, such as a shadow on an x-ray film that is caused by unnatural objects or by manipulation.

articulate To unite or join the teeth of one arch in the proper position with the teeth of the opposing arch.

articulator An instrument for holding the casts of jaws or teeth in the proper relationship to one another.

artificial stone A plasterlike substance used for making dental casts. The base of artificial stone is a gypsum material, hydrocal.

asepsis A method of treatment that creates an antiseptic condition by the exclusion of microorganisms.

asphyxia Suspension of breathing and animation because the body is deprived of oxygen, as in drowning or suffocation.

atrophy The wasting away of tissue or parts, through lack of use or disease.

attrition Normal wearing away by friction. In dentistry, it refers to wearing down the surfaces of the teeth by mastication of food.

autoclave A sterilizer that performs its function by the generation of high temperatures which, in turn, are created by steam under pressure.

auxiliary personnel Persons, such as the dental hygienist, dental assistant, and dental laboratory technician, who work under the supervision or direction of the dentist.

axial The long or vertical dimension of the tooth, or the axis of the tooth.

bacillus A microorganism that is rod-shaped.

bacteria Microscopic, typically unicellular plants whose undifferentiated rigid cells occur as spheres, rods, or spirals.

bacteremia Bacteria in the blood.

bacterial plaque A film-like covering on the teeth, which is often very difficult to see in a well-kept mouth.

bactericide A substance or agent that destroys bacteria.

bacteriastatic A substance that inhibits the growth of bacteria.

baseplate A sheet of wax, metal, or other material that is used for making trial denture setups.

benign Not malignant.

Bennett movement The sliding of the rotational center of the condyle laterally, while the mandible is in movement. The lateral movement of the mandible is the result of the movement of the heads of the condyle along the lateral inclines of the mandibular or glenoid fossa.

bicuspids Teeth with 2 cusps, situated between the cuspids and molars. There are 8 in the full complement of permanent teeth; also called "premolars."

bifurcation Division into 2 parts or branches, as in the case of 2 roots of a tooth.

biology The science of substances or organisms that either are alive or have been alive.

biopsy Surgical removal of tissue for microscopic examination, primarily for the purpose of diagnosing the possibility of benign or malignant tumors.

bite-wing radiograph (or x-ray) A specific type of x-ray picture that shows, simultaneously, the crowns of upper and lower posterior teeth and a portion of their roots and supporting structures. Generally used to diagnose the presence of dental decay in adjoining tooth surfaces.

boxing The construction of a retaining wall (usually in wax) around a dental impression, so as to hold modeling material until it sets.

bruxism The clenching or grinding of the teeth.

buccal Pertaining to the cheek, The buccal surface of a tooth is located toward the cheek.

bur A small rotary instrument of steel for cutting tooth structure, metal, and cement. Burs are operated by a dental engine or lathe.

burnishing Polishing by friction. Tinfoil is burnished for the purpose of adapting it to the cast.

calcareous Pretaining to a compound of calcium, such as calcium carbonate or calcium phosphate.

calculus A hard, calcareous (calcium compound) material that is deposited on the surfaces of the crowns or roots of the teeth. Calculus may also be deposited in other parts of the body. The deposit of calculus on tooth structure is dependent upon an organic compound or matrix.

canine eminence A noticeable bulge over the cuspid tooth on the upper jaw, just below and to the outside of the nose.

capsule A mucoid or gelatinous case that surrounds some bacteria and protects them from destruction.

carborundum An abrasive that is extremely hard (harder than emery). It is a registered trade name for silicon carbide.

Carborundum stones and wheels are used in dentistry to polish restorations and teeth. They mount in the handpiece, and the unit motor makes them spin as a bur spins.

carcinoma A malignant tumor.

cardiac Pertaining to the heart.

cardiovascular Pertaining to the heart and the blood vessels.

caries Decay in tooth structure.

carious Relating to decay in tooth structure.

carious lesion An area of tooth structure exhibiting caries, as identified by clinical or radiographic examination.

case history All the information the dentist is able to gather about a patient that will help in diagnosing and treating that patient. This information is strictly confidential.

cassette A rigid film holder, in which are mounted 2 intensifying screens.

casting A process by which a reproduction is formed by forcing or pouring a liquid into a mold and permitting it to solidify, so that it will be of the desired shape when it has hardened.

catalyst A substance or agent that speeds up a chemical action but presumably does not enter into the chemical action itself. A so-called *negative catalyst* would slow down a chemical action.

cathode A negative terminal or electrode. In the x-ray tube, the filament is the cathode and emits the negative electrons that are attracted toward the target, which is the positive anode (see *anode*).

cavities

one surface Occlusal, buccal, labial, or lingual. A carious lesion that involves a single surface of a tooth.

two surfaces Distal occlusal, mesial occlusal. A carious lesion that involves 2 adjacent tooth surfaces of an individual tooth, either the distal and occlusal surfaces (DO) or the mesial and occlusal surfaces (MO).

three surfaces Mesial, occlusal, distal. A carious lesion that involves 3 tooth surfaces on an individual tooth, the mesial, occlusal, and distal surfaces (MOD).

cavity A hollow, hole, or lesion produced by dental caries.

cavity liner Material, usually a varnish, used to line the preparation in a tooth before the tooth is fitted or crowned or has an inlay placed.

cc. Abbreviation for cubic centimeter.

C.D.A. Abbreviation for Certified Dental Assistant.

cementum A bonelike tissue that forms the outer surface of the roots of the tooth.

centigrade thermometer A thermometer on which there are 100 degrees divisions between the freezing and boiling points of water; the freezing point of water is 0 degrees and the boiling point of water is 100 degrees. Temperatures are recorded in the centigrade scale for most scientific studies, whereas the Fahrenheit scale is commonly used in the United States for all nonscientific references to temperature (see *Fahrenheit thermometer*).

centimeter A measurement of length. There are 100 cm. in 1 meter; 2.54 cm. equals 1 inch.

centric relation A relationship between the upper and lower jaws when the associated muscles are in balance, and one that must be considered when artificial teeth are positioned in the artificial denture.

cervical Pertaining to the neck of a tooth or that portion near the junction of the crown and root of a tooth.

cervical line The line or landmark formed by the junction of the enamel and the cementum on a tooth.

cheilitis Inflammation of the lip.

chronic Of long duration; the opposite of acute, which means of short duration.

cingulum The lingual lobe of an incisor tooth.

clasp An integral part of a removable partial denture constructed of metal and used as a stabilizing and retaining device to keep both tooth and denture in passive apposition.

clinic, dental A physical facility to which patients are admitted for diagnosis, evaluation, and treatment of dental defects by 2 or more dentists practicing dentistry together.

cocci Bacteria that are spherical in shape and appears in chains or clusters.

cold sterilization A process of sterilization through the use of chemical agents as a disinfectant. It is an unreliable procedure for destroying organisms and spores, and when used for sterilization, it is necessary to follow a rigid regime. The use is usually limited to instruments that do not lend themselves to other methods of sterilization or to instruments that have sharp cutting surfaces that must be maintained.

colloid A mixture in which the dispersed particles are aggregates of molecules, which makes them larger than the particles or molecules that characterize the substance of a solution.

coma Prolonged loss of consciousness that does not reverse by itself.

compound A chemical compound is one that has been formed as a result of a chemical reaction between 2 or more elements. The term "compound" is frequently employed in dental laboratories and clinics to refer to the wax-like substances that can be molded when heated.

congenital Existing at the time of birth.

contact point The area of a tooth's surface that touches a neighboring tooth.

contra-angle Attachment for straight handpiece that permits burs, stones, and disks to be used at a more effective angle in the mouth.

coronal Referring to the crown or visible portion of a tooth, as seen in the mouth.

corrode To wear away, as by the chemical action that occurs on the surface of a metal, as rusting and tarnishing.

C.P. An abbreviation used on labels for chemicals, which means that the substance meets the standards that permits it to be labeled as "chemically pure."

crown The portion of a tooth that is normally covered with enamel and that projects from the tissues in which the root is fixed. The portion that is visible under any normal or abnormal conditions is the *clinical crown,* but the portion that meets the basic definition is called the *anatomic crown.* An *artificial crown* is a cap of metal or plastic that acts as a restoration for the *natural crown.*

crown and bridge That branch of dental science primarily concerned with the replacement of missing or naturally destroyed teeth or tooth structures by use of permanent nonremovable dental prostheses or restorations.

curve of Spee An imaginary curve passing through the condyles and the cuspid teeth to the incisal edge of the lower centrals. Compensating curve, an imaginary line that contacts the tips of the buccal cusps of the bicuspids and molars and extends to the condyles.

cusp A pronounced elevation, or point, on or near the masticating or occlusal surface of the tooth.

cuspid A tooth with one point or cusp. There are 4 cuspids in the permanent dentition—one on either side in each jaw, situated at the corners of the mouth.

cutaneous Relating to the skin.

cutting edge See *incisal edge.*

cyst A saclike structure containing liquid or other materials, which may be normal or pathologic.

cytology, oral exfoliative The microscopic diagnostic study of cells that have desquamated (fallen away) from the external or internal surfaces of the body. A diagnostic procedure used to assist in the detection of oral tumors.

D.D.S. Abbreviation of *Doctor of Dental Surgery,* the academic degree given for the completion of the 4 years of formal study in an accredited dental school. The curriculum is essentially the same as that for the degree of D.M.D. (see *D.M.D.*).

debilitant An agent for inducing weakness; a remedy that allays excitement.

deciduous See *primary.*

DEF rate Similar to the DMF rate, but used for primary dentition (baby teeth); the letter D, which stands for decayed primary teeth, is indicated for filling, and the letter F, which represents filled primary teeth, have the same meaning as in DMF. The symbol E, however, stands only for decayed teeth indicated for extraction. Missing teeth are not counted for this rate, since they often cannot be differentiated from teeth lost through natural exfoliation.

dental assistant A person employed by a dentist to perform chairside duties and any other duties assigned and supervised by the dentist.

- ***certified dental assistant*** A dental assistant who has received formal training in dental assisting and who has met all requirements of the Certification Board of the American Dental Assistants Association.
- ***chairside assistant*** Specifically, a dental assistant who assists the dentist in the performance of rendering dental treatment.
- ***coordinating assistant*** A dental assistant who assists the dentist and the chairside assistant, and in general coordinates the work procedures in the dental operating room.
- ***currently certified dental assistant*** A dental assistant who has met the requirements of the Certification Board of the American Dental Assistants Association and has renewed her certificate annually.

dental health education A term commonly used in dentistry for instructing the patient in preventive and corrective methods.

dental health team A relatively new concept to the practice of dentistry, composed of the dentist, as the pivotal member, and a group of specially trained persons whom he employs and supervises in the performance of certain clearly defined duties. These persons are referred to as auxiliary personnel.

dental hygienist A person trained in and practicing the art of dental prophylaxis. Generally, the only licensed person, other than a dentist, who receives specific training in dental health education and who is permitted to work directly within the oral cavity.

dental stone Materials that have essentially the same composition as *plaster of Paris,* $(CaSO_4)_2 \cdot H_2O$; however, their crystals differ physically, and they are much stronger and harder. They are used to make dies and models, from which inlays, crowns, and other dental appliances can be fabricated. *Hydrocal* is another name for *dental stone.*

dental technician A person self-employed or employed by a dentist or dental laboratory company who is essentially concerned with the fabrication of dental appliances or devices on the direct prescription or work order of the licensed practitioner.

dentifrice A substance, such as tooth powder or toothpaste, used with a toothbrush for the purpose of cleansing the accessible surfaces of the teeth.

dentin (dentine) The tissue that constitutes the chief substance of the tooth.

dentition A term used to designate the general character and arrangement of the teeth, taken as a whole.

dentoenamel junction That junction of the inner surface of the enamel crown with the dentin. Same as amelodentinal junction.

dentofacial deformities Disabling abnormalities of the teeth, oral cavity, and face, usually congenital in origin, such as oral clefts, severe malocclusion.

denture An artificial substitute for missing natural teeth and adjacent structures.

- ***complete denture*** A dental prosthesis that replaces the lost natural dentition and associated structures of the entire maxilla or mandible.
- ***fixed partial denture*** A restoration of 1 or more missing teeth that cannot be readily removed by the patient or dentist; it is permanently attached to natural teeth or roots which furnish the primary support to the appliance, generally referred to as a bridge.
- ***immediate denture*** A dental prosthesis constructed for insertion immediately following the extraction of natural teeth.
- ***partial denture*** An artificial replacement of 1 or more but less than all of the natural teeth and associated structures.
- ***removable partial denture*** A prosthetic appliance that artificially replaces missing teeth and associated structures in a partially edentulous jaw and that can be removed from the mouth and replaced at will; it depends in part on the oral mucosa for its support.

detergent A cleansing agent.

developmental grooves Fine, depressed lines in the enamel of a tooth, which mark the junction of its lobes.

diabetes An inheritable, constitutional disease of unknown cause, characterized by the failure of the body tissues to oxidize carbohydrate at a normal rate. It manifests itself in an excess of sugar in the blood, presence of sugar in the urine, and in more advanced stages, acidosis and coma, with symptoms of intense thirst and hunger, weakness, and loss of weight.

diagnosis The procedures involved in determining the nature or the cause of a disease. Also, the identification of the disease.

diagnostic services Procedures, such as radiographs, clinical examinations, biopsies, blood tests, study models, and vitality tests, that assist the dentist in determining the disease conditions present and the treatment required.

die An exact replica or model of an article or object, usually fabricated from metal or stone.

direct technique A procedure for the preparation of casting of gold inlays or crowns. In this technique, the wax pattern is formed and carved directly on the tooth that is being restored (see *indirect technique*).

direct-flame sterilization A procedure in which an open flame is used to sterilize needles and other metal materials.

disease A deviation from a state of good health; a disturbance in the function of any organ of the body.

disinfectant An agent that effectively kills pathogenic microorganisms, including bacteria, viruses, and fungi.

distal Pertaining to a distant location or position. The distal surface of a tooth is the surface most distant from the median line.

D.M.D. Abbreviation for *Doctor of Dental Medicine* (see *D.D.S.*).

DMF rate For an individual, the number of permanent teeth (or for a group, the average number) that are decayed (D), missing (M), or indicated for extraction, and filled (F). The DMF rate is a measure of the cummulative effects of dental caries and a useful means for comparing the lifetime dental decay experience of groups of comparable age.

dram (or drachm) A unit weight. One dram equals ⅛ apothecaries' ounce, or 60 grains.

dry-heat sterilization A method of sterilization

that utilizes elevated temperature (about 160 degrees C., or 320 degrees F.), created in an oven.

ductile Description of the physical nature of a metal, which indicates that it can be drawn into thin wires or hammered into thin sheets.

dysfunction Lack or impairment of function.

edema Excessive accumulation of fluid in the tissues, which causes swelling.

edentulous Without teeth.

electron Negatively charged particle; a unit of negative electricity. The arrangement and number of electrons revolving about the nucleus of an atom determine many of the physical and chemical properties of the element.

embolus A clot or bit of foreign substance that obstructs the flow of blood in a vessel.

embrasure The opening with sloping sides formed by the adjacent surfaces of teeth.

employee A person who, acting under the direction and control of the person by whom he is hired, performs services for an employer in return for remuneration.

emulsion A mixture of 2 liquids, neither of which is soluable in the other, as in the case of minute oil globules dispersed throughout water.

emulsion, photographic A gelatinous solution containing silver salts.

enamel The hard, calcified tissue that covers the dentin of the crown portion of a tooth.

endocrine glands Glands that secrete internally.

endodontics A branch of dentistry that deals with the treatment of pulpless teeth.

enzyme A complex chemical substance that acts to expedite and to catalyze the digestive process.

epidemiology The scientific study of diseases from the standpoint of their distribution and frequency of occurrence.

epithelium The covering of the skin and mucous membranes.

erosion In dentistry, the destruction of superficial layers of the tooth at the neck, beginning with the enamel and working inward. It is probably due to a combination of chemical action and abrasion. The cavities have dense and polished surfaces.

eruption The process of a new tooth entering the mouth from its place of formation.

erythema Redness of the skin.

esthetic Appreciation of the beautiful in nature and art.

ethics The science of right conduct.

etiology The study or science related to the cause of any disease.

exfoliation The shedding of a horny layer or the shedding of a tooth, as in the case of a child losing his deciduous teeth.

exodontics A branch of dentistry that deals with the extraction of teeth (see *extraction*).

exposure 1. An opening into the pulp chamber of a tooth, usually the result of injury or decay, whereby the pulp is brought into contact with the oral environment (including bacteria and saliva). 2. The time that ionization produced by an x-ray machine is permitted to come in contact with the object being radiographed. 3. A procedure whereby surgical removal of tissue permits an unerupted tooth to be visible within the oral cavity.

extraction The separation and surgical removal of a tooth from its natural state.

extraoral Outside the mouth.

F.A.C.D. Abbreviation for Fellow of American College of Dentists.

face-bow An instrument or caliper-like device used to record the relationship of the maxillae to the temporomandibular joint.

facial surface Term used to collectively designate the buccal and labial surfaces of the teeth.

Fahrenheit thermometer An instrument for measuring the temperature or the degree of heat. The Fahrenheit thermometer carries the name of its originator, G. D. Fahrenheit (1686-1736). On this thermometer, the freezing point of water is 32 degrees, the average normal body temperature is 98.6 degrees, and the boiling point of water is 212 degrees. This temperature scale is used widely in the United States by weather bureaus and housewives, as well as by dentists and physicians in measuring the temperature of the human body. The centigrade scale is used for most scientific experiments in the United States and is widely used for all purposes outside the United States.

febrile Pertaining to fever; feverish.

F.I.C.D. Abbreviation for Fellow of International College of Dentists.

fissure A fault in the surface of a tooth, caused by imperfect joining; a deep ditch or cleft; commonly the result of the imperfect fusion of the enamel of the adjoining dental lobes.

fistula A deep sinuous ulcer or canal-like tube into the cavity of an alveolar abscess.

five-handed dentistry The new concept in the practice of dentistry to increase the efficiency of 4-handed dentistry. The chairside assistant utilizes the left hand for both delivering and receiving instruments, which leaves the right hand free to manipulate air, water, oral evacuator, and so on. This technique is also called the "3-handed dental assistant concept."

flora Bacteria living in various parts of the digestive tract.

flow The change in the shape of a material, when placed under a stationary load. This may generally be considered a measure of plasticity. It is usually associated with noncrystalline substances, although there is an outstanding exception in amalgam.

fluorescence The property that certain bodies manifest when irradiated; such bodies emit light of a different wavelength from the light they absorb.

fluoridation The addition of fluoride to a community water supply as an aid in the control of dental caries; usually in quantities of 1 part per million.

fluoride, topical—application of The direct application of a solution of fluoride, usually sodium fluoride or stannous fluoride, to the crowns of the teeth, as a measure for partially preventing the incidence of dental caries. Application is recommended on a routine basis through childhood and adolescence.

fluorosis A result of consuming excessive amounts of fluorine, as in the case of the enamel surface becoming mottled from drinking excessively fluoridated water.

focal infection A type of infection in which the bacteria are localized primarily in one place, as in the tonsils or periodontal tissue, and sent into the blood supply from that focal point.

foil, gold Small pellets of rolled gold foil, which are malleted into a cavity preparation to restore the function and shape of the tooth. A type of dental restoration.

foramen A hole or perforation, such as the foramen in bone through which nerves or vessels pass.

formaldehyde solution A colorless, volatile fluid, used as a surgical and general antiseptic and preservative.

fossa A round or angular depression in the surface of a tooth. Fossae occur mostly in the occlusal surfaces of the molars and in the lingual surfaces of the incisors.

four-handed dentistry The new concept in the practice of dentistry, which utilizes the chairside assistant as the dentist's second pair of hands to perform dental treatment.

fracture The breaking of a cartilage or a bone.

frenectomy Surgical removal of the labial or lingual frenum (frena).

frenum Labial, the band of tissue that passes from the inside of the lip to a point midway between the central incisors; lingual, the band of tissue that passes from under the tongue to the lingual aspect of the midpoint of the lower jaw.

fringe benefits Benefits, such as health insurance, vacations, and disability income, provided either as a result of collective bargaining or unilaterally by the employer.

fulcrum The point of a lever system that is stationary. Being stationary, the "rest" finger position used in prophylactic techniques acts as a fulcrum to provide security and surety of lever movement.

fumigation Exposure to the fumes of sulfur or to the action of a disinfectant gas. (This method of sanitation of premises is presently believed to be ineffective.)

fungicide An element or compound capable of inducing the destruction of fungi.

fusion The act of melting; uniting, as by melting together.

general anesthetic An agent, such as ether or nitrous oxide, that produces anesthesia throughout the entire body, as opposed to a "local anesthetic," which produces anesthesia in 1 portion of the body or around 1 area of tissue.

germicide Any substance that kills germs.

gingiva The portion of tissue enveloping the necks of the teeth crownwise from the attachment at the gingival line.

glossitis Inflammation of the tongue.

gram A unit of weight; 454 grams equal 1 pound, and 1,000 grams equal 1 kilogram.

groove A long depression in the surface of a tooth.

guards The position assumed by the thumb and fingers of the left hand to steady the parts operated upon and protect them from injury in case of accidental slipping of an instrument.

gutta-percha A sticky gumlike material obtained from the juice of various trees found in the Malayan peninsula (temporary stopping).

hepatitis, infectious A disease of the liver. Its incidence is related to close communal living, and its virus is very resistant to heat, cold, chlorine, and alcohol. The incubation period is approximately 30 days. Prevention of disease depends upon maintenance of high levels of sanitation and personal hygiene. The only safe method of sterilizing instruments, as far as this disease is concerned, is boiling and autoclaving for 15 minutes.

histology The scientific study of the structure and composition of the tissues.

homogeneous Uniform, similar in makeup throughout.

hormone A chemical substance produced in an organ that, when carried to an associated organ by the bloodstream, influences its functional activity.

horn, pulpal A slender or blunt-pointed process

of the pulp of a tooth, extending toward the point of a cusp.

hot-water sterilization Most widely used method of sterilizing inanimate objects; immersion of articles in boiling water (100 degrees C. or 212 degrees F.) for 10 to 20 minutes. This method is quick and economical, requires no special apparatus, leaves no toxic residue, has great penetrating power, and is harmless to a wide variety of materials, but it should not be used for sterilizing cutting instruments.

hydrated Combined with water.

Hydrocal See *dental stone.*

hypercementosis An excessive formation of cementum, usually at the apical portion of the root of a tooth, giving a bulbous appearance.

hyperplasia Abnormal increase in number of cells.

hypersecretion Excessive secretion.

hypertrophy Abnormal increase in the size of cells.

hypnotic Inducing sleep.

hypothyroidism Morbid state produced by deficient secretion by the thyroid gland.

immunity The condition of an organism that permits it to resist disease.

impacted tooth Commonly, a tooth embedded in either the soft or bony tissues of the jaw in such a way that it has not erupted or has erupted only partially.

impression A negative likeness of a form or model. Impressions are made of tissues, in order to produce models of the original tissues.

incisal edge The surface of an incisor or a cuspid that is the cutting edge.

incisor A tooth with a cutting edge. There are 4 incisors in the upper jaw and four in the lower jaw, called the upper and lower right and left central incisors and the upper and lower right and left lateral incisors.

inclination of a tooth—the deviation of the long axis of a tooth from the perpendicular line, as the mesial inclination of the incisors; of a surface—the deviation of a portion of the surface of a tooth from the general plane of that surface.

indirect technique A technique in which an impression is taken of the tooth or teeth after the cavity preparations have been made. Models, generally stone, are then made, and the wax patterns are fabricated on this die outside the mouth (see *direct technique*).

infectious disease An impairment of function that an organism suffers because of the activities of some other organism that lives within or upon it.

inlay, dental A dental inlay is generally a cast-gold restoration, prepared by making a wax pattern to fit the cavity preparation, carved to restore the missing anatomy of the tooth. This pattern is reproduced in gold by casting and is then cemented in the tooth.

instrument exchange The passing and receiving of hand and rotary instruments between the dentist and the chairside assistant.

instrument exchange area The designated place where the dentist and chairside assistant exchange hand and rotary instruments. The exchange area is directly in front of the patient's chin, never more than 2 to 4 inches from the operating zone. In children or apprehensive patients, the exchange area may be directly behind the patient's head.

instrument grasps The manner of grasping and holding instruments to their work. The 4 fundamental instrument grasps are palm and thumb, palm-thrust, pen, and inverted pen grasps.

palm and thumb grasp The handle of the instrument rests in the palm of the hand and is grasped by the 4 fingers, while the thumb usually rests on some adjoining surface.

palm-thrust grasp The end of the large handle is grasped in the center of the palm, the shank being held between the balls of the thumb and first and second fingers.

pen grasp The instrument is held like a pen, the shank being in contact with the thumb and first and second fingers.

inverted pen grasp Similar to the pen grasp, except that the position of the instrument is reversed, so that the working part points toward instead of away from the operator.

interdental Situated between the teeth.

interdigitation Meshing of upper and lower cusps in occlusion.

interproximal space The v-shaped space bounded by the proximate surfaces of the adjoining teeth and the border of the septum of the alveolar process. Normally, this space is filled with gum tissue.

investing The utilization of a substance (investment material) for covering an object, such as a tooth, in order to produce the mold that will be used to fabricate artificial crowns, inlays, and so on.

investment A material for enveloping or embedding a cast or denture in a flask.

in vivo Refers to vital processes occurring in the living being.

ion An atom or group of atoms having a charge of positive or negative electricity.

ionize To render a substance electrically conductive by the production in it of small electrified particles or ions. Ionization takes place when a substance (such as a compound) breaks up into its ions, which in turn have an electrical charge, thus rendering the material conductive.

jacket A specific type of crown, generally fabricated of porcelain or acrylic resin, or a combination of precious metal and porcelain or acrylic resin. Often called a "cap."

kilovolt A unit of 1,000 volts.

labial Pertaining to the lips, as a position toward the lips. The labial surface of a tooth (incisor or cuspid) is that surface that is close to the lips.

laboratory stone See *dental stone.*

Lactobacillus A rod-shaped organism that has been isolated from the alimentary tract of man and animals, from carious teeth, and from milk that has undergone fermentation.

lamina dura Thin, hard bone lining the tooth socket.

lesion Any change in continuity of a tissue due to disease or injury, or the loss of function of a part.

ligature A cord, thread, or wire used to tie off or bind. One type is used to hold rubber dam in place. Another type is used in an orthodontic appliance.

lingual Pertaining to the tongue, as a position toward the tongue. The lingual surface of a tooth is the surface that is close to the tongue. All teeth have lingual surfaces.

lobe A part of a tooth formed by any one of the separate points of the beginning of calcification.

local anesthetic A drug that produces anesthesia in 1 portion of the body or around 1 area of tissue, as opposed to a general anesthetic, which produces anesthesia throughout the entire body.

malaise The French word for *illness.* Any indisposition, discomfort, or distress.

malar Referring to the cheek or cheekbone.

malignant Tending to go from bad to worse; the opposite of benign.

malocclusion Deviation from the normally acceptable contact of the teeth in the opposing arches.

mammelons The 3 rounded prominences seen on the cutting edges of the incisors when they first erupt through the gums into the mouth.

mandible The lower jawbone.

mandibular Pertaining or referring to the mandible.

marginal ridge A ridge or elevation of enamel, forming the margin of a surface of a tooth; specifically, at the mesial and distal margins of the lingual surfaces of incisors and canines.

mastication The act of chewing.

maxilla The upper jawbone.

maxillary Pertaining or referring to the maxillae.

median line The periphery of the median plane; the vertical, central line dividing the body into right and left.

medication Administration of remedies; a medical agent.

membrane A thin layer of tissue that covers a surface or divides a space or organ.

mesial Toward or situated in the middle, as toward the median line of the dental arch. Those surfaces of the teeth that, as they stand in the arch and, following its curve, are toward the median line, are called mesial surfaces.

metastasis The transfer of disease from 1 organ or body part to another, as in the case of a transfer of cells through blood vessels or lymph channels.

microorganisms Animal or vegetable organisms too small to be seen without a microscope.

microscope Instrument with a lens or combination of lenses for making small things look large.

milliampere One thousandth part of an ampere.

milliampere-second The product of the number of milliamperes of tube current, multiplied by the number of seconds of the exposure; used to designate the factors of a roentgenogram.

milliroentgen One thousandth part of a roentgen.

molar A grinding tooth.

morphology A branch of biology that deals with the form and structure of animals or plants during any stage of their life.

mucin A glycoprotein found in the secretions of the mucous glands.

mucous membrane The moist, pink membrane that lines the mouth, nasal cavities, and alimentary canal.

narcotic A drug that relieves pain and tends to produce stupor or sleep at the same time, depending on the dosage.

nausea Sickness at the stomach, together with a tendency to vomit.

necrosis Deadness of a certain portion of tissue, not the entire body. Dental necrosis is decay of a tooth.

neoplasm A new growth, such as a tumor.

nitrous oxide A gas used in some general anesthetics; same as "laughing gas." Its first use in dentistry was by Dr. Horace Wells in 1844.

nomenclature Terminology. A system of names in a particular science, art, or field of knowledge.

oblique ridge A ridge running obliquely across the occlusal surface of the upper molars. It is formed by the union of the triangular ridge of the distobuccal cusp with the distal portion of the ridge forming the mesiolingual cusp.

obturator An artificial appliance that closes an opening in the palate, prescribed for patients with cleft palates.

occlude To shut, close (see *occlusion*).

occlusal The chewing or grinding surface of a tooth.

occlusion The natural closure and fitting together of upper and lower teeth; the relation of the mandibular and maxillary teeth when closed or during those excursive movements of the mandible by which masticating efficiency is obtained.

odontology The science that deals with the teeth, their structure, and their development; used frequently as a synonym for dentistry.

onlay An inlay that is built upon the occlusal or incisal edges of the tooth. Often used to restore lost tooth structure and to increase the height of the tooth.

operative dentistry The branch of dentistry primarily concerned with restoring carious, diseased, or damaged natural teeth to a satisfactory state of health, function, and aesthetics.

oral examination Those procedures performed by a dentist that aid in making diagnostic conclusions about the oral health of an individual patient.

oral medicine The branch of dentistry that deals with the diagnosis and treatment of diseases of the oral cavity in the perspective of their relationship to diseases or conditions in other parts of the body.

oral pathology The branch of dentistry concerned with the study of disease processes of the hard and soft tissues of the oral cavity.

oral surgery The branch of dentistry concerned with operative procedures in and about the oral cavity and jaws.

organism A plant or animal having organs or an organized structure.

orthodontics The branch of dentistry that deals with the prevention and correction of irregularities of the teeth and malocclusion.

osmosis The passage of solvents or solutions through a semipermeable membrane that is selective in the substances it will permit to pass.

osteology The scientific study of bones and their structures.

oxidation The act of oxidizing or combining with oxygen.

oxidizing agent Anything which produces oxidation (such as the excess of oxygen in the flame of a blowtorch applied to casting gold).

oxygen A colorless, odorless, gaseous element, which combines readily with most elements. It is necessary to all animal and vegetable life and for combustion. It makes up 20% by weight of the atmosphere and about 88% of water.

palate The roof of the mouth. Cleft palate—a palate with a fissure in the median line of the roof of the mouth, present at birth; hard palate—the anterior part of the roof of the mouth, the bony palate; soft palate—the posterior part of the palate near the uvula.

palliative Treatment of pain or discomfort affording relief from the primary concern of pain, but not necessarily effecting cure.

papilla A small nipple-shaped elevation. Incisive papilla—a rounded projection at the anterior end of the palate; interdental papilla—the triangular pad of gum that fills the space between the necks of the teeth; lingual papilla—any one of the papillae of the tongue.

paradental personnel Term coming into usage for reference to the auxiliary dental personnel, such as dental hygienists, dental assistants, and dental laboratory technicians.

pasteurization sterilization Process used in food sterilization. Fluid held at 143 degrees F. for 30 minutes or 160 degrees F. for 15 minutes is pasteurized. This process kills all vegetable cells of pathogenic bacteria; its purpose is to disinfect and to postpone spoilage.

pathogenic Disease-producing.

pathology The science that deals with the nature of disease and its causes and effects.

pedodontics The branch of dentistry that deals with dental conditions of children.

periapical Pertaining to that area of the tooth around the apex (tip) of the root.

periodontal Surrounding a tooth, as the periodontal membrane.

periodontics The branch of dentistry that deals with the prevention and treatment of diseases of the bone and soft tissues surrounding the teeth.

periphery The outward part or the surface or border. A term frequently used to describe the border of a denture or an impression.

permanent teeth The teeth of adult age, as distinguished from the deciduous (temporary or primary) teeth.

pH The symbol of a value that denotes the degree of acidity of a material. It is dependent upon the amount of ionizable hydrogen present. A pH of 7 is considered neutral; a value of less than 7 is acidic; a value greater than 7 is basic or alkaline, with a pH of 14 being the upper limit of alkalinity.

pharmacology The scientific study of drugs.

phenol coefficient Germicidal power of a chemical; represents the strength of an antiseptic, relative to that of phenol; a measure of antibacterial activity that can be quantitated readily and expressed mathematically.

phonetics The study of the production and understanding of speech sounds, including variations by individuals and groups. Phonetics also includes the classification of the sounds produced.

pit A sharp, pointed depression in the enamel. Pits occur mostly where several developmental grooves join, as in the occlusal surfaces of the molars and at the endings of the buccal grooves on the buccal surfaces of the molars.

plaster of Paris See *dental stone.*

pontic The portion of a dental bridge that replaces the missing tooth.

porte-polisher A hand instrument in which an orangewood point has been inserted. The point is dipped into a polishing agent and then placed on the tooth and moved up and down with a wrist movement to polish the teeth.

post-dam A raised ridge ⅛ inch wide at the posterior border of the denture, designed to seal the denture against the palate.

posterior teeth Those teeth of either jaw that are to the rear of the incisors and cuspids.

preprepared tray system A system whereby the armamentarium for a specific dental procedure is prepared in advance of usage and stored until needed.

preventive dentistry The branch of dentistry devoted primarily to averting oral diseases and inhibiting the progress of diseases already present. Some elements of prevention are inherent in all branches of dental practice.

primary Specifically, the first dentition of man or animal.

prognosis The act of predicting the course or outcome, as of a disease.

prophylactic Given for the purpose of preventing disease.

prophylaxis The removal of calculus (tartar) and stains from the exposed and unexposed surfaces of the teeth by scaling and polishing.

prosthesis The replacement of an absent part of the body by one that is artificial.

prosthodontics The branch of dentistry that deals with the replacement of missing teeth and adjacent structures by artificial teeth and devices.

proximal Nearest, next, immediately preceding, or following; same as proximate.

ptyalin An enzyme found in the saliva of man and some of the lower animals, which changes starch into dextrin, maltose, and glucose.

public health dentistry That branch of dentistry concerned primarily with the prevention and control of dental diseases and the promotion of dental health through organized community efforts.

pulp The soft tissue that fills the pulp chambers and root canals of the teeth.

pulpectomy The complete surgical removal of the pulp of a tooth.

pulpotomy The partial removal of the pulp of a tooth, usually performed on children as a treatment after dental caries or a fracture has penetrated to the pulp.

pus A liquid made up of white blood cells (leukocytes) and a thin fluid called liquor puris. It is the product of inflammation.

pyogenic Refers to the production of pus.

radiation Divergence from a center. The emission of radiant energy. A structure made up of divergent elements. Energy propagated through space, as in the case of radiation from x-rays or radiation of heat.

radiograph A roentgenogram, an image produced on a sensitized film by roentgen rays.

radiology The science of radiant energy and radiant substances, especially the branch of medical and dental science that deals with the use of radiant energy.

ramus (ramus mandibuli) The ramus of the lower jaw—the bone back of the posterior teeth, which reaches upward to the head of the condyle.

R.D.H. Abbreviation for Registered Dental Hygienist.

rebase A process of refitting a denture by the replacement of the denture-base material without changing the occlusal relations of the teeth.

recall system Any method for periodically reminding patients to return for examination.

referral Sending a patient to another dentist or a member of another health profession, usually a specialist, for diagnosis or treatment.

rehabilitation (oral) The complete reconstruction of the masticatory apparatus to as nearly a normal condition as possible; includes the replacement of lost teeth and tissue parts and the restoration of aesthetics and function.

reline To resurface the tissue side of a denture with new base material to make it fit more accurately.

removable denture See *denture, removable, partial.*

resin Certain plastic materials. Some types are used in dentistry for denture bases, artificial teeth, and filling materials.

resorption Gradual destruction of tooth root.

restoration Broad term referring to artificial structures that are constructed to replace missing structures.

restorative dentistry See *operative dentistry.*

rests A position of the third and fourth fingers to steady the right hand, in order that the instrument may be held securely to its work without slipping.

retromolar pad Area behind the lower molar teeth.

ridge A long elevation on the surface of a tooth.

R.N. Abbreviation for Registered Nurse.

roentgen The international unit quantity of x-radiation or gamma radiation; the associated corpuscular emission per 0.001 grams of air produces, in air, ions carrying 1 electrostatic quantity of electricity of either sign.

roentgen ray Short-wave, high-energy radiation produced when electrons traveling at high speed impinge on various substances, especially the heavy metals.

roentgenogram See *radiograph*.

roentgenology The branch of radiology that deals with the diagnostic and therapeutic uses of roentgen rays.

root The portion of the tooth that is fixed in the bony walls of the alveolus, or socket, and is covered with cementum.

root canal The space within the root of a tooth containing pulp tissue and connecting the pulp chamber with the apex of the root.

R.Ph. Abbreviation for Registered Pharmacist.

saddle Pertaining to the base. The part of the base of a denture that contacts and covers the soft tissue of the edentulous bony arch.

scaling A dental procedure performed to remove calculus (tartar) and necrotic tissue from around the necks and roots of the teeth. Commonly performed in the "cleaning" of the teeth or in periodontal treatment.

screening (applicant) Any examination of individuals or their records to ascertain their abilities or talents for a respective position.

sedative An agent that quiets activity and, hence, produces a state of sedation.

sepsis A poisoned state caused by the absorption into the blood stream of pathogenic bacteria and their products from a region of infection.

septum A partition; the portion of the alveolar process that lies between the roots of the teeth, separating their alveoli.

silicate cement A type of dental restorative material, used primarily to restore anterior teeth to their proper form, function, and aesthetic coloring. Occasionally referred to as "synthetic porcelain," a misnomer.

solubility The degree to which a substance (the solute) will dissolve in a given amount of another substance (the solvent).

solute The dissolved substance.

solution A homogeneous mixture with no definite composition. The molecules of the dissolved substance (the solute) are dispersed among those of the dissolving medium (the solvent).

solvent The dissolving substance; a substance, usually a liquid, that can dissolve other substances.

space maintainer An appliance constructed for the purpose of preventing adjacent and opposing teeth from moving into the space left by teeth lost prematurely; a method of preventing malocclusion.

spasm A sudden, violent, involuntary muscular contraction.

spatulation The act of mixing or spreading with a spatula.

specialist One who has acquired special skill and knowledge beyond that acquired in either dental or medical school. In some cases, the dentist will announce to the public his area of special interest, and, in some cases, he may restrict his practice to this single area. The dental profession permits the use of the term "specialist" only in connection with those specialities that are officially recognized by the American Dental Association—oral surgery, orthodontics, prosthodontics, periodontics, pedodontics, oral pathology, and dental public health. Other groups are applying for similar recognition.

spirillum A form of bacteria, cylindrical in shape and characterized by a number of bends or spirals along the long axis.

spirochete An elongated, flexible organism, twisted spirally around its long axis and exhibiting motility without possessing flagella.

splint A rigid or flexible appliance for fixation of displaced or movable parts, such as broken jaws.

spore A single cell capable of growing into a new plant or animal.

sprue An attachment of metal or wax to the wax pattern that produces the funnel or channel for the molten metal after the wax pattern with sprue is invested.

staphylococci Normal body parasites; arranged in small groups or clusters.

sterilization Making incapable of reproduction; destruction or removal of all forms of life, with particular reference to organisms.

stomatology The branch of science that deals with the diseases of the mouth.

strain Used in connection with dental materials; the deformation that results when the external forces exerted become greater than the internal forces that resist them.

streptococci A group of spherical bacteria that multiply by dividing in only 1 direction, usually forming chains and causing serious infections.

stress The internal resistance of a body, opposing deformation, when it is subjected to mechanical force.

study model A reproduction of an organ or part in plaster, clay, wax, stone, metal, or other material; used as an aid in diagnosis and in planning treatment of certain conditions.

sulcus, gingival The space between the free gingiva and the tooth.

supernumerary tooth A tooth in excess of the regular or normal number.

suture 1. A surgical stitch. 2. The line of junction of bones in the head. 3. The material used to sew up a wound.

syncope The act of fainting. It is directly caused by an insufficient supply of blood to the brain.

synthetic A substance that has been prepared by artificial means, as opposed to a substance formed naturally.

target In radiography, the target is the tungsten button in the anode at which the electrons produced by the cathode are directed.

temporomandibular joints The joints, just ahead of each ear, upon which the lower jaw swings open and shut and can slide forward.

terminology The complete system of scientific or technical words applying to a science, art, or subject.

therapeutic Pertaining to the treatment of disease.

therapy Treatment; specifically, the treatment of disease.

three-handed dental assisting A term used when the chairside assistant uses the left hand to pass and receive hand instruments, thereby leaving the right hand free to perform other duties.

tincture A solution in which alcohol is the solvent.

topical Pertaining to a specific location, as in the case of topical application of fluoride solutions on the teeth.

torus A bulging projection. Torus palatinus—a bony prominence often found in the center of the palate; torus mandibularis—a bony prominence found in the region between the first and second bicuspids.

toxin Any poisonous product of animal or vegetable metabolism, especially one of those produced by bacteria and constituting the causative agents in certain diseases.

transformer An electrical instrument, composed of coils, that transforms or transfers electrical energy from one circuit to another, usually changing high voltage to low voltage or changing low voltage to high voltage.

traumatic Pertaining to that which has been caused by injury.

treatment plan A series of operations or procedures that are proposed to treat a specific dental disorder or disease or used for the attainment of a given state of oral health.

trituration The process of producing a powder from solid substances by rubbing.

tubercle bacillus A parasite that produces tuberculosis.

tuberosity, maxillary A broad, rough platform or eminence on the bone, located at the end of the maxillary ridge.

tumor A swelling or enlargement, especially one due to morbid growth of a tissue not normal to the part.

typhoid bacillus A microorganism that causes typhoid fever.

U.S.P. An abbreviation for *United States Pharmacopeia,* which is a volume of formulas that are recognized as standards.

vascular Pertaining to vessels, as blood vessels.

vasoconstrictor A substance or a nerve that causes the constriction of blood vessels.

virulence The relative infectiousness of a microorganism, or its ability to overcome the body defenses of the host.

virus One of several living agents or substances of submicroscopic size that causes certain diseases.

volt A unit of electricity that is the electric force or pressure necessary to push electric current at the rate of 1 ampere through a resistance of 1 ohm.

x-ray See *roentgen ray.*

zoology The branch of biology concerned with the animal kingdom and its members as individuals as well as classes.

zygomatic arch An arch of bone commonly known as the "cheekbone." It begins just in front of the ear, arches slightly outward and forward, and then curves slightly inward to an area just below the outer corner of the eye. The "arch" portion of this bone is just above the ramus of the mandible; it is blocked by muscles.

Index

Boldface numerals indicate that a term or concept appears in an illustration.